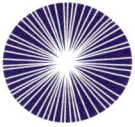

AMERICAN ACADEMY
OF OPHTHALMOLOGY®

Protecting Sight. Empowering Lives.

CW01472311

4 | Ophthalmic Pathology and Intraocular Tumors

2020-2021
BCSC
Basic and Clinical Science Course™

EB⬤ Published after collaborative
review with the European Board
of Ophthalmology subcommittee

The American Academy of Ophthalmology is accredited by the Accreditation Council for Continuing Medical Education (ACCME) to provide continuing medical education for physicians.

The American Academy of Ophthalmology designates this enduring material for a maximum of 10 *AMA PRA Category 1 Credits*™. Physicians should claim only the credit commensurate with the extent of their participation in the activity.

CME expiration date: June 1, 2023. *AMA PRA Category 1 Credits*™ may be claimed only once between June 1, 2020, and the expiration date.

BCSC® volumes are designed to increase the physician's ophthalmic knowledge through study and review. Users of this activity are encouraged to read the text and then answer the study questions provided at the back of the book.

To claim *AMA PRA Category 1 Credits*™ upon completion of this activity, learners must demonstrate appropriate knowledge and participation in the activity by taking the posttest for Section 4 and achieving a score of 80% or higher. For further details, please see the instructions for requesting CME credit at the back of the book.

The Academy provides this material for educational purposes only. It is not intended to represent the only or best method or procedure in every case, nor to replace a physician's own judgment or give specific advice for case management. Including all indications, contraindications, side effects, and alternative agents for each drug or treatment is beyond the scope of this material. All information and recommendations should be verified, prior to use, with current information included in the manufacturers' package inserts or other independent sources, and considered in light of the patient's condition and history. Reference to certain drugs, instruments, and other products in this course is made for illustrative purposes only and is not intended to constitute an endorsement of such. Some material may include information on applications that are not considered community standard, that reflect indications not included in approved FDA labeling, or that are approved for use only in restricted research settings. **The FDA has stated that it is the responsibility of the physician to determine the FDA status of each drug or device he or she wishes to use, and to use them with appropriate, informed patient consent in compliance with applicable law.** The Academy specifically disclaims any and all liability for injury or other damages of any kind, from negligence or otherwise, for any and all claims that may arise from the use of any recommendations or other information contained herein.

All trademarks, trade names, logos, brand names, and service marks of the American Academy of Ophthalmology (AAO), whether registered or unregistered, are the property of AAO and are protected by US and international trademark laws. These trademarks include AAO; AAOE; AMERICAN ACADEMY OF OPHTHALMOLOGY; BASIC AND CLINICAL SCIENCE COURSE; BCSC; EYENET; EYEWIKI; FOCAL POINTS; FOCUS DESIGN (logo shown on cover); IRIS; ISRS; OKAP; ONE NETWORK; OPHTHALMOLOGY; OPHTHALMOLOGY GLAUCOMA; OPHTHALMOLOGY RETINA; PREFERRED PRACTICE PATTERN; PROTECTING SIGHT. EMPOWERING LIVES; and THE OPHTHALMIC NEWS & EDUCATION NETWORK.

Cover image: Photomicrograph depicting adenoid cystic carcinoma of the lacrimal gland. *(Courtesy of Vivian Lee, MD.)*

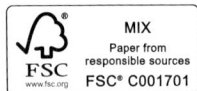

MIX
Paper from
responsible sources
FSC
www.fsc.org   FSC® C001701

Printed in China.

Basic and Clinical Science Course

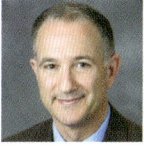

Christopher J. Rapuano, MD, Philadelphia, Pennsylvania
Senior Secretary for Clinical Education

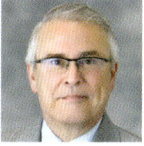

J. Timothy Stout, MD, PhD, MBA, Houston, Texas
Secretary for Lifelong Learning and Assessment

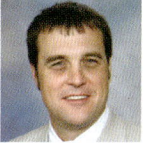

Colin A. McCannel, MD, Los Angeles, California
BCSC Course Chair

Section 4

Faculty for the Major Revision

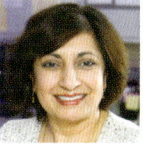

Nasreen A. Syed, MD
Chair
Iowa City, Iowa

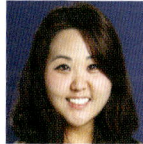

Vivian Lee, MD
Philadelphia, Pennsylvania

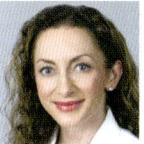

Jesse L. Berry, MD
Los Angeles, California

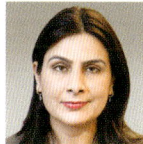

Kirtee Raparia, MBBS
Santa Clara, California

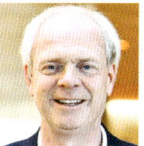

Steffen Heegaard, MD
Copenhagen, Denmark

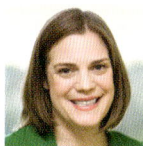

Alison H. Skalet, MD, PhD
Portland, Oregon

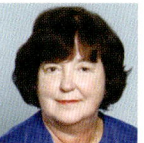

Theresa Retue Kramer, MD
Baltimore, Maryland

The Academy acknowledges the *American Association of Ophthalmic Oncologists and Pathologists* for recommending faculty members to the BCSC Section 4 committee.

The Academy also acknowledges the following committees for review of this edition:

Committee on Aging: Patricia Chévez-Barrios, MD, Houston, Texas

Vision Rehabilitation Committee: William M. McLaughlin Jr, DO, Scranton, Pennsylvania

BCSC Resident/Fellow Reviewers: Sharon L. Jick, MD, *Chair,* St Louis, Missouri; Gordon S. Crabtree, MD; Lindsay De Andrade, MD; Lilangi S. Ediriwickrema, MD; Brittni A. Scruggs, MD, PhD; Duo (David) Xu, MD

Practicing Ophthalmologists Advisory Committee for Education: Stephen R. Klapper, MD, *Primary Reviewer,* Carmel, Indiana; Bradley D. Fouraker, MD, *Chair,* Tampa, Florida; Cynthia S. Chiu, MD, Oakland, California; George S. Ellis Jr, MD, New Orleans, Louisiana; Gaurav K. Shah, MD, Town and Country, Missouri; Rosa A. Tang, MD, MPH, MBA, Houston, Texas; Troy M. Tanji, MD, Waipahu, Hawaii; Michelle S. Ying, MD, Ladson, South Carolina

In addition, the Academy acknowledges the following committee for assistance in developing Study Questions and Answers for this BCSC Section:

Resident Self-Assessment Committee: Robert A. Beaulieu, MD, Royal Oak, Michigan; Benjamin W. Botsford, MD, Pittsburgh, Pennsylvania; Olga M. Ceron, MD, Worcester, Massachusetts; Ian P. Conner, MD, PhD, Pittsburgh, Pennsylvania; Kimberly A. Crowder, MD, Jackson, Missouri; James Andrew David, MD, New Orleans, Louisiana; Claire E. Fraser, MD, PhD, Lexington, Kentucky; Kevin Halenda, MD, Augusta, Georgia; Rola N. Hamam, MD, Beirut, Lebanon; Amanda D. Henderson, MD, Baltimore, Maryland; Joshua Hendrix, MD, Dalton, Georgia; Matthew B. Kaufman, MD, Portland, Oregon; Sangeeta Khanna, MD, St Louis, Missouri; Chandrasekharan Krishnan, MD, Boston, Massachusetts; Ajay E. Kuriyan, MD, Pittsford, New York; Kevin E. Lai, MD, Indianapolis, Indiana; Kenneth C. Lao, MD, Temple, Texas; Ken Y. Lin, MD, Irvine, California; Kelly T. Mitchell, MD, Lubbock, Texas; Yasha S. Modi, MD, New York, New York; Matthew S. Pihlblad, MD, McDonald, Pennsylvania; Lorraine A. Provencher, MD, Cincinnati, Ohio; Jamie B. Rosenberg, MD, New York, New York; Syed Mahmood Shah, MD, Pittsburgh, Pennsylvania; Ann Shue, MD, Palo Alto, California; Misha F. Syed, MD, Galveston, Texas; Parisa Taravati, MD, Seattle, Washington; Sarah Van Tassel, MD, New York, New York; Evan L. Waxman, MD, PhD, Pittsburgh, Pennsylvania; Jules A. Winokur, MD, Great Neck, New York

EB

European Board of Ophthalmology: Tero T. Kivelä, MD, *Chair,* Helsinki, Finland; Edoardo Midena, MD, PhD, *Liaison,* Padua, Italy; Nikolaos E. Bechrakis, MD, FEBO, Innsbruck, Austria; Sarah E. Coupland, MBBS, PhD, FRCPath, Liverpool, United Kingdom; Laurence Desjardins, MD, Paris, France; Steffen Heegaard, MD, DMSc, Copenhagen, Denmark; Elisabeth M. Messmer, MD, PhD, FEBO, Munich, Germany; Fiona Roberts, MBChB, MD, FRCPath, Glasgow, United Kingdom

Financial Disclosures

The other authors and reviewers state that within the 12 months prior to their contributions to this CME activity and for the duration of development, they have had no financial interest in or other relationship with any entity discussed in this course that produces, markets, resells, or distributes ophthalmic health care goods or services consumed by or used in patients, or with any competing commercial product or service.

Recent Past Faculty

Michele M. Bloomer, MD
Dan S. Gombos, MD
Tero T. Kivelä, MD
Tatyana Milman, MD
Heather A. D. Potter, MD
Robert H. Rosa Jr, MD

In addition, the Academy gratefully acknowledges the contributions of numerous past faculty and advisory committee members who have played an important role in the development of previous editions of the Basic and Clinical Science Course.

American Academy of Ophthalmology Staff

Dale E. Fajardo, EdD, MBA, *Vice President, Education*
Beth Wilson, *Director, Continuing Professional Development*
Ann McGuire, *Acquisitions and Development Manager*
Stephanie Tanaka, *Publications Manager*
Susan Malloy, *Acquisitions Editor and Program Manager*
Jasmine Chen, *Manager, E-Learning*
Teri Bell, *Production Manager*
Beth Collins, *Medical Editor*
Eric Gerdes, *Interactive Designer*
Lynda Hanwella, *Publications Specialist*
Naomi Ruiz, *BCSC Projects Specialist*
Debra Marchi, *Permissions Assistant*

American Academy of Ophthalmology
655 Beach Street
Box 7424
San Francisco, CA 94120-7424

Contents

Introduction to the BCSC xv

Objectives 1

PART I   Ophthalmic Pathology 3

1   Introduction to Part I 5
Highlights 5
Overview 5
Organizational Framework and Basic Pathologic Concepts 6
   Topography 7
   Disease Processes 7
   Differential Diagnosis 16

2   Specimen Handling 19
Highlights 19
Overview 19
Communication 20
Fixatives for Tissue Preservation 21
Specimen Orientation 21
Gross Examination and Dissection 24
Processing and Staining 24
   Tissue Processing 24
   Slide Preparation and Tissue Staining 26

3   Special Testing and Procedures in Pathology 29
Highlights 29
Introduction 29
Immunohistochemistry 29
Flow Cytometry, Molecular Pathology, and
   Diagnostic Electron Microscopy 33
   Flow Cytometry 33
   Molecular Pathology 33
   Diagnostic Electron Microscopy 39
Special Procedures 39
   Fine-Needle Aspiration Biopsy 39
   Frozen Section 40

4   Wound Repair 43
Highlights 43
General Aspects of Wound Repair 43

Wound Repair in Specific Ocular Tissues 44
    Cornea 45
    Conjunctiva 45
    Sclera 47
    Uveal Tract 47
    Lens 47
    Retina 48
    Vitreous 48
    Orbit and Ocular Adnexa 48
    Optic Nerve 49
Pathologically Apparent Sequelae of Ocular Trauma 49

5 Conjunctiva **55**
Highlights 55
Topography 55
Developmental Anomalies 57
    Choristomas 57
    Hamartomas 57
Inflammation 57
    Acute or Chronic Conjunctivitis 59
    Infectious Conjunctivitis 59
    Noninfectious Conjunctivitis 60
    Papillary Versus Follicular Conjunctivitis 61
    Granulomatous Conjunctivitis 61
    Pyogenic Granuloma 63
Degenerations 64
    Pinguecula and Pterygium 64
    Amyloid Deposits 67
    Epithelial Inclusion Cyst 68
    Conjunctivochalasis 68
Neoplasia 69
    Squamous Epithelial Lesions 69
    Melanocytic Lesions 74
    Lymphoid Lesions 85
    Glandular Neoplasms 88
    Other Neoplasms 88

6 Cornea **89**
Highlights 89
Topography 89
Developmental Anomalies 91
    Dermoid 91
    Peters Anomaly 91
Inflammation 91
    Infectious Keratitis 91
    Noninfectious Keratitis 98
Degenerations, Depositions, and Ectasias 98

Salzmann Nodular Degeneration 98
Calcific Band Keratopathy 99
Actinic Keratopathy 100
Pinguecula and Pterygium 101
Pannus 101
Bullous Keratopathy 101
Corneal Graft Failure 102
Corneal Pigment Deposits 104
Ectatic Disorders 104
Dystrophies 106
Epithelial and Subepithelial Dystrophies 107
Epithelial–Stromal *TGFBI* Dystrophies 107
Stromal Dystrophies 110
Descemet Membrane and Endothelial Dystrophies 111
Neoplasia 116

7 Anterior Chamber and Trabecular Meshwork **117**
Highlights 117
Topography 117
Developmental Anomalies 118
Primary Congenital Glaucoma 119
Anterior Segment Dysgenesis 119
Inflammation 120
Degenerations 120
Iridocorneal Endothelial Syndrome 120
Secondary Glaucoma 122
Neoplasia 128

8 Sclera **129**
Highlights 129
Topography 129
Developmental Anomalies 130
Choristoma 130
Nanophthalmos 130
Microphthalmia 131
Inflammation 131
Episcleritis 131
Scleritis 131
Degenerations 134
Senile Calcific Plaque 134
Scleral Staphyloma 134
Melanoma-Associated Spongiform Scleropathy 134
Neoplasia 135

9 Lens **137**
Highlights 137
Topography 137

Capsule 137
Epithelium 137
Cortex and Nucleus 139
Zonular Fibers 139
Developmental Anomalies 140
Congenital Aphakia 140
Anterior Lenticonus and Lentiglobus 140
Posterior Lenticonus and Lentiglobus 140
Inflammation 141
Propionibacterium acnes Endophthalmitis 141
Phacoantigenic Uveitis 141
Phacolytic Uveitis 143
Degenerations 143
Cataract and Other Lens Abnormalities 143
Neoplasia and Associations With Systemic Disorders 147
Pathology in Intraocular Lenses 147

10 Vitreous **149**
Highlights 149
Topography 149
Developmental Anomalies 150
Persistent Fetal Vasculature 150
Bergmeister Papilla 151
Mittendorf Dot 151
Vitreous Cysts 151
Inflammation 152
Degenerations 153
Syneresis and Aging 153
Posterior Vitreous Detachment 153
Hemorrhage 156
Asteroid Hyalosis 157
Vitreous Amyloidosis 158
Neoplasia 159
Intraocular Lymphoma 159

11 Retina and Retinal Pigment Epithelium **163**
Highlights 163
Topography 163
Neurosensory Retina 164
Retinal Pigment Epithelium 167
Developmental Anomalies 167
Albinism 167
Myelinated Nerve Fibers 168
Vascular Anomalies 169
Congenital Hypertrophy of the RPE 170
Inflammation 171
Infectious Etiologies 171
Noninfectious Etiologies 174

Degenerations 174
    Typical and Reticular Peripheral Cystoid Degeneration
       and Retinoschisis 174
    Lattice Degeneration 175
    Sequelae of Retinal Detachment 176
    Paving-Stone Degeneration 176
    Ischemia 177
    Abusive Head Trauma 189
    Age-Related Macular Degeneration 191
    Polypoidal Choroidal Vasculopathy 195
    Macular Dystrophies 196
    Diffuse Photoreceptor Dystrophies 198
Neoplasia 202
    Retinoblastoma 202
    Retinocytoma 207
    Medulloepithelioma 209
    Fuchs Adenoma 210
    Combined Hamartoma of the Retina and RPE 210
    Adenomas and Adenocarcinomas of the RPE 211

12 Uveal Tract **213**
Highlights 213
Topography 213
    Iris 213
    Ciliary Body 215
    Choroid 215
Developmental Anomalies 216
    Aniridia 216
    Coloboma 217
Inflammation (Uveitis) 218
    Infectious Uveitis 218
    Noninfectious Uveitis 219
Degenerations 222
    Rubeosis Iridis 222
    Hyalinization of the Ciliary Body 222
    Choroidal Neovascularization 222
Neoplasia 223
    Iris 223
    Choroid and Ciliary Body 225
    Metastatic Tumors 232
    Other Uveal Tumors 233

13 Eyelids **237**
Highlights 237
Topography 237
Developmental Anomalies 239
    Distichiasis 239

Phakomatous Choristoma 239
Dermoid Cyst 240
Inflammation 240
Infectious Inflammatory Disorders 240
Noninfectious Inflammatory Disorders 241
Degenerations and Deposits 243
Xanthelasma 243
Amyloidosis 243
Cysts 245
Epidermoid Cysts 245
Ductal Cysts 245
Neoplasia 245
Epidermal Neoplasms 245
Dermal Neoplasms 252
Neoplasms and Proliferations of the Dermal Appendages 252
Merkel Cell Carcinoma 256
Melanocytic Neoplasms 257

14 Orbit and Lacrimal Drainage System **261**
Highlights 261
Topography 261
Bony Orbit and Soft Tissues 261
Developmental Anomalies 262
Cysts 262
Inflammation 263
Noninfectious Inflammation 263
Infectious Inflammation 266
Degenerations 269
Amyloid 269
Neoplasia 269
Lacrimal Gland Neoplasia 270
Lymphoproliferative Lesions 272
Soft-Tissue Tumors 274
Vascular Tumors 274
Tumors With Fibrous Differentiation 275
Tumors With Muscle Differentiation 278
Peripheral Nerve Sheath and Central Nervous System Tumors 280
Adipose Tumors 282
Bony Lesions of the Orbit 282
Secondary Tumors 282
Lacrimal Sac Neoplasia 283

15 Optic Nerve **285**
Highlights 285
Topography 285
Developmental Anomalies 287
Colobomas 287
Optic Pits 287

Inflammation 287
    Infectious Optic Neuritis 288
    Noninfectious Optic Neuritis 289
Degenerations 291
    Optic Atrophy 291
    Optic Nerve Head Drusen 292
Neoplasia 294
    Melanocytoma 294
    Glioma 295
    Meningioma 296

PART II   Intraocular Tumors: Clinical Aspects 299

16 **Introduction to Part II** 301

17 **Melanocytic Tumors** 303
Highlights 303
Introduction 303
Iris Nevus 304
Iris Melanoma 304
Ciliary Body and Choroidal Nevi 305
Melanocytoma of the Iris, Ciliary Body, and Choroid 309
Melanoma of the Choroid and Ciliary Body 312
    Clinical Characteristics 313
    Diagnostic Evaluation 314
    Differential Diagnosis 318
    Classification 323
    Metastatic Evaluation 324
    Treatment 327
    Prognosis and Prognostic Factors 330
Epithelial Tumors of the Uveal Tract and Retina 331
    Adenoma and Adenocarcinoma 331
    Acquired Hyperplasia 332
    Simple Hamartoma 333
    Combined Hamartoma 333
Fine-Needle Aspiration Biopsy 334

18 **Vascular Tumors** 335
Highlights 335
Introduction 335
Choroidal Vascular Tumors 335
    Choroidal Hemangiomas 335
Retinal Vascular Tumors 339
    Prenatal Retinal Vascular Tumors: Non-Leaking Lesions 339
    Postnatal Retinal Vascular Tumors: Leaking Lesions 341

19 Retinoblastoma 347

Highlights 347
Introduction 347
Diagnostic Evaluation 348
    Clinical Examination 348
    Ancillary Imaging 350
    Differential Diagnosis 354
Retinoblastoma Classification 357
Treatment 358
    Enucleation 360
    Chemotherapy 361
Local Consolidation Therapy 363
    Laser Photocoagulation 363
    Cryotherapy 363
    Plaque Radiotherapy 363
    Intravitreal Chemotherapy 364
    External Beam Radiotherapy 364
Spontaneous Regression 365
Genetic Counseling 365
Associated Conditions 367
    Retinocytoma 367
    Primitive Neuroectodermal Tumor 367
Prognosis 368

20 Ocular Involvement in Systemic Malignancies 371

Highlights 371
Secondary Tumors of the Eye 371
    Metastatic Carcinoma 371
    Direct Intraocular Extension 380
Lymphoid Tumors 380
    Primary Intraocular Lymphoma 380
    Primary Uveal Lymphoma 383
    Secondary Involvement of Systemic Lymphoma 386
Ocular Manifestations of Leukemia 386

Additional Materials and Resources 389
Requesting Continuing Medical Education Credit 391
Study Questions 393
Answers 401
Index 409

Introduction to the BCSC

The Basic and Clinical Science Course (BCSC) is designed to meet the needs of residents and practitioners for a comprehensive yet concise curriculum of the field of ophthalmology. The BCSC has developed from its original brief outline format, which relied heavily on outside readings, to a more convenient and educationally useful self-contained text. The Academy updates and revises the course annually, with the goals of integrating the basic science and clinical practice of ophthalmology and of keeping ophthalmologists current with new developments in the various subspecialties.

The BCSC incorporates the effort and expertise of more than 90 ophthalmologists, organized into 13 Section faculties, working with Academy editorial staff. In addition, the course continues to benefit from many lasting contributions made by the faculties of previous editions. Members of the Academy Practicing Ophthalmologists Advisory Committee for Education, Committee on Aging, and Vision Rehabilitation Committee review every volume before major revisions, as does a group of select residents and fellows. Members of the European Board of Ophthalmology, organized into Section faculties, also review volumes before major revisions, focusing primarily on differences between American and European ophthalmology practice.

Organization of the Course

The Basic and Clinical Science Course comprises 13 volumes, incorporating fundamental ophthalmic knowledge, subspecialty areas, and special topics:

1 Update on General Medicine
2 Fundamentals and Principles of Ophthalmology
3 Clinical Optics
4 Ophthalmic Pathology and Intraocular Tumors
5 Neuro-Ophthalmology
6 Pediatric Ophthalmology and Strabismus
7 Oculofacial Plastic and Orbital Surgery
8 External Disease and Cornea
9 Uveitis and Ocular Inflammation
10 Glaucoma
11 Lens and Cataract
12 Retina and Vitreous
13 Refractive Surgery

References

Readers who wish to explore specific topics in greater detail may consult the references cited within each chapter and listed in the Additional Materials and Resources section at the back of the book. These references are intended to be selective rather than exhaustive, chosen by the BCSC faculty as being important, current, and readily available to residents and practitioners.

Multimedia

This edition of Section 4, *Ophthalmic Pathology and Intraocular Tumors,* includes videos related to topics covered in the book. The videos were selected by members of the BCSC faculty to present important topics that are best delivered visually. This edition also includes an interactive feature, or "activities," developed by members of the BCSC faculty. Both the videos and the activities are available to readers of the print and electronic versions of Section 4 (https://www.aao.org/bcscvideo_section04 and https://www.aao.org/bcscactivity_section04). Mobile-device users can scan the QR codes below (you may need to install a QR-code reader on the device) to access the videos and activities.

Videos

Activities

Self-Assessment and CME Credit

Each volume of the BCSC is designed as an independent study activity for ophthalmology residents and practitioners. The learning objectives for this volume are given on page 1. The text, illustrations, and references provide the information necessary to achieve the objectives; the study questions allow readers to test their understanding of the material and their mastery of the objectives. Physicians who wish to claim CME credit for this educational activity may do so by following the instructions given at the end of the book.

This Section of the BCSC has been approved as a Maintenance of Certification (MOC) Part II self-assessment CME activity and also is approved by the American Board of Pathology as an MOC CME activity.

Conclusion

The Basic and Clinical Science Course has expanded greatly over the years, with the addition of much new text, numerous illustrations, and video content. Recent editions have sought to place greater emphasis on clinical applicability while maintaining a solid foundation in basic science. As with any educational program, it reflects the experience of its authors. As its faculties change and medicine progresses, new viewpoints emerge on controversial subjects and techniques. Not all alternate approaches can be included in this series; as with any educational endeavor, the learner should seek additional sources, including Academy Preferred Practice Pattern Guidelines.

The BCSC faculty and staff continually strive to improve the educational usefulness of the course; you, the reader, can contribute to this ongoing process. If you have any suggestions or questions about the series, please do not hesitate to contact the faculty or the editors.

The authors, editors, and reviewers hope that your study of the BCSC will be of lasting value and that each Section will serve as a practical resource for quality patient care.

Objectives

Upon completion of BCSC Section 4, *Ophthalmic Pathology and Intraocular Tumors*, the reader should be able to

- describe a structured approach to understanding major ocular conditions based on a hierarchical framework of topography, disease process, and differential diagnosis

- list the steps for handling ocular specimens for pathologic study, including obtaining, dissecting, processing, and staining tissues

- explain the basic principles of special procedures and diagnostic testing used in ophthalmic pathology, such as immunohistochemistry, flow cytometry, molecular genetic techniques, and diagnostic electron microscopy

- describe the types of specimens, processing, and techniques appropriate to the clinical situation

- list the steps in wound healing in ocular tissues

- state the main histologic features of common ocular conditions

- describe the relationship between clinical and pathologic findings in various ocular conditions

- discuss current information about the most common primary tumors of the eye and ocular adnexa

- identify those ophthalmic lesions that indicate systemic disease and are potentially life threatening

- describe the methodologies used for diagnosing intraocular tumors

- describe current treatment modalities for ocular tumors in terms of patient prognosis and ocular function

- describe the genetic information that would be important to provide to families affected by retinoblastoma

PART I

Ophthalmic Pathology

CHAPTER **1**

Introduction to Part I

This chapter includes related activities. Go to www.aao.org/bcscactivity_section04 or scan the QR codes in the text to access this content.

Highlights

- Ophthalmic pathology is a subspecialty recognized by the American Academy of Ophthalmology, as well as other North American and international ophthalmology organizations.
- Understanding the disorders and diseases that affect the eye and periocular structures requires an understanding of normal ocular structures and functions.
- Pathologic entities are generally divided into the following major categories: developmental anomaly, inflammation, degeneration and dystrophy, and neoplasia.
- The degeneration of a blind, traumatized eye involves a range of tissue alterations, including atrophia bulbi without shrinkage, atrophia bulbi with shrinkage, and phthisis bulbi.

Overview

Ophthalmic pathology is recognized as a subspecialty by the American Academy of Ophthalmology, the American Board of Ophthalmology, the Association of University Professors of Ophthalmology, and the International Council of Ophthalmology. The study of ophthalmic pathology has contributed significantly to our understanding of the pathogenesis of diseases of the eye and ocular adnexa. In the United States, ophthalmologists and pathologists may receive subspecialty fellowship training in ophthalmic pathology after completion of an ACGME (Accreditation Council for Graduate Medical Education)-accredited residency in ophthalmology or pathology; some ophthalmic pathologists are board certified in both ophthalmology and pathology.

BCSC Section 4, *Ophthalmic Pathology and Intraocular Tumors,* provides a general overview of ophthalmic pathology and oncology: common practices and pathologic processes, as well as some less common, but important, entities, are discussed. For more comprehensive reviews of these entities, please refer to the references listed in the Basic Texts section at the end of this volume.

This chapter describes the organizational framework used in Chapters 5 through 15. Chapter 2 discusses specimen handling and processing and emphasizes the importance of communication between the ophthalmologist and the pathologist for providing good patient care. Chapter 3 covers special testing modalities such as immunohistochemical staining, flow cytometry, polymerase chain reaction (PCR), and frozen sections. Chapter 4 covers basic principles and specific aspects of wound repair. The remainder of Part I, Chapters 5 through 15, is dedicated to specific anatomical regions and pathology.

Organizational Framework and Basic Pathologic Concepts

As stated previously, Chapters 5 through 15 focus on specific ocular structures and disease processes. In these chapters, the text is organized from general to specific, with the following topics as the framework for the discussion:

- topography
- disease process
- differential diagnosis

Thus, the text also provides an organizational paradigm for the study of ophthalmic pathology (Table 1-1).

Table 1-1 Organizational Paradigm for Ophthalmic Pathology

Topography
    Conjunctiva
    Cornea
    Anterior chamber/trabecular meshwork
    Sclera
    Lens
    Vitreous
    Retina
    Uveal tract
    Optic nerve
    Eyelids
    Orbit

Disease process
    Developmental anomaly
      Choristoma vs hamartoma
    Inflammation
      Acute or chronic
      Focal or diffuse
      Granulomatous or nongranulomatous
      Infectious or noninfectious
    Degeneration and dystrophy
    Neoplasia
      Benign or malignant
      Epithelial, mesenchymal, hematopoietic, or melanocytic

Differential diagnosis
    Identification of index feature
    Formulation of a focused list of conditions resulting from the pathologic processes identified above

Topography

Topography refers to the description of the anatomical location and structural features of a particular tissue. Topographic identification is the first step in analysis of a pathologic specimen. Recognizing normal tissue in a specimen helps to define abnormal areas and narrow the differential diagnosis. This requires knowledge of the general landscape of normal ocular structures. For example, collagenous tissue lined by keratinized stratified squamous epithelium with dermal appendages is typical of eyelid skin, whereas organized layers, including nonkeratinized stratified squamous epithelium, Bowman layer, collagenous stroma, Descemet membrane, and endothelium, are typical of the cornea. Using the topographic features of the specimen, an examiner can then orient and identify the tissue in question. Recognition of characteristic features, such as the presence or absence of an epithelium, can be particularly helpful. See BCSC Section 2, *Fundamentals and Principles of Ophthalmology,* for a review of ophthalmic anatomy.

Disease Processes

The major disease processes discussed in Chapters 5 through 15 include

- developmental anomaly
- inflammation
- degeneration and dystrophy
- neoplasia

In the evaluation of a pathologic specimen, the examiner should attempt to determine the general disease process after surveying the topography (Activity 1-1).

ACTIVITY 1-1   Identify the disease process.
Developed by Vivian Lee, MD.
Go to www.aao.org/bcscactivity_section04 to access all activities in Section 4.

Developmental anomaly

Developmental anomalies are structural or functional anomalies that develop in utero or during early childhood, as the body is developing. They may be detected prenatally, at birth, or later in life. Developmental anomalies usually involve abnormalities in size, location, organization, or amount of tissue, such as congenital hypertrophy of the retinal pigment epithelium or eyelid coloboma. Often, they may be classified as choristomas or hamartomas. A *choristoma* consists of normal, mature tissue (1 or 2 embryonic germ layers) at an abnormal location. An *epibulbar dermoid* is classified as a choristoma because it consists of normal, mature skin structures at an atypical location, the limbus. In contrast, *hamartoma* describes hypertrophy and hyperplasia (abnormal amount) of mature tissue in a normal location. An *orbital cavernous hemangioma* is an example of a hamartoma, as it is an encapsulated mass of mature venous channels in the orbit. A tumor made up of tissue derived from all 3 embryonic germ layers is called a *teratoma* (Fig 1-1).

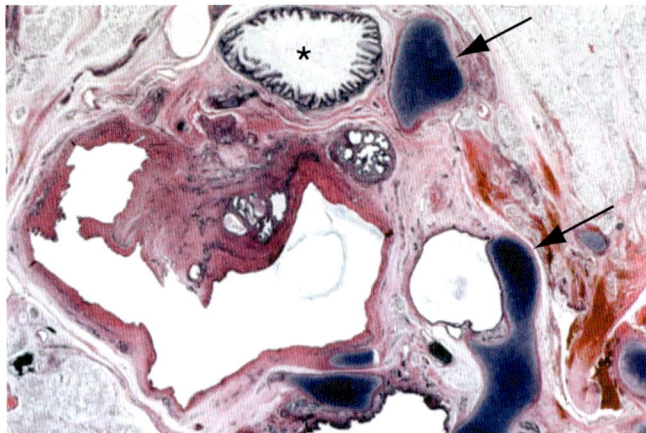

Figure 1-1 Orbital teratoma with tissue from the 3 germ layers. Note gastrointestinal mucosa *(asterisk)* and cartilage *(arrows)* in the tumor. *(Courtesy of Hans E. Grossniklaus, MD.)*

Inflammation

Inflammation can be classified in several ways: for example, as acute or chronic in regard to onset; focal or diffuse regarding location; infectious or noninfectious with respect to etiology; and granulomatous or nongranulomatous regarding predominant cell type (see Table 1-1). A bacterial corneal ulcer, for instance, is generally an acute, focal, nongranulomatous inflammatory process, whereas sympathetic ophthalmia is a chronic, diffuse, granulomatous inflammatory disease.

In the early phases of the inflammatory process, polymorphonuclear leukocytes, which include neutrophils, eosinophils, and basophils, typically predominate and can be found in tissues (Fig 1-2). *Neutrophils* typify the acute inflammatory response and can be recognized by their multisegmented nuclei and intracytoplasmic granules (Fig 1-3). They are often associated with bacterial infections and may be found in blood vessel walls in some forms of vasculitis. *Eosinophils* are commonly found in allergic reactions but may also be present in chronic inflammatory processes such as sympathetic ophthalmia. They have bilobed nuclei and prominent intracytoplasmic eosinophilic granules (Fig 1-4). *Basophils* contain basophilic intracytoplasmic granules; when found in tissues, they are referred to as *mast cells* (Fig 1-5).

Inflammatory cells that are characteristic of a chronic inflammatory response include lymphocytes, plasma cells, and monocytes (see Fig 1-2B). *Lymphocytes* are small cells with round, hyperchromatic nuclei and scant cytoplasm (Fig 1-6). Lymphocytes mature either in the thymus *(T cells)* or the bone marrow *(B cells)*. To distinguish T cells from B cells in tissue sections, specific immunohistochemical stains are required, as it is not possible to distinguish between B and T lymphocytes with routine histologic stains. T cells can be classified into several subtypes based on their surface markers, with each subtype having a different function. B cells can differentiate into *plasma cells* that produce immunoglobulins. Plasma cells are characterized by eccentric nuclei with a "cartwheel" or "clock-face" chromatin pattern and a perinuclear halo corresponding to the Golgi apparatus (Fig 1-7A, B). These

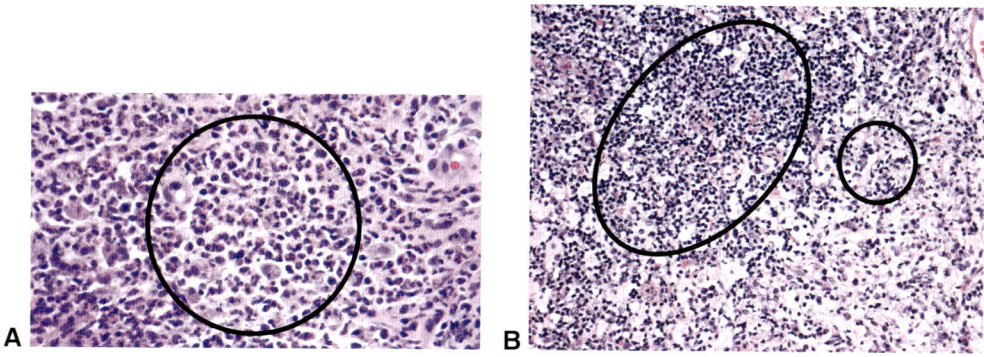

Figure 1-2 Acute and chronic inflammation. **A,** Acute inflammatory infiltrate, composed predominantly of neutrophils *(circle)*. **B,** Chronic inflammatory infiltrate, composed predominantly of lymphocytes *(oval)* and plasma cells *(circle)*. *(Part A courtesy of Vivian Lee, MD; part B courtesy of Nasreen A. Syed, MD.)*

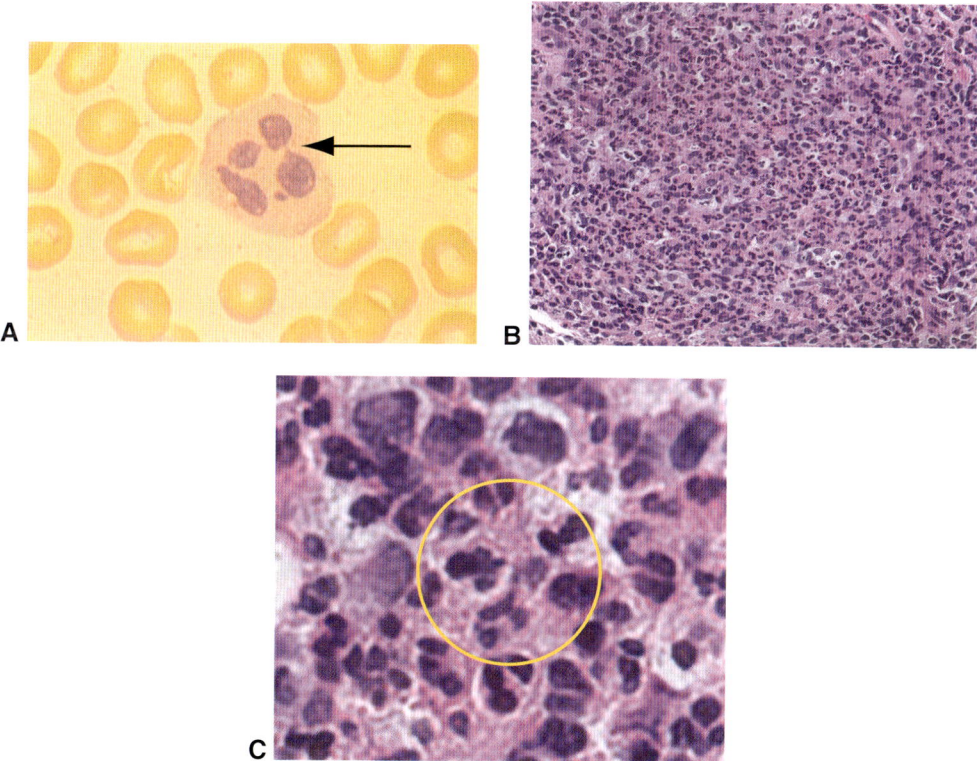

Figure 1-3 **A,** Blood smear showing a polymorphonuclear leukocyte (PMN) with multisegmented nucleus *(arrow)*. **B,** Tissue section demonstrating PMNs (neutrophils) at low magnification. **C,** Tissue section (same as in part B) showing PMNs *(circle)* at high magnification. *(Part A courtesy of Hans E. Grossniklaus, MD; parts B and C courtesy of Vivian Lee, MD.)*

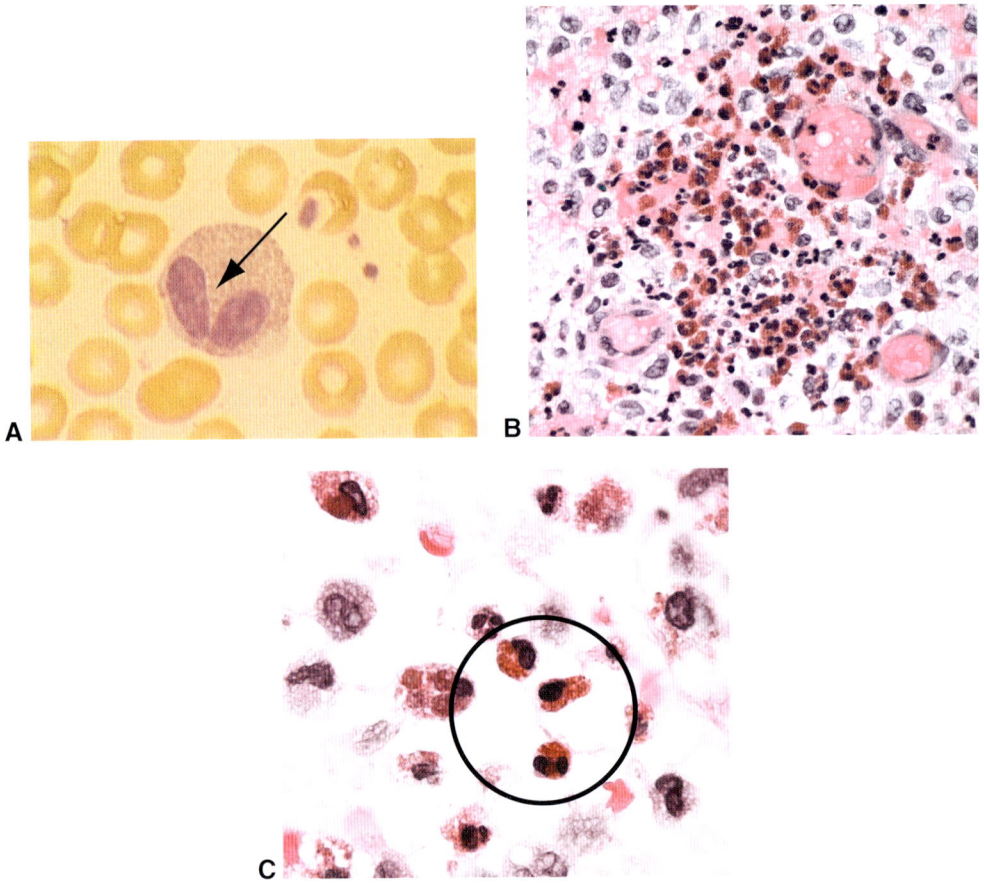

Figure 1-4 **A,** Blood smear showing an eosinophil with bilobed nucleus *(arrow)* and granular cytoplasm. **B,** Tissue section demonstrating eosinophils at low magnification. **C,** Tissue section (same as in part B) showing eosinophils *(circle)* at high magnification. *(Part A courtesy of Hans E. Grossniklaus, MD; parts B and C courtesy of Nasreen A. Syed, MD.)*

Figure 1-5 Blood smear demonstrates a basophil with intracytoplasmic basophilic granules *(arrows)*. Basophils (mast cells) are difficult to identify in tissue sections without the assistance of special stains. *(Courtesy of Hans E. Grossniklaus, MD.)*

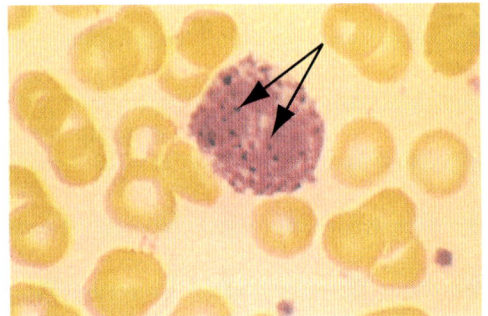

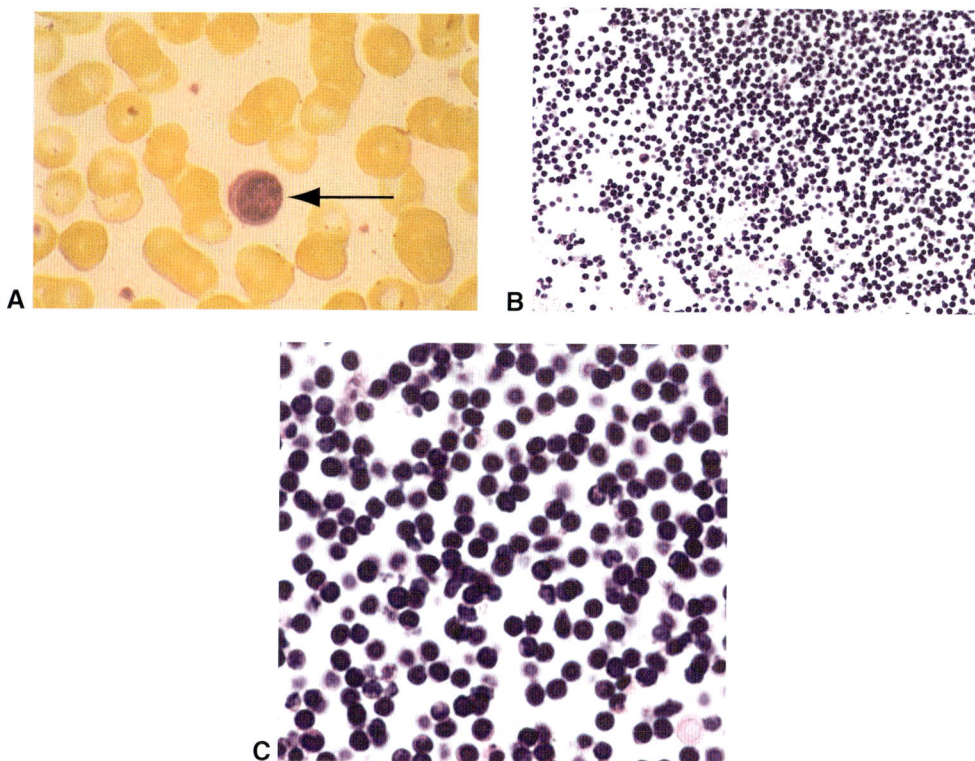

Figure 1-6 **A,** Blood smear showing a lymphocyte *(arrow)* with a small, hyperchromatic nucleus and scant cytoplasm. **B,** Tissue section demonstrating lymphocytes at low magnification. **C,** Higher magnification of lymphocytes shown in part **B.** Note again the small, round uniformly staining nuclei with minimal cytoplasm. *(Part A courtesy of Hans E. Grossniklaus, MD; parts B and C courtesy of Vivian Lee, MD.)*

cells may become completely distended with immunoglobulin and form *Russell bodies* (Fig 1-7C). See BCSC Section 9, *Uveitis and Ocular Inflammation*, for in-depth discussion of the mechanisms involved in inflammatory processes.

Monocytes consist primarily of histiocytes (also known as *macrophages*) when they migrate from the intravascular space into tissue (Fig 1-8). *Histiocytes* have eccentrically located, indented nuclei and abundant eosinophilic cytoplasm (see Fig 1-8C). Histiocytes activated by an antigen are referred to as *epithelioid histiocytes* because of their resemblance to epithelial cells. Epithelioid histiocytes are the hallmark of granulomatous inflammation and may aggregate into a spheroid formation known as a *granuloma*. Granulomas may consist completely of viable epithelioid histiocytes ("hard" tubercles; Fig 1-9A), or they may exhibit necrotic centers ("caseating" granulomas; Fig 1-9B). Epithelioid histiocytes may coalesce to form a *multinucleated giant cell,* of which there are several varieties:

- Langhans cells, characterized by a horseshoe arrangement of the nuclei (Fig 1-10A)
- Touton giant cells, characterized by an annulus of nuclei surrounded by a foamy, lipid-filled pale zone (Fig 1-10B)
- foreign body giant cells, characterized by haphazardly arranged nuclei (Fig 1-10C)

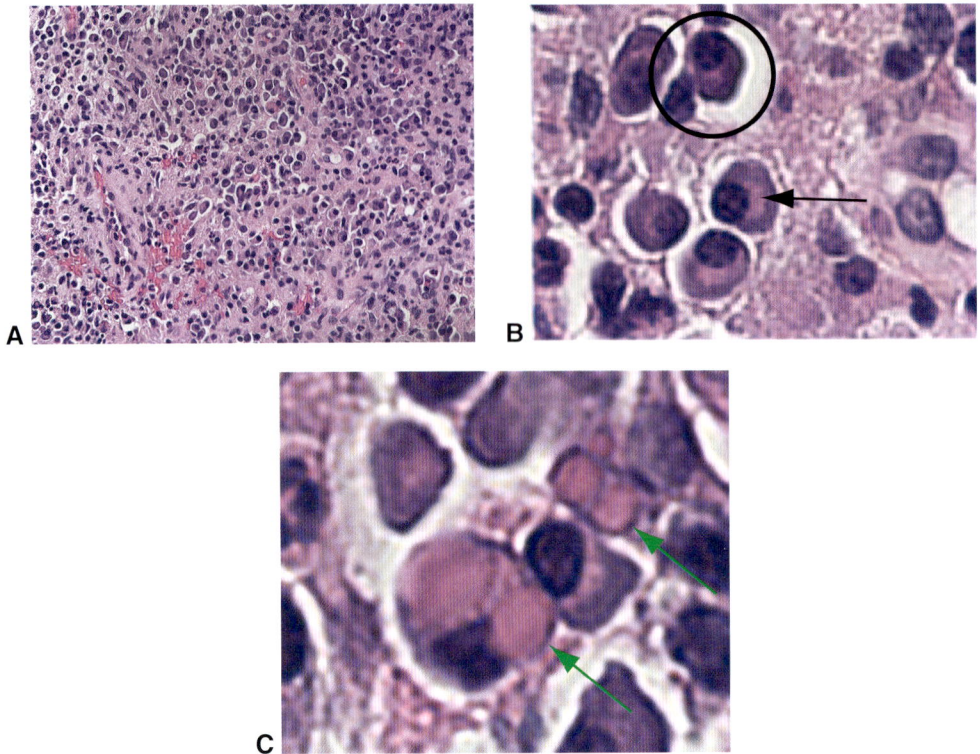

Figure 1-7 **A,** Plasma cell–rich infiltrate in tissue. **B,** High magnification highlights eccentric nuclei and the clock-face arrangement of nuclear chromatin *(circle).* The lucent curvilinear area adjacent to the nucleus is the Golgi apparatus *(arrow).* Plasma cells are typically found in soft tissue and are rarely found in the blood. **C,** Plasma cell with intracellular accumulation of immunoglobulin (Russell bodies) *(arrows). (Courtesy of Vivian Lee, MD.)*

For more on cells that are part of the inflammatory response, see Activity 1-2.

ACTIVITY 1-2 Identify the cell type.
Developed by Vivian Lee, MD.

Degeneration and dystrophy

Degeneration refers to a wide variety of changes that may occur in tissue over time. It is usually characterized by accumulation of acellular material or loss of tissue mass rather than proliferation of cells. Extracellular deposits may result from cellular overproduction of normal material or metabolically abnormal material. These findings may occur in response to injury or inflammation or as part of a systemic process. Examples include calcification of the lens in congenital cataract (developmental anomaly) and corneal amyloid deposition in trachoma (inflammatory process). As used in this book, the concept of degeneration encompasses a wide range of tissue alterations in order to streamline the discussion and avoid using multiple subcategories, such as aging, trauma, and vasculopathies.

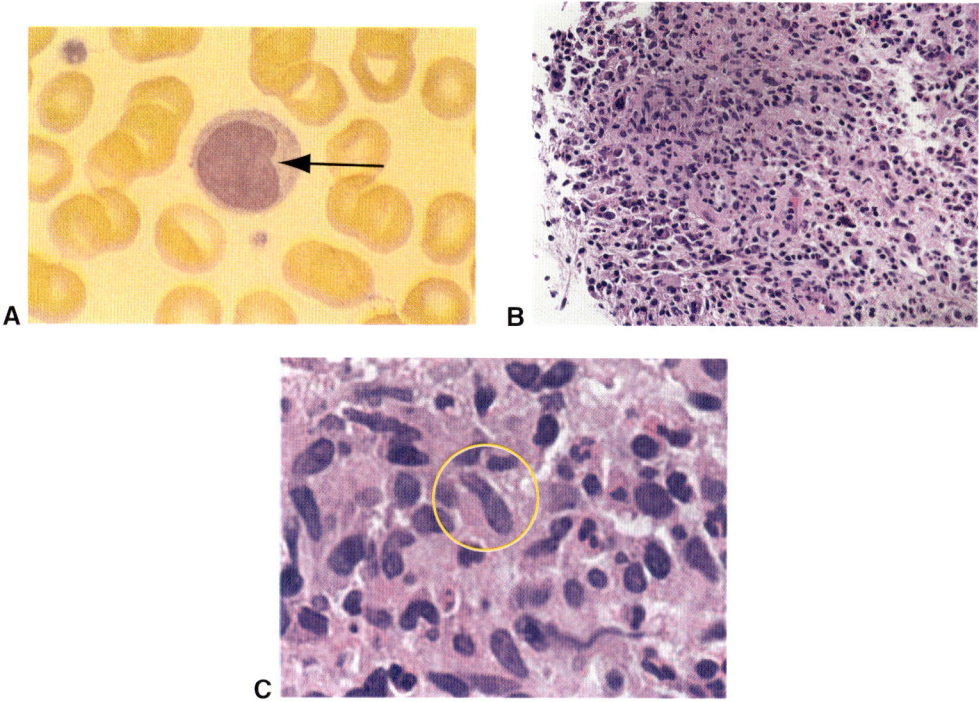

Figure 1-8 **A,** Blood smear demonstrating a monocyte with indented nucleus *(arrow).* **B,** Tissue section showing monocytes (histiocytes) in soft tissue at low magnification. **C,** Tissue section (same as in part B) showing monocytes *(circle)* in soft tissue at high magnification. *(Part A courtesy of Hans E. Grossniklaus, MD; parts B and C courtesy of Vivian Lee, MD.)*

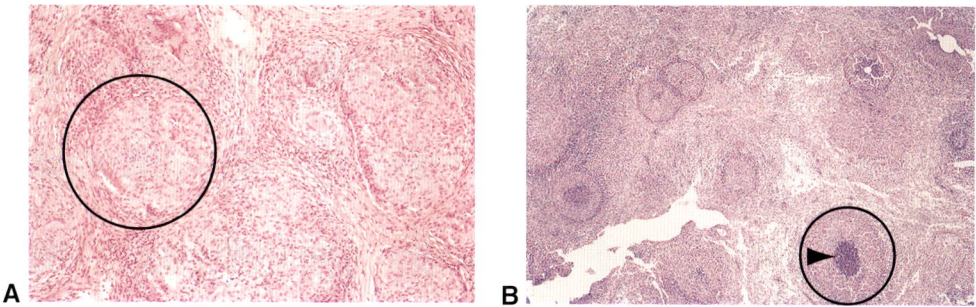

Figure 1-9 Granulomas. **A,** Numerous noncaseating granulomas *(example circled)*, or "hard" tubercles, formed by aggregates of epithelioid histiocytes surrounded by a cuff of lymphocytes. **B,** Caseating granuloma *(circle)* with necrotic center *(arrowhead). (Courtesy of Hans E. Grossniklaus, MD.)*

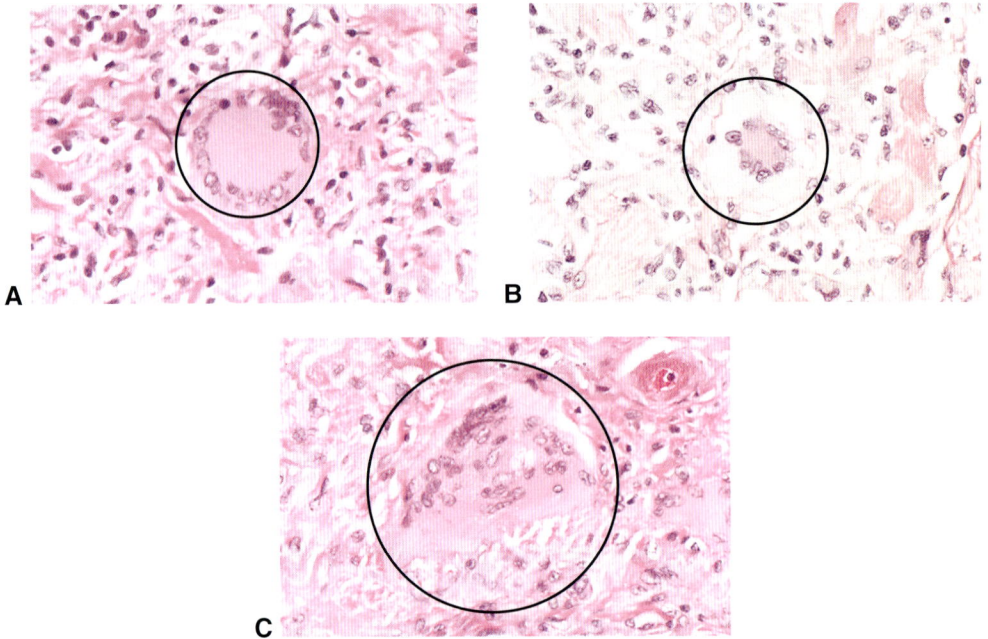

Figure 1-10 Types of multinucleated giant cells. **A,** Langhans *(circle)*. Note the peripheral arrangement of nuclei. **B,** Touton giant cell *(circle)*. Note the central eosinophilic cytoplasm and annulus of nuclei surrounded by a foamy, lipid-filled pale outer ring. **C,** Foreign body giant cell *(circle)*. Note the haphazardly arranged nuclei.

Dystrophies are defined as bilateral, often symmetric, inherited conditions that appear to have little or no relationship to environmental or systemic factors. Dystrophies affecting the eye typically involve abnormal deposition of material in ocular tissues or characteristic patterns of degeneration.

Degeneration of the eye The globe can undergo a unique range of tissue alterations secondary to trauma and chronic disease processes. *Phthisis bulbi* is defined as atrophy, shrinkage, and disorganization of the eye and intraocular contents. Not all eyes rendered sightless by trauma become phthisical. If the nutritional status of the eye and near-normal intraocular pressure (IOP) are maintained during the repair process, the globe will remain clinically stable. However, blind eyes are at high risk for repeated trauma, with cumulative destructive effects. Slow, progressive functional decompensation may also prevail.

STAGES OF OCULAR DEGENERATION Many blind eyes pass through several stages of atrophy and disorganization before progressing to the end stage of phthisis bulbi:

- *Atrophia bulbi without shrinkage.* In this initial stage, the size and shape of the eye are maintained despite the atrophy of intraocular tissues. The following structures are most sensitive to loss of nutrition: the lens, which becomes cataractous; the retina, which atrophies and becomes separated from the retinal pigment epithelium (RPE) by serous fluid accumulation; and the aqueous outflow tract, where anterior and posterior synechiae develop.

- *Atrophia bulbi with shrinkage.* In this stage, the eye becomes soft because of ciliary body dysfunction and progressive reduction of IOP. The globe becomes smaller and assumes a squared-off configuration as a result of the influence of the 4 rectus muscles. The anterior chamber collapses. Associated corneal endothelial cell damage initially results in corneal edema, followed by opacification with degenerative pannus, stromal scarring, and vascularization. Most of the remaining internal structures of the eye will be atrophic but recognizable histologically.

- *Phthisis bulbi* (Fig 1-11). In this end stage, the size of the globe shrinks from a normal average diameter of 23–25 mm to an average diameter of 16–19 mm. Most of the ocular contents become disorganized. In areas of preserved uvea the RPE proliferates, and nodular drusen may develop. In addition, extensive dystrophic calcification of the Bowman layer, lens, retina, and drusen usually occurs. Osseous metaplasia of the RPE with bone formation may be a prominent feature. Finally, the sclera becomes markedly thickened, particularly posteriorly.

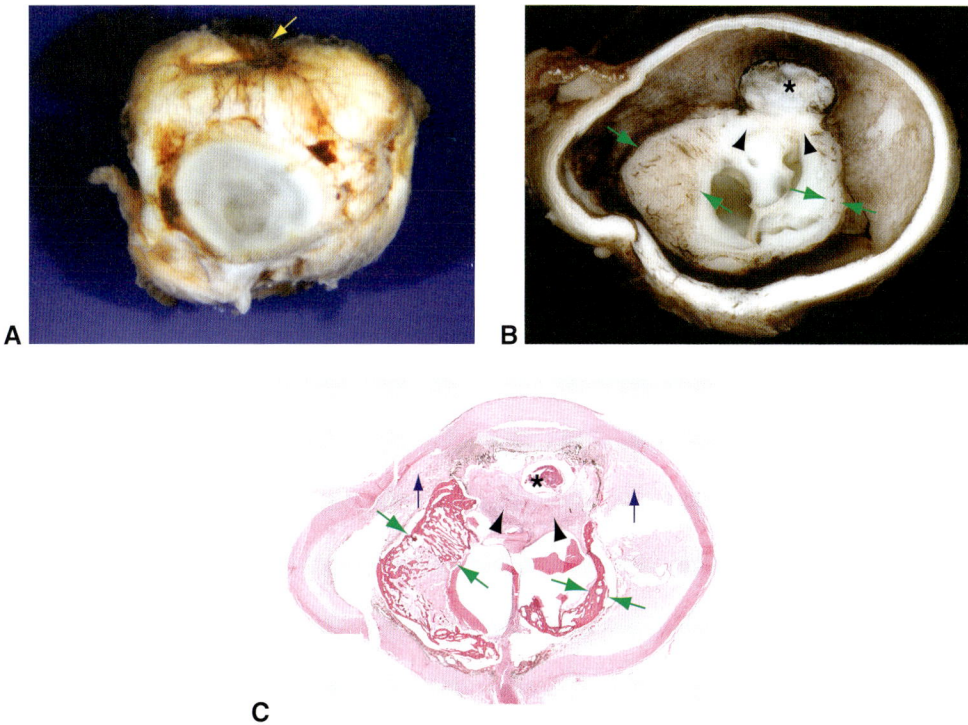

Figure 1-11 Phthisis bulbi. **A,** Gross photograph of a whole globe. Note the squared-off shape of the globe *(arrow),* resulting from hypotony and the force of the 4 rectus muscles on the sclera. **B,** Gross photograph of a phthisical globe that has been opened. Note the irregular contour, cataractous lens with calcification *(asterisk),* cyclitic membrane with adherent retina *(arrowheads),* and bone formation *(between green arrows).* **C,** Photomicrograph demonstrating the histopathologic correlation with the gross photograph shown in part **B.** In addition, organized ciliochoroidal effusions are apparent histologically *(blue arrows). (Part A courtesy of Ralph C. Eagle, MD; parts B and C courtesy of Robert H. Rosa Jr, MD.)*

Neoplasia

A *neoplasm* is a new, often monotonous, growth of a specific tissue phenotype and can be either benign or malignant. General histologic signs of malignancy include nuclear hyperchromatism and pleomorphism; prominent nucleoli; necrosis; hemorrhage; and increased, sometimes atypical, mitoses. Some neoplastic proliferations are called *borderline* or *indeterminate* because they exhibit both malignant and nonmalignant characteristics. Many examples in this book are presented as definitively benign or malignant, but for some cases in clinical practice, the diagnosis is less certain or may evolve over time. Table 1-2 summarizes the origin and general classification of neoplasms and includes clinical examples of neoplasms found in various tissues. See Figure 1-12 for illustrations of neoplastic growth patterns.

Differential Diagnosis

Formulating a differential diagnosis begins after evaluation of the topography of the specimen and determination of the disease process. Recognizing an *index feature,* a morphological characteristic that helps define a disease process more specifically, can be extremely useful in establishing the correct diagnosis. For example, a tumor in the uveal tract composed of atypical cells containing cytoplasmic pigment is suggestive of uveal melanoma, whereas a small, round, blue cell tumor at the posterior pole of the eye of an infant or child is highly suggestive of retinoblastoma. The index feature should differentiate the specimen from others demonstrating the same general disease process. Returning to the example above, both uveal melanoma and retinoblastoma are malignant intraocular tumors, but the former is characterized by atypical pigmented cells while the latter is characterized by small blue cells. Although very basic index features can be recognized without great difficulty, recognition of other index features requires familiarity and experience.

Table 1-2 Classification of Neoplasia

| Tissue Origin | Terminology | | Clinical Examples |
	Benign	Malignant	
Epithelial	Papilloma Adenoma	Carcinoma Adenocarcinoma	Squamous papilloma, squamous cell carcinoma
Mesenchymal	Cell type + -*oma*	Cell type + *sarcoma*	Schwannoma, leiomyoma, rhabdomyosarcoma *Note:* This nomenclature is not always consistent. For example, although the term *melanoma* contains the suffix -*oma*, this tumor is malignant.
Hematopoietic	Hyperplasia Infiltrate	Leukemia Lymphoma	Lymphoid hyperplasia, extranodal marginal zone B-cell lymphoma
Melanocytic	Nevus Melanosis/melanocytosis	Melanoma	Primary acquired melanosis, melanoma

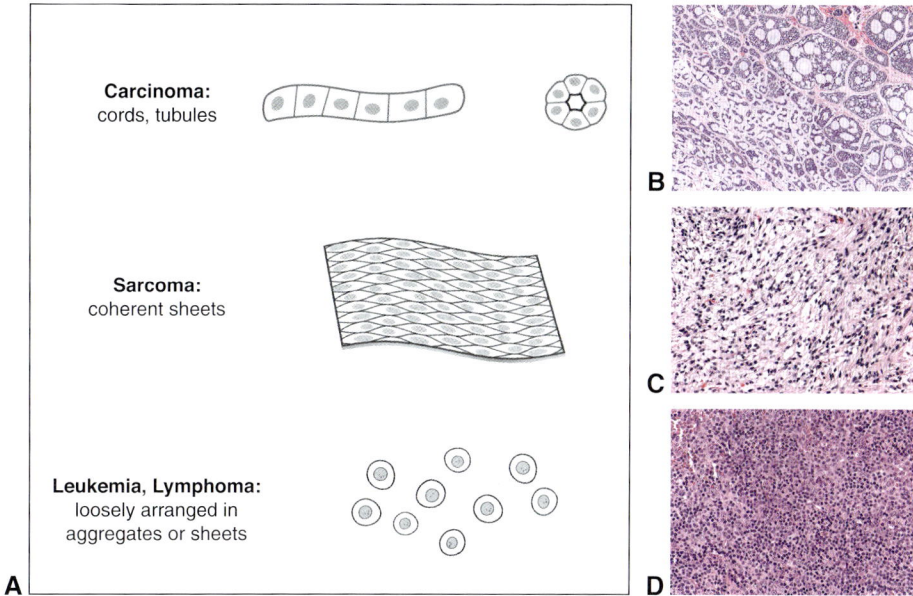

Figure 1-12 General classification and growth patterns of malignant tumors **(A)** with photomicrographs depicting adenoid cystic carcinoma of the lacrimal gland **(B),** rhabdomyosarcoma **(C),** and large B-cell lymphoma **(D).** *(Illustration by Christine Gralapp; parts B and D courtesy of Vivian Lee, MD; part C courtesy of Nasreen A. Syed, MD.)*

For example, the differential diagnosis for a melanocytic proliferation of the conjunctiva includes nevus, primary acquired melanosis, and melanoma. Narrowing the differential diagnosis in this case requires recognition of the key histologic features of each of these entities.

If a key index feature is absent, forming a focused differential diagnosis based on the topography of the specimen and the disease process is necessary before a definitive or specific diagnosis can be established. Special stains or other ancillary pathology studies may provide information that focuses the differential. For instance, the differential diagnosis that can be constructed from the features of noncaseating granulomatous inflammation of the conjunctiva includes sarcoidosis, foreign body, and fungal and mycobacterial infections. Some of these entities can be excluded from the differential with the use of special stains for acid fast and fungal organisms.

Readers are encouraged to practice using the hierarchical framework presented in this chapter by reviewing each step in sequence when they examine histologic images and pathologic specimens. Chapters 5 through 15 of this book provide tissue-specific examples of the differential diagnoses for each of the major disease process categories. See Table 1-1 for the expanded organizational paradigm.

CHAPTER 2

Specimen Handling

This chapter includes a related video. Go to www.aao.org/bcscvideo_section04 or scan the QR code in the text to access this content.

Highlights

- Direct and personal communication between the ophthalmologist and pathologist is essential for accurate diagnosis, particularly in special circumstances, such as suspicion of malignancy or determination of a critical diagnosis.
- Tissues for pathologic examination typically require some type of fixation to arrest tissue decomposition and preserve cellular morphology.
- Histologic stains allow contrasting color staining of various cellular and extracellular elements and/or identification of specific material in tissue sections.

Overview

This chapter covers the methods that pathology laboratories use to process tissue specimens with the final product being glass slides. These specimens include globes and ocular adnexal biopsy tissues, as well as specimens requiring evaluation of surgical margins. The main steps for processing of specimens are

- communication with the pathologist regarding specimen orientation (as indicated)
- fixation to preserve the tissue
- gross dissection to prepare the specimen for histologic sectioning
- tissue processing, typically into paraffin
- slide preparation and tissue staining

The most common method used to make the tissue firm enough to be cut into thin sections is embedding in paraffin and cutting sections (permanent sections), which is discussed in this chapter. Another method used, typically for evaluation of surgical margins of resection, is frozen section, which is discussed in Chapter 3. Permanent sections are always preferred in ophthalmic pathology because this technique allows better preservation of morphological features than do frozen sections, which are prone to artifact.

Discussion between the ophthalmologist and the pathologist prior to the biopsy or surgery is important, as it enables them to determine the best way to collect a specimen and submit it to the laboratory. The following section discusses this topic.

Communication

Communication with the pathologist before, during, and after surgical procedures is an essential aspect of quality patient care. Standards for the technical handling of specimens and reporting of results have been developed; a few are available online at no cost. The ophthalmologist is responsible for providing relevant details regarding the clinical history when submitting the specimen to the laboratory. This history facilitates clinicopathologic correlation and enables the pathologist to provide the most accurate interpretation of the specimen. The final histologic diagnosis reflects successful collaborative work between clinician and pathologist.

In general, communication can usually be accomplished via the pathology request form and the pathology report. However, if there are any special circumstances, such as suspicion of malignancy or identification of a critical diagnosis, direct and personal communication between the ophthalmologist and the pathologist is essential. Discussion prior to surgery allows these physicians to consider the best way to collect a specimen and submit it to the laboratory. For example, the pathologist may wish to have fresh tissue for immunofluorescent staining and molecular diagnostic studies, glutaraldehyde-fixed tissue for electron microscopy, and formalin-fixed tissue for routine paraffin embedding. If the tissue is simply submitted in formalin, the opportunity to perform certain studies may be lost, resulting in a less definitive diagnosis. Communication between clinician and pathologist is especially important in ophthalmic pathology, in which specimens are often very small and require particularly careful handling. In some cases, careful selection of the surgical facility is necessary to ensure proper specimen handling. See Chapter 3, Table 3-1, for a preoperative checklist addressing the handling of ophthalmic pathology specimens.

Anytime a previous biopsy has been performed at the site of the present pathology, the clinician should request a review of the prior biopsy slides if possible, especially if there is a history of malignancy, so that the pathologist can compare the current and prior morphological features and diagnoses. The surgical plan may be altered substantially if the initial biopsy was thought to represent, for example, a basal cell carcinoma when in fact the disease was sebaceous carcinoma. In addition, when the case is reviewed in advance, the pathologist is able to interpret intraoperative frozen sections more accurately.

If there is a significant discrepancy between the clinical diagnosis and the histologic diagnosis, the ophthalmologist should promptly contact the pathologist directly to resolve the discrepancy. For example, merely correcting the patient age on the pathology request form may change the interpretation of melanocytic lesions of the conjunctiva from benign to malignant, or vice versa.

College of American Pathologists. Cancer protocol templates. Accessed September 17, 2019. https://www.cap.org/protocols-and-guidelines/cancer-reporting-tools/cancer-protocol-templates

Grossniklaus HE, Hyrcza M, Jain D, et al. Eye. PathologyOutlines.com. Accessed September 17, 2019. www.pathologyoutlines.com/eye.html

Table 2-1 **Fixatives Used in Ophthalmic Pathology**

Fixative	Color	Examples of Use
10% neutral-buffered formalin (NBF)	Clear	Routine fixation of all tissues (eg, eyelid, conjunctiva, globe, orbital)
Bouin solution	Yellow	Small biopsy specimens (eg, gastrointestinal tissue, conjunctiva)
Absolute ethanol or methanol	Clear	Crystals (eg, corneal urate crystals)
Cytology fixatives (ethanol, methanol, or Saccomanno fixative)	Variety of colors	Liquid specimens or smears (eg, vitreous, aqueous humor, fine-needle aspirates, corneal smears)
Glutaraldehyde	Clear	Electron microscopy (eg, corneal microsporidia)
Michel or Zeus transport medium[a]	Clear	Immunofluorescence (eg, conjunctival biopsy for mucous membrane pemphigoid)
Roswell Park Memorial Institute (RPMI) tissue culture medium[a]	Pink, salmon	Tissue culture (eg, orbital tumor for cytogenetics or flow cytometry) or transport medium for molecular studies

[a] Not a true fixative but prolongs tissue decomposition.

Fixatives for Tissue Preservation

Table 2-1 lists many of the fixatives and transport media used by pathology laboratories for various forms of analysis. The most commonly used fixative is 10% neutral-buffered formalin. Formalin is a 40% solution of formaldehyde that stabilizes proteins, lipids, and carbohydrates and prevents enzymatic destruction of the tissue (autolysis) by crosslinking proteins. In general, the volume of the fixative in which tissue is immersed should be at least 10 times the volume of the tissue. Formalin diffuses fairly quickly through tissue. Tissue fixation time varies depending on the size and composition of the specimen. When a globe is to be sent for pathologic evaluation, it is not necessary or desirable to open the eye, inject fixative, or create windows in the sclera, despite the relatively large size and volume of the globe. Furthermore, opening an eye before fixation may damage or distort sites of pathology, making histologic interpretation difficult or impossible. To ensure adequate fixation, an eye should be suspended in formalin (at least a 10:1 ratio of fixative to tissue) for at least 24–48 hours before processing. As different institutions may use different protocols, preoperative consultation with the pathologist is critical.

Specimen Orientation

Globes may be oriented according to the location of the extraocular muscles and of the long posterior ciliary arteries and nerves, which are located in the horizontal meridian. The medial, inferior, lateral, and superior rectus muscles insert progressively farther from

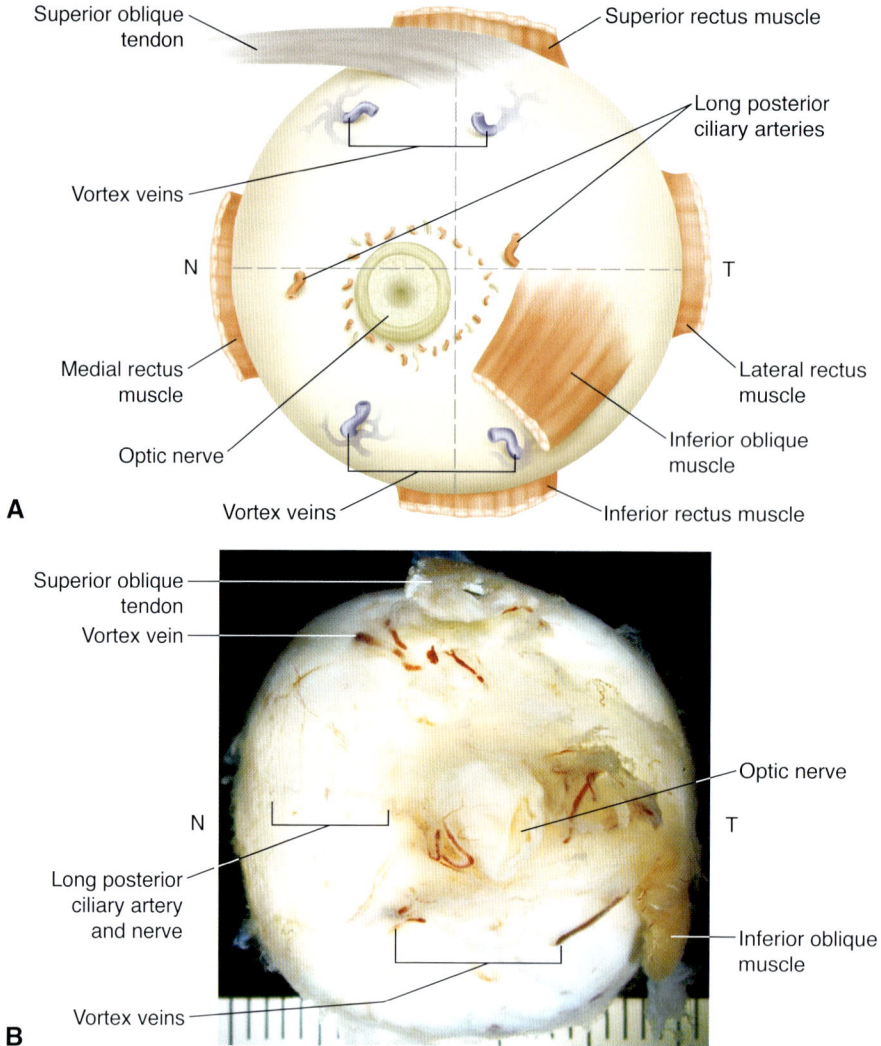

Figure 2-1 Posterior view of the right globe. N = nasal; T = temporal. **A,** Diagram. **B,** Macroscopic photograph. Note that the posterior ciliary artery and nerve appear as a subtle blue-gray line as they pass through the sclera. This marks the horizontal meridian of the globe. Also note that the rectus muscle insertions are not present. The rectus muscles are typically incised at their scleral insertion during enucleation so that they may be attached to the orbital implant. *(Part A modified by Cyndie C. H. Wooley from an illustration by Thomas A. Weingeist, MD, PhD; part B courtesy of Nasreen A. Syed, MD.)*

the limbus. Locating the inferior oblique muscle insertion relative to the optic nerve is helpful in distinguishing between a right eye and a left eye. The inferior oblique inserts on the sclera temporally over the macula, with its fibers running inferiorly (Fig 2-1). Once the laterality of the eye is determined, accurate location of ocular lesions is possible.

When eyelid or conjunctival tissue is sent for pathologic evaluation, it may be important in some clinical situations to evaluate the resection margins (ie, determine whether

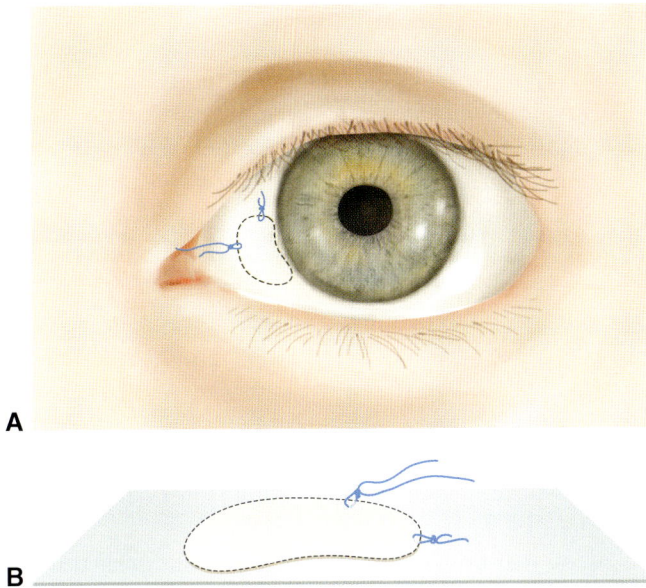

Figure 2-2   Marking the orientation of excised tissue for analysis of surgical margins. **A,** Sutures, 1 long and 1 short, are placed 90° apart. **B,** The tissue is carefully placed on a piece of filter paper and allowed to adhere for several seconds before it is placed in a container of formalin. *(Illustration by Cyndie C. H. Wooley.)*

the lesion is present in the margins of resection). Note that the smaller a tissue sample is, the more difficult it will be to accurately assess the surgical margins. If the tissue rolls up or bunches, it can be difficult to orient. Furthermore, once the tissue is fixed in formalin, it cannot be reshaped. For these reasons, when the biopsy specimen is obtained, it should be unrolled and placed on a dry piece of filter paper or similar absorptive to keep it flat. The tissue should be allowed to adhere to the paper for several seconds, and then the paper with the tissue can be floated in a container of formalin.

To properly orient a specimen, the pathologist needs landmarks. Therefore, before the biopsy tissue is placed in formalin, it must be marked in some way to enable correct orientation of the surgical margins; a corresponding diagram indicating the meaning of the marks must also be created. The best way to mark tissue is to use sutures (long and short) positioned 90° apart (Fig 2-2). Small sutures may look large with surgical magnification, but they are difficult to see in the pathology laboratory; thus, sutures that are visible with the naked eye should be used. Ink is not a good way to mark tissue because most types of ink, including permanent marker and surgical marking ink, dissolve in formalin.

Labeling both the specimen container and the paperwork with 2 patient identifiers is mandatory before submission to the pathology laboratory. The diagram should be submitted along with the specimen.

Gross Examination and Dissection

The objective of gross examination and dissection is to prepare the specimen for histologic sectioning. This typically includes describing the physical appearance of the tissue; measuring it; orienting the tissue as clinically indicated; and possibly cutting the tissue into smaller, more manageable pieces. All types of tissues submitted to the pathology laboratory undergo some type of gross examination and/or dissection prior to tissue processing into paraffin. The remainder of this discussion is focused on gross examination and dissection of a globe.

Dissection of a globe includes opening it in such a way as to display as many of the pathologic changes as possible on a single slide. Before gross dissection, the globe is *transilluminated* with bright light. This helps identify intraocular lesions such as tumors, which block the transilluminated light and cast a shadow (Fig 2-3A). The shadow can be outlined on the sclera with a marking pencil (Fig 2-3B). This outline can then be used to guide the dissection so that the center of the section includes the maximum extent of the area of interest (Fig 2-3C–E).

Most eyes are cut so that the pupil and optic nerve are present in the same section, called the *pupil–optic nerve (PO) section.* The meridian, or clock-hour, of the section is determined by the unique features of the case, such as the presence of an intraocular tumor or a history of previous surgery or trauma. In routine cases, globes with no prior surgery or intraocular neoplasm are typically opened in the horizontal meridian, which includes the macula in the same section as the pupil and optic nerve (Fig 2-4). Globes with a surgical or nonsurgical wound should be opened such that the wound is perpendicular to, and included in, the PO section. Globes with intraocular tumors are opened horizontally, vertically, or obliquely to place the center of the tumor, as outlined by transillumination, in the PO section (Video 2-1).

VIDEO 2-1 Gross dissection of the eye.
Courtesy of Ralph C. Eagle Jr, MD.
Go to www.aao.org/bcscvideo_section04 to access all Section 4 videos.

The globe can also be opened coronally with separation of the anterior and posterior segments, allowing a clinician's view of posterior segment pathology.

Processing and Staining

Tissue Processing

Tissue processing involves dehydration of the specimen to allow infiltration of the tissue with paraffin. The tissue is then embedded in a paraffin block, which mechanically stabilizes the tissue, enabling it to be cut into very thin sections.

The organic solvents used in tissue processing—for example, ethanol and xylene—dissolve lipids and may dissolve some synthetic materials. Routine processing usually dissolves intraocular lenses made of acrylic or silicone but does not dissolve sutures made of silk, nylon, or other synthetic materials.

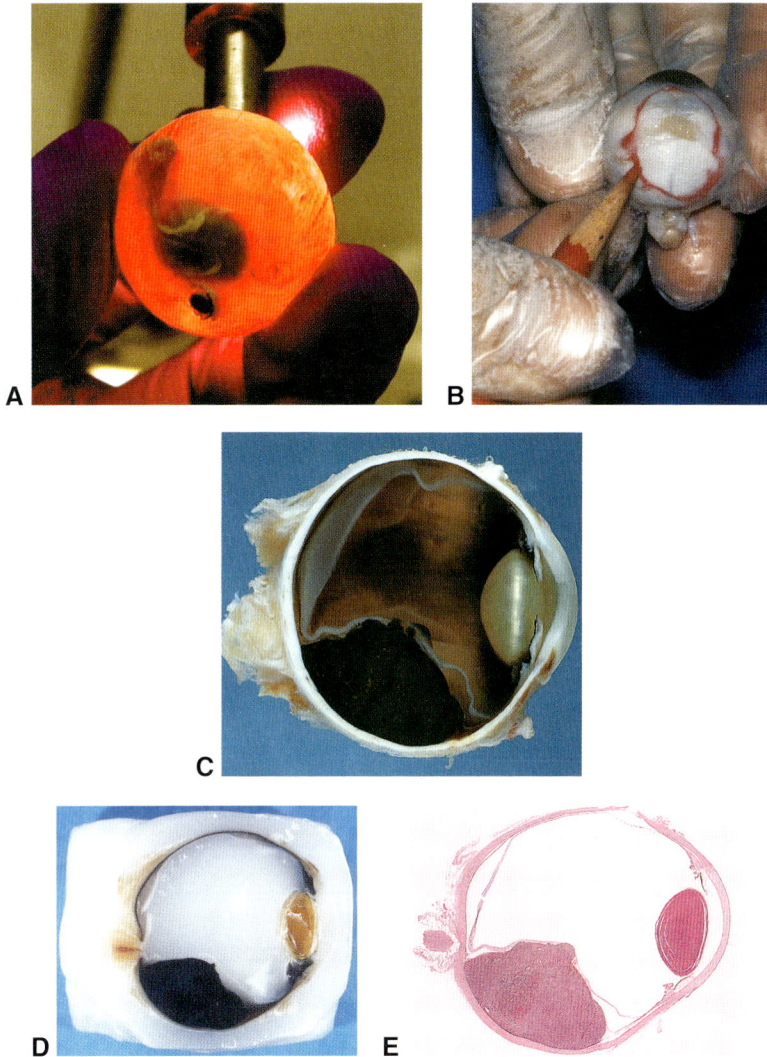

Figure 2-3 Preparation of an intraocular tumor enucleation specimen. **A,** Transillumination shows blockage of light due to an intraocular tumor. **B,** The shadow is traced with a marking pencil. **C,** The opened eye shows the intraocular tumor that was demonstrated by transillumination. **D,** The paraffin-embedded eye shows the intraocular tumor. **E,** The hematoxylin-eosin (H&E)–stained section shows that the maximum dimension of the tumor, demonstrated by transillumination grossly, is in the center of the section, which also includes the pupil–optic nerve (PO) section. *(Part A courtesy of Nasreen A. Syed, MD; part B courtesy of Hans E. Grossniklaus, MD.)*

The processing of a routine specimen usually takes a day. Techniques for the rapid processing of special surgical pathology material are generally reserved for small biopsy specimens that require urgent handling. Rapid processing usually results in inferior tissue preparations and therefore should not be requested routinely. Surgeons should communicate directly with their pathologists about the availability and shortcomings of these techniques.

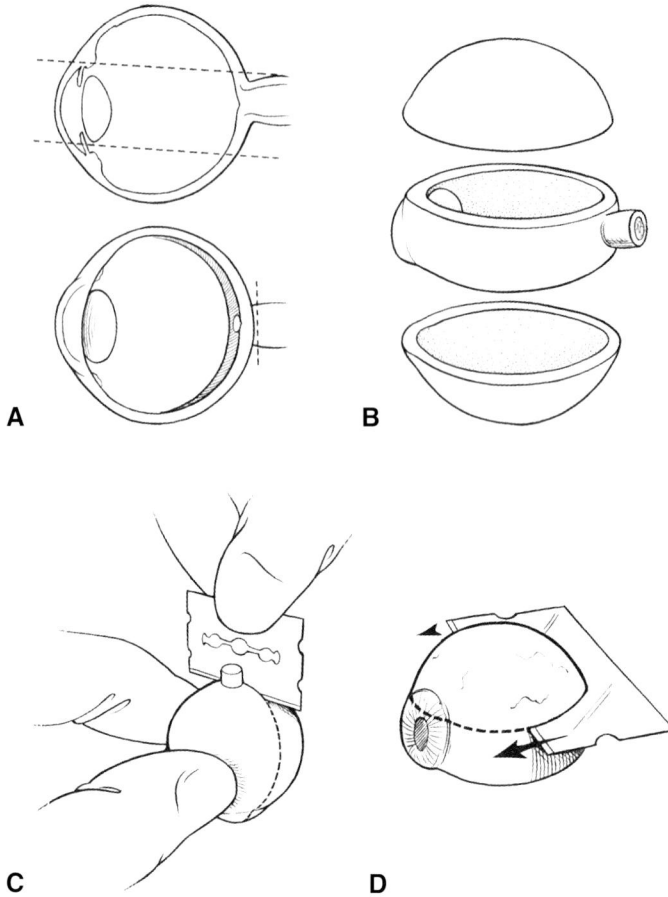

Figure 2-4 Gross dissection of a globe. **A,** The goal of sectioning is to obtain a PO section that contains the maximum area of interest. **B,** Two caps, or calottes, are removed to obtain a PO section. **C,** The first cut is generally performed from posterior to anterior. **D,** The second cut yields the PO section. *(Illustration by Christine Gralapp.)*

Slide Preparation and Tissue Staining

Tissue sections in paraffin are usually cut at 4–6 µm. The cut section is colorless except for areas of indigenous pigmentation. Various tissue dyes—principally hematoxylin and eosin (H&E) and periodic acid–Schiff (PAS)—are used to stain the tissue section in order to visualize the tissue under the microscope. The stains provide contrast and color, making it possible for pathologists to identify cellular elements (nuclear versus cytoplasmic). They also highlight various cellular and extracellular structures, depending on their chemical composition (Table 2-2). A small amount of resin is placed over the stained section and covered with a thin glass coverslip to protect and preserve it.

Special histochemical stains

Pathologists employ special histochemical stains to identify organisms and constituent substances present in tissue, supplementing the information available through examination of

Table 2-2 Histochemical Stains Commonly Used in Ophthalmic Pathology

Stain	Material Stained: Color	Examples of Use
Hematoxylin-eosin (H&E)	Nucleus: blue Cytoplasm: pink	General tissue stain (see Fig 2-3E)
Periodic acid–Schiff (PAS)	Glycogen and proteoglycans: magenta	Descemet membrane (see Fig 6-14C, D), lens capsule, Bruch membrane, goblet cells
Alcian blue	Acid mucopolysaccharide: blue	Cavernous optic atrophy (see Fig 15-10B)
Alizarin red	Calcium: red	Band keratopathy
Colloidal iron	Acid mucopolysaccharide: blue	Macular dystrophy (see Fig 6-23C, D)
Congo red	Amyloid: red orange, apple green with polarized light (dichroism)	Lattice corneal dystrophy (see Fig 6-20C, D)
Fite-Faraco	Some acid-fast organisms: red	*Mycobacterium leprae*
Giemsa, Wright-Giemsa	Some bacteria and parasites: blue	Conjunctival *Chlamydia* (eg, trachoma), corneal *Acanthamoeba*
Gomori or Grocott methenamine silver (GMS)	Fungal elements: black	Fungal *Fusarium* (see Fig 6-5B)
Gram stain for tissue (Brown and Brenn [B&B], Brown and Hopps [B&H])	Gram-positive bacteria: blue Gram-negative bacteria: red	Bacterial infection (see Fig 6-7B)
KOH with calcofluor white	Fungal elements	Fungal infections (Stain usually performed in microbiology laboratory)
Masson trichrome	Collagen: blue Muscle: red	Granular corneal dystrophy (see Fig 6-21C) Red deposits
Oil red O	Lipid: red	Sebaceous carcinoma of eyelid
Perls Prussian blue	Iron: blue	Fleischer ring
Thioflavin T (ThT)	Amyloid: fluorescent yellow-white	Lattice corneal dystrophy
Verhoeff–van Gieson (elastin)	Elastic fibers: black	Temporal artery elastic layer (see Fig 15-6B)
von Kossa	Calcium phosphate salts: black	Band keratopathy (see Fig 6-10C)
Ziehl-Neelsen	Acid-fast organisms: red	*Mycobacterium tuberculosis* and most other mycobacteria

tissue using routine stains such as H&E. Special stains are typically performed on the basis of changes identified by the pathologist on routine stains or when a particular diagnosis is suspected clinically. These stains are performed on permanent sections, with the exception of oil red O, which requires a frozen tissue section instead of paraffin-processed tissue. See Table 2-2, which lists the histochemical stains commonly used in ophthalmic pathology.

CHAPTER 3

Special Testing and Procedures in Pathology

Highlights

- Special procedures such as immunohistochemistry and flow cytometry, as well as molecular genetic and cytogenetic techniques, have led to improvements in the diagnosis of eye diseases.
- The ophthalmic surgeon is responsible for submitting tissue in a manner that allows special studies to be performed when needed. Appropriate submission requires preoperative consultation with the pathologist.
- Frozen section pathology should be used when the pathologic results would alter the surgical procedure, as with evaluation of surgical margins when a malignancy is excised.

Introduction

New methodologies in pathologic analysis of tissue specimens have contributed to improvements in the diagnosis of infectious agents, dystrophies, degenerations, and neoplasms, as well as to the classification of neoplasms, particularly the non-Hodgkin lymphomas and sarcomas. Refinements in immunohistochemical (IHC) staining and in flow cytometric, molecular genetic, and cytogenetic techniques lead to more accurate diagnoses and to more precise identification of biomarkers of value in risk stratification, prognostication, and targeted therapeutics.

If special studies are anticipated, the ophthalmic surgeon is responsible for consulting with the pathologist prior to the procedure and then appropriately obtaining and submitting tissue for evaluation. See Table 3-1 for a checklist of important considerations when submitting tissue for pathologic consultation.

Immunohistochemistry

A given cell type can express specific antigens. Pathologists take advantage of this property to identify the cell type or cell of origin, typically in tumors. In the IHC stains commonly used in ophthalmic pathology, a primary antibody binds to a specific antigen in or

---

Table 3-1 Checklist for Requesting an Ophthalmic Pathology Consultation

Routine Specimens
1. Fill out requisition form or electronic order, providing
   a. Two patient identifiers
   b. Sex and age of patient
   c. Location of lesion (laterality and exact location)
   d. Previous biopsies of the site and diagnosis
   e. Pertinent clinical history
   f. Clinical differential diagnosis
   g. Ophthalmologist phone, pager, and/or fax numbers
2. Submit specimen in adequately sealed container with
   a. Ample amount of 10% formalin (at least 10 times the volume of the biopsy specimen)
   b. Label with 2 patient identifiers and location of biopsy site
3. Include diagram for indicating the biopsy site and landmarks for orientation of resection margins (eg, complete resection of eyelid or conjunctival malignancies, ciliary body/iris tumors).

Frozen Sections
1. If possible, initiate communication with pathologist before requesting the section.
2. Fill out frozen section requisition form or electronic order, specifying the reason for submitting tissue, such as
   a. Margins
   b. Diagnosis
   c. Adequacy of sampling
   d. Determining whether tissue should be submitted for molecular testing (eg, retinoblastoma, rhabdomyosarcoma, metastatic neuroblastoma)
3. Include map/diagram of the lesion for indicating resection margins and orientation.
4. Label the tissue with landmarks (eg, sutures) to orient according to the diagram (for analysis of margins).

Fine-Needle Aspiration Biopsy and Cytology
1. Initiate communication with pathologist prior to the procedure to discuss goals and logistics.
   a. Logistics of the biopsy
      i. Possible adequacy check during the biopsy (intraocular tumors)
      ii. Fixative to be used
      iii. Fresh tissue for possible molecular testing
   b. Specific cytology form or electronic order to be filled out

Flow Cytometry
1. Unfixed, unfrozen tissue is critical.
2. Initiate communication with pathologist before the biopsy to discuss
   a. Recommendations on fresh tissue transport (no media vs nutrient media, such as RPMI)
   b. Size of the sample needed
   c. Geographic proximity to the laboratory and transportation of tissue to laboratory

Molecular Techniques and Electron Microscopy
1. Initiate communication with pathologist before the biopsy to discuss
   a. Differential diagnosis
   b. Fixative or transport medium (fresh vs alcohol vs glutaraldehyde vs other)
   c. Logistics of the biopsy
      i. Time and date (availability of specialized personnel)
      ii. Geographic proximity to laboratory and transportation of tissue to laboratory

---

on a cell, and a secondary antibody linked to a chromogen (a compound that produces a particular color as a result of a chemical reaction) then binds to the primary antibody (Fig 3-1). The most common chromogen color product is brown (see Fig 3-1C) or red (see Fig 3-5B). A red chromogen color product is especially helpful in working with pigmented

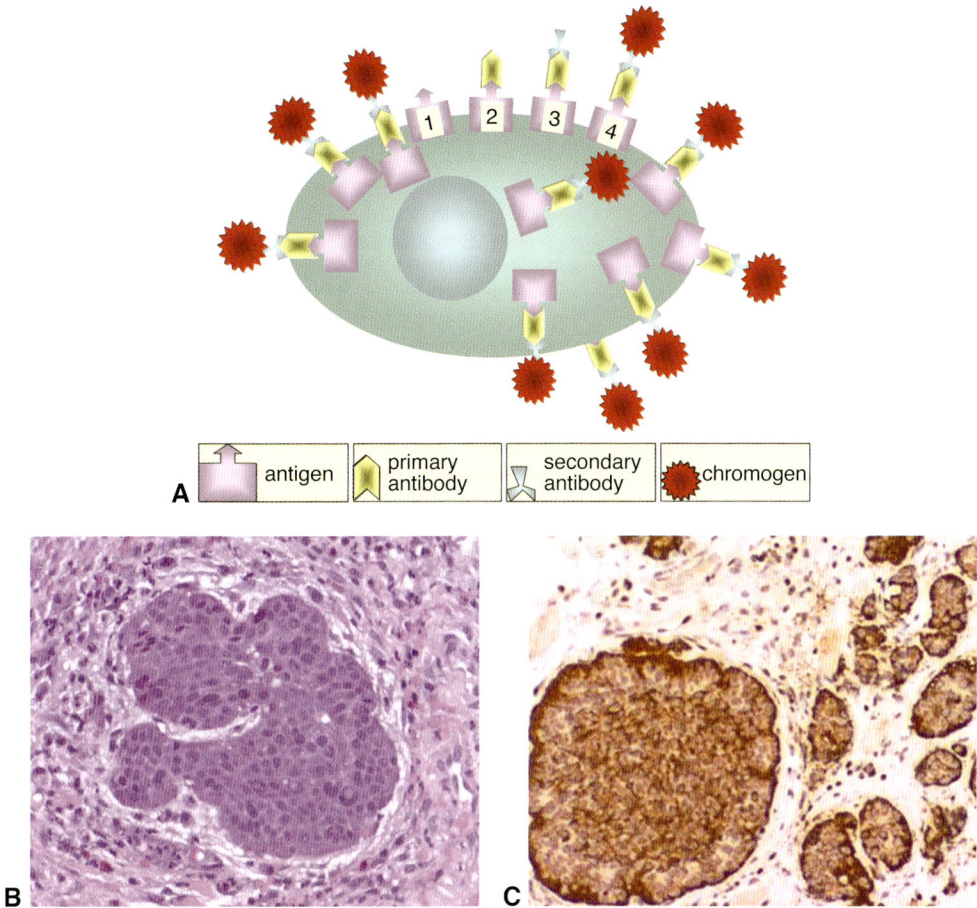

Figure 3-1 Immunohistochemistry. **A,** Schematic representation of the general immuno-histochemistry method. (1) The cellular antigen is recognized by the specific primary antibody; (2) a secondary antibody targeting the primary antibody is added and attaches to the primary antibody; (3) the secondary antibody reacts with the enzymatic complex, thereby activating the chromogen; (4) the final product allows visualization of the cell containing the antigen based on identification of the color product of the activated chromogen in the tissue section. **B–C,** A metastatic carcinoid to the orbit seen with hematoxylin-eosin (H&E) staining **(B)** shows bland epithelial characteristics. In **C,** an antibody directed against chromogranin highlights the neuro-endocrine nature of the cells. *(Courtesy of Patricia Chévez-Barrios, MD.)*

ocular tissues and with melanomas, because it contrasts with the brown melanin pigment in the uveal tissue or tumor.

A specific antigen can be identified using this method, and depending on the antigen profile, the specific cell type that expresses this antigen(s) can be ascertained. Many antibodies are routinely used for diagnosis, treatment, and prognosis. The following are some common antibodies used in IHC stains; a more comprehensive list can be found in Table 3-2:

- cytokeratins (many different antibodies) for diagnosis of lesions that are derived from epithelial cells (eg, adenoma, carcinoma)

Table 3-2 Common Immunohistochemical Stains in Ophthalmic Pathology

Associated Condition	Antibodies
Primary tumors	
Carcinomas	Various cytokeratins
Melanoma and melanocytic lesions	Melan A, HMB-45, S-100, SOX-10
Lymphoma and reactive lymphoid hyperplasia	CD3, CD20, kappa and lambda light chains, CD43, CD5, CD10, BCL-2
• B lymphocytes	CD19, CD20, PAX-5
• T lymphocytes	CD3, CD4, CD8
Schwannoma	S-100
Rhabdomyosarcoma	Muscle-specific actin, desmin, myogenin, myoglobin, Myo-D1
Neuroblastoma	Neuron-specific enolase
Retinoblastoma	Synaptophysin, neuron-specific enolase, high proliferative index (Ki-67)
Meningioma	Epithelial membrane antigen, somatostatin receptor 2a
Optic nerve glioma	Glial fibrillary acidic protein (GFAP)
Metastatic tumors	
Carcinoma (nonspecific)	Cytokeratin AE1/AE3, cytokeratin 7, cytokeratin 20, CAM5.2, cytokeratin 5/6, EMA
Lung carcinoma	Thyroid transcription factor 1 (TTF-1), napsin A
Breast carcinoma	Estrogen and progesterone receptors (ER and PR), GATA-binding protein 3
Prostate carcinoma	Prostate-specific antigen (PSA)
Gastrointestinal tract carcinomas	CDX2
Neuroendocrine tumors	Chromogranin, synaptophysin
Infections	
Retinitis	Herpes simplex virus, herpes zoster virus, cytomegalovirus

- desmin, myoglobin, or actin for diagnosis of lesions with smooth muscle or skeletal muscle features (eg, rhabdomyosarcoma, leiomyoma)
- S-100 protein for diagnosis of lesions of neuroectodermal origin (eg, schwannoma, neurofibroma, melanoma)
- Melan A and HMB-45 for diagnosis of melanocytic lesions (eg, nevus, melanoma)
- chromogranin and synaptophysin for diagnosis of neuroendocrine lesions (eg, metastatic carcinoid [see Fig 3-1C], small cell carcinoma)
- leukocyte common antigen for diagnosis of lesions of hematopoietic origin (eg, leukemia, lymphoma)
- CD (cluster of differentiation) antigens for subtyping white blood cells, particularly lymphocytes
- BAP1 for prognosis of neoplasia (eg, uveal melanoma)

Antibodies used for IHC vary in their specificity and sensitivity, which will affect interpretation. Interpretation of IHC stains includes comparing the results of the tissue being tested with appropriate standardized controls. The specificities and sensitivities of new antibodies are continually being evaluated. In addition, automated equipment and antigen retrieval techniques are currently used to increase sensitivity and decrease turnaround time.

Flow Cytometry, Molecular Pathology, and Diagnostic Electron Microscopy

Flow Cytometry

Pathologists use flow cytometry to analyze the physical and chemical properties of cells moving in single file in a fluid stream (Fig 3-2A, a). The most common use of flow cytometry in clinical practice is for immunophenotyping hematopoietic proliferations. This procedure may be performed on ocular adnexal tissue, aqueous humor, or vitreous. One example of flow cytometry is leukocyte immunophenotyping. For this procedure, the cells need to be fresh (unfixed, unfrozen). Fluorochrome-labeled antibodies targeted against various leukocyte antigens bind to the surface of lymphoid cells, and a suspension of labeled cells is sequentially illuminated by a light source (usually an argon laser) for approximately 10^{-6} second (Fig 3-2A, b). As the excited fluorochrome returns to its resting energy level, a specific wavelength of light is emitted (Fig 3-2A, c), which is sorted by wavelength stream (Fig 3-2A, d) and received by a photodetector (Fig 3-2A, e). The flow cytometer then converts this signal to electronic impulses, which are analyzed by computer software. The results may be represented by a multicolored dot-plot histogram (Fig 3-2B, C).

An advantage of flow cytometry is that it shows the proportion of particular cells in a specimen in histogram format. In addition, multiple antibodies and cellular size can be analyzed simultaneously. For example, the proportion of CD4 (helper T cells), CD8 (suppressor T cells), both CD4$^+$ and CD8$^+$, or either CD4$^+$ or CD8$^+$ may be displayed for a given lymphocytic infiltrate. The disadvantages of flow cytometry are its failure to show the location and distribution of these cells in tissue and the possibility of sampling error. Depending on the number of cells in the sample and on clinical information, the flow cytometrist chooses the panel of antibodies to be tested. Flow cytometric data should therefore be used as an adjunct to routine light microscopy and immunohistochemistry.

The ability of a laboratory to test small and viscous specimens such as vitreous with flow cytometry varies on an individual basis. Consultation with the pathologist is recommended before tissue is submitted for this type of testing.

Molecular Pathology

Molecular biology techniques are used increasingly in diagnostic ophthalmic pathology and extensively in experimental pathology (Table 3-3). More recently, the use of these techniques has expanded to include disease prognostication and treatment selection. Molecular pathology is employed to identify tumor-promoting or tumor-inhibiting genes, such as the retinoblastoma gene (eg, via comparative genomic hybridization [CGH], polymerase chain reaction [PCR], or array CGH), and viral DNA or RNA strands, such as those seen in herpesviruses and Epstein-Barr virus (eg, via PCR or in situ hybridization [ISH]). Molecular pathology techniques have made it possible not only to recognize the presence or absence of a strand of nucleic acid but also to localize precise DNA sequences within specific cells (eg, via fluorescence in situ hybridization [FISH] or ISH). Two major techniques have markedly advanced our knowledge of developmental biology and tumorigenesis: PCR (and its variations) and microarray (and its subtypes).

A

B   CD5 APC ->

C   mKAPPA FITC ->

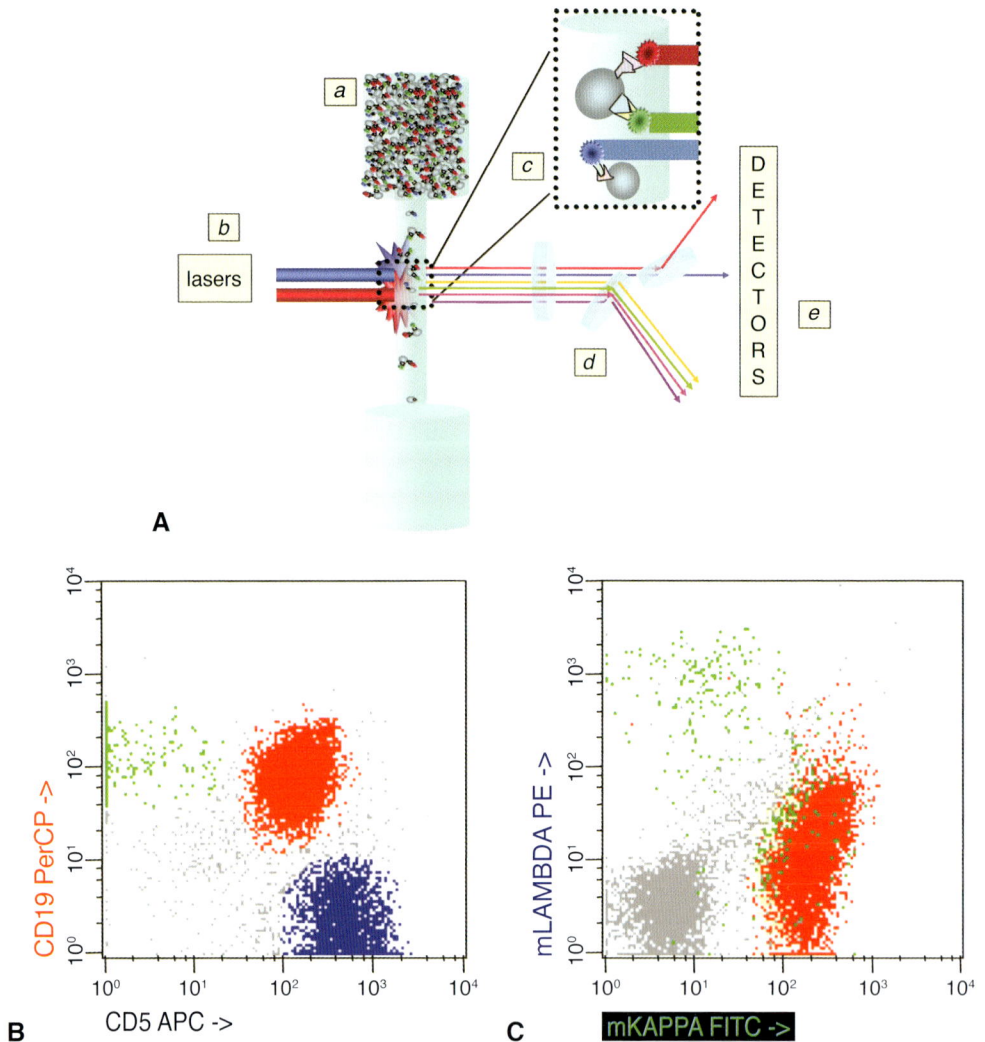

Figure 3-2 Flow cytometry. **A,** Flow cytometry analyzes cells moving in single file in a fluid stream *(a)*. Solid tissue is enzyme digested to separate cells for this procedure. Specific antibodies that are fluorochrome (PerCP and APC) tagged bind to the surface of the cells, and a suspension of labeled cells is sequentially illuminated/excited by a laser *(b)*. As the excited fluorochrome returns to its resting energy level, a specific wavelength of light is emitted *(c)*, which is sorted by wavelength *(d)* and received by a photodetector *(e)*. This signal is then converted to electronic impulses, which are in turn analyzed by computer software. **B–C,** Flow cytometry scatter graphs showing a clonal population of CD19+ kappa-restricted lymphocytes. Note that most of the CD19+ cells *(red in part **B**)* fail to express lambda light chains; however, the cells do exhibit strong kappa expression *(red in part **C**)*. *(Courtesy of Patricia Chévez-Barrios, MD.)*

Polymerase chain reaction

A common molecular biology technique is the PCR method, which amplifies a single strand of nucleic acid by several orders of magnitude, generating thousands to millions of copies of a particular DNA sequence (Fig 3-3). This method relies on thermal cycles of

Table 3-3 Summary of Molecular Techniques Used in Diagnostic Pathology

Technique	Description	Advantages	Disadvantages/Limitations
Comparative genomic hybridization (CGH)	Molecular cytogenetic method for analysis of copy number changes (gains/losses) in the DNA content of an individual, often in tumor cells	1. Detects and maps alterations in copy number of DNA sequences 2. Analyzes all chromosomes in a single experiment and does not require division of cells	Inability to detect mosaicism, balanced chromosomal translocations, inversions, or whole-genome ploidy changes
Polymerase chain reaction (PCR)	Amplification of a single strand of DNA (nucleic acid) of known sequence. Used clinically for early detection of cancer, hereditary diseases, and infectious diseases	Quality snap-frozen tissue (optimal) and archival paraffin-embedded tissue in some cases	1. Variable success rate of DNA extraction 2. Contamination with other nucleic acid material
Fluorescence in situ hybridization (FISH)	Chromosome region-specific, fluorescently labeled DNA probes (cloned pieces of genomic DNA) able to detect their complementary DNA sequences	Microfluidic chip allows automation and clinical use	Need to know type and location of expected aberrations
Reverse transcriptase-PCR (RT-PCR)	Amplifies DNA from RNA. Clinically used to determine the expression of a gene	Quality snap-frozen tissue (optimal) and archival paraffin-embedded tissue in some cases	1. Variable success rate of RNA extraction 2. Contamination with other nucleic acid material
Real-time, or quantitative, PCR	Measurement of PCR-product accumulation during the exponential phase of DNA amplification using a dual-labeled fluorogenic probe	Direct detection of PCR-product formation by measuring the increase in fluorescent emission continuously during the PCR reaction	Variable success rate of RNA extraction
Multiplex ligation-dependent probe amplification (MLPA)	Amplification of multiple targets using only a single primer pair within a single PCR mixture to produce amplicons of varying sizes that are specific to different DNA sequences	Additional information may be gained from a single test run.	Targets must be different enough to form distinct bands when visualized by gel electrophoresis.

(Continued)

Table 3-3 *(continued)*

Technique	Description	Advantages	Disadvantages/Limitations
Next-generation sequencing (massively parallel sequencing)	Parallelization of the sequencing process, producing thousands or millions of sequences concurrently. Used in genome sequencing and resequencing, transcriptome profiling (RNA-seq), DNA-protein interactions (ChIP-sequencing), and epigenome characterization	1. Ability to rapidly sequence the entire genome 2. Reduced reagent costs 3. Small amounts of starting material required 4. High precision with some methodologies	1. Short sequencing read lengths and higher error rates with some methodologies 2. Equipment can be expensive
SNP oligonucleotide microarray analysis (SOMA)	Type of DNA microarray used to detect single nucleotide polymorphisms (SNPs), the most frequent type of variation in the genome, within a population. Uses an array containing immobilized nucleic acid sequences and 1 or more labeled allele-specific oligonucleotide probes	1. SNPs, which are highly conserved between species and within a population, serve as a genotypic marker for research. 2. Able to detect copy-neutral loss of heterozygosity to uniparental disomy 3. Has huge potential in cancer diagnostics	Unable to detect mosaicism, balanced chromosomal translocations, inversions, or whole-genome ploidy changes

repeated heating and cooling of the DNA sample for thermal denaturation (DNA melting) and enzymatic replication. The components required for selective and repeated amplification are *primers,* which are short DNA fragments that contain sequences complementary to the target region (cDNA), DNA polymerase, and nucleotides. The selectivity of PCR is due to the use of these primers. Successful DNA extraction from various tissues and fluids with PCR techniques is dependent on the condition of the specimen.

PCR techniques have advanced considerably in recent years, and there are now approximately 20 PCR variants. The clinical relevance of detecting a PCR product depends on numerous variables, including the primers selected, laboratory controls, and demographic considerations. Thus, for clinicians making a clinicopathologic diagnosis, PCR is best used as an adjunct to routine pathologic diagnostic techniques. See also Part III, Genetics, in BCSC Section 2, *Fundamentals and Principles of Ophthalmology.*

Microarray

Scientists and clinicians use microarrays to survey the expression of thousands of genes in a single assay, the output of which is called a *gene expression profile (GEP).* Microarray

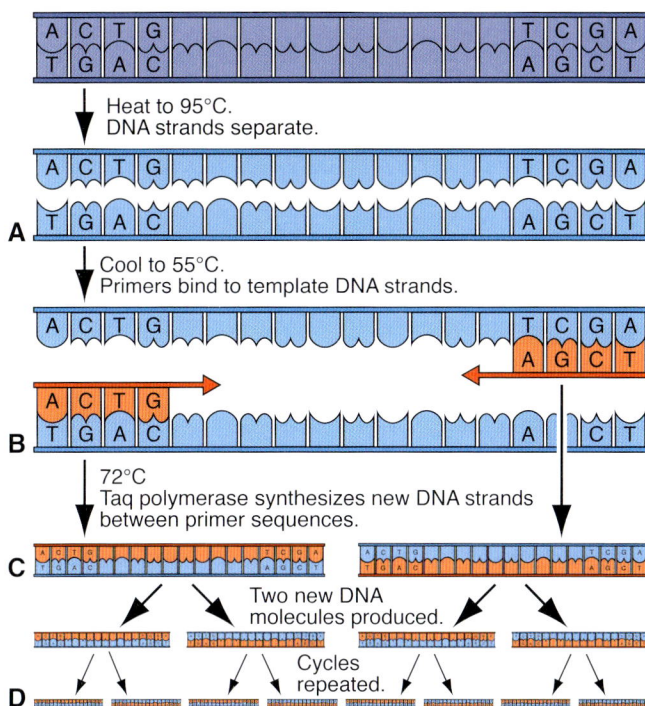

Figure 3-3 Polymerase chain reaction (PCR). **A,** PCR starts with a denaturing step in which DNA samples are heated to 95°C to separate the target double-stranded DNA into single strands. **B,** The temperature is then lowered to 55°C to allow the primers to anneal to their complementary sequences. The primers are designed to bracket the DNA region to be amplified. **C,** The temperature is raised to 72°C to allow polymerase to attach at each priming site and extend or synthesize a new DNA strand between primer sequences, producing 2 new DNA molecules. **D,** Step C is repeated numerous times to generate thousands to millions of copies. *(Courtesy of Theresa R. Kramer, MD.)*

technology can be used to further our understanding of fundamental aspects of human growth and development, explore the molecular mechanisms underlying normal and dysfunctional biological processes, and elucidate the genetic causes of many human diseases. Different types of microarrays are available, including DNA microarrays (the most common type), microRNA microarrays (MMChips), protein microarrays, tissue microarrays (Fig 3-4), cellular (or transfection) microarrays, antibody microarrays, and carbohydrate (glycoarray) microarrays.

The basic process underlying all of the DNA microarray platforms is straightforward: a glass slide or chip is spotted or "arrayed" with oligonucleotides or DNA fragments (called *probes*) that represent specific gene-coding regions. Fluorescently or chemiluminescently labeled purified cDNA or cRNA (called *target*) is hybridized to the arrayed slide or chip. After the chip is washed, the raw data are obtained by laser scanning, entered into a database, and analyzed with statistical methods.

Although DNA microarrays were initially developed to quantify the expression of a limited number of genes of clinical relevance, the technology has also been applied to

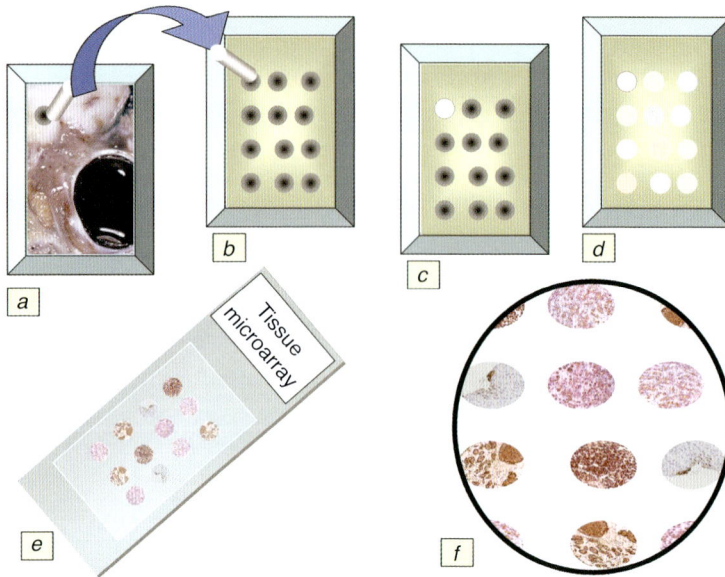

Figure 3-4 Tissue microarrays are constructed with small core biopsies of different tumors/tissues. A core is trephined from the donor paraffin block of the tumor *(a)*. A recipient paraffin block is prepared, creating empty cores *(b)*. The cores are incorporated into the slots *(c)* until all are occupied *(d)*. Glass slides are prepared and stained from the paraffin block containing the cores with a selected antibody *(e)*. Microscopic examination reveals the different staining patterns of each core *(f)*. *(Courtesy of Patricia Chévez-Barrios, MD.)*

tumor diagnosis and drug resistance in malignancies. Validating the results of microarray experiments is a critical step in the analysis of gene expression. Quantitative (real-time) PCR is the preferred method for validating gene expression profiling.

Clinical use of PCR and microarray

Routine clinical use of PCR and microarray was traditionally limited to the diagnosis of leukemias, lymphomas, soft-tissue neoplasms, and tumors with nondiagnostic histopathology results. These procedures are now increasingly used in the detection of infectious agents (eg, the herpesvirus family), in tumor prognostication (eg, uveal melanoma), and in detection of genetic alterations that are amenable to targeted therapies (eg, cutaneous melanoma and hematologic malignancies). Some current commercial microarray and PCR platforms can be used to stratify biopsy-sized tumor samples based on the metastatic potential of the tumor.

The selection of commercially available microarray and PCR kits continues to grow. The ongoing refinement and wider commercial availability of molecular genetic techniques will likely lead to wider integration of these modalities into clinical practice and the pathologic evaluation of biopsy specimens. However, the cost of these testing modalities is often significantly higher than that of other, more traditional, diagnostic modalities and should be discussed with patients before tests are ordered. See Part III, Genetics, in BCSC Section 2, *Fundamentals and Principles of Ophthalmology,* for further discussion of molecular genetics.

Khong JJ, Moore S, Prabhakaran VC, Selva D. Genetic testing in orbital tumors. *Orbit.* 2009; 28(2–3):88–97.

Liu L, Li Y, Li S, et al. Comparison of next-generation sequencing systems. *J Biomed Biotechnol.* 2012;2012:251364.

Vaziri K, Schwartz SG, Kishor K, Flynn HW Jr. Endophthalmitis: state of the art. *Clin Ophthalmol.* 2015;9:95–108.

Diagnostic Electron Microscopy

Historically, diagnostic electron microscopy (DEM) was used to indicate the cell of origin of a tumor of questionable differentiation rather than to distinguish between benign and malignant processes. DEM is now used in selected cases to complement immunopathologic studies when IHC is not sufficient for accurate diagnosis. However, DEM is less widely available and more expensive than IHC. The surgeon should consult with the pathologist before surgery to determine whether DEM could play a role in the study of a particular tissue specimen and to ensure that the tissue is fixed appropriately.

Special Procedures

Fine-Needle Aspiration Biopsy

Diagnostic intraocular fine-needle aspiration biopsy (FNAB) may be useful in distinguishing between primary uveal tumors and metastases. The procedure is performed under direct visualization through a dilated pupil, transvitreally or transsclerally (see Chapter 17, Videos 17-1 and 17-2, respectively). Iris tumors may be accessible for FNAB via sampling through the anterior chamber.

Special cytology fixatives, typically alcohol-based, are used for FNAB specimens. The cells obtained through FNAB can be processed using various cytopathologic techniques, such as a cytospin preparation, in which cells are centrifuged onto a glass slide, or when enough cells are present, they can be centrifuged and processed into a paraffin block (cell block) (Fig 3-5). A cell block allows the pathologist to employ special stains, IHC, ISH, microarray, and gene expression profiling if needed and as cellular material permits. In cases of suspected uveal melanoma, biopsy specimens can undergo genetic analysis to identify prognostic chromosomal abnormalities and gene expression profiling patterns. Intraocular FNAB has also been utilized in the diagnosis of primary intraocular lymphoma (PIOL). In cases of suspected PIOL, the biopsy specimen can undergo flow cytometric analysis, immunocytologic analysis, cytokine analysis, or molecular biological analysis (using PCR on both fixed and nonfixed material), depending on the sample volume. See also Chapters 17 and 20.

Intraocular FNAB has been postulated to increase the risk of tumor spread outside the eye, although this is controversial. In general, when properly performed, FNAB does not pose a major risk for tumor seeding. However, retinoblastoma is a notable exception, as FNAB can definitely increase the risk of local and distant tumor spread.

Some orbital surgeons have used FNAB to diagnose orbital lesions, especially optic nerve tumors and presumed metastases to the orbit. However, FNAB of an orbital mass

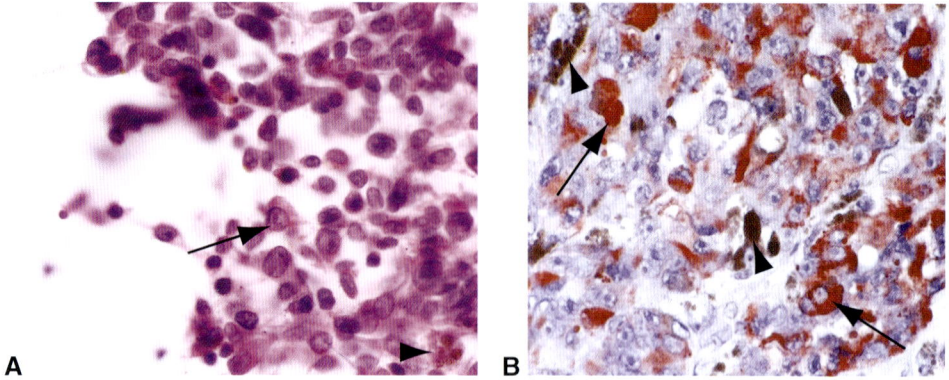

Figure 3-5 Fine-needle aspiration biopsy (FNAB) of a choroidal tumor. **A,** Cytologic liquid-based preparation displays prominent nucleoli *(arrow)* and some brown pigment *(arrowhead)* suggestive of melanoma. **B,** Sections from a cell block of the aspirated cells, stained with HMB-45 immunohistochemical stain using a red chromogen, is positive, confirming the diagnosis of melanoma. Notice the difference between the red chromogen color product *(arrows)* and the brown melanin *(arrowheads)*. *(Courtesy of Patricia Chévez-Barrios, MD.)*

may not adequately sample all representative areas of the tumor because it is difficult for the surgeon to make several passes at different angles through an intraorbital tumor without risking complications. Specific indications for performing intraocular or intraorbital FNAB are beyond the scope of this discussion, but some of these indications are discussed in Chapters 17 and 20 of this book. Ophthalmic FNAB should be performed with the assistance of an ophthalmic pathologist or cytopathologist experienced with these cases, because of the small amount of tissue/cells often obtained.

> Eide N, Walaas L. Fine-needle aspiration biopsy and other biopsies in suspected intraocular malignant disease: a review. *Acta Ophthalmol.* 2009;87(6):588–601.
> McCannel TA. Fine-needle aspiration biopsy in the management of choroidal melanoma. *Curr Opin Ophthalmol.* 2013;24(3):262–266.

Frozen Section

A *frozen section,* tissue that is snap-frozen and immediately sectioned in a cryostat, is indicated when the results of the study will affect intraoperative management of the patient. *Permanent sections,* tissue that is processed into paraffin prior to sectioning, are always preferred in ophthalmic pathology because of the inherent small size of the samples and the superior morphological preservation achieved with this technique (see Chapter 2). If the tissue sample is too small, it could be lost during frozen sectioning.

The most frequent indication for a frozen section is to determine whether the resection margins are free of tumor, especially in eyelid carcinomas. When tissue is submitted for margin evaluation, appropriate orientation of the specimen, correlated with documentation (through drawings of the excision site, labeled margins, or margins of the excised tissue that are tagged with sutures or other markers), is crucial; see Figure 2-2 in

Frozen section technique

Mohs technique

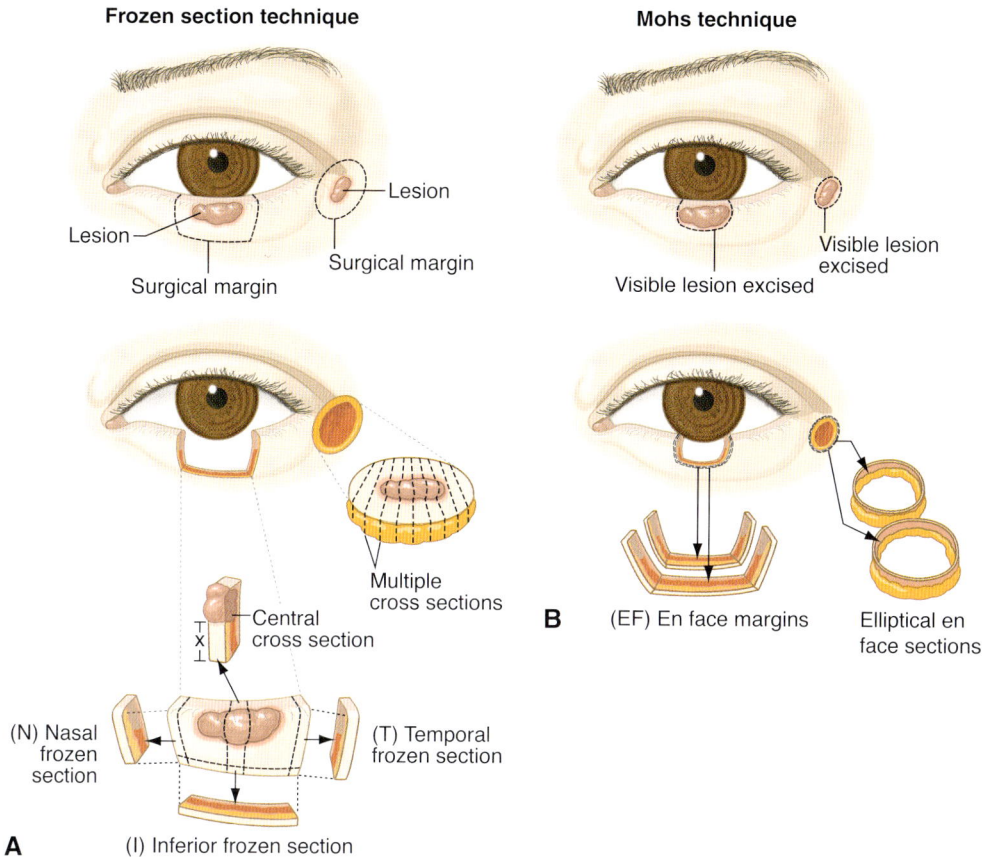

Figure 3-6 Frozen section and Mohs micrographic surgery techniques. **A,** To prepare a frozen section, the surgeon excises the lesion, typically a malignancy, with surgical margins denoted for the pathologist. For an eyelid margin lesion, the surgeon often performs a pentagonal wedge eyelid resection. The pathologist samples the nasal, temporal, and inferior margins to assess for the presence of tumor. A central cross section may be performed to demonstrate the distance of the tumor from the inferior surgical margin. An elliptical excision of a skin tumor can be evaluated by frozen section using the bread-loaf technique, in which multiple cross sections are prepared. **B,** In Mohs micrographic surgery performed on an eyelid margin tumor, the surgeon excises the visible lesion. Then, additional thin shavings of tissue are prepared by frozen section from the bed of the residual defect, allowing the surgeon to evaluate en face margins. In another variation of Mohs surgery, the surgeon performs an elliptical excision of the visible tumor. Frozen en face sections are obtained from the undersurface and the edges of the excised lesion. The tumor locations are marked on a map for a subsequent second-stage excision. *(Illustration developed by Tatyana Milman, MD, and rendered by Mark Miller.)*

Chapter 2. Two techniques can be used for assessing the margins in eyelid carcinomas (eg, basal cell carcinoma, squamous cell carcinoma): (1) routine frozen sections (as discussed previously); and (2) Mohs micrographic surgery (Fig 3-6), which preserves normal tissue while obtaining clear margins. Eyelid lesions, especially those located in the canthal areas, require tissue conservation in order to maintain adequate cosmetic and functional results.

Another indication for obtaining frozen sections is to determine whether adequate diagnostic tissue has been obtained by the surgeon. As frozen sections are a time-intensive and costly process, they should be used with discretion.

See the section on eyelid disorders in BCSC Section 7, *Oculofacial Plastic and Orbital Surgery,* for more information.

Chévez-Barrios P. Frozen section diagnosis and indications in ophthalmic pathology. *Arch Pathol Lab Med.* 2005;129(12):1626–1634.

CHAPTER 4

Wound Repair

Highlights

- Wound healing involves an acute inflammatory phase, a proliferative phase, and a remodeling phase.
- In the eye, scarring from wound healing can result in decreased vision.
- The tensile strength of wounds in the cornea and sclera is less than that of native, undisturbed tissue, because these tissues are relatively avascular.
- In most circumstances, wounds of the uveal tissues (ie, iris, ciliary body, and choroid) do not stimulate a healing response.
- The retina is made of terminally differentiated cells that typically do not regenerate when injured.
- Injury to the optic nerve may result in irreversible axonal degeneration and vision loss.

General Aspects of Wound Repair

The purpose of wound healing is to restore the anatomical and functional integrity of an organ or tissue as quickly as possible. Although it is a common physiologic process, wound healing involves a complicated sequence of tissue events. The process may take many months, and the end result is typically a scar (Fig 4-1). When wound healing occurs in the eye, it can interfere with vision. There are 3 general phases of wound healing:

1. Inflammatory phase: The *acute inflammatory phase* may last from minutes to hours. Blood clots quickly in adjacent vessels in response to tissue activators. Neutrophils and fluid enter the extravascular space. Histiocytes (also called *macrophages*) remove debris from the damaged tissues, and new vessels form. Fibroblasts begin to produce collagen, the main structural protein in connective tissues. Collagen plays multiple roles in wound healing, including interacting with platelets to initiate the inflammatory phase and functioning as a scaffold or guide for fibroblast migration.
2. Proliferative phase: *Regeneration* is the replacement of lost cells and occurs only in tissues composed of cells capable of undergoing mitosis throughout life (eg, epithelial cells, fibroblasts).
3. Remodeling phase: *Repair* is the process of restructuring of tissues to recapitulate normal tissue and typically results in a fibrous scar. In this final phase, *contraction*

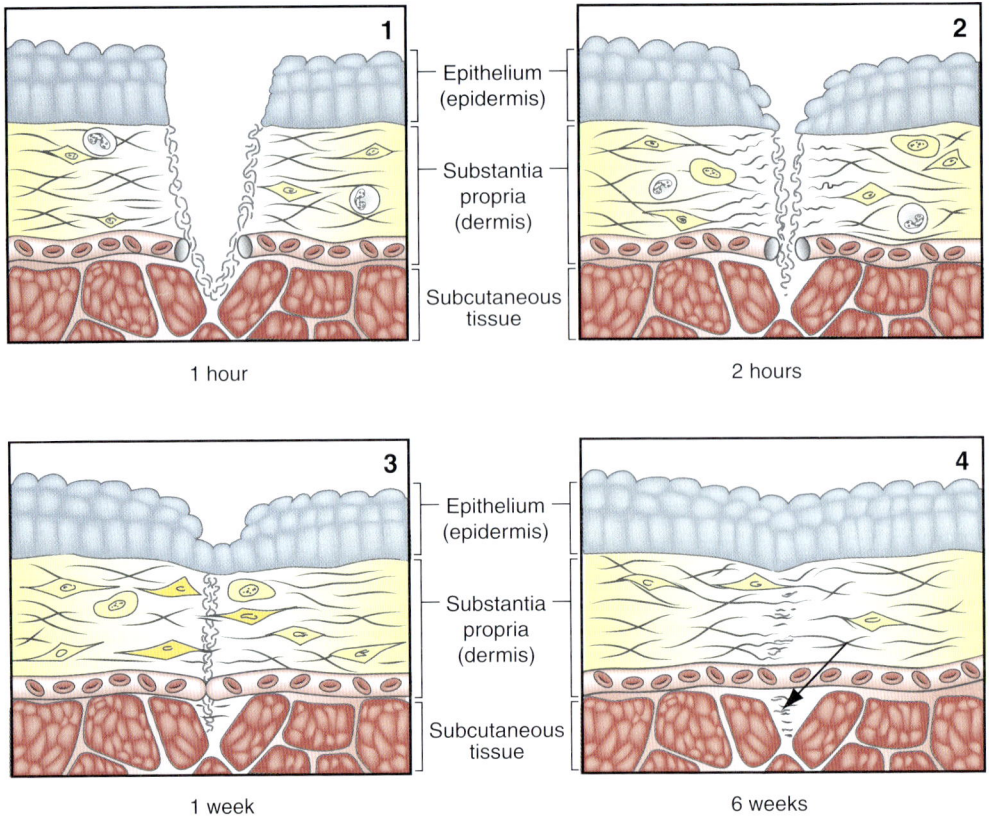

Figure 4-1 Sequence of general wound healing with an epithelial surface. **1,** The wound is created. Blood clots in the vessels; neutrophils migrate to the wound; the wounded edges begin to disintegrate. **2,** The wound edges are reapposed with the various tissue planes in good alignment. The epithelium is lost over the wound but starts to migrate. The stromal/dermal fibroblasts enlarge and become activated. Fibronectin is deposited at the wound edges. The blood vessels begin to produce buds. **3,** The epithelium seals the surface. Fibroblasts and blood vessels enter the wound and lay down new collagen. Much of the debris is removed by histiocytes. **4,** As the scar matures, the fibroblasts subside. Newly formed blood vessels canalize. New collagen strengthens the wound, which contracts. Note that the striated muscle cells in the subcutaneous tissue do not regenerate and are replaced by a scar *(arrow)*. *(Illustration by Cyndie C. H. Wooley.)*

causes the reparative tissues to shrink so that the scar is smaller than the surrounding uninjured tissues. This process may affect adjacent tissues and structures. Both repair and contraction of wounds are highly dependent on fibroblasts.

Wound Repair in Specific Ocular Tissues

Wound healing has variable mechanisms and consequences in different ocular tissues. The processes summarized in the following sections are also discussed in other volumes of the BCSC. Also see the appropriate chapters in this volume for the topography of a specific ocular tissue.

Cornea

A corneal *abrasion,* or corneal epithelial defect, refers to a wound that is limited to the surface corneal epithelium, although Bowman layer and superficial stroma may also be involved. Within an hour of injury, the parabasilar epithelial cells begin to migrate across the denuded area until they touch other migrating cells; then *contact inhibition* stops further migration. Simultaneously, the surrounding basal cells undergo mitosis to supply additional cells to cover the defect. Reepithelialization occurs at a rate of 2 mm per day, on average. Although a large corneal abrasion is usually covered by migrating epithelial cells within 24–48 hours, complete healing, which includes restoration of the full thickness of epithelium (5–8 layers) and re-formation of the anchoring fibrils, takes 4–6 weeks. If a thin layer of anterior corneal stroma is lost with the abrasion, epithelial cells will fill the shallow crater, forming a *facet.* The Bowman layer is not replaced when it is incised or destroyed.

Corneal stromal healing is avascular and occurs via the process of fibrosis rather than by the fibrovascular proliferation seen in other tissues (Fig 4-2). Following a central corneal wound, neutrophils arrive at the site via the tears (Fig 4-3), and the edges of the wound swell. The corneal matrix glycosaminoglycans, keratan sulfate and chondroitin sulfate, disintegrate at the edge of the wound. The stromal keratocytes (fibroblast-like cells) are activated and eventually migrate across the wound, laying down collagen and fibronectin. The spacing of the keratocytes is not regular, and collagen fibers are not parallel to the stromal lamellae. Hence, cells are directed anteriorly and posteriorly across a wound that will always be visible microscopically as an irregularity in the stroma and clinically as an opacity. If the wound edges are not well-apposed, the gap will not be completely filled by the proliferating keratocytes, resulting in focal stromal thinning.

Both the epithelium and the endothelium are critical to good central wound healing. If the epithelium does not cover the wound within a few days of injury, healing of the subjacent stroma will be limited and the wound will be weak. In addition, growth factors from the epithelium stimulate and sustain healing. The surface of a healed ulceration is covered by epithelium, but little of its lost stroma is replaced by fibrous tissue. The endothelial cells adjacent to the wound slide across the posterior cornea; a few cells are replaced through mitosis. The endothelial cells lay down a new thin layer of Descemet membrane. If the internal aspect of the wound is not covered by Descemet membrane, stromal keratocytes may continue to proliferate onto the posterior surface of the membrane as fibrous ingrowth, or the posterior wound may remain open permanently. In the late months of healing, the initial fibrillar collagen is replaced by stronger, thicker collagen fibers.

Conjunctiva

The conjunctiva is composed of nonkeratinized stratified squamous epithelium with goblet cells overlying a stroma called the *substantia propria.* The substantia propria is composed of blood vessels, lymphatic channels, and collagen fibers that are randomly distributed in a relatively loose configuration. In response to a wound, activated platelets form hemostatic plugs within the vessels, and neutrophils migrate to the surface of the wound edges (see Fig 4-1). The epithelium migrates to cover the wound. Meanwhile,

Figure 4-2 A full-thickness corneal wound *(arrows)* from cataract surgery. Note the mild hypercellularity of the wound due to fibrosis. There are no blood vessels in or around the wound. *(Courtesy of Nasreen A. Syed, MD.)*

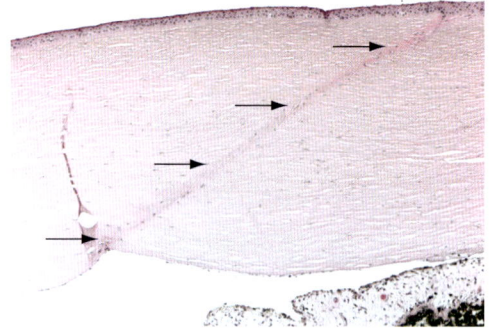

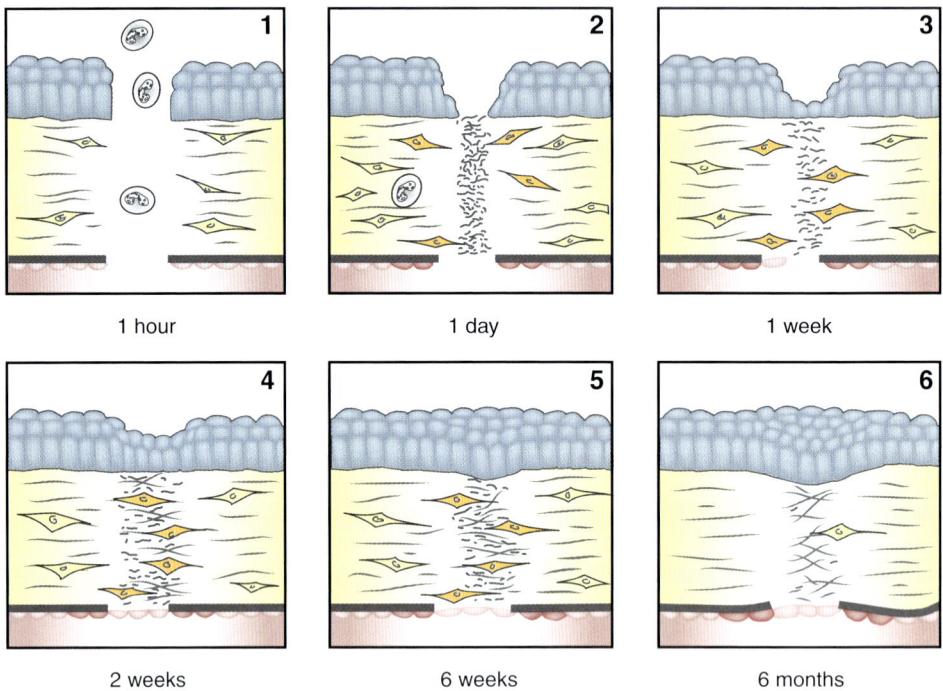

1 hour	1 day	1 week

2 weeks	6 weeks	6 months

Figure 4-3 Clear corneal wound. **1,** Tears carry neutrophils *(white cells)* with lysozymes to the wound within an hour. **2,** Immediately after closure of the incision, the wound edge shows early disintegration and edema. The glycosaminoglycans at the edge are degraded. The nearby keratocytes are activated. **3,** At 1 week, migrating epithelial and endothelial cells partially seal the wound; keratocytes begin to migrate and supply collagen and fibronectin. **4,** Fibrocyte activity and collagen and matrix deposition continue. The endothelium, sealing the inner wound, lays down a new layer of Descemet membrane. **5,** Epithelial regeneration is complete. Keratocytes fill the wound with type I collagen and repair slows. **6,** The final wound contracts. The collagen fibers are not parallel with the surrounding lamellae, resulting in a wound that appears microscopically as scarring and clinically as an opacity. The number of keratocytes decreases. *(Illustration by Cyndie C. H. Wooley.)*

stromal fibroblasts begin to proliferate and deposit fibronectin at the wound edges. Fibroblasts and blood vessels enter the wound and lay down new collagen. The final phase of remodeling is associated with canalization of new blood vessels and scarring due to contraction of collagen.

Sclera

The sclera differs from the cornea in that its collagen fibers vary in thickness and are randomly distributed rather than laid down in orderly lamellae. As the sclera is relatively avascular and hypocellular, the episclera, when stimulated by injury, migrates into the scleral wound, supplying vessels, fibroblasts, and activated histiocytes. The final wound contracts, creating a puckered appearance. If the adjacent uveal tract (also called *uvea*) is damaged, uveal fibrovascular tissue may enter the scleral wound, resulting in a scar with dense adhesion between the uvea and the sclera. Indolent episcleral fibrosis produces a dense coat around an extrascleral foreign body such as an encircling scleral buckling element or a glaucoma tube shunt.

Because the wound healing processes in the cornea and sclera are relatively avascular, the tensile strength of wounds in these parts of the eye is less than that of the native, undisturbed tissue. In certain clinical situations, such as glaucoma filtering procedures, modifying the healing process through the use of topical antimetabolites such as 5-fluorouracil or mitomycin C may be desirable to prevent scar tissue from forming between the conjunctiva and the sclera at the surgical site (see BCSC Section 10, *Glaucoma*, Chapter 13). In keratoconus, modification of healing via collagen crosslinking is used in the cornea to prevent progressive thinning.

Uveal Tract

In most circumstances, wounds of the iris do not stimulate a healing response in either the stroma or the epithelium. Though richly endowed with blood vessels and fibroblasts, the iris stroma does not produce granulation tissue to close a defect. In some circumstances, the pigmented epithelium may be stimulated to migrate, but that migration is usually limited to the subjacent surface of the lens capsule, where subsequent adhesion of epithelial cells occurs (posterior synechia). When fibrovascular tissue forms, it usually does so on the anterior surface of the iris as a neovascular membrane that may cover iridectomy or pupillary openings. This fibrovascular tissue may arise from the iris, the anterior chamber angle, or the peripheral cornea. Lack of wound healing in the iris is exploited when iridotomies, both surgical and laser, are performed.

The stroma and melanocytes of the ciliary body and choroid do not regenerate after injury. Histiocytes remove debris, and a thin fibrous scar, which appears white and atrophic clinically, develops.

Lens

Small tears in the anterior lens capsule are sealed by nearby lenticular epithelial cells. In circumstances that make the lenticular epithelium anoxic or hypoxic, such as posterior synechiae or markedly elevated intraocular pressure, a metaplastic response may occur, producing fibrous plaques intermixed with basement membrane.

Retina

The retina is made of terminally differentiated cells that typically do not regenerate when injured. Because the retina is part of the central nervous system (CNS), glial cells (eg, Müller cells, astrocytes), rather than fibroblasts, proliferate in response to retinal injury. Surgical techniques to close holes or tears in the neurosensory retina are successful when the retina and retinal pigment epithelium (RPE) are injured (eg, as a result of cryotherapy, photocoagulation), forming an adhesive, atrophic scar between the neurosensory retina and Bruch membrane (see Chapter 11, Fig 11-27).

The internal limiting membrane (ILM) and Bruch membrane provide the architectural anchors for glial scarring; adhesions between the ILM and Bruch membrane may incorporate a rare residual glial cell, and variable numbers of retinal and RPE cells may be present between the membranes. If the wound has damaged Bruch membrane, choroidal fibroblasts and vessels may participate in the formation of the final scar. The end result is a metaplastic fibrous or fibrovascular plaque in the sub–neurosensory retina and sub-RPE regions. The RPE usually undergoes hyperplasia in such scars, causing the dense pigmented clumps seen clinically on fundus examination.

Vitreous

The vitreous has few cells and no blood vessels. However, the collagen fibrils of the vitreous can provide a scaffold for glial and fibrovascular tissue from the retina and uveal tract to grow and extend into the vitreous to proliferate as membranes. These membranes usually have a contractile component, which can lead to traction on the retina and ciliary body.

Orbit and Ocular Adnexa

The rich blood supply to the eyelid skin supports rapid healing. Approximately the third day after an injury to the skin, myofibroblasts derived from vascular pericytes migrate around the wound and actively contract, decreasing the size of the wound. The eyelid and orbit are compartmentalized by intertwining fascial membranes that enclose muscular, tendinous, fatty, lacrimal, and ocular tissues; these tissues can become distorted by scarring. Exuberant contraction distorts muscle action, producing dysfunctional scars. The striated muscles of the orbicularis oculi and extraocular muscles are made of terminally differentiated cells that do not regenerate after injury, but the viable cells may hypertrophy.

Extraocular muscles

The extraocular muscles are composed of 2 different types of muscle fibers: slow, tonic type and fast, twitch type. The ratio of nerve fibers to muscle fibers is very high, which allows precise movements of the eye. Each extraocular muscle attaches to the sclera at a specific anatomical location via a tendinous insertion, allowing coordinated movement of the eyes. As a response to injury or inflammation, strabismus may occur because of atrophy of the muscle belly itself or from scarring of the tendon to the sclera, which results in muscle restriction.

Optic Nerve

The optic nerve is part of the CNS, and like the brain and spinal cord, it is vulnerable to traumatic injury. Injury to the optic nerve may result in irreversible axonal degeneration and vision loss. There is ongoing research to evaluate and modulate the innate immune response to injury, as well as to promote axonal regeneration and remyelination, but effective therapies for optic nerve injury are not currently available.

Pathologically Apparent Sequelae of Ocular Trauma

Ocular trauma can lead to a variety of pathologically apparent sequelae involving different parts of the eye, depending on the nature of the trauma. *Rupture of Descemet membrane* may occur after minor trauma (eg, in keratoconus; Fig 4-4) or major trauma (eg, forceps delivery; Fig 4-5).

The anterior chamber angle structures, especially the trabecular beams, are vulnerable when the anterior segment is distorted during trauma. *Traumatic recession of the anterior chamber angle* occurs when there is a tear in the anterior ciliary body between the longitudinal fibers and the circular fibers of the ciliary muscle with posterior displacement of the iris root (Fig 4-6). Concurrent damage to the trabecular meshwork with subsequent fibrosis may lead to glaucoma.

Iridodialysis is a tear in the iris at the thinnest portion of the diaphragm, the iris root, where it inserts into the supportive tissue of the ciliary body (Fig 4-7). Only a small amount of supporting tissue surrounds the iris sphincter. If the sphincter muscle is torn, contraction of the remaining muscle will create a notch at the pupillary border.

Cyclodialysis results from disinsertion of the longitudinal ciliary muscle fibers from the scleral spur (Fig 4-8). This condition can lead to hypotony because the aqueous humor of the anterior chamber now has free access to the suprachoroidal space, resulting in increased outflow; in addition, because the blood supply to the ciliary body is reduced, the production of aqueous humor is decreased.

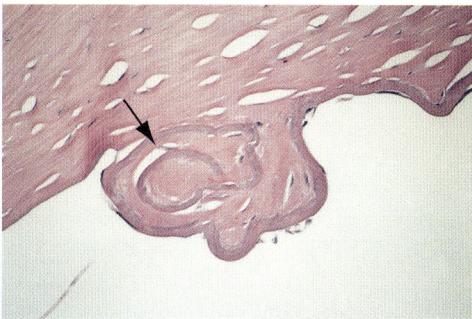

Figure 4-4 A break in Descemet membrane in keratoconus shows anterior curling of Descemet membrane toward the corneal stroma *(arrow)*. *(Courtesy of Hans E. Grossniklaus, MD.)*

Figure 4-5 A break in Descemet membrane as a result of forceps injury shows anterior curling of the original membrane *(arrow)* and production of a secondary thickened membrane. *(Courtesy of Hans E. Grossniklaus, MD.)*

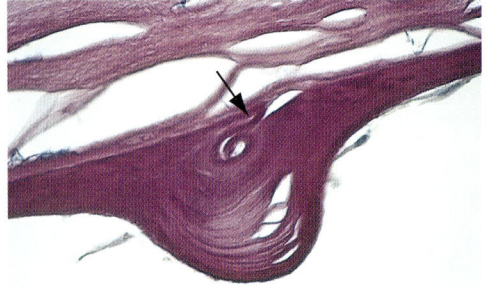

Figure 4-6 Angle recession due to a tear in the ciliary body in the plane between the external longitudinal muscle fibers and the internal circular and oblique fibers *(arrow);* the iris root is displaced posteriorly *(arrowhead).* Note the scleral spur *(asterisk).*

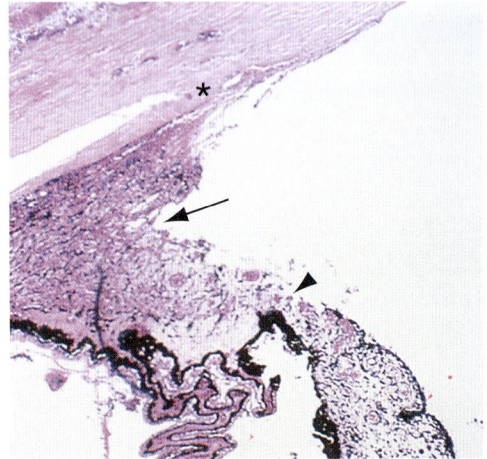

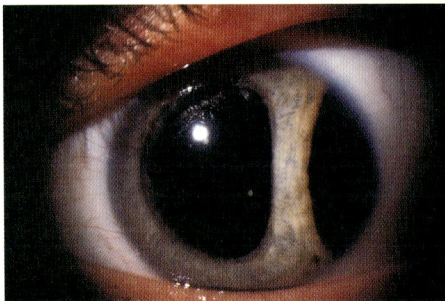

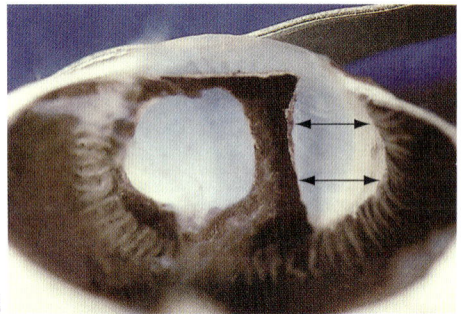

Figure 4-7 Iridodialysis. **A,** Clinical photograph of an eye showing iridodialysis, a disinsertion of the iris root from the ciliary body. **B,** Gross photograph showing a posterior view of iridodialysis *(arrows). (Part A courtesy of Hans E. Grossniklaus, MD.)*

The uveal tract is attached to the sclera at 3 points: the scleral spur, the internal ostia of the vortex veins, and in the peripapillary region. This anatomical arrangement is the basis of the evisceration technique and explains the vulnerability of the eye to expulsive choroidal hemorrhage. The borders of a dome-shaped suprachoroidal hemorrhage are delimited by the position of the vortex veins and the scleral spur (Fig 4-9).

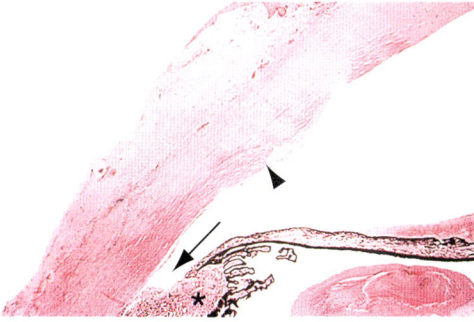

Figure 4-8 Cyclodialysis *(arrow)* resulting from the disinsertion of the ciliary muscle *(asterisk)* from the scleral spur *(arrowhead)*. *(Courtesy of Hans E. Grossniklaus, MD.)*

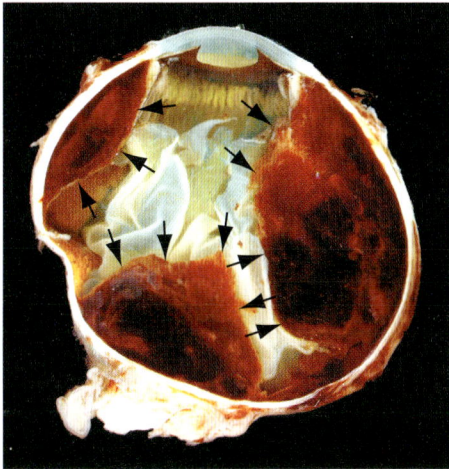

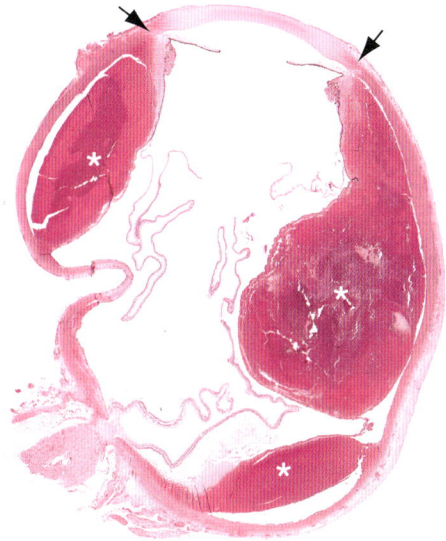

A

B

Figure 4-9 Suprachoroidal hemorrhage. **A,** Macroscopic image demonstrating multiple areas of suprachoroidal hemorrhage *(arrows)*. **B,** Microscopic image of the same eye with multiple areas of suprachoroidal hemorrhage *(asterisks)*. The anterior edge of the hemorrhages is delineated by the insertion of the choroid at the scleral spur *(arrows)*. *(Courtesy of Nasreen A. Syed, MD.)*

A *Vossius ring* appears when iris pigment epithelial cells are compressed against the anterior surface of the lens, depositing a ring of melanin pigment concentric with the pupil.

If the lens capsule is disrupted, a *cataract* may form immediately. The capsule is thinnest at the posterior pole, the point farthest from the lens epithelial cells. The epithelium of the lens may be stimulated by trauma to form an anterior fibrous plaque just inside the capsule. The lens zonular fibers are points of relative weakness; if they rupture, lens displacement occurs, either partial (subluxation) or complete (luxation). Focal areas of zonular rupture may allow formed vitreous to enter the anterior chamber.

Commotio retinae (Berlin edema) often complicates blunt trauma to the eye. Although it is most prominent in the macula, commotio retinae can affect any portion of the retina. The retinal opacification seen clinically results from disruption in the architecture of the photoreceptor outer segments and the RPE, which can be seen with optical coherence tomography (OCT) or on histologic examination.

Retinal dialysis is most likely to develop in the inferotemporal or superonasal quadrant. The retina is anchored anteriorly to the nonpigmented epithelium of the ciliary pars plana. This union is reinforced by the attachment of the vitreous base, which straddles the ora serrata. Deformation of the eye can result in a circumferential retinal tear at the point of attachment of the ora serrata or immediately posterior to the point of attachment of the vitreous base (Fig 4-10). The interface between necrotic and normal neurosensory retina is also vulnerable to retinal tears.

After a penetrating injury, intraocular *fibrous* or *fibrovascular proliferation* may occur. This proliferation may lead to vitreous, subretinal, and/or choroidal hemorrhage; tractional retinal detachment; proliferative vitreoretinopathy (PVR), including anterior PVR (Fig 4-11); hypotony; and phthisis bulbi (discussed in Chapter 1). Formation of proliferative intraocular membranes may affect the timing of vitreoretinal surgery. Sequelae of intraocular hemorrhage include hemosiderosis bulbi secondary to iron deposition from breakdown of red blood cells, and cholesterolosis, also from red blood cell breakdown.

Rupture of Bruch membrane or a *choroidal rupture* may occur after direct or indirect injury to the globe. Choroidal neovascularization, granulation tissue proliferation, and

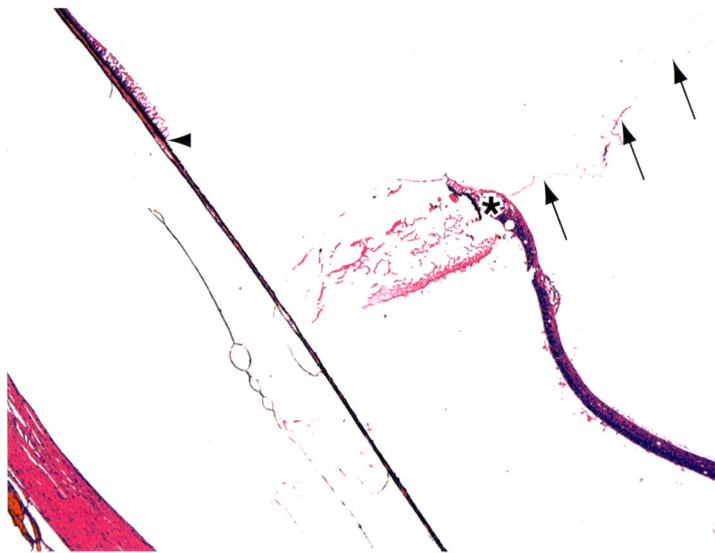

Figure 4-10   Retinal dialysis. This photomicrograph illustrates the separation of the retina from its normal attachment to the posterior edge of the nonpigmented epithelium of the pars plana *(arrowhead)* at the ora serrata *(asterisk)*. The vitreous base is still attached to the ora serrata *(arrows)*. *(Courtesy of Tatyana Milman, MD.)*

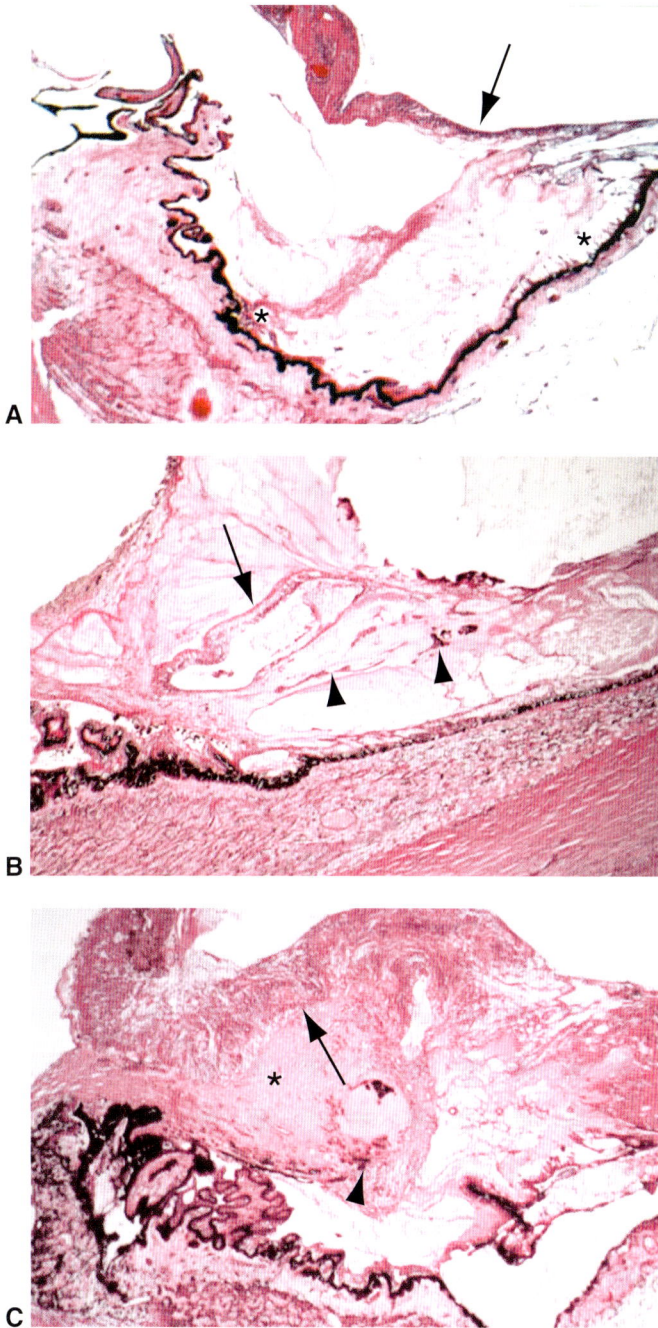

Figure 4-11 Anterior proliferative vitreoretinopathy (PVR). **A,** Traction of the vitreous base on the peripheral retina *(arrow)* and ciliary body epithelium *(asterisks)*. **B,** Incorporation of peripheral retinal *(arrow)* and ciliary body tissue *(arrowheads)* into the vitreous base. **C,** A condensed vitreous base *(asterisk)*, adherent retina *(arrow)*, and RPE hyperplasia *(arrowhead)*. *(Courtesy of Hans E. Grossniklaus, MD.)*

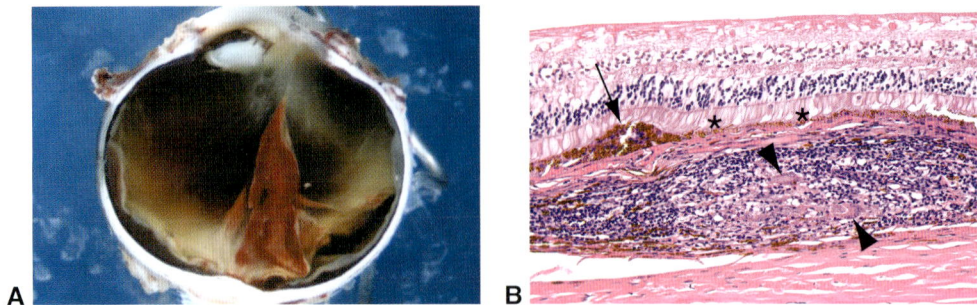

Figure 4-12 Focal posttraumatic choroidal granulomatous inflammation. **A,** An enucleated eye in which a projectile caused a perforating limbal injury that extends to the posterior choroid. **B,** Photomicrograph shows chronic inflammation with multinucleated giant cells *(arrowheads)* in the choroid, focal RPE hyperplasia *(arrow)*, and attenuation of photoreceptor outer segments *(asterisks)*. *(Part A courtesy of Hans E. Grossniklaus, MD; part B courtesy of Vivian Lee, MD.)*

scar formation may occur in areas where the choroid has ruptured or where there are disruptions in the Bruch membrane. A subset of direct choroidal ruptures, usually those occurring after a projectile injury, may result in *focal posttraumatic choroidal granuloma-tous inflammation* (Fig 4-12). This inflammation may be related to foreign material intro-duced into the choroid. A chorioretinal rupture and necrosis is known as *chorioretinitis sclopetaria.*

CHAPTER 5

Conjunctiva

Highlights

- Developmental lesions such as dermoids and dermolipomas of the conjunctiva can occur in the bulbar or forniceal conjunctiva.
- Inflammation of the conjunctiva is common and may be infectious or noninfectious. Histologic examination may be helpful in some cases of inflammation.
- Pinguecula and pterygium share the histologic feature of elastotic degeneration in the conjunctival stroma.
- Ocular surface squamous neoplasia typically affects the interpalpebral limbal zone and involves varying amounts of epithelial dysplasia and cellular atypia, ranging from mild dysplasia to invasive squamous cell carcinoma.
- Pigmentation of the conjunctiva can result from a variety of processes. These lesions may involve epithelial cells or melanocytes and often require biopsy to determine the clinical course and treatment options.

Topography

The conjunctiva is a mucous membrane that lines the posterior surface of the eyelids and the anterior surface of the globe up to the limbus. It can be divided into 3 regions: palpebral, forniceal, and bulbar. The conjunctiva consists of nonkeratinized stratified squamous epithelium with goblet cells and a delicate basement membrane that rests on the underlying stroma (substantia propria) (Fig 5-1A–D). Elements of the stroma include loosely arranged collagen fibers; blood vessels and lymphatic channels; nerves; occasional accessory lacrimal glands; and resident lymphocytes, plasma cells, histiocytes, and mast cells. In places, the lymphocytes are organized into lymphoid follicles, referred to as *conjunctiva-associated lymphoid tissue (CALT),* which is a subtype of mucosa-associated lymphoid tissue (MALT).

Two specialized areas of the conjunctiva are the caruncle and the plica semilunaris. The *caruncle,* the most medial area of the bulbar conjunctiva, histologically is a transitional zone between skin and conjunctiva. Its surface consists of nonkeratinized squamous epithelium and, like skin, the caruncle contains adnexal structures such as hair follicles, sebaceous glands, and sweat glands (Fig 5-1E). The *plica semilunaris,* a fold of bulbar conjunctiva just temporal to the caruncle, is a vestige of the nictitating membrane found in many other species. The epithelium is rich in goblet cells, and smooth muscle fibers are often present in the stroma.

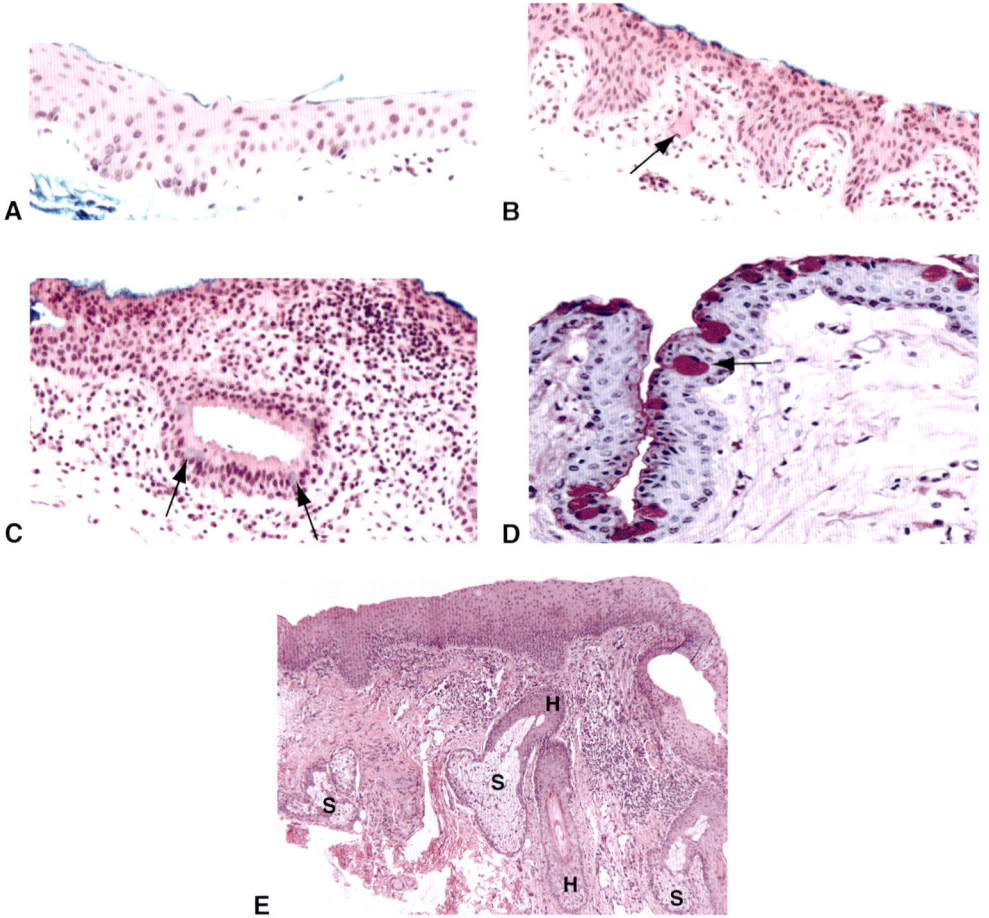

Figure 5-1 **A,** Bulbar conjunctiva with nonkeratinized stratified squamous epithelium. **B,** Palpebral conjunctiva with epithelial ridges. The stroma contains lymphatic and blood vessels *(arrow)* and inflammatory cells. **C,** Conjunctiva in the fornices contains pseudoglands of Henle (infoldings of conjunctival epithelium with abundant goblet cells *[arrows]*). **D,** Periodic acid–Schiff (PAS) stain highlights the mucin in goblet cells *(arrow).* **E,** Caruncular conjunctiva, containing sebaceous glands (S) and hair follicles (H). *(Parts A–D courtesy of Patricia Chévez-Barrios, MD; part E courtesy of George J. Harocopos, MD.)*

Tenon capsule (fascia bulbi) is a fascial sheath composed of collagen that surrounds the globe and the anterior portions of the extraocular muscles, separating them from the orbital fat. The capsule lies between the conjunctiva and the sclera and is separated from the outer surface of the sclera by a potential space, the episcleral (Tenon) space. Anteriorly, Tenon capsule is connected to the sclera by fine bands of connective tissue posterior to the sclerocorneal junction. Posterior to the globe, the capsule fuses with the optic nerve sheath. See BCSC Section 2, *Fundamentals and Principles of Ophthalmology*, and Section 8, *External Disease and Cornea*, for further discussion of these structures.

Developmental Anomalies

Choristomas

A *choristoma* is a benign developmental proliferation of histologically mature tissue in an abnormal location. On the ocular surface, choristomatous lesions range from simple to complex forms.

Epibulbar dermoids are firm, dome-shaped, noncystic (solid) white-yellow nodules typically found at or straddling the limbus, most commonly in the inferotemporal quadrant (Fig 5-2A, B). Dermoids may occur in isolation or, particularly when bilateral, as a manifestation of a developmental syndrome such as linear nevus sebaceous syndrome (ie, an oculoneurocutaneous disorder) or Goldenhar syndrome (ie, oculoauriculovertebral dysgenesis). The latter is characterized by upper eyelid coloboma, preauricular skin tags, and vertebral anomalies in addition to epibulbar dermoid.

Dermolipomas are choristomas containing a substantial amount of mature adipose tissue, which makes them softer and yellower than dermoids. Like dermoids, dermolipomas may be associated with Goldenhar syndrome or linear nevus sebaceous syndrome. Unlike dermoids, dermolipomas occur more commonly in the superotemporal quadrant, toward the fornix; they may also extend posteriorly into the orbit.

The common histologic feature of epibulbar dermoids and dermolipomas is dense, obliquely arranged bundles of collagen in the substantia propria. Dermal adnexal structures are often present, and the surface epithelium may or may not be keratinized (Fig 5-2C, D). However, in dermolipomas, adipose tissue is present deep to the dense collagenous tissue in the stroma.

Clinically, *complex choristomas* are often indistinguishable from dermoids or dermolipomas. They may also be associated with linear nevus sebaceous syndrome. The histologic features of complex choristomas overlap with those of epibulbar dermoids or dermolipomas. However, complex choristomas contain other tissues such as bone (osseous choristoma), cartilage, lacrimal tissue, or neural tissue (Fig 5-2E). See also BCSC Section 6, *Pediatric Ophthalmology and Strabismus.*

Hamartomas

Like choristomas, hamartomas are benign developmental proliferations; however, in contrast to choristomas, they represent abnormal overgrowths of mature tissue normally present at a given location (hence the derivation from the Greek word *hamartia* for "defect or error"). In the conjunctiva, the most common variety of hamartoma is the capillary hemangioma, although this mass most often involves the eyelid (see Chapter 13).

Inflammation

Because the conjunctiva is an exposed surface, it can be affected by a variety of organisms, allergens, and toxic agents, which can initiate an inflammatory response referred to as *conjunctivitis.* Depending on the onset and duration, etiology, constituents of the

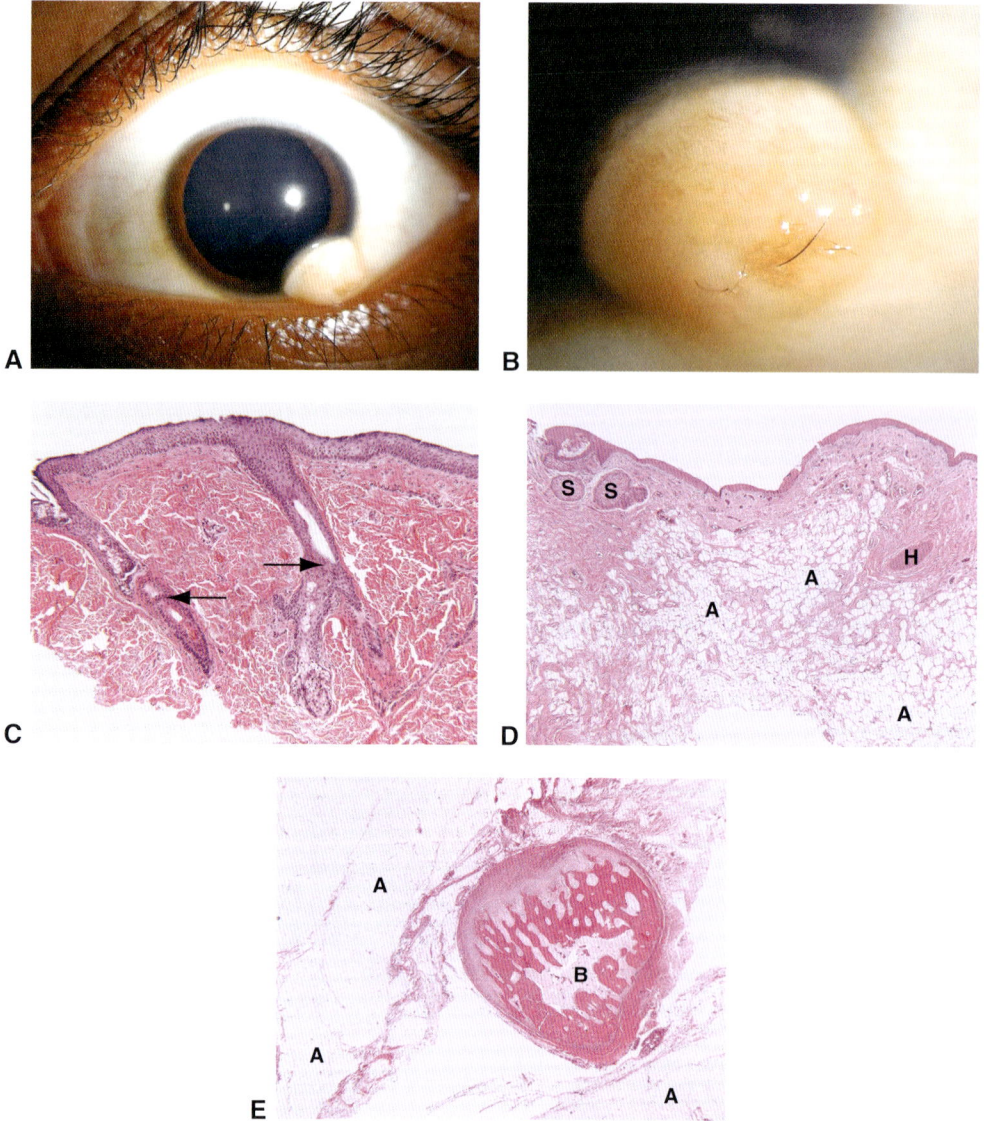

Figure 5-2 Ocular surface choristomas. **A,** Clinical photograph of a solid limbal dermoid. **B,** Higher magnification shows hairs emanating from the dermoid. **C,** Histology of the dermoid shows keratinized epithelium, dense bundles of collagen in the stroma, and hair follicles with associated sebaceous glands *(arrows).* **D,** A dermolipoma differs from a dermoid in that it also contains a significant amount of mature adipose tissue (A). This dermolipoma also contains dermal adnexal structures, including a hair follicle (H) and sebaceous glands (S). **E,** Complex choristomas combine features of multiple types of choristomas, in this case osseous, with the presence of bone (B), and dermolipoma, with the presence of adipose tissue (A). *(Parts A and B courtesy of Morton E. Smith, MD; parts C–E courtesy of George J. Harocopos, MD.)*

inflammatory infiltrate, or macroscopic and microscopic appearance of the conjunctiva, this response may be categorized as

- acute or chronic
- infectious or noninfectious
- papillary, follicular, or granulomatous

See BCSC Section 6, *Pediatric Ophthalmology and Strabismus,* and Section 8, *External Disease and Cornea,* for additional discussion of conjunctivitis.

Acute or Chronic Conjunctivitis

Most cases of conjunctivitis are not biopsied; they are diagnosed on the basis of the acute nature of the clinical presentation or the chronicity of the case, as well as the ophthalmologist's clinical acumen. See BCSC Section 8, *External Disease and Cornea,* for additional discussion on the clinical distinction between acute and chronic conjunctivitis.

Infectious Conjunctivitis

A wide variety of pathogens can infect the conjunctiva, including viruses, bacteria, atypical bacteria (eg, Chlamydiae), fungi, and parasites. Bacterial infection is more common in children (eg, *Haemophilus influenzae, Streptococcus pneumoniae*), whereas adenovirus and other viruses tend to be more common in adults. Infectious conjunctivitis may be diagnosed on the basis of clinical history and examination findings (typically sufficient for viral disease), or it may require laboratory studies such as biopsy with special stains (eg, Gram, Giemsa), culture, polymerase chain reaction analysis, or serology depending on the suspected organism. In cases of diagnostic uncertainty or nonresponsiveness to initial treatment, cytologic evaluation of the ocular surface epithelium (Fig 5-3) or tissue biopsy may help establish a definitive diagnosis.

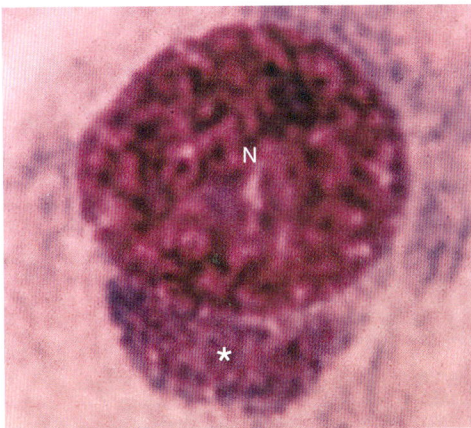

Figure 5-3 *Chlamydia,* conjunctival scraping for cytologic examination for infectious conjunctivitis, Giemsa stain. The cytoplasmic inclusion body *(asterisk),* composed of chlamydial organisms, can be seen capping the epithelial cell nucleus (N). A distinct space separates the inclusion body from the nuclear chromatin. Since this finding is often difficult to identify in conjunctival samples, other methods such as polymerase chain reaction are usually used to identify chlamydial infection.

Noninfectious Conjunctivitis

Toxic exposure, allergy/atopy, and autoimmune disease are a few of the many etiologies of noninfectious conjunctivitis. Often, the inflammation found in these conditions is histologically nonspecific, although the presence of eosinophils in the tissue suggests an allergic/atopic etiology.

Mucous membrane pemphigoid (MMP; also known as *ocular cicatricial pemphigoid*) is a form of cicatrizing conjunctivitis of autoimmune etiology. Typically, it involves not only the conjunctiva (Fig 5-4A) but also other mucous membranes; in approximately 25% of affected patients, MMP involves the skin. When this diagnosis is suspected clinically, conjunctival biopsy is performed to establish the diagnosis. Half of the specimen is submitted in formalin for routine histologic examination, and half is submitted in a special medium (eg, Michel or Zeus) or saline for direct immunofluorescence analysis. Histologic findings are generally nonspecific but typically show a subepithelial, bandlike, mixed inflammatory cell infiltrate rich in plasma cells. The overlying epithelium may demonstrate squamous metaplasia with keratinization and loss of goblet cells. Bullae are occasionally present (Fig 5-4B). Immunofluorescence is the gold standard for diagnosis of MMP and demonstrates linear deposition of immunoglobulins (IgG, IgM, and/or IgA) and/or complement (C3) along the epithelial basement membrane (Fig 5-4C). The clinician must bear in mind that the sensitivity of immunofluorescence may be as low as 50%

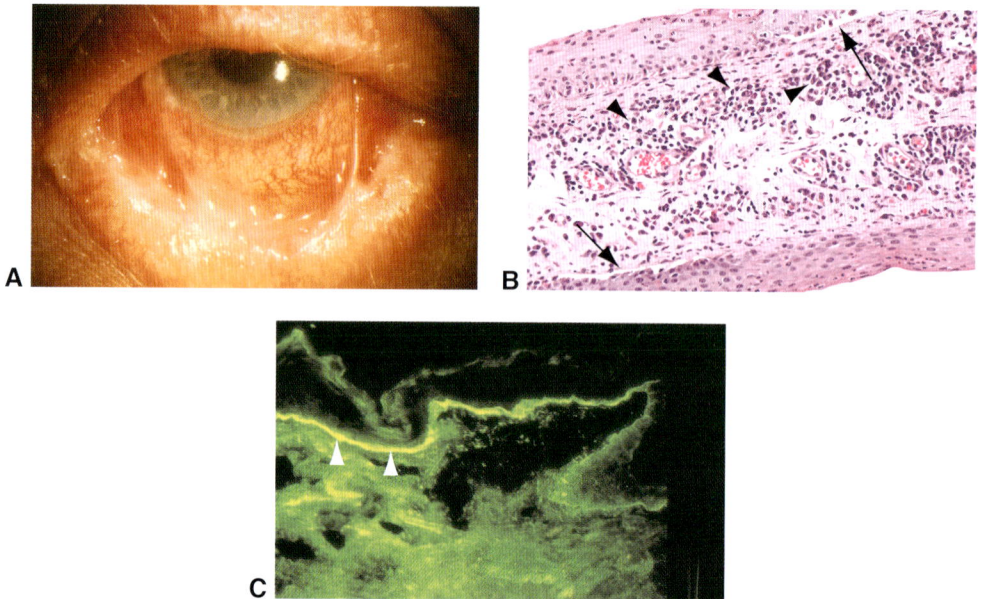

Figure 5-4 Mucous membrane pemphigoid (MMP). **A,** Clinical photograph. Note the conjunctival injection, symblepharon formation, shortening of the inferior fornix, and conjunctival/eyelid cicatrization. **B,** Histology shows epithelial bullae *(arrows)* and a dense chronic inflammatory cell infiltrate in the stroma *(arrowheads)*. **C,** Direct immunofluorescent staining of unfixed tissue demonstrates immunoglobulin deposition along the epithelial basement membrane *(arrowheads)* in MMP. *(Part A courtesy of Andrew J.W. Huang, MD; part B courtesy of George J. Harocopos, MD.)*

(particularly in long-standing cases with severe cicatrization). Thus, a negative result does not rule out MMP.

Labowsky MT, Stinnett SS, Liss J, Daluvoy M, Hall RP, Sheih C. Clinical implications of direct immunofluorescence findings in patients with ocular mucous membrane pemphigoid. *Am J Ophthalmol.* 2017;183:48–55.

Queisi MM, Zein M, Lamba N, Mees H, Foster CS. Update on ocular cicatricial pemphigoid and emerging treatments. *Surv Ophthalmol.* 2016;61(3):314–317.

Papillary Versus Follicular Conjunctivitis

Most cases of conjunctivitis are diagnosed as either papillary or follicular according to the macroscopic and microscopic appearances of the conjunctiva (Fig 5-5). Neither type is pathognomonic. Clinically, *papillary conjunctivitis* shows a cobblestone arrangement of small nodules with central vascular cores (Fig 5-6A). Histologically, papillae appear as closely packed, flat-topped epithelial projections, with inflammatory cells in the stroma surrounding a central vascular channel (Fig 5-6B). *Follicular conjunctivitis* is characterized clinically by the presence of follicles (Fig 5-7A): small, pink, dome-shaped nodules with overlying vessels but without a prominent central vessel. Histologically, a follicle appears as a dense oval aggregate of lymphocytes in the superficial stroma. The lymphocytes are occasionally arranged into reactive follicles with germinal centers composed of large proliferating B cells, surrounded by a mantle of smaller, more differentiated B cells (Fig 5-7B).

Granulomatous Conjunctivitis

Granulomatous conjunctivitis is less common than papillary and follicular conjunctivitis and has both infectious and noninfectious causes. Clinically, the nodular elevations of granulomatous conjunctivitis may be difficult to distinguish from follicles, but the clinical history and systemic symptoms may point to the diagnosis. See BCSC Section 8, *External Disease and Cornea,* and Section 9, *Uveitis and Ocular Inflammation,* for additional discussion of granulomatous conjunctivitis.

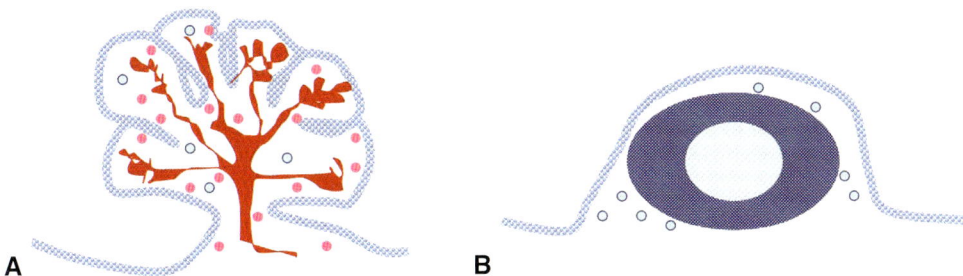

Figure 5-5 Schematic representations of papillary and follicular conjunctivitis. **A,** In papillary conjunctivitis, the conjunctival epithelium *(blue line)* extends over fine projections of blood vessels *(red)* and fibrous tissue, and the stroma contains eosinophils *(pink circles)*, lymphocytes, and plasma cells *(blue circles)*. **B,** In follicular conjunctivitis, the conjunctival epithelium *(blue line)* overlies lymphoid follicles in the superficial stroma that have a paler germinal center surrounded by a darker corona *(central pale blue surrounded by purple)*. The surrounding stroma contains lymphocytes and plasma cells *(small blue circles)*. *(Courtesy of Patricia Chévez-Barrios, MD.)*

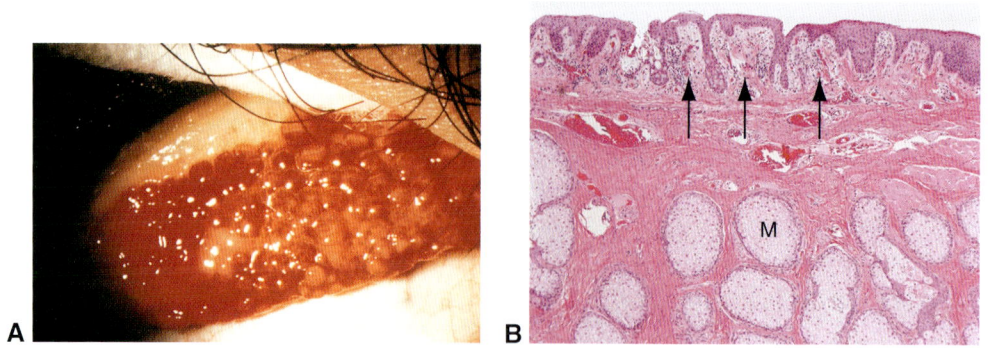

Figure 5-6 Papillary conjunctivitis. **A,** Clinical photograph. Papillae efface the normal palpebral conjunctival surface and form a confluent cobblestone pattern. **B,** Low-magnification photomicrograph shows the characteristic closely packed, flat-topped papillae with central fibrovascular cores *(arrows)*. The normal meibomian glands (M) of the tarsus are also shown. *(Part A courtesy of Harry H. Brown, MD; part B courtesy of George J. Harocopos, MD.)*

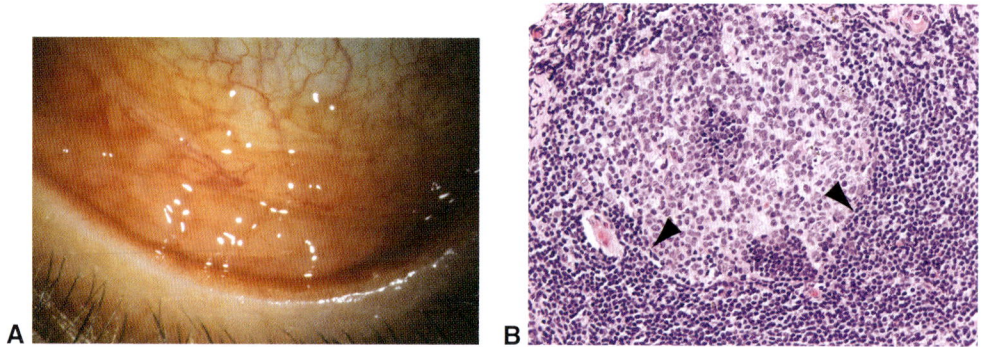

Figure 5-7 Follicular conjunctivitis. **A,** Clinical photograph showing follicles, which occur only in the fornix. **B,** High-magnification photomicrograph shows a lymphoid follicle and the boundary between the germinal center and the mantle zone *(arrowheads)*. Note the paler, relatively larger, immature lymphocytes in the germinal center compared with the darker, small, mature lymphocytes in the corona. *(Part A courtesy of Anthony J. Lubniewski, MD; part B courtesy of George J. Harocopos, MD.)*

Granulomatous conjunctivitis occurring in association with ipsilateral regional lymphadenopathy is known as *Parinaud oculoglandular syndrome.* Many organisms, often atypical ones such as *Bartonella henselae,* can cause this syndrome. The diagnosis can be made by using cultures, serologic testing, polymerase chain reaction analysis, or a combination of these. In some cases, special stains such as Gram, acid-fast, or silver stain may be useful for identifying organisms in biopsy tissue. When conjunctival biopsy is performed, the granulomas in infectious granulomatous conjunctivitis typically show central necrosis (caseating granulomas).

A presumably noninfectious cause of granulomatous conjunctivitis is *sarcoidosis,* a systemic disease that may involve all the ocular tissues, including the conjunctiva. It manifests as small tan nodules without overt inflammatory signs, primarily in the lower forniceal conjunctiva (Fig 5-8A). Conjunctival biopsy can be a simple, minimally invasive way of providing diagnostic confirmation of this systemic disease. Histologically, noncaseating

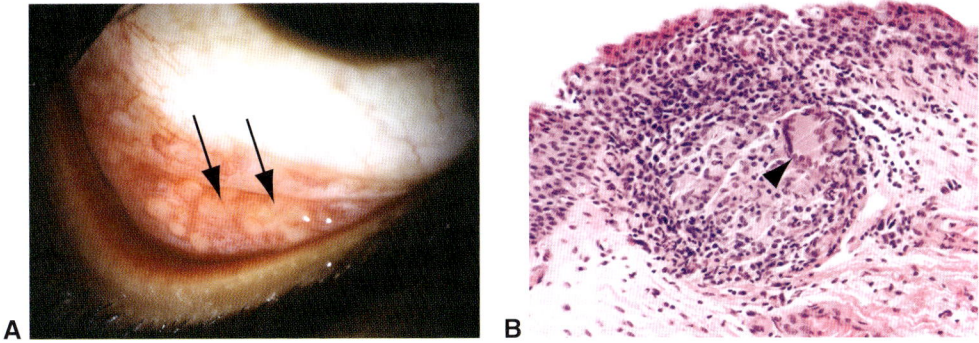

Figure 5-8 Sarcoidosis. **A,** Clinical photograph shows granulomas *(arrows)* of the conjunctiva in a patient with sarcoidosis. **B,** Histology shows a noncaseating granuloma with pale-staining histiocytes, including a multinucleated giant cell *(arrowhead)*. Note the small cuff of lymphocytes and plasma cells. *(Courtesy of George J. Harocopos, MD.)*

granulomatous nodules (round to oval aggregates of epithelioid histiocytes with or without multinucleated giant cells) are present within the conjunctival stroma, typically with a cuff of lymphocytes and plasma cells (Fig 5-8B). Central necrosis is not characteristic and, if present, suggests an infectious etiology. To ensure that granulomas are not missed in the biopsy tissue, step-sectioning of the paraffin block is done, similar to a temporal artery biopsy. The histologic findings are not pathognomonic for sarcoidosis and must be correlated with clinical findings after infectious causes of granulomatous inflammation have been excluded by special stains and/or cultures.

Foreign bodies are another cause of granulomatous conjunctivitis, as the surface of the eye is continually exposed to dust, hair, or other foreign material. Some foreign bodies may be transient and/or inert, whereas others may become embedded and incite a foreign-body reaction, identifiable histologically as epithelioid histiocytes and multinucleated giant cells surrounding the foreign material. Viewing the tissue section under polarized light may help reveal the presence of foreign material (Fig 5-9).

Bui KM, Garcia-Gonzalez JM, Patel SS, Lin AY, Edward DP, Goldstein DA. Directed conjunctival biopsy and impact of histologic sectioning methodology on the diagnosis of ocular sarcoidosis. *J Ophthalmic Inflamm Infect.* 2014;4(1):1–5.

Pyogenic Granuloma

Pyogenic granuloma (exuberant granulation tissue) appears as a fleshy, red, pedunculated, nodular elevation on the conjunctival surface, typically occurring in association with a chalazion (on the palpebral conjunctiva) or a punctum or at a site of prior accidental or surgical trauma. Granulation tissue is a reparative process that is necessary for wound healing after inflammation or injury. The term "pyogenic granuloma" is a misnomer because the lesion is not pus producing and is not granulomatous. Rather, pyogenic granuloma is an exuberant proliferation (overgrowth) of granulation tissue composed of acute and chronic inflammatory cells and radially arranged, proliferating capillaries within a loose connective tissue framework (Fig 5-10).

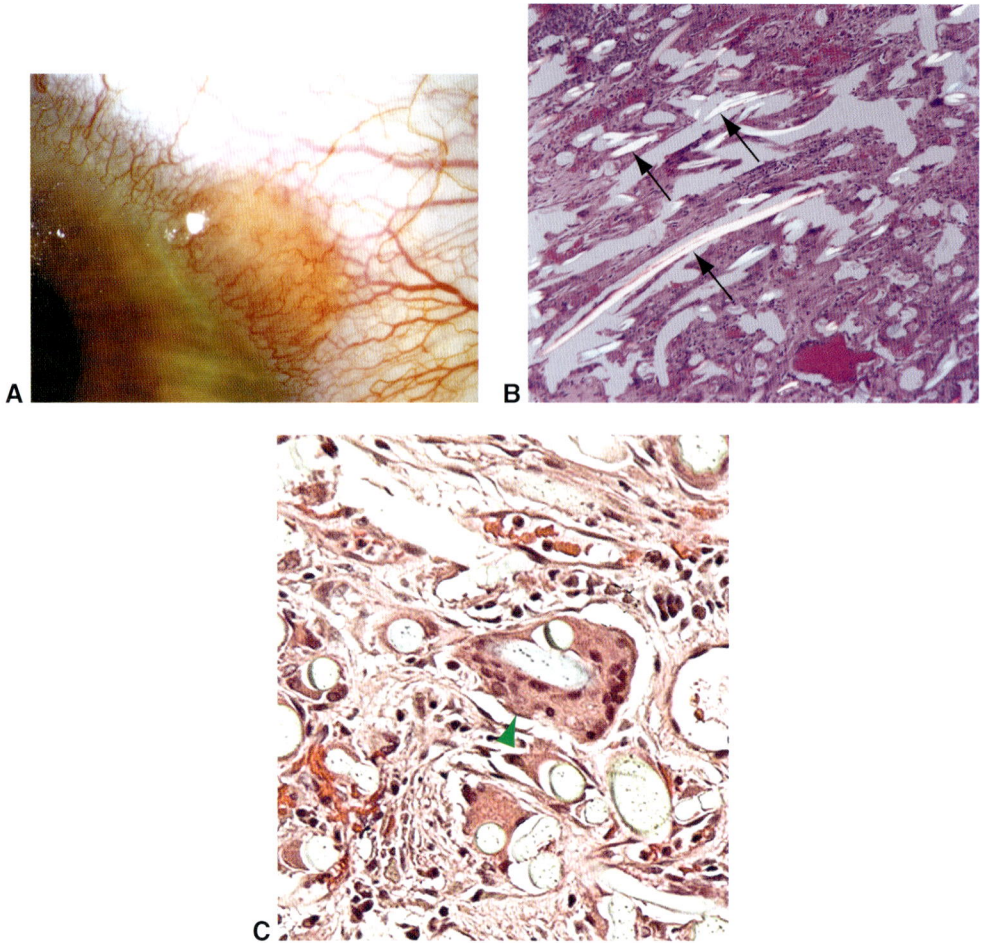

Figure 5-9 Conjunctival foreign-body granuloma. **A,** Clinical appearance on the bulbar conjunctiva. **B,** Histologic analysis of the specimen (from a different patient) under polarized light shows multiple refractile foreign fibers *(arrows).* **C,** Hematoxylin-eosin (H&E) stain demonstrates fibers with surrounding foreign-body granulomatous reaction, including multiple giant cells *(arrowhead).* *(Part A courtesy of Anthony J. Lubniewski, MD; part B courtesy of George J. Harocopos, MD; part C courtesy of Tatyana Milman, MD.)*

Degenerations

See BCSC Section 8, *External Disease and Cornea,* for discussion of the clinical aspects of many of the topics covered in the following sections.

Pinguecula and Pterygium

A *pinguecula* is a small, yellow-tan bulbar conjunctival nodule typically located at the nasal and/or temporal limbus, often bilaterally (Fig 5-11A). A manifestation of actinic damage (ie, exposure to sunlight) or other environmental trauma, such as that caused by dust and

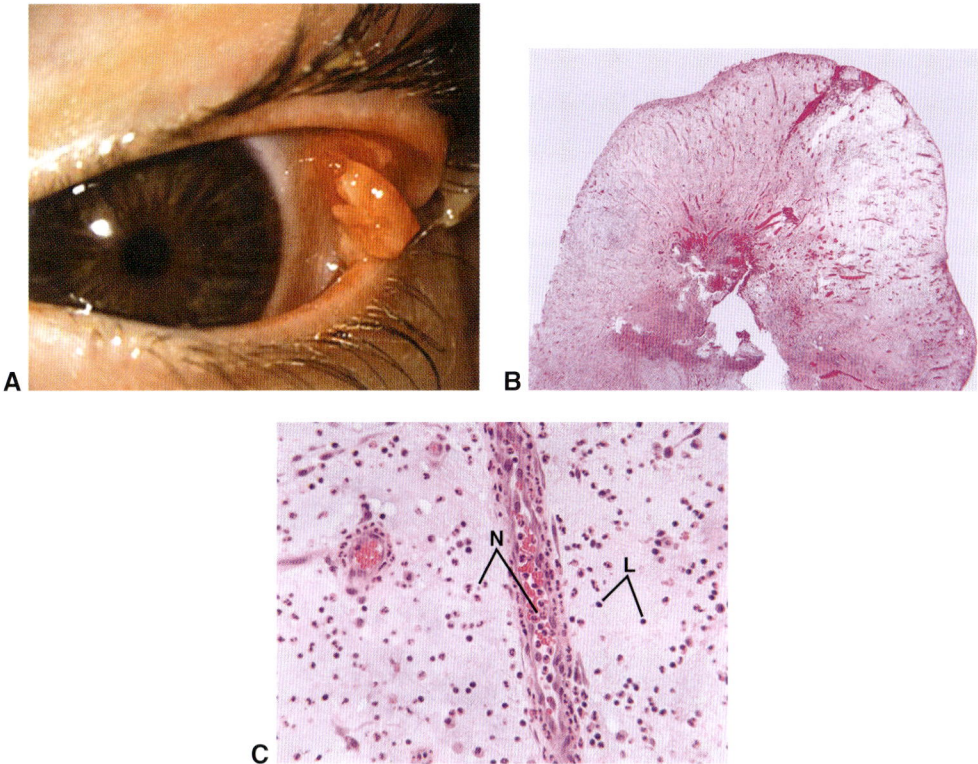

Figure 5-10 Pyogenic granuloma. **A,** Clinical appearance at a site of prior strabismus surgery. **B,** Low-magnification photomicrograph illustrates a pedunculated mass composed of granulation tissue with a "spoke-wheel" vascular pattern. **C,** High magnification shows a mixture of acute and chronic inflammatory cells. Note the neutrophils (N) both within the lumen of the blood vessels and infiltrating the tissue. Chronic inflammatory cells, predominantly lymphocytes (L), are present in this field. *(Part A courtesy of Gregg T. Lueder, MD; parts B and C courtesy of George J. Harocopos, MD.)*

wind, this growth is more common with advancing years. On histologic examination, the stromal collagen shows fragmentation and basophilic degeneration, referred to as *elastotic degeneration* (also known as *pseudoelastosis* or *solar elastosis*). These terms refer to the staining of the degenerated collagen with stains for elastin, such as Verhoeff–van Gieson, even after tissue has been treated with elastase for digestion of true elastin (Fig 5-11B, C).

A *pterygium* is similar to a pinguecula in etiology and location but differs from the latter in its invasion of the superficial cornea as a fibrovascular, wing-shaped growth (Fig 5-12A). Histologic examination typically shows elastotic degeneration, as in a pinguecula, as well as prominent blood vessels that correlate with the vascularity seen clinically (Fig 5-12B, C), fibrosis, and variable degrees of chronic inflammation. A *recurrent pterygium* may lack the histologic feature of elastotic degeneration and is thus more accurately classified as pannus (discussed in Chapter 6) or a fibrovascular connective tissue response.

In pingueculae and pterygia, the overlying epithelium may exhibit mild squamous metaplasia, for example, loss of goblet cells and surface keratinization. Some studies have

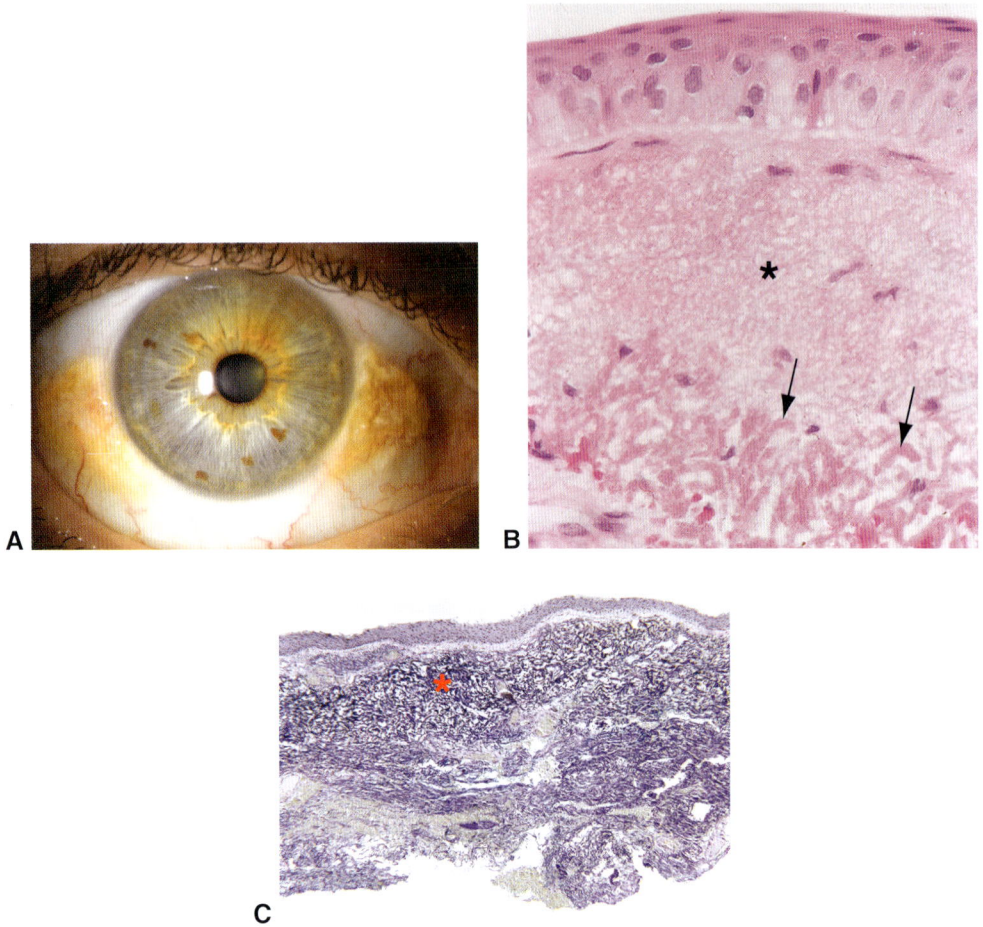

Figure 5-11 Pinguecula. **A,** Clinical appearance adjacent to the nasal and temporal limbus. **B,** Histologic examination demonstrates the acellular, amorphous, slightly basophilic material in the stroma *(asterisk)* and thick, curly fibers *(arrows)* indicative of elastotic degeneration. **C,** With Verhoeff–van Gieson stain for elastin, the basophilic material stains black *(asterisk).* *(Parts A and C courtesy of George J. Harocopos, MD; part B courtesy of Hans E. Grossniklaus, MD.)*

demonstrated abnormal expression of Ki-67 (a proliferation marker); dysregulation of tumor suppressor genes such as *p53* and *p63,* and other genes associated with DNA repair; cell proliferation, migration, and angiogenesis; loss of heterozygosity; and microsatellite instability. Thus, as with actinic damage to the skin, there is the possibility of malignant transformation of the epithelium, although this occurs rarely. When conjunctival squamous neoplasia arises, it often overlies an area of preexisting elastotic degeneration; therefore, it is important to examine these specimens histologically when they are excised (see the section "Ocular surface squamous neoplasia" later in this chapter).

Liu T, Liu Y, Xie L, He X, Bai J. Progress in the pathogenesis of pterygium. *Curr Eye Res.* 2013; 38(12):1191–1197.

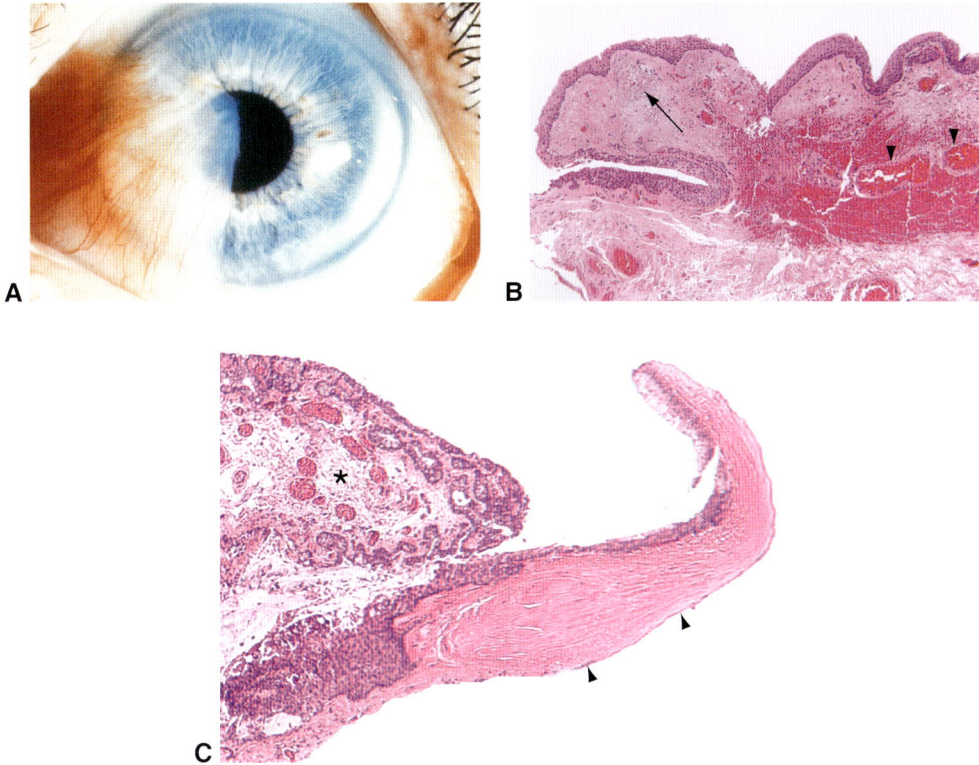

Figure 5-12 Pterygium. **A,** Clinical photograph. **B,** Histologically, a focus of elastotic degeneration is present *(arrow)*, as well as prominent blood vessels *(arrowheads)*, with surgically induced hemorrhage. **C,** In this case, the conjunctival and corneal portions of the pterygium are
evident. Note the prominent blood vessels in the conjunctival portion *(asterisk)* and destruction
of Bowman layer by ingrowth of fibroconnective tissue *(arrowheads)* in the corneal portion.
(Part A courtesy of Hans E. Grossniklaus, MD; parts B and C courtesy of George J. Harocopos, MD.)

Amyloid Deposits

Amyloid deposition in the conjunctiva is most commonly a localized idiopathic process
seen in healthy young and middle-aged adults. The deposits are typically composed of
monoclonal immunoglobulin (AL amyloid) secreted by local clonal plasma cells. Conjunctival amyloidosis may also be induced by long-standing inflammation, as with trachoma (ie, secondary localized amyloidosis, AA amyloid). In rare cases, conjunctival
amyloidosis may occur in the setting of primary conjunctival lymphoma or plasmacytoma
or secondary to systemic lymphoma or plasma cell myeloma.

Clinically, conjunctival amyloidosis typically presents as a salmon-colored nodular
elevation that may be associated with hemorrhage (Fig 5-13A). Histologically, amyloid
appears as a glassy pink, extracellular deposit within the stroma, sometimes in a perivascular distribution. On Congo red stain under standard light, amyloid deposits appear red
orange. When viewed with polarized light, they exhibit birefringence with dichroism; that
is, they change from red orange to apple green (Fig 5-13B–D). Other useful stains include
crystal violet and the fluorescent stain thioflavin T.

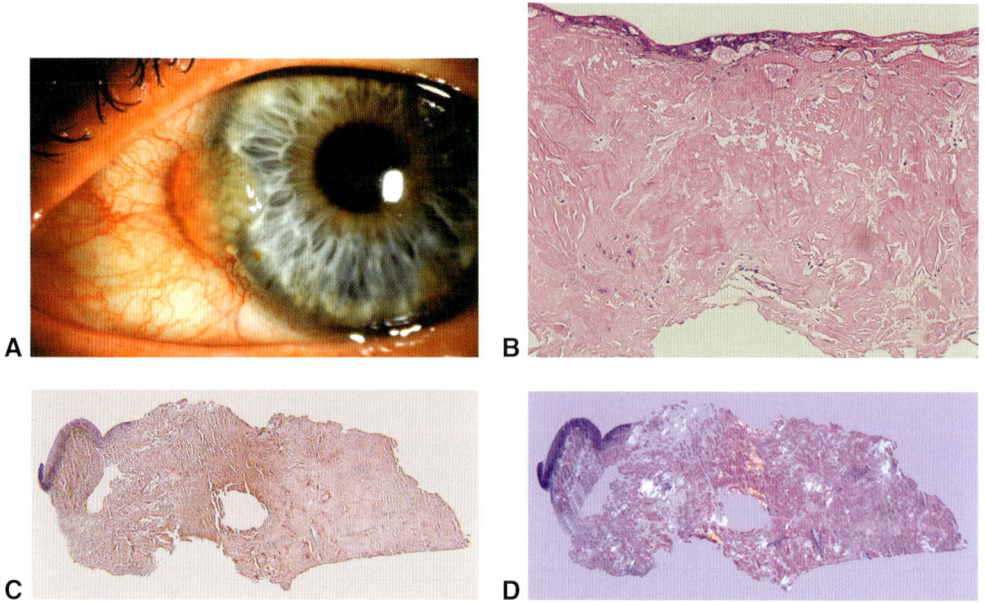

Figure 5-13 Conjunctival amyloidosis. **A,** Clinical appearance at the limbus and adjacent bulbar conjunctiva. **B,** Histologic examination reveals diffuse, amorphous, extracellular eosinophilic material throughout the stroma. **C,** Congo red stain under standard light stains the amyloid red orange. **D,** On Congo red stain under polarized light, amyloid exhibits apple-green birefringence (dichroism). *(Parts A, C, and D courtesy of George J. Harocopos, MD; part B courtesy of Shu-Hong Chang, MD.)*

Electron microscopy shows characteristic fibrils. Immunohistochemical (IHC) methods, sequencing, and mass spectrometry–based proteomic analysis are some of the techniques used in amyloid subtyping. Mass spectrometry is particularly sensitive.

Picken MM. Amyloidosis—where are we now and where are we heading? *Arch Pathol Lab Med.* 2010;134(4):545–551.

Epithelial Inclusion Cyst

A conjunctival epithelial inclusion cyst may form at a site of prior accidental or surgical trauma (eg, after strabismus surgery, retinal surgery, or enucleation). Clinically, the lesion appears as a clear, translucent cystic elevation on the ocular surface. There may be associated prominent vascularity. Histologic examination shows a cystic space in the stroma lined by nonkeratinized stratified squamous epithelium with or without goblet cells (Fig 5-14A). The lumen may be empty or may contain proteinaceous material and cellular debris (Fig 5-14B).

Conjunctivochalasis

Conjunctivochalasis is a chronic condition characterized by loose, redundant, nonedematous, bulbar conjunctival folds that may overhang the lower eyelid margin and is often associated with aging. Some histologic studies have revealed stromal inflammation and/or dilated lymphatic vessels in this condition.

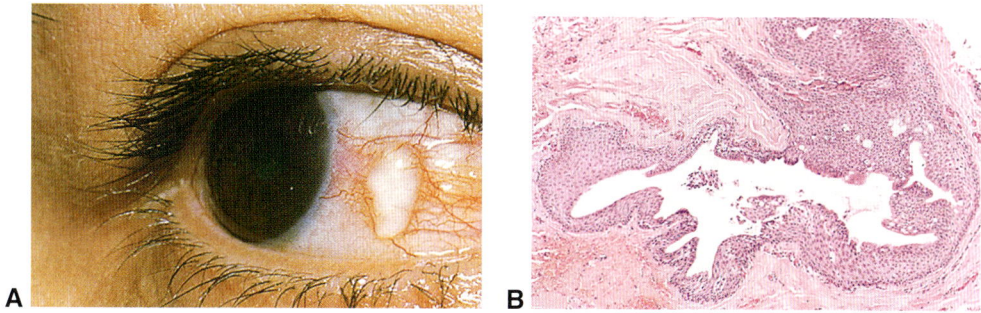

Figure 5-14 Epithelial inclusion cyst. **A,** Clinical photograph. **B,** Histologically, the cyst is lined by nonkeratinized stratified squamous epithelium with goblet cells, characteristic of the conjunctiva.

Marmalidou A, Kheirkhah A, Dana R. Conjunctivochalasis: a systematic review. *Surv Ophthalmol.* 2018;63(4):554–564.

Neoplasia

Conjunctival specimens, particularly those involving potential malignancies, require special submission procedures along with excellent communication between the clinician and the pathologist to optimize prognosis and treatment. Techniques such as immunohistochemistry (IHC), flow cytometry, and in situ hybridization, as well as molecular studies, may be required for an accurate diagnosis and prognostication or for determining whether targeted therapy may be appropriate for the patient. See also Chapter 3.

Squamous Epithelial Lesions

Squamous papilloma

The most common ocular surface neoplasms are those of the squamous family. Of these, the most common benign variant is squamous papilloma. Clinically, squamous papilloma may be divided into pedunculated and sessile subtypes.

Pedunculated papilloma is an exophytic, pink-red, strawberry-like frond frequently localized to the caruncle (Fig 5-15A), plica semilunaris, or forniceal conjunctiva. It occurs most commonly in children and young adults, with multiple lesions sometimes present in affected patients. Pedunculated papilloma is associated with human papillomavirus (HPV) infection, subtypes 6 and 11. Histologic examination of a pedunculated papilloma demonstrates fingerlike projections of hyperplastic squamous epithelium with a central fibrovascular core (Fig 5-15B). Goblet cells may be present as in normal conjunctival epithelium. When overlying tear film disruption results in exposure, the number of goblet cells may become reduced and the surface keratinized. Neutrophils may be seen within the epithelium, and a chronic inflammatory infiltrate is frequently present in the stroma. Pedunculated papillomas typically exhibit benign behavior and rarely undergo malignant transformation.

A *sessile papilloma* generally arises on the bulbar conjunctiva, especially at the limbus, and occurs more commonly in adults. This type of papilloma is also associated with HPV

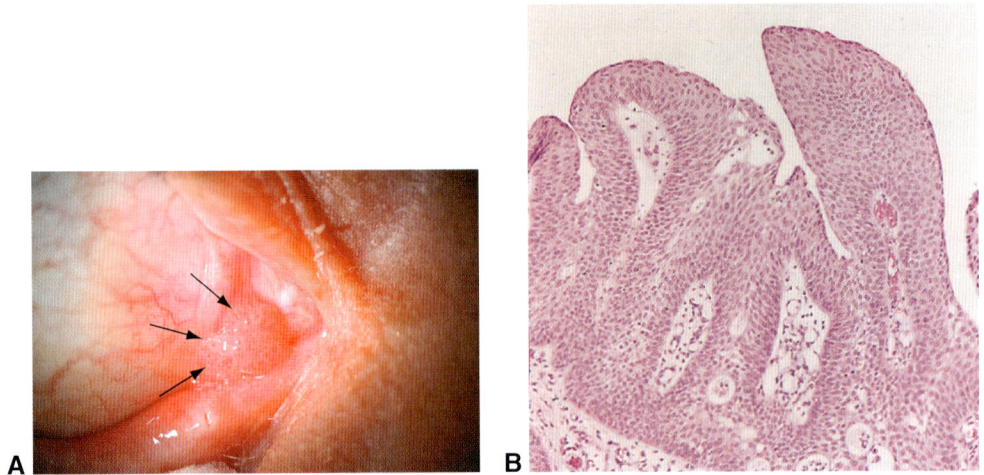

Figure 5-15 Squamous papilloma. **A,** Clinical photograph shows squamous papilloma located at the caruncle *(arrows)*. **B,** The epithelium is hyperplastic with fingerlike projections surrounding fibrovascular cores. *(Part A courtesy of George J. Harocopos, MD.)*

infection, subtypes 16 and 18—the same subtypes associated with squamous malignancies. Clinical features worrisome for malignant transformation include leukoplakia (ie, white patches indicative of keratinization), inflammation, atypical vascularity, and corneal involvement. Histologically, a sessile papilloma exhibits a broad base and lacks the prominent fingerlike projections seen in a pedunculated papilloma. The epithelium is hyperplastic with intervening fibrovascular cores but is otherwise normal. The presence of nuclear hyperchromatism and pleomorphism, altered maturation (dysplasia), dyskeratosis, and frequent mitotic figures suggests a diagnosis of ocular surface squamous neoplasia.

Ocular surface squamous neoplasia

Ocular surface squamous neoplasia (OSSN) comprises a wide spectrum of dysplastic changes of the ocular surface epithelium, including conjunctival and corneal intraepithelial neoplasia (CIN), squamous cell carcinoma in situ, and squamous cell carcinoma (SCC), which, by definition, invades through the epithelial basement membrane (Fig 5-16).

The prevalence of OSSN is increased in equatorial regions of the world. Ultraviolet (UV) light exposure is a known risk factor for the condition, especially in individuals with light skin pigmentation. Some reports have shown mutations in tumor suppressor genes such as *p53* secondary to UV light exposure. A hereditary impairment of DNA repair (as in xeroderma pigmentosum) also increases the risk of OSSN. In addition, OSSN occurs more frequently in patients who are immunosuppressed, such as those with HIV infection/AIDS, and in those with ocular surface HPV infection (subtypes 16 and 18). OSSN is commonly the first presenting sign of HIV/AIDS in regions where HIV infection is endemic. HIV-associated OSSN may demonstrate rapid growth and aggressive behavior, and HIV infection should be suspected in any patient with OSSN who is younger than 50 years.

OSSN typically arises in the interpalpebral limbal zone. It usually presents as a unilateral vascularized, gray, gelatinous limbal mass located medially or laterally in the

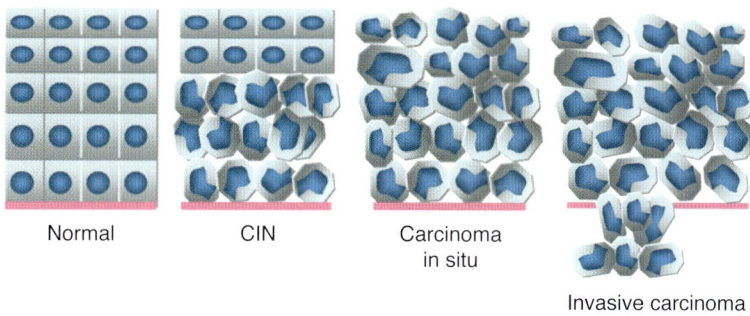

Figure 5-16 Schematic representation of the degrees of ocular surface squamous neoplasia (OSSN). The first panel represents normal epithelium with a basement membrane *(pink line)*. In conjunctival intraepithelial neoplasia (CIN), the deeper layers of the epithelium are replaced with disorganized, often atypical cells that are not maturing normally (dysplasia). Carcinoma in situ is full-thickness replacement of epithelium by dysplastic cells, with the basement membrane still intact. In invasive squamous cell carcinoma, note the invasion through the basement membrane into the stroma. *(Courtesy of Patricia Chévez-Barrios, MD.)*

sun-exposed interpalpebral fissure; the lesion may extend onto the peripheral cornea. Other features such as overlying leukoplakia (white plaque) and tortuous dilated "corkscrew" feeder vessels may be present (Figs 5-17, 5-18A, B). Clinical features overlap with those of other ocular surface lesions, making diagnosis of OSSN based solely on clinical assessment difficult. Other entities in the clinical differential diagnosis of OSSN include pannus, benign papilloma, pinguecula, pterygium, vitamin A deficiency, benign intraepithelial dyskeratosis, and nevus.

Anterior segment optical coherence tomography (AS-OCT), ultrasound biomicroscopy (UBM), and impression cytology (IC) are less invasive options for possible diagnosis of CIN and OSSN. AS-OCT imaging has been reported to correlate with histologic findings in distinguishing noninvasive and invasive OSSN (Fig 5-18C, D). However, these diagnostic techniques are not routinely used for this purpose, and biopsy remains the standard for accurate diagnosis of these entities.

Conjunctival biopsy and handling of these specimens require special care and attention for accurate diagnosis of OSSN and evaluation of the margins of excision (see Chapter 3 for more information on specimen preparation). Histologically, the epithelium often demonstrates an abrupt transition to an area of hyperplasia, loss of goblet cells, loss of polarity (loss of normal maturation from basal to superficial layers), nuclear hyperchromatism and pleomorphism, and mitotic figures that may be atypical. Dyskeratosis, including surface keratinization (resulting in the clinical appearance of leukoplakia) and formation of keratin pearls within the epithelium, may be present. Often, there is chronic inflammation and increased vascularity in the underlying superficial stroma. Elastotic degeneration is also often present in the stroma (Fig 5-18E, F; see also Fig 5-17B).

The most important histologic assessment in OSSN is determining whether the neoplasia is contained by the epithelial basement membrane (ie, intraepithelial or in situ) or whether neoplastic cells have breached the basement membrane and invaded the stroma (see Figs 5-17, 5-18). The term *conjunctival intraepithelial neoplasia (CIN)* is often used for

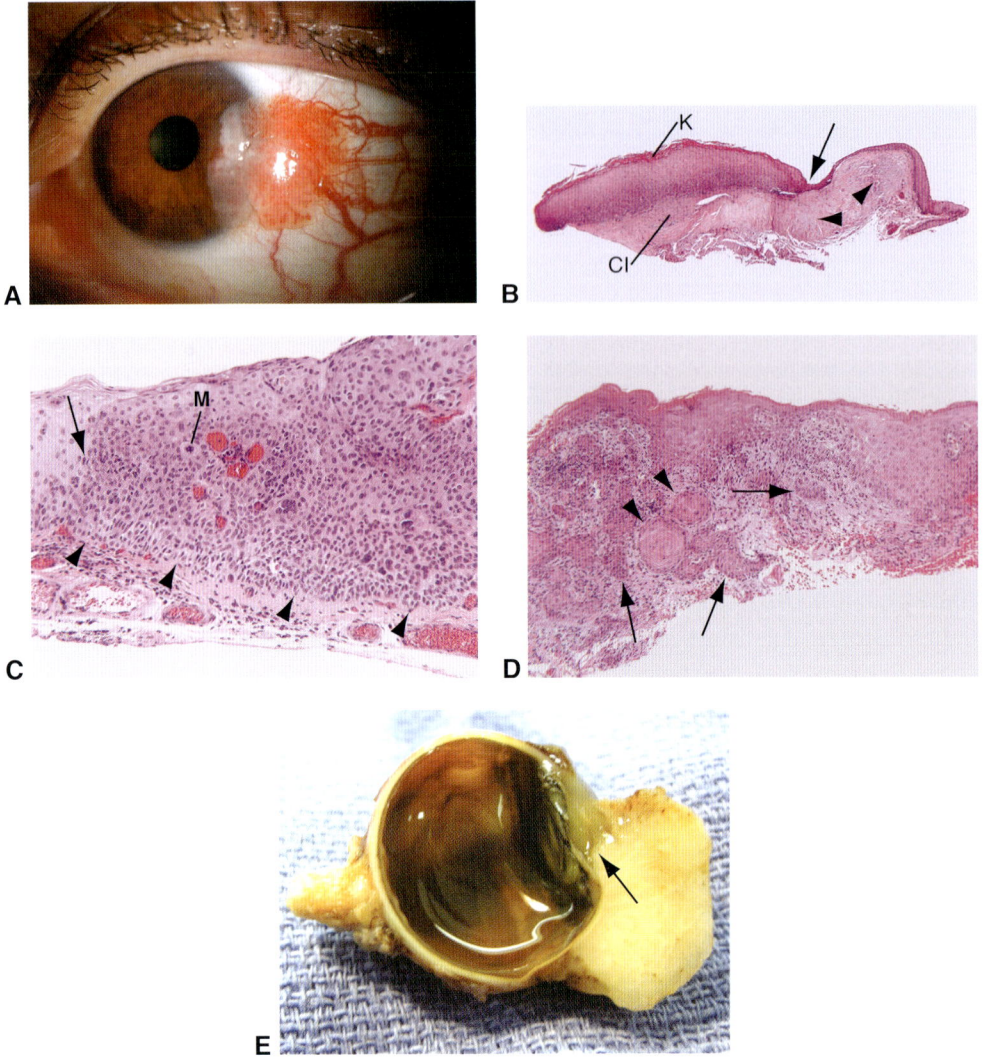

Figure 5-17 Ocular surface squamous neoplasia (OSSN). **A,** Clinical photograph. Note the vascular tortuosity of the conjunctival portion and the gelatinous appearance with focal leukoplakia of the corneal portion. Also note the prominent feeder vessels. **B,** Histologic examination shows the sharp demarcation *(arrow)* between normal and abnormal epithelia in OSSN. The epithelium is hyperplastic, with surface keratinization (K). Because the basement membrane is intact and there is partial-thickness dysplasia of the epithelium, a diagnosis of CIN is made. There is a chronic inflammatory response in the stroma (CI). Also note areas of elastotic degeneration in the stroma *(arrowheads),* indicating that the lesion arose over a pinguecula. **C,** High magnification (image from a different patient) shows the transition zone where neoplasia begins *(arrow).* To the right of the arrow, the epithelium exhibits mild surface keratinization, hyperplasia, nuclear hyperchromatism and pleomorphism, goblet cell loss, altered cell polarity, full-thickness involvement, and mitotic figures (M). The basement membrane is intact *(arrowheads),* making this a squamous cell carcinoma (SCC) in situ. **D,** In SCC, tongues of epithelium violate the basement membrane and invade the stroma *(arrows),* with whorls of epithelial cells known as *squamous eddies (arrowheads).* **E,** Gross photograph of a large ocular surface squamous carcinoma that invaded the limbus and anterior chamber angle through a previous surgical incision *(arrow). (Part A courtesy of Vahid Feiz, MD; parts B–E courtesy of George J. Harocopos, MD.)*

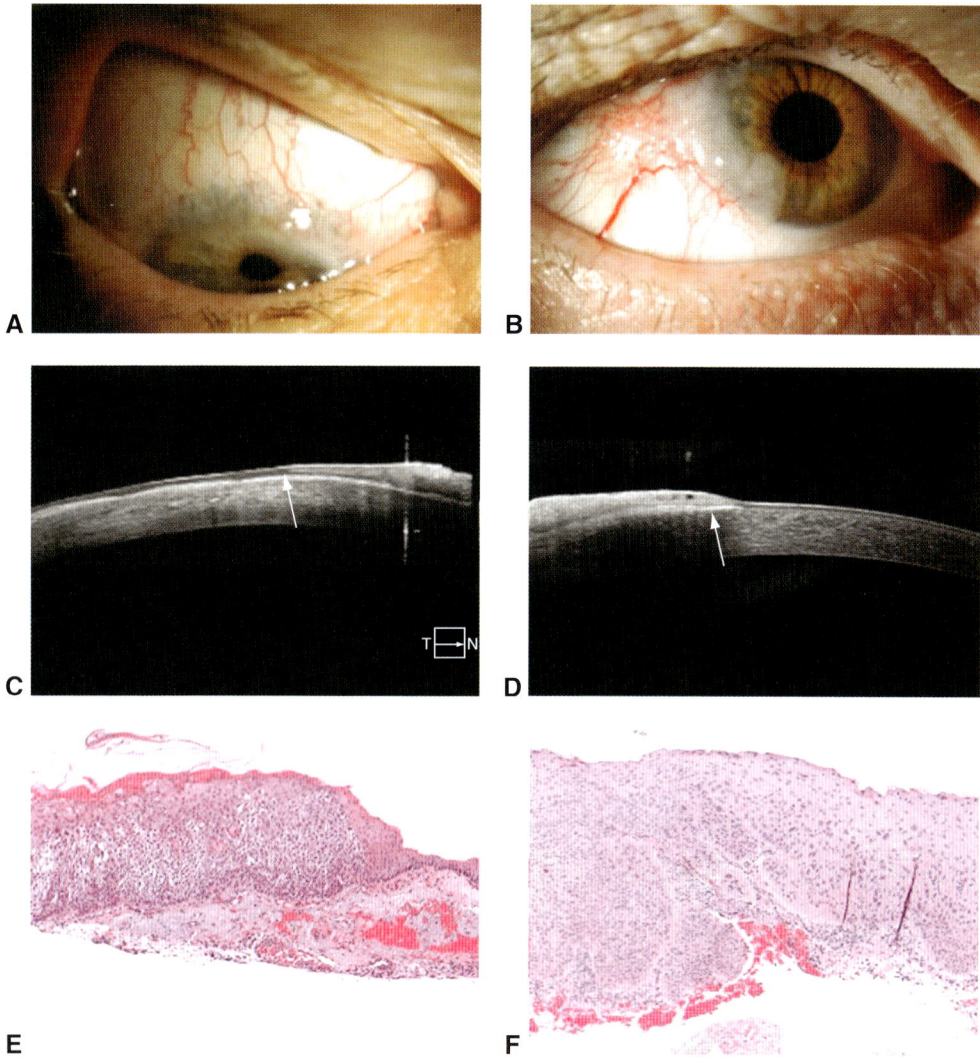

Figure 5-18 Noninvasive and invasive ocular surface squamous neoplasia (OSSN). **A,** Slit-lamp photograph of a superior limbal gelatinous, grayish lesion with vascularity and extension onto the cornea. **B,** Slit-lamp photograph of a temporal limbal gelatinous lesion with large feeder vessels and extension onto the cornea. **C,** Anterior segment optical coherence tomography (AS-OCT) image of the lesion depicted in part **A,** demonstrating epithelial thickening and hyperreflectivity consistent with OSSN; in addition, there is hyperreflectivity at the epithelial base *(arrow),* possibly suggestive of more superficial epithelial disease. **D,** AS-OCT image of the lesion depicted in part **B,** demonstrating epithelial thickening and hyperreflectivity as well as prominent subepithelial hyperreflectivity *(arrow),* possibly suggestive of deeper invasion. **E,** Histology of the lesion depicted in parts **A** and **C,** demonstrating moderate to severe epithelial dysplasia consistent with noninvasive OSSN. **F,** Histology of the lesion depicted in parts **B** and **D,** demonstrating superficially invasive squamous cell carcinoma consistent with invasive OSSN. *(Reproduced with permission from Polski A, Sibug Saber M, Kim JW, Berry JL. Extending far and wide: the role of biopsy and staging in the management of ocular surface squamous neoplasia. Clin Exp Ophthalmol. 2019;47(2):193–200.)*

lesions contained by the basement membrane. The neoplasia is graded as mild, moderate, or severe according to the degree of cellular atypia. In cases of the most severe dysplasia, there is full-thickness involvement of the epithelium, often with squamous eddies or keratin whorls or pearls (see Figs 5-17C, D and 5-18E). For full-thickness dyplastic lesions, the term *squamous carcinoma in situ* is used.

Invasion of the stroma by neoplastic cells is diagnostic of *invasive SCC* (see Figs 5-17D, E, and 5-18F). Invasion of the sclera or cornea with intraocular spread is an uncommon complication of invasive SCC that typically occurs at the site of a previous surgical procedure or in patients whose immune response is suppressed. In addition, *mucoepidermoid carcinoma* and *spindle cell carcinoma,* rare variants of conjunctival carcinoma, may demonstrate aggressive behavior, with higher rates of recurrence, intraocular spread, and orbital invasion. Although regional lymph node metastasis and distant metastasis are less common with conjunctival SCC than with squamous carcinomas of the skin or other sites, dissemination and death occur in a small percentage of cases.

Conway RM, Graue GF, Pelayes DE, et al. Conjunctival carcinoma. In: American Joint Committee on Cancer (AJCC). *AJCC Cancer Staging Manual.* 8th ed. Springer; 2017: 787–793.

Moyer AB, Roberts J, Olsen RJ, Chévez-Barrios P. Human papillomavirus-driven squamous lesions: high-risk genotype found in conjunctival papillomas, dysplasia, and carcinoma. *Am J Dermatopathol.* 2018;40(7):486–490.

Polski A, Sibug Saber M, Kim JW, Berry JL. Extending far and wide: the role of biopsy and staging in the management of ocular surface squamous neoplasia. *Clin Exp Ophthalmol.* 2019;47(2):193–200.

Melanocytic Lesions

About half of all conjunctival lesions in adults are pigmented and/or melanocytic in nature. Conjunctival melanocytes are normally dendritic and located exclusively in the basal layer of the epithelium alongside basal squamous cells, which also contain melanin. The melanocytes produce and secrete melanin into the adjacent epithelium, providing protection from UV light. The amount of conjunctival melanin in the epithelium is usually insufficient to be visible to the naked eye. Thus, the presence of clinically apparent pigmentation of the conjunctiva may necessitate further investigation, including developing a differential diagnosis and performing a biopsy when there is suspicion of malignancy. Although not all of the entities discussed in this section are neoplasms, they are covered here because all are forms of ocular surface pigmentation.

Pigmented conjunctival epithelial lesions, melanocytic neoplasms of the conjunctiva and caruncle, and other pigmented lesions of the ocular surface include the following:

- conjunctival junctional, compound, and stromal nevi, including
  - inflamed juvenile conjunctival nevus (inflamed juvenile nevus of childhood and adolescence)
  - blue nevus of the conjunctiva
- congenital ocular or oculodermal melanocytosis (nevus of Ota)
- secondary acquired melanosis or reactive melanosis of the conjunctiva
- complexion-associated melanosis (benign epithelial melanosis of the conjunctiva)

- primary acquired melanosis (PAM) with or without atypia (conjunctival melanocytic intraepithelial neoplasia [C-MIN])
- conjunctival melanoma

Melanocytic nevi

Melanocytic nevi (also called *nevocellular nevi, nevus cell nevi*) are classified as hamartomas or neoplasms depending on whether the lesions are congenital or acquired. Conjunctival melanocytic nevi usually become clinically apparent in childhood, appearing as unilateral circumscribed pigmented lesions on the perilimbal interpalpebral bulbar conjunctiva, frequently incorporating small, clear epithelial cysts (Fig 5-19A). Melanocytic nevi are also common in the caruncle. They occur in the palpebral conjunctiva only in rare instances; pigmented lesions in this area are typically intraepithelial acquired melanosis or melanoma.

Amelanotic nevi of the conjunctiva are melanocytic nevi containing no pigment, meaning they have a pinkish appearance, which makes clinical diagnosis more challenging. The pigmentation and size of a nevus may increase during puberty, at which point the lesion may become noticeable.

Histologically, conjunctival melanocytic nevi are neoplasms composed of nests or sheets of nevus cells (specialized melanocytes) with benign features, including round to oval, uniformly staining nuclei and a moderate amount of cytoplasm. Epithelial cysts are often encountered within the stromal component of a nevus. The presence of these cysts within the stromal component of a nevus is typically indicative of a benign lesion.

Like cutaneous melanocytic nevi, conjunctival nevi undergo evolutionary changes with age. In the initial, junctional phase (usually in the first and second decades of life), nevus cells are arranged in nests (theques) at the interface (junction) between the epithelium and the stroma (Fig 5-19B). As the nevus evolves and proliferates, the nests descend

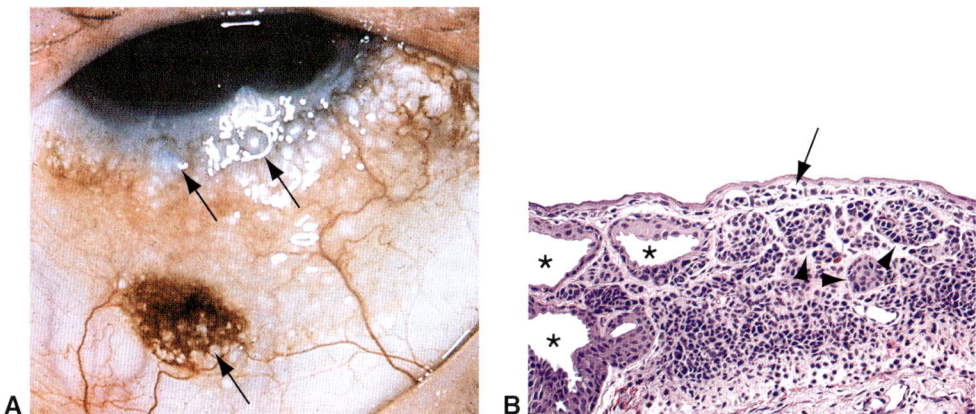

Figure 5-19 Conjunctival melanocytic nevus. **A,** Clinical appearance with characteristic cystic areas *(arrows)*. **B,** Histologically, the nevus cells have round, oval, or pear-shaped nuclei with a moderate amount of cytoplasm, mostly arranged in nests *(arrowheads)*. Nevus cells are also present at the epithelial–stromal junction *(arrow)*; hence, this is a compound nevus. Note the epithelial inclusion cysts *(asterisks)* within the lesion, correlating with the clinical appearance. *(Part B courtesy of George J. Harocopos, MD.)*

into the stroma and eventually may lose connection with the epithelium. Nevus cells residing exclusively at the epithelial–stromal junction are called *junctional nevi*, whereas nevi located exclusively in the stroma are termed *subepithelial* or *stromal nevi*; nevi with both junctional and subepithelial components are designated as compound nevi. In an older individual, the presence of a junctional component in a conjunctival nevus may represent malignant transformation.

An *inflamed juvenile conjunctival nevus* is a compound nevus that typically becomes apparent in childhood or adolescence and clinically often appears to grow rapidly, which is suggestive of malignancy. Histologically, the aggregates of nevus cells are surrounded and invaded by lymphocytes, plasma cells, and often eosinophils. This lesion may be misinterpreted histologically as malignant if the pathologist is not familiar with it.

Another form of melanocytic nevi that may occur in the conjunctiva is a *blue nevus*. Clinically, it appears as a dark blue–gray to blue-black nodule. Its melanocytes have a spindle cell morphology, similar to that of nevus cells seen in the uveal tract, and tend to contain a large amount of cytoplasmic melanin. *Ocular* and *oculodermal melanocytosis,* which is more often seen in dark-complexioned individuals, occurs deep to the conjunctiva, in the episclera and sclera, and consists of aggregates of dendritic melanocytes (Fig 5-20).

Intraepithelial melanosis

Conjunctival melanosis is a clinical term for localized or diffuse acquired pigmentation of the conjunctiva that occurs within the epithelium. Histologically, the term *melanosis* can be confusing, as it does not make a distinction between increased melanin content in epithelial cells and proliferation of melanocytes. These different etiologies of conjunctival pigmentation are more appropriately referred to as *intraepithelial nonproliferative melanocytic pigmentation* (a condition in which usually a small number of conjunctival basal dendritic melanocytes synthesize increased amounts of melanin that is transferred to surrounding basal epithelial cells) and *intraepithelial melanocytic proliferation* without atypia (a condition in which increased numbers of normal-appearing dendritic melanocytes—hyperplasia or early neoplasia—are generally confined to the basal epithelial layers in a linear arrangement).

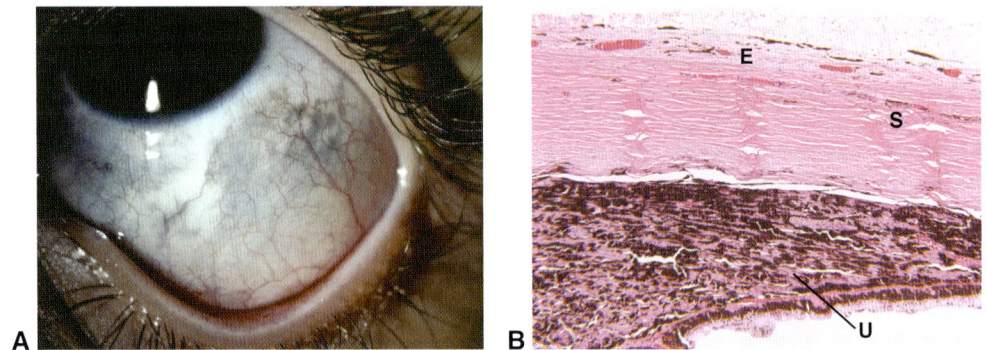

Figure 5-20 Ocular melanocytosis. **A,** Clinical photograph illustrating slate-gray patches of pigmentation of the scleral surface. **B,** Histologic examination shows an increased population of intensely pigmented spindle and dendritic melanocytes in the deep episclera (E), sclera (S), and uveal tract (U). *(Part A courtesy of Gabriela M. Espinoza, MD; part B courtesy of George J. Harocopos, MD.)*

The classification of and terminology used for various forms of melanosis are the subjects of debate. Conjunctival melanosis can be divided into primary, secondary, and complexion-associated forms (Fig 5-21). Secondary and complexion-associated melanoses generally do not involve melanocytic proliferation, only increased pigment production. PAM involves melanocytic proliferation and thus has a risk of progression to malignancy.

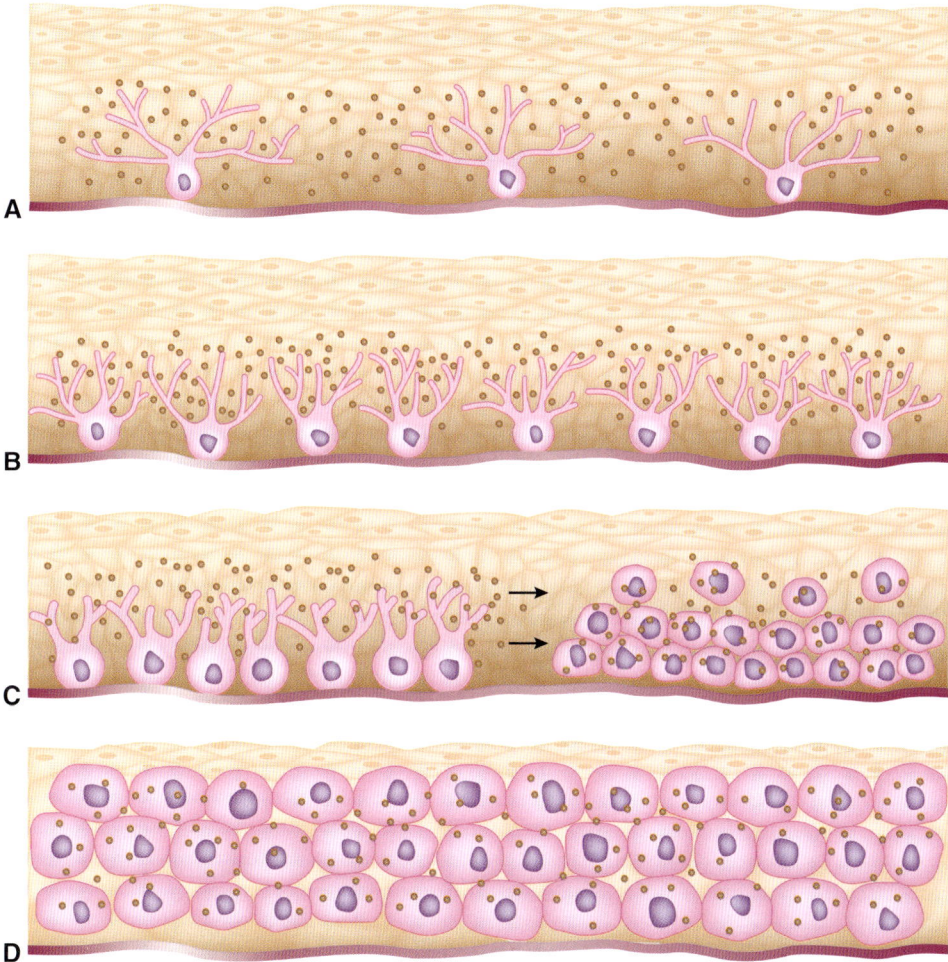

Figure 5-21 Schematic representation of the spectrum of non-nevoid pigmented lesions of the conjunctiva. Small brown dots denote melanin. **A,** Complexion-associated melanosis represents a nonproliferative melanocytic process in which a normal number of melanocytes produce an increased amount of melanin that is transferred to the surrounding basal epithelial cells. There is an increase in pigment but no change in cell numbers or morphology. **B,** Primary acquired melanosis (PAM) without atypia or with mild atypia (conjunctival melanocytic intraepithelial neoplasia [C-MIN] 1, 2) refers to low-grade lesions in which there is both increased pigment production and an increased number of melanocytes but no or very mild change in melanocyte morphology. **C,** PAM with moderate to severe atypia (C-MIN 3, 4, 5). There is increased pigment production, an increased number of melanocytes, and migration of melanocytes into the more superficial epithelial layers. Morphology of melanocytes is atypical. **D,** Melanoma in situ (C-MIN >5) with full-thickness replacement of the epithelium by morphologically atypical melanocytes shows an increased nucleocytoplasmic ratio. *(Illustration by Cyndie C. H. Wooley.)*

An understanding of the nomenclature and processes that apply to pathologic diagnosis is important when management of these lesions is considered. Equally important is communicating the suspected clinical diagnosis to the pathologist, as proper interpretation of histologic findings is greatly enhanced by that knowledge.

Secondary acquired melanosis *Conjunctival pigmentation with mild increase in normal melanocytes* (reactive melanosis of the conjunctiva) may be triggered by another conjunctival lesion (eg, squamous papilloma or carcinoma) or by underlying conjunctival inflammation.

Complexion-associated melanosis Complexion-associated melanosis (also called *benign epithelial melanosis, racial melanosis, primary conjunctival melanosis*) appears as bilateral flat patches of brown pigmentation with irregular margins, typically involving the bulbar conjunctiva in individuals with dark skin pigmentation (Fig 5-22A; see pp. 80–81). Streaks and whorls of melanotic pigmentation may extend onto the peripheral cornea, a condition called *striate melanokeratosis*. The caruncle and palpebral conjunctiva may also be involved. Histologically, there is increased pigmentation primarily in the basal epithelial cells, and the epithelial melanocytes are normal in number and cytomorphology (hence the proposed new term *hypermelanosis*) (Fig 5-22B).

Primary acquired melanosis PAM is divided into *PAM without atypia* and *PAM with atypia*. PAM characteristically presents as a unilateral melanotic macule or patch in middle-aged light-skinned individuals. The lesion may remain stable, or it may wax and wane over a number of years. It is impossible to clinically distinguish PAM without atypia from PAM with atypia; these lesions can be distinguished only histologically. The recommendations regarding when to observe PAM versus when to perform biopsy are controversial. However, clinical findings such as larger size (3 clock-hours or more) and a caruncular, forniceal, or palpebral location portend a worse prognosis. Recommendations for incisional/excisional biopsy of PAM are discussed in BCSC Section 8, *External Disease and Cornea*.

The terminology and classification used for *non-nevoid intraepithelial melanocytic proliferations* are unique to the conjunctiva and have been subjects of ongoing debate. Specifically, the terms *PAM with* and *without atypia* are not used to describe other tissues. Also, the grading of mild, moderate, and severe atypia is somewhat subjective. To mirror the terminology used for cutaneous lesions and perhaps more accurately predict prognosis, several other classification schemes have been suggested for these intraepithelial melanocytic proliferations. The other main classification scheme is the conjunctival melanocytic intraepithelial neoplasia (C-MIN) scoring system, which is more complex and assigns a score of 1–10 according to the horizontal and vertical extent of epithelial involvement. PAM with atypia and C-MIN are considered synonymous terms for describing intraepithelial melanocytic neoplasia. The recently published World Health Organization (WHO) Classification of Tumours of the Eye proposes a simplified classification that grades intraepithelial melanocytic neoplasia as either low grade or high grade.

The PAM with/without atypia classification is familiar to most ophthalmologists and has generated more published information linked to prognosis and risk of metastasis than have other classification systems. Thus, despite the histologic ambiguity of the term *melanosis*, this classification is still the most commonly used system for grading and prognostication of intraepithelial melanocytic proliferations and is described here (see Figs 5-21, 5-22).

PAM without atypia is characterized by an increased number of cytologically unremarkable melanocytes arranged linearly along the basal epithelial layer, with the pigment localized mainly to the epithelial cells (see Fig 5-22E, F). In *PAM with atypia*, melanocytes are increased in number and may be cytologically atypical with a bloated appearance or pleomorphic nuclei. The melanocytes migrate into the superficial layers of the epithelium (see Fig 5-22H–J). These melanocytes form discohesive intraepithelial nests and migrate as individual cells or small clusters into the more superficial epithelium (ie, pagetoid spread). They may completely replace the epithelium (ie, melanoma in situ). Migration of melanocytes into the more superficial layers of the epithelium and cytologic atypia occur to varying degrees and are graded by the pathologist as mild, moderate, or severe (see Fig 5-22). Features of *severe cytologic atypia* include mitotic activity, nesting, pagetoid spread, cellular enlargement, epithelioid cell morphology, prominent nucleoli, and enlarged hyperchromatic nuclei. IHC stains for melanocytes, such as Melan A, HMB-45, and MITF, ideally complexed with a red chromogen, often highlight the presence and extent of melanocytic proliferation.

PAM with mild atypia carries minimal, if any, risk of malignant transformation. In contrast, PAM with moderate or severe atypia (see Fig 5-22G–J) and melanoma in situ (see Fig 5-22G, K, L) carry a significant risk (approximately 10%–15%) of progression to melanoma.

Table 5-1 summarizes the clinical features of common nonmalignant melanocytic conjunctival lesions. Table 5-2 summarizes the histology of non-nevoid pigmented lesions of the conjunctiva and correlations with the clinical nomenclature and histologic classification schemes. See also BCSC Section 8, *External Disease and Cornea*.

Conway RM, Graue GF, Pelayes DE, et al. Conjunctival melanoma. In: American Joint Committee on Cancer (AJCC). *AJCC Cancer Staging Manual*. 8th ed. Springer; 2017: 803–813.

Damato B, Coupland SE. Conjunctival melanoma and melanosis: a reappraisal of terminology, classification and staging. *Clin Exp Ophthalmol*. 2008;36(8):786–795.

Margo C, Coupland SE, Moulin A, Roberts F. Melanocytic tumours of the conjunctiva and caruncle. In: Grossniklaus HE, Eberhart CG, Kivelä TT, eds. *WHO Classification of Tumours of the Eye*. 4th ed. International Agency for Research on Cancer (IARC); 2018.

Shields JA, Shields CL, Mashayekhi A, et al. Primary acquired melanosis of the conjunctiva: risks for progression to melanoma in 311 eyes. The 2006 Lorenz E. Zimmerman lecture. *Ophthalmology*. 2008;115(3):511–519.e2.

Conjunctival melanoma

Approximately 50%–70% of cases of conjunctival melanoma arise from PAM with atypia (Fig 5-23); the remainder develop from a nevus or are de novo. Melanomas are usually nodular and can involve any portion of the conjunctiva. The nodule may be pigmented or amelanotic (15%–25% of conjunctival melanomas). Conjunctival melanomas metastasize

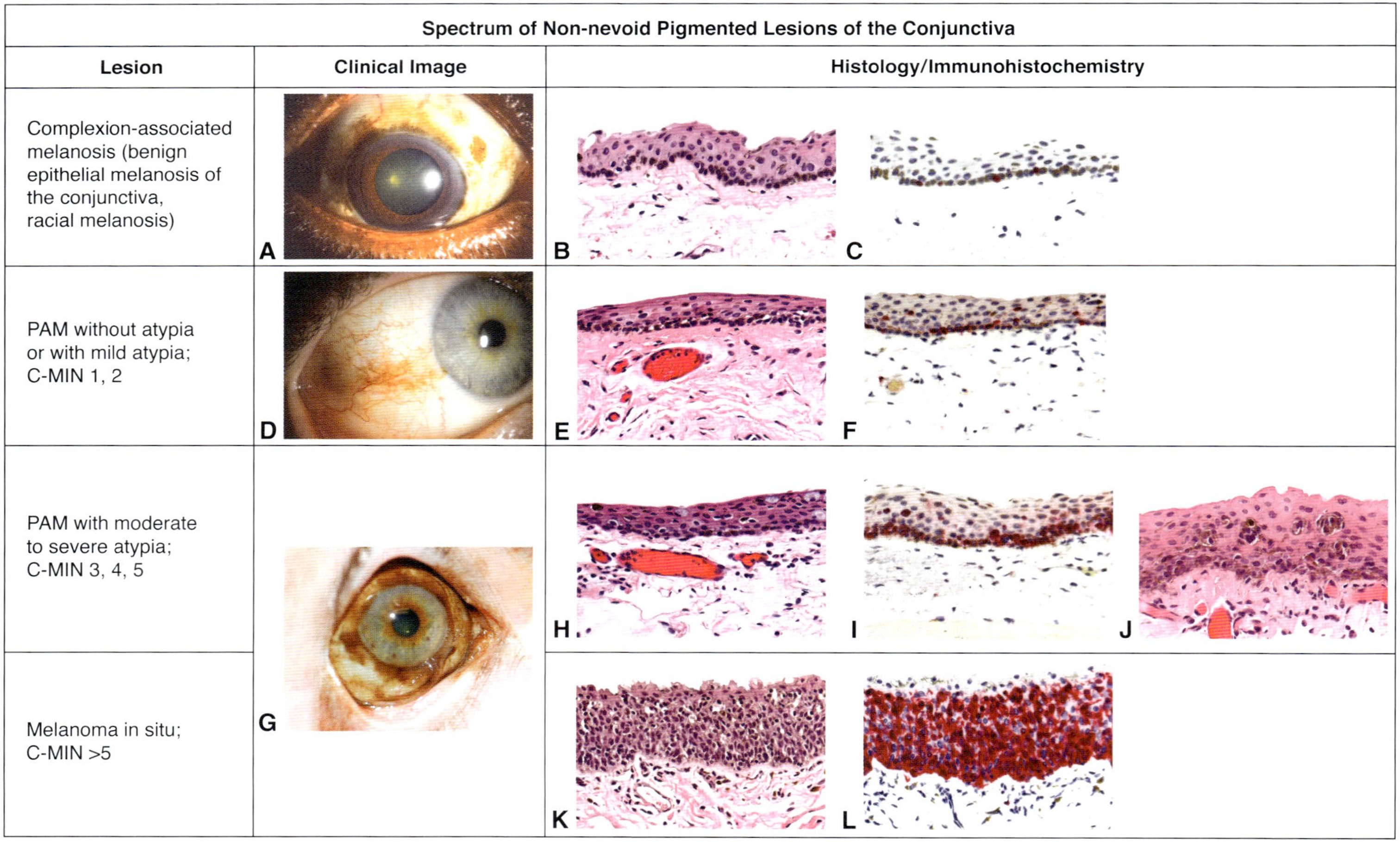

Spectrum of Non-nevoid Pigmented Lesions of the Conjunctiva

Lesion	Clinical Image	Histology/Immunohistochemistry	
Complexion-associated melanosis (benign epithelial melanosis of the conjunctiva, racial melanosis)	A	B	C
PAM without atypia or with mild atypia; C-MIN 1, 2	D	E	F
PAM with moderate to severe atypia; C-MIN 3, 4, 5	G	H	I, J
Melanoma in situ; C-MIN >5		K	L

Figure 5-22 *(see legend on next page)*

Figure 5-22 Spectrum of non-nevoid pigmented lesions of the conjunctiva. **A,** Clinical appearance of complexion-associated melanosis (benign epithelial melanosis). **B,** Histology of complexion-associated melanosis with morphologically unremarkable melanocytes confined to the basal epithelial layer. **C,** Immunohistochemical (IHC) staining for SOX-10, a melanocyte marker, demonstrates a normal number of melanocytes. **D,** Clinical photograph of PAM without atypia or with mild atypia (C-MIN 1, 2). **E,** Histology of PAM without atypia demonstrating a linear pattern of morphologically typical pigmented melanocytes in the basal layer of the epithelium. **F,** SOX-10 IHC stain demonstrates an increase in the number of melanocytes restricted to the deeper epithelial layers. **G,** Clinical photograph demonstrating the appearance of PAM with moderate to severe atypia (C-MIN 3, 4, 5) involving many clock-hours and/or melanoma in situ (C-MIN >5). These 2 degrees of atypical melanosis cannot be distinguished clinically. **H,** Histology of PAM with moderate atypia (C-MIN 3, 4, 5). Note the cells with round dark nuclei in the more superficial epithelial layers. **I,** MITF-1 IHC stain, another marker of melanocytes, stains melanocytes red and highlights the atypical pattern of melanocytic growth. **J,** Histology of PAM with severe atypia (C-MIN 5) with nests of atypical pigmented melanocytes in the more superficial layers of the epithelium. **K,** Histology of melanoma in situ (C-MIN >5). Note the full-thickness replacement of conjunctival epithelium with atypical, largely nonpigmented melanocytes with small, dark nuclei. **L,** Melan-A IHC stain, also a marker for melanocytes, demonstrates full-thickness replacement of conjunctival epithelium with atypical melanocytes (red-staining cells). *Note:* The clinical appearance of PAM/C-MIN of various stages can be indistinguishable; thus, these lesions usually require biopsy for a definitive diagnosis. *(Parts A and D courtesy of George J. Harocopos, MD; part G courtesy of Vahid Feiz, MD; all other parts courtesy of Tatyana Milman, MD.)*

Table 5-1 **Clinical Comparison of Nonmalignant Melanocytic Lesions of the Conjunctiva**

Lesion (Alternative Terminology)	Onset	Characteristics	Location	Malignant Potential
Nevus	Childhood or adolescence	Circumscribed brown or pink patch with small cysts; usually unilateral	Bulbar conjunctiva Caruncle	Yes, but low (conjunctival melanoma)
Ocular and oculodermal melanocytosis	Congenital	Patchy or diffuse slate-gray patches; usually unilateral	Episclera/sclera (deep to the conjunctiva)	Yes (uveal melanoma)
Complexion-associated melanosis (benign epithelial melanosis, racial melanosis)	Young adulthood, often increase with age	Flat brown patches with irregular margins; usually bilateral but not symmetric	Conjunctiva, typically bulbar	None
Primary acquired melanosis (PAM) (conjunctival melanocytic intraepithelial neoplasia [C-MIN])	Middle age	Flat, brown, sometimes granular patches with irregular margins; usually unilateral	Anywhere on the conjunctiva	Yes (conjunctival melanoma), when atypia is present

Table adapted with permission from Tatyana Milman, MD.

Table 5-2 **Non-nevoid Pigmented Lesions of the Conjunctiva**

Clinical Nomenclature	Histology
Non-neoplastic Lesions	
Secondary acquired melanosis of the conjunctiva	Depends on specific etiology (ie, related to systemic disease or reactive)
Complexion-associated melanosis (benign epithelial melanosis, racial melanosis)	Increased *melanin production* by melanocytes, transferred and localized to the basal epithelial cells *without increase in number or change in morphology of melanocytes*

Clinical Nomenclature		Histology
Neoplastic Lesions		
Primary Acquired Melanosis (PAM) or Conjunctival Melanocytic Intraepithelial Neoplasia (C-MIN)		
PAM Classification System	C-MIN Classification System	
PAM without atypia	C-MIN score=1	Increase in pigment production and proliferation of *normal-appearing melanocytes* (hyperplasia) arranged in a linear fashion and *localized* to the basal epithelial basement membrane
PAM with mild atypia	C-MIN score=2	Proliferation of melanocytes with *low-grade cytologic atypia* and abnormal patterns of intraepithelial spread *above* the basal epithelial layers
PAM with moderate atypia	C-MIN score=3	Proliferation of melanocytes with *moderate cytologic atypia* and abnormal patterns of intraepithelial spread *above* the basal epithelial layers
PAM with severe atypia (<75% of epithelial thickness)	C-MIN score=4–5	Intraepithelial proliferation of melanocytes with *high-grade or severe-grade atypia*: abnormal patterns of intraepithelial spread infiltrating up to *75% of the epithelial thickness;* severe cytologic atypia is present, including mitotic activity, nesting, pagetoid spread, cellular enlargement, epithelioid cells, hyperchromatic nucleoli, and enlarged hyperchromatic nuclei
Conjunctival melanoma in situ	C-MIN score >5	*Full-thickness* intraepithelial proliferation of melanocytes with *severe cytologic atypia*
Invasive conjunctival melanoma	Invasive conjunctival melanoma	Proliferation of various combinations of atypical melanocytes, including spindle cells, polyhedral cells, and epithelioid cells; atypical melanocytes *break through the epithelial basement membrane* and invade the stroma, and *severe cytologic atypia* is typically present

Courtesy of Tatyana Milman, MD.

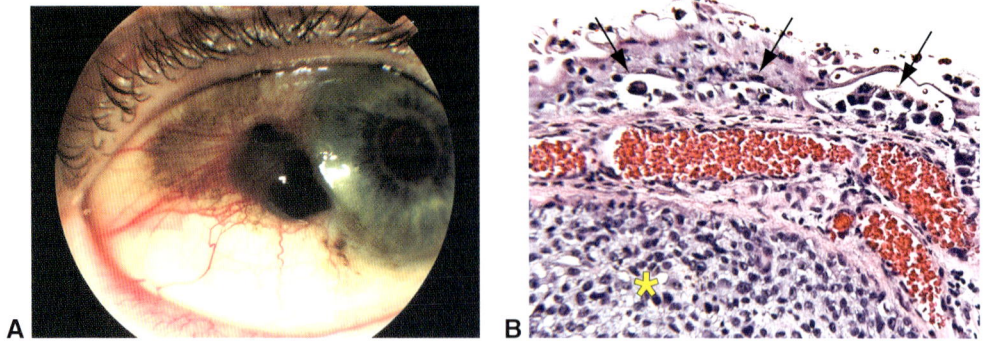

Figure 5-23 Melanoma arising from PAM with atypia. **A,** Clinical photograph. Note the elevated melanoma nodule adjacent to the limbus, arising from a background of PAM (diffuse, flat, brown pigmentation). Also note the prominent vascularity. **B,** Histologic examination shows melanoma *(asterisk)* arising from PAM *(arrows). (Part A courtesy of Morton E. Smith, MD; part B courtesy of Tatyana Milman, MD.)*

to regional lymph nodes in 25% of patients, as well as to the lungs, liver, brain, bone, and skin. The overall mortality rate in these cases ranges from 15% to 30%. Clinical features associated with a worse prognosis include

- nonbulbar conjunctival location (ie, plica semilunaris/caruncle, forniceal or palpebral conjunctiva)
- increased tumor thickness (>1.8 mm)
- involvement of the eyelid margin

When clinical suspicion for melanoma is high, referral to a surgeon with extensive experience in excision and treatment of ocular surface tumors should be considered because the outcome for the patient with incomplete excision is poor.

Occasionally, extrascleral extension of an anterior uveal melanoma presents as an episcleral/conjunctival mass that may mimic a primary conjunctival melanoma. Extrascleral extension of anterior uveal melanoma should be included in the differential diagnosis, particularly for a nonmobile pigmented or amelanotic episcleral nodule overlying the ciliary body that has sentinel vessels but without surrounding PAM (Fig 5-24). A complete eye examination, including gonioscopy and dilated ophthalmoscopy, should always be performed in any patient with a conjunctival mass. In individuals with darker complexions, conjunctival SCC is occasionally associated with reactive pigmentation masquerading as melanoma.

Histologically, the atypical melanocytes in melanoma range from spindle to polyhedral to epithelioid. The atypical cells may replace the epithelium only with an intact basement membrane *(melanoma in situ, C-MIN >5)*, involve both the epithelial layer and the stroma, or involve just the stroma *(invasive melanoma)*. The morphological cell types present in conjunctival melanoma do not have the same prognostic significance that they have in uveal melanoma. Rather, as in cutaneous melanoma, depth of invasion has a stronger correlation with prognosis. Mitotic figures may be present and are more frequent in more aggressive lesions.

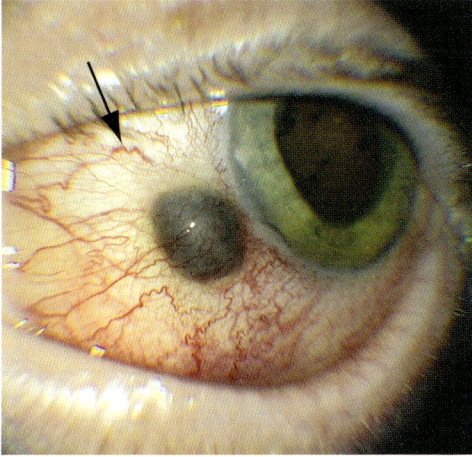

Figure 5-24 Melanoma of the ciliary body with extrascleral extension, presenting as an ocular surface mass. Note that there is no PAM surrounding the nodule, a clue that the lesion might have an intraocular origin. Also note that the lesion is associated with deep episcleral/scleral vessels (sentinel vessels, *arrow*) and does not obscure the overlying conjunctival vessels. This indicates that the lesion is deep to the conjunctiva. *(Courtesy of J. William Harbour, MD.)*

IHC stains for melanocytes, such as Melan A, HMB-45, and MITF, may be helpful in diagnostically challenging cases. In addition, identification of tumor-specific biomarkers has enhanced the assessment of conjunctival melanoma. For example, mutations in the *BRAF* gene, present in 30%–50% of conjunctival melanomas, can be a predictor of metastasis. Identification of melanoma biomarkers is also important in treating disease that has spread beyond the ocular surface, as targeted therapies against biomarkers are currently available. See also BCSC Section 8, *External Disease and Cornea.*

Shields CL, Chien JL, Surakiatchanukul T, Sioufi K, Lally SE, Shields JA. Conjunctival tumors: review of clinical features, risks, biomarkers, and outcomes—the 2017 J. Donald M. Gass Lecture. *Asia-Pac J Ophthalmol.* 2017;6(2):109–120.

Lymphoid Lesions

Both benign and malignant lymphoid proliferations can occur in the conjunctiva. Normal conjunctiva contains mucosa-associated lymphoid tissue (MALT), including a few small lymphoid follicles that are often visible clinically in the normal inferior fornix. However, lymphoid tissue may proliferate abnormally in the conjunctiva, often in the absence of inflammatory signs; this lymphoid hyperplasia may be benign (reactive) or malignant. Clinically, both benign and malignant lymphoid conjunctival lesions appear as soft, mobile, salmon-pink masses with a smooth surface, characteristically localized to the forniceal and bulbar conjunctivae (Fig 5-25A, B). The condition may be unilateral (more common) or bilateral. An orbital component may also be present.

Benign lymphoid hyperplasia consists of a polyclonal proliferation of lymphocytes, often with a follicular pattern demonstrating germinal centers. *Lymphoma,* a malignant neoplasm derived from a monoclonal proliferation of B or T lymphocytes and, less frequently, natural killer cells (NK cells), is divided into 2 major groups: Hodgkin lymphoma and non-Hodgkin lymphoma (NHL). The NHLs, a large heterogeneous group of neoplasms, can be divided into those originating from B lymphocytes and those developing from their precursors, T cells, and NK cells. Non-Hodgkin B-cell lymphoma is the most common type of lymphoma observed in the ocular adnexa.

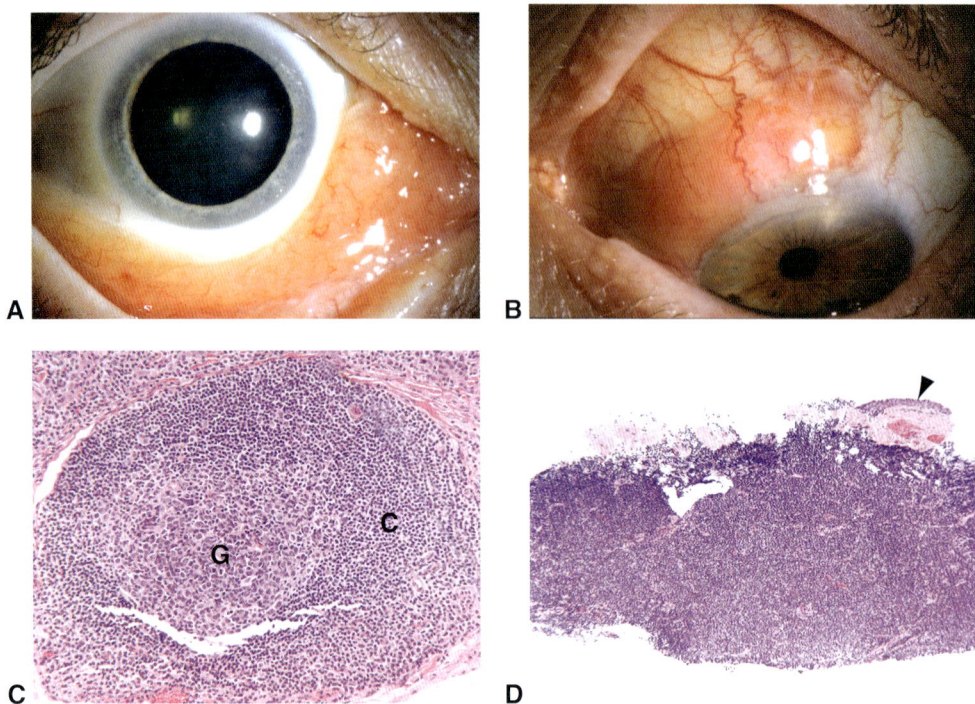

Figure 5-25 Lymphoid proliferations of the conjunctiva. Clinical photographs show a salmon-pink mass in the inferior fornix **(A)** and in the bulbar conjunctiva **(B)**. **C,** Histologic examination of benign lymphoid hyperplasia reveals normal follicular architecture with a well-defined germinal center (G) and corona (C). **D,** Histologic examination of lymphoma shows a monotonous sheet of lymphocytes infiltrating the stroma, without well-defined follicles. Note the conjunctival epithelium *(arrowhead)*. *(Part A courtesy of Anthony J. Lubniewski, MD; part B courtesy of Anjali K. Pathak, MD; parts C and D courtesy of George J. Harocopos, MD.)*

Conjunctival lymphoid lesions require biopsy in order to determine the nature of the neoplasm (ie, benign vs malignant). Because the pathologic evaluation of these lesions is limited by the size of the biopsy specimen obtained, communication with the pathologist regarding optimal specimen submission (including handling and fixation) is essential. Histologic examination and IHC are routinely used to evaluate conjunctival lymphoid lesions. IHC analysis includes staining for a variety of lymphocyte antigens. When the submitted tissue is sufficient for additional studies, flow cytometry and molecular genetic studies can also be performed. Flow cytometry can be especially useful in identifying clonality, which is typical of lymphoid malignancies (see Chapters 2 and 3).

On routine hematoxylin-eosin sections, histologic features favoring a diagnosis of benign lymphoid hyperplasia include the presence of normal-appearing lymphoid follicles with distinct germinal centers and with small, mature coronal lymphocytes (Fig 5-25C). In contrast, lymphoma frequently demonstrates a diffuse monomorphic sheet of lymphocytes in the stroma, without well-defined follicles (Fig 5-25D). IHC stains typically show a predominance of B lymphocytes that are often kappa or lambda light chain restricted. The most common type of lymphoma involving the conjunctiva is extranodal marginal zone B-cell lymphoma (MALT type) (Fig 5-26).

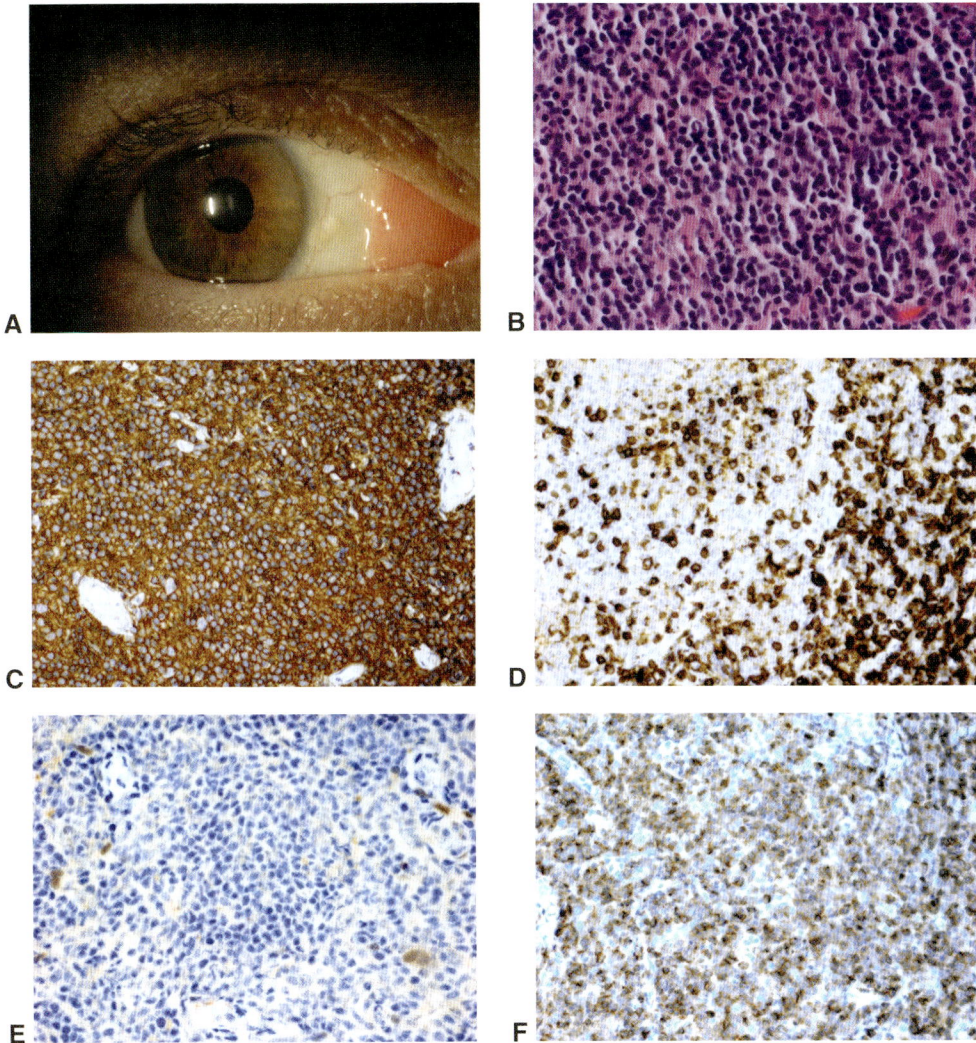

Figure 5-26 Histology of conjunctival extranodal marginal zone B-cell lymphoma of mucosa-associated lymphoid tissue (MALT) type. **A,** Clinical photograph of a salmon-patch conjunctival lesion. **B,** H&E-stained preparation demonstrates a diffuse proliferation of small lymphocytes with mildly irregular nuclear contours, inconspicuous nucleoli, and scant cytoplasm. **C,** IHC staining shows that nearly all lymphocytes are CD20+, indicating the presence of mainly B cells. **D,** Scattered reactive T cells are positive with CD3. **E,** The lymphocytes are cyclin-D1 negative, and **(F)** show diffuse expression of BCL-2, a regulator of the cell cycle. *(Courtesy of Hans Grossniklaus, MD.)*

Of all ocular adnexal lymphomas, a conjunctival tumor has the most favorable prognosis, as approximately 70%–75% of these lymphomas are localized to the conjunctiva, with the remainder associated with systemic disease. When a conjunctival lymphoma is diagnosed, systemic evaluation is necessary in order to exclude other sites of involvement (tumor staging). See BCSC Section 8, *External Disease and Cornea,* and Section 7, *Oculofacial Plastic and Orbital Surgery,* for additional discussion.

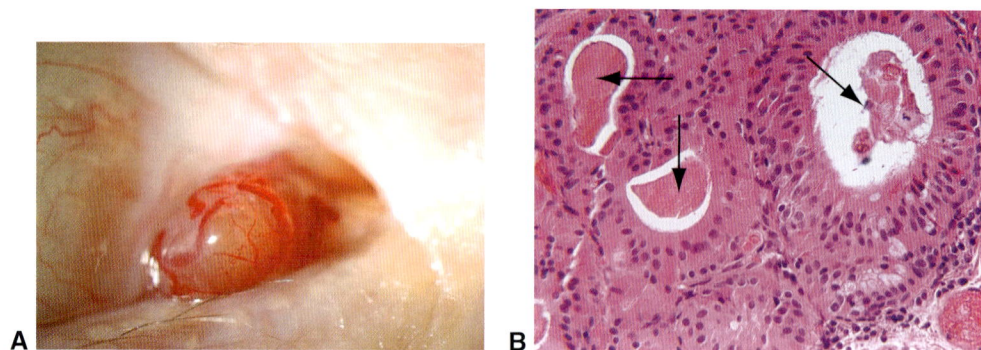

Figure 5-27 Oncocytoma. **A,** Clinical photograph of a mass in the caruncle. **B,** Histology shows cystadenomatous proliferation of large polygonal epithelial cells with abundant, deeply eosinophilic cytoplasm. Some of the cells surround protein-filled lumina *(arrows). (Part A courtesy of Mark J. Mannis, MD; part B courtesy of George J. Harocopos, MD.)*

Kirkegaard MM, Coupland SE, Prause JU, Heegaard S. Malignant lymphoma of the conjunctiva: a major review. *Surv Ophthalmol.* 2015;60(5):444–458.

Shields CL, Chien JL, Surakiatchanukul T, Sioufi K, Lally SE, Shields JA. Conjunctival tumors: review of clinical features, risks, biomarkers, and outcomes—the 2017 J. Donald M. Gass Lecture. *Asia-Pac J Ophthalmol.* 2017;6(2):109–120.

Swerdlow SH, Campo E, Harris NL, et al. *WHO Classification of Tumours of Haematopoietic and Lymphoid Tissues.* 4th ed. International Agency for Research on Cancer (IARC); 2008.

Glandular Neoplasms

Oncocytoma (oxyphilic adenoma) is a benign proliferation of metaplastic apocrine or accessory lacrimal gland epithelium (ie, an adenoma). It typically arises in the caruncle, but it occasionally occurs elsewhere on the conjunctiva. Oncocytoma most commonly occurs in elderly women. Clinically, it appears as a tan to reddish vascularized nodule (Fig 5-27). Histologically, the lesion shows a multicystic proliferation of enlarged polygonal, somewhat columnar, epithelial cells with abundant, intensely eosinophilic granular cytoplasm (reflecting the presence of numerous mitochondria) and periodic acid–Schiff–positive material in the lumen.

Other Neoplasms

Virtually any neoplasm that can occur in the orbit and eyelid skin can occur, although less frequently, in the conjunctiva, including sebaceous, neural, muscular, vascular, and fibrous tumors. Metastasis of lesions to the conjunctiva is rare. Orbital neoplasms are discussed in Chapter 14. See also BCSC Section 8, *External Disease and Cornea,* and Section 7, *Oculofacial Plastic and Orbital Surgery.*

CHAPTER 6

Cornea

Highlights

- The precise structure and normal function of each of the 5 layers of the cornea are essential for maintaining its transparency. Disruption of any of these layers may result in vision loss due to lack of corneal clarity.
- Infectious keratitis can be due to a variety of organisms and may result in significant scarring, ulceration, and even perforation of the cornea.
- Degeneration of corneal structures and stromal ectasias may be primary or may be secondary to other ocular conditions.
- Corneal dystrophies are bilateral, typically progressive, inherited conditions that often interfere with visual function.

Topography

The normal cornea is avascular and is composed of 5 layers (Fig 6-1):

- epithelium
- Bowman layer
- stroma
- Descemet membrane
- endothelium

The corneal *epithelium* is nonkeratinized stratified squamous epithelium without goblet cells; it ranges from 5 to 8 cell layers in thickness. The epithelial basement membrane is thin and indistinct and is best seen with periodic acid–Schiff (PAS) stain.

Located immediately beneath the epithelial basement membrane is the *Bowman layer,* an acellular layer of the anterior stroma that is composed of densely packed, randomly arranged collagen fibrils.

The corneal *stroma* makes up 90% of the total corneal thickness and consists of collagen-producing keratocytes (fibroblast-like cells), collagenous lamellae, and proteoglycan ground substance. The collagen lamellae are uniform in size and periodicity, resulting in corneal transparency. The posterior-most stroma is acellular and strongly adherent to the underlying Descemet membrane. This results in a surgical cleavage plane between the posterior-most stroma and the remainder of the stroma (the pre-Descemet *Dua layer*), which can be exploited in deep lamellar keratoplasty.

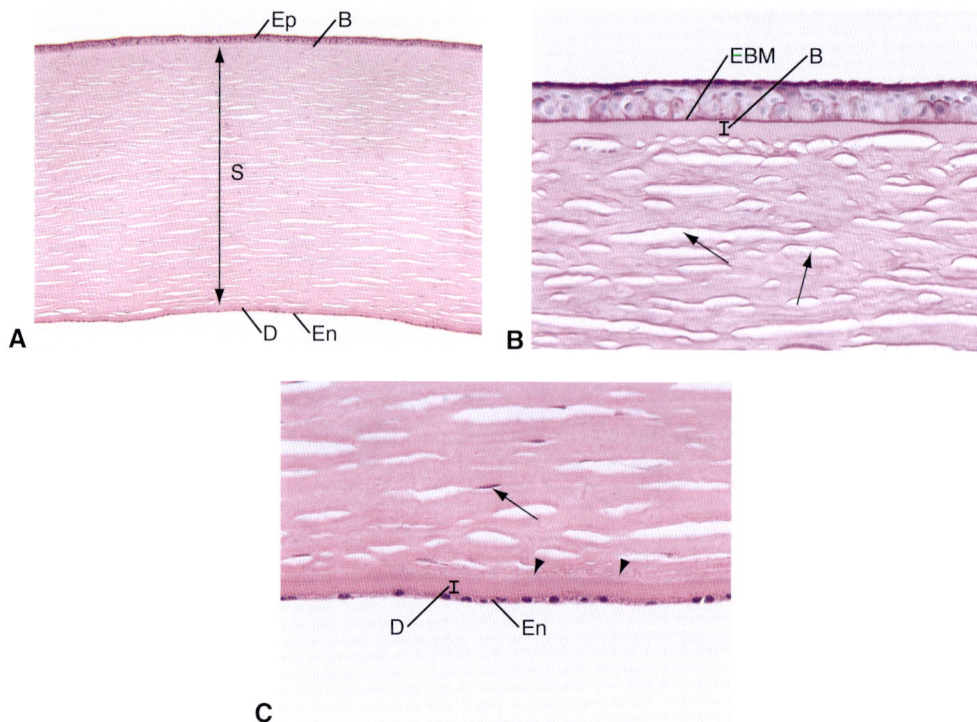

Figure 6-1 Normal cornea. **A,** The cornea is composed of epithelium (Ep), Bowman layer (B), stroma (S), Descemet membrane (D), and endothelium (En). **B,** On higher magnification, periodic acid–Schiff (PAS) stain highlights the epithelial basement membrane (EBM), distinguishing it from Bowman layer (B). Because of dehydration of the tissue during processing for paraffin embedding, multiple areas of separation (clefts) between the stromal lamellae are evident on normal histology *(arrows).* If the stromal clefts are absent, corneal edema or scarring is likely. This is an example of a meaningful artifact. **C,** Higher magnification (hematoxylin-eosin [H&E] stain) also delineates Descemet membrane (D); endothelium (En); and a thin acellular layer of pre-Descemet stroma *(arrowheads).* The keratocyte nuclei *(arrow)* are apparent. Note that the Descemet membrane is best visualized with PAS stain as this membrane is the basement membrane of the endothelium. *(Courtesy of George J. Harocopos, MD.)*

Descemet membrane is a PAS-positive true basement membrane that is produced by the corneal endothelium. The anterior portion of Descemet membrane (known as the *anterior banded layer* ultrastructurally) is formed during embryogenesis. The membrane slowly thickens throughout life because of the production of additional basement membrane material by endothelial cells (posterior banded layer).

The corneal *endothelium* is composed of a single layer of cells. The cells appear hexagonal *en face* (eg, on confocal microscopy). In a histologic cross section of the cornea, the endothelial cells have a low cuboidal appearance. The endothelium is primarily responsible for corneal deturgescence. See BCSC Section 2, *Fundamentals and Principles of Ophthalmology,* and Section 8, *External Disease and Cornea,* for discussion of the embryology, structure, and physiology of the cornea.

DelMonte DW, Kim TK. Anatomy and physiology of the cornea. *J Cataract Refract Surg.* 2011; 37(3):588–598.

Dua HS, Faraj LA, Said DG, Gray T, Lowe J. Human corneal anatomy redefined: a novel pre-Descemet's layer (Dua's layer). *Ophthalmology.* 2013;120(9):1778–1785.

Developmental Anomalies

Dermoid

Dermoid, a type of choristoma that may involve the cornea, is discussed in Chapter 5 (see Fig 5-2). See also BCSC Section 6, *Pediatric Ophthalmology and Strabismus.*

Peters Anomaly

Peters anomaly represents the severe end of the spectrum of *anterior segment dysgenesis* syndromes, in which neural crest cells do not properly migrate or differentiate during embryologic development. This disrupts anterior segment development and, in severe cases, prevents cleavage of the lens from the corneal endothelium. This condition is typically bilateral and sporadic, but autosomal dominant and recessive modes of inheritance have been reported. Studies suggest that mutations in genes, including paired box protein 6 *(PAX6),* paired-like homeodomain transcription factor 2 *(PITX2),* and forkhead box C1 *(FOXC1),* cause anterior segment dysgenesis, including the heritable form of Peters anomaly.

In this anomaly, a localized defect of the endothelium and Descemet membrane, known as *internal ulcer of von Hippel,* appears centrally or paracentrally. At the edges of the defect, iris strands typically adhere to the posterior corneal surface. In the most severe form of Peters anomaly, the lens also adheres to the posterior corneal surface. The anterior chamber angle may be malformed, predisposing to congenital glaucoma. Associated findings can include *sclerocornea,* which is characterized by peripheral corneal stromal opacification and vascularization, and *cornea plana,* in which the curvature of the cornea is flattened (Fig 6-2). In vivo confocal microscopy or anterior segment optical coherence tomography (AS-OCT) can be helpful in distinguishing the different forms of anterior segment dysgenesis. See Chapter 7 in this volume for additional discussion of this entity. See also BCSC Section 8, *External Disease and Cornea,* and Section 6, *Pediatric Ophthalmology and Strabismus.*

Reis LM, Semina LM. Genetics of anterior segment dysgenesis. *Curr Opin Ophthalmol.* 2011; 22(5):314–324.

Inflammation

Infectious Keratitis

Infectious processes caused by a number of microbial agents may result in inflammation of the cornea. Severe inflammation can lead to corneal necrosis, ulceration, and perforation. See also BCSC Section 8, *External Disease and Cornea.*

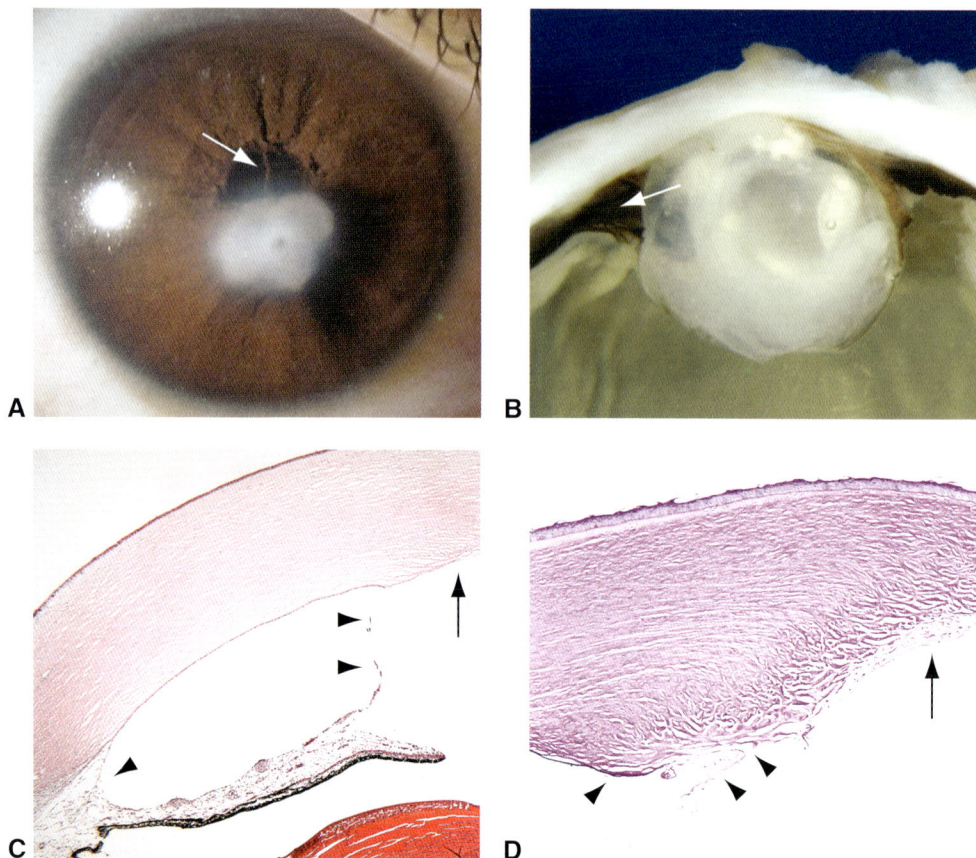

Figure 6-2 Peters anomaly. **A,** Clinical photograph. Note the central corneal opacity (leukoma) with attached iris strands *(arrow).* The lens is uninvolved. **B,** Gross photograph of a more severe form of Peters anomaly demonstrates attachment of a cataractous lens to the opacified cornea (adherent leukoma). Note the accompanying peripheral flattening of the corneal curvature (cornea plana) and opacification (sclerocornea). The iris and anterior chamber angle structures are malformed *(arrow).* **C,** Low-magnification photomicrograph demonstrates internal ulcer of von Hippel *(arrow)* with attached iris strands *(double arrowhead).* Incomplete cleavage of the anterior chamber angle structures (fetal angle deformity) is also present *(single arrowhead).* **D,** PAS stain highlights peripheral Descemet membrane *(single arrowhead).* The central cornea is fibrotic and demonstrates absence of posterior stroma and Descemet membrane *(arrow).* A fibrotic iris strand *(double arrowhead)* is attached to the edge of the corneal defect. *(Courtesy of Tatyana Milman, MD.)*

Bacterial infections

Bacterial infections of the cornea often follow a disruption in corneal epithelial integrity resulting from contact lens wear, trauma, alteration in immunologic defenses (eg, use of topical or systemic immunosuppressive agents), preexisting corneal disease (eg, dry eye disease, exposure keratopathy), ocular medication toxicity, or contamination of ocular medications. Bacterial organisms commonly involved in corneal infections include *Pseudomonas aeruginosa, Staphylococcus aureus,* and *Streptococcus pneumoniae,* as well as members of the family Enterobacteriaceae.

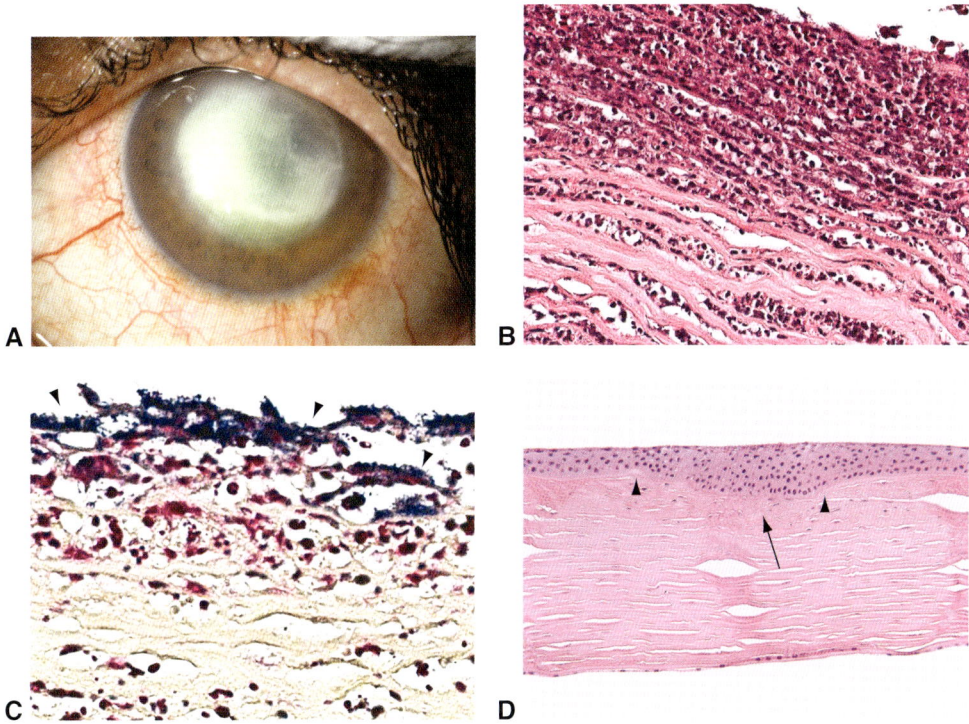

Figure 6-3 Bacterial corneal ulcer. **A,** Clinical photograph. **B,** H&E stain demonstrates acute necrotizing ulcerative keratitis, with necrosis and numerous neutrophils infiltrating the corneal stromal lamellae. **C,** Gram stain shows numerous gram-positive cocci *(arrowheads).* **D,** Keratoplasty specimen shows a scar from healed keratitis. Note the loss of Bowman layer *(between arrowheads),* stromal thinning with fibrosis *(arrow),* and compensatory epithelial thickening. *(Part A courtesy of Andrew J.W. Huang, MD; parts B and C courtesy of Tatyana Milman, MD; part D courtesy of George J. Harocopos, MD.)*

Scrapings from infected corneas show collections of neutrophils admixed with necrotic debris. Gram stain may demonstrate the presence of microorganisms (Fig 6-3). A culture is helpful for accurate identification of specific organisms and for assessment of antibiotic sensitivities.

Herpes simplex virus keratitis

Herpes simplex virus (HSV) keratitis is usually a self-limited corneal epithelial infection, but it may have recurrent or chronic forms. HSV epithelial keratitis is characterized by a linear arborizing pattern of shallow ulceration and swelling of epithelial cells, known as a *dendrite* (Fig 6-4A), that reflects viral reactivation in the corneal nerves. Corneal scrapings obtained from a dendrite and prepared using Giemsa or hematoxylin-eosin (H&E) stain may reveal intranuclear viral inclusions. Viral culture and, especially, polymerase chain reaction (PCR) techniques are useful for confirmation of viral infection. Like the dendritic ulcer, a geographic ulcer is caused by replicating virus; however, it has a much larger epithelial defect, similar in appearance to a map. Metaherpetic (trophic) ulcer is the only form of epithelial ulceration that does not contain any live virus. These ulcers result

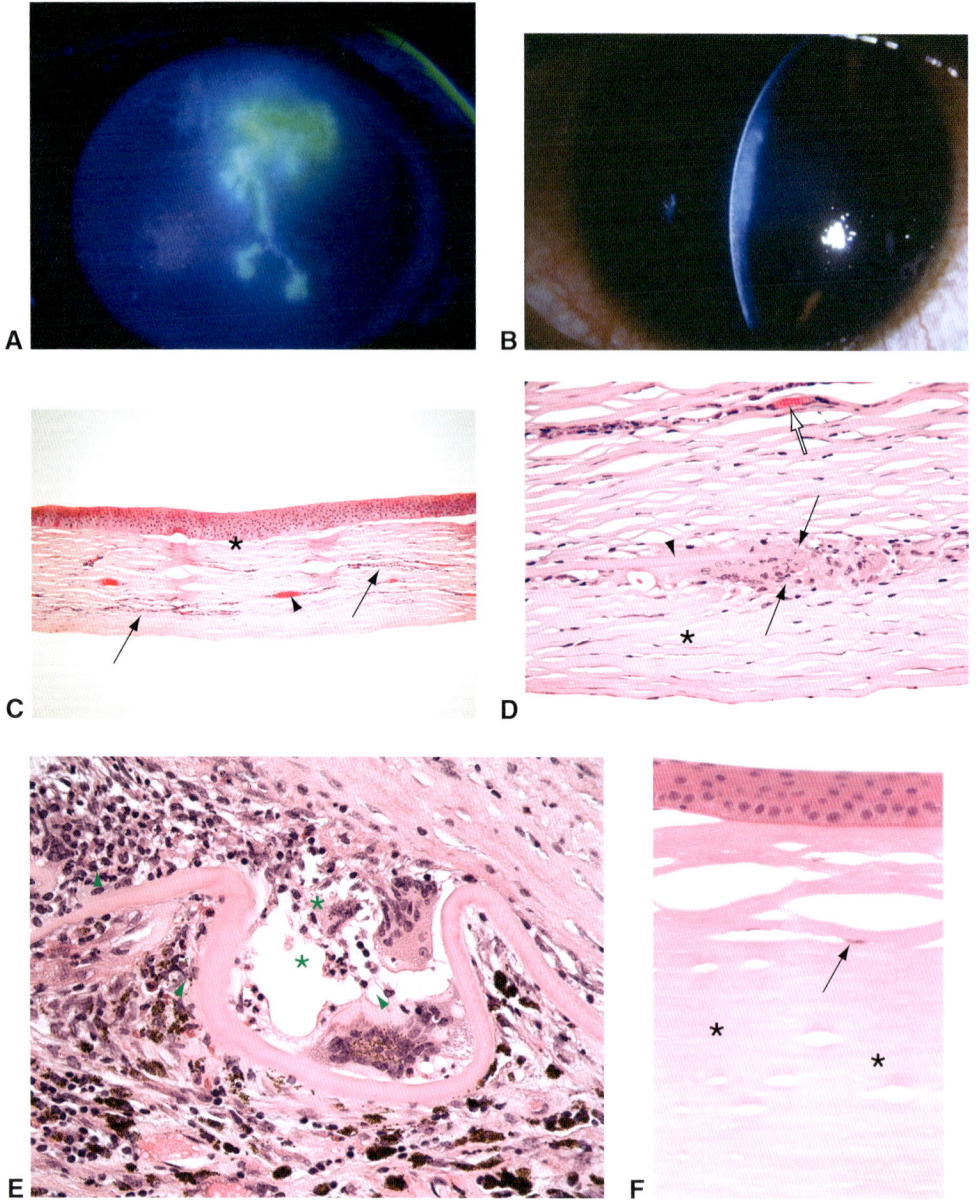

Figure 6-4 Herpes simplex virus keratitis. Clinical photographs depicting dendritic **(A)** and stromal (disciform) **(B)** keratitis. Note the central stromal haze and thickening in **B. C,** Histology of a corneal button illustrating stromal keratitis with loss of Bowman layer *(asterisk)*, stromal scarring and vascularization *(arrowhead)*, and scattered chronic inflammatory cells *(arrows).* **D,** Higher-magnification photomicrograph shows a granulomatous reaction *(area between arrows)* in the region of Descemet membrane *(arrowhead).* Note the fibrous retrocorneal membrane *(asterisk)*, scattered chronic inflammatory cells, and blood vessel *(open arrow).* **E,** Multinucleated giant cells *(asterisks)* located just anterior to Descemet membrane *(arrowheads).* **F,** Postherpetic neurotrophic keratopathy. Photomicrograph shows a featureless corneal stroma *(asterisks)* with very few keratocytes *(arrow). (Parts A and B courtesy of Anthony J. Lubniewski, MD; parts C and D courtesy of Tatyana Milman, MD; part E courtesy of Ralph C. Eagle Jr, MD; part F courtesy of Robert H. Rosa Jr, MD.)*

from the inability of the epithelium to heal. Stromal and/or disciform keratitis (Fig 6-4B) may accompany or follow epithelial infection as an immune-mediated response directed against viral antigens but not necessarily with the presence of active replicating virus. Histologically, chronic inflammatory cells and blood vessels may be seen tracking between stromal lamellae, a phenomenon known as *interstitial keratitis (IK)* (Fig 6-4C), which is discussed later in this chapter. In some cases, stromal keratitis may demonstrate significant necrosis, resulting in stromal thinning and even full-thickness perforation. Endotheliitis may also occur, with a granulomatous reaction at the level of Descemet membrane (Fig 6-4D, E). Postherpetic neurotrophic keratopathy may result from corneal hypoesthesia or anesthesia; it is characterized histologically by marked loss of stromal keratocytes (Fig 6-4F).

Fungal keratitis

Fungal (mycotic) keratitis is often a complication of trauma, especially trauma involving plant or vegetable matter or microtrauma related to contact lens wear. Corticosteroid use, especially topical, is another major risk factor. Unlike most bacteria, some fungi can penetrate the cornea and extend through the Descemet membrane into the anterior chamber. The most common fungal organisms are the septate, filamentous fungi *Aspergillus* and *Fusarium,* and the yeast *Candida.* Cultures, particularly on Sabouraud agar, are helpful for accurate identification of specific fungi and for assessment of antifungal sensitivities. When cultures are negative and organism identity remains elusive, corneal biopsy may be considered. Histologic evaluation can demonstrate the presence of fungal microorganisms with the use of special stains such as Gomori or Grocott methenamine silver (GMS) (Fig 6-5) or PAS with diastase. Identification of the exact fungal species solely on the basis of histology is often difficult.

Acanthamoeba *keratitis*

Acanthamoeba protozoa most commonly cause infection in soft contact lens wearers who do not take appropriate precautions in cleaning and disinfecting their lenses or whose lenses come into contact with contaminated stagnant water (eg, as found in hot tubs or ponds). Tap water may also harbor *Acanthamoeba* in small numbers. Patients presenting with *Acanthamoeba* keratitis usually have severe eye pain caused by radial keratoneuritis. In the late stages of the disease, a corneal ring infiltrate may be present (Fig 6-6A). Special culture techniques and media, including nonnutrient blood agar layered with *Escherichia coli,* are required to grow *Acanthamoeba* but are not widely available. The microorganisms penetrate the deeper layers of the stroma and may be difficult to isolate from a superficial scraping. Because of these challenges, PCR-based methods for diagnosis of *Acanthamoeba* keratitis are becoming more widely used. Histologically, corneal epithelial scrapings, biopsy specimens, or corneal buttons may show cysts and trophozoites (Fig 6-6B). The organisms are generally visualized with routine H&E sections but may also be highlighted with PAS and GMS stains. Calcofluor white or acridine orange fluorescent stains may also be used.

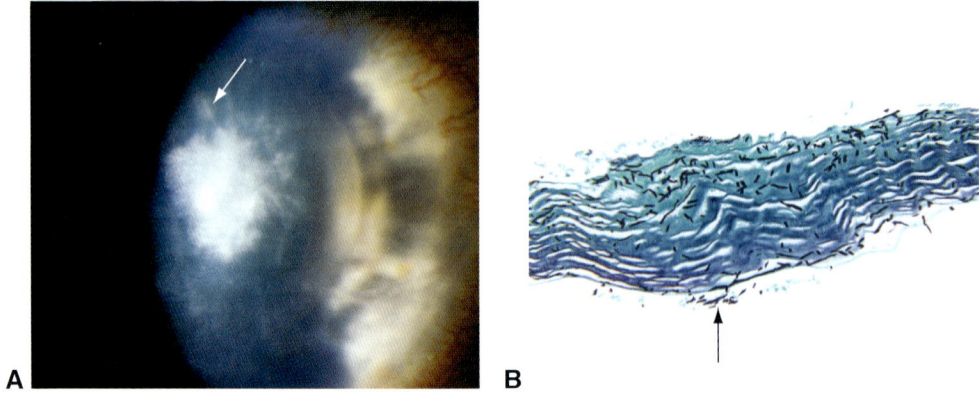

Figure 6-5 *Fusarium* keratitis. **A,** Clinical photograph shows gray-white stromal infiltrate with feathery margins and satellite lesions *(arrow)*. **B,** Grocott methenamine silver (GMS) stain of a corneal button demonstrates frequent fungal hyphae *(black)*. Note that fungal hyphae have penetrated through Descemet membrane *(arrow)*. *(Part A courtesy of Andrew J.W. Huang, MD; part B courtesy of George J. Harocopos, MD.)*

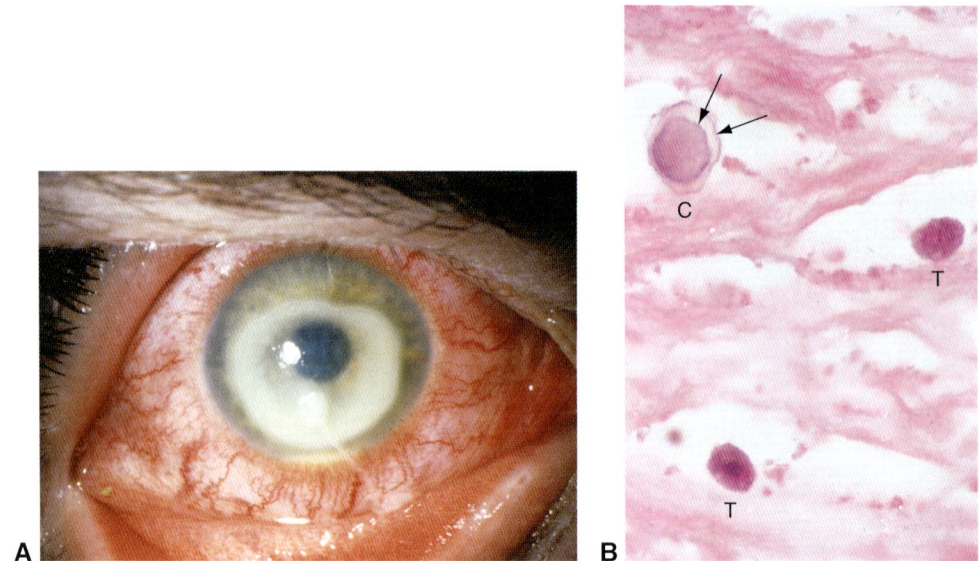

Figure 6-6 *Acanthamoeba* keratitis. **A,** Clinical photograph depicting a corneal ring infiltrate and a small hypopyon. **B,** Histology of stromal organisms. Note the cyst (C) and trophozoite (T) forms. The cyst has a double wall (ie, endocyst and exocyst) *(arrows)*. *(Part A courtesy of Sander Dubovy, MD.)*

Infectious crystalline keratopathy

Infectious crystalline keratopathy (ICK) typically occurs in patients who are on long-term topical corticosteroid therapy—for example, following penetrating keratoplasty (PK). The infection typically arises along a suture track or a surgical wound. The most common etiologic microorganism is *Streptococcus viridans* (α-hemolytic Strep), but many other

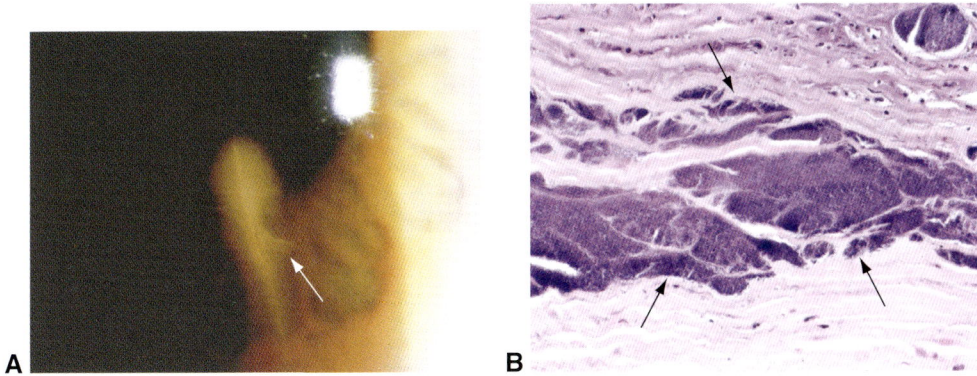

Figure 6-7 Infectious crystalline keratopathy. **A,** Clinical photograph depicting crystalline-appearing, feathery stromal infiltrate *(arrow)*, with intact overlying epithelium. The infection arose along a suture track following repair of a corneal laceration. **B,** Gram stain demonstrates sequestrations of gram-positive cocci interposed between stromal collagen lamellae *(arrows)* without an appreciable inflammatory response. *(Part A courtesy of Anthony J. Lubniewski, MD; part B courtesy of Morton E. Smith, MD.)*

organisms have been reported, including bacteria, mycobacteria, and fungi. Chronic immunosuppression, when combined with properties of the organism's glycocalyx (a glycoprotein and glycolipid covering that surrounds the cell membranes of some bacteria and sequesters the organism from the immune system), may promote growth of the organism in this condition. No true crystals are involved; rather, this condition derives its name from the crystalloid, feathery clinical appearance of the opacity (Fig 6-7A).

In many cases, the diagnosis is missed clinically and is made histologically after failure of a corneal graft. Histologically, sequestrations of organisms are present within the interlamellar spaces of the stroma. Typically, the inflammatory cell infiltrate is insignificant. The organisms are sometimes apparent on H&E stain; they may also be highlighted with Gram, PAS, GMS, or acid-fast stain, depending on the etiologic agent (Fig 6-7B).

Porter AJ, Lee GA, Jun AS. Infectious crystalline keratopathy. *Surv Ophthalmol.* 2018;63(4): 480–499.

Interstitial keratitis

In interstitial keratitis (IK), nonsuppurative inflammatory cells infiltrate the interlamellar spaces of the corneal stroma, often with vascularization. Typically, the overlying epithelium remains intact. The changes observed in IK are thought to result from an immunologic response to infectious microorganisms or their antigens. Transplacental infection of the fetus by *Treponema pallidum* (congenital syphilis) may cause IK (Fig 6-8A). Histologically, chronic syphilis-related (luetic) IK is characterized by the presence of stromal ghost vessels devoid of erythrocytes with surrounding stromal fibrosis and a variable degree of chronic inflammation. The Bowman layer and Descemet membrane are characteristically intact. In addition, the Descemet membrane may demonstrate focal multilaminated excrescences (Fig 6-8B) that are reminiscent of *guttae* (Latin for *drops*), droplike excrescences of Descemet membrane, observed in Fuchs endothelial corneal dystrophy (discussed later in this chapter).

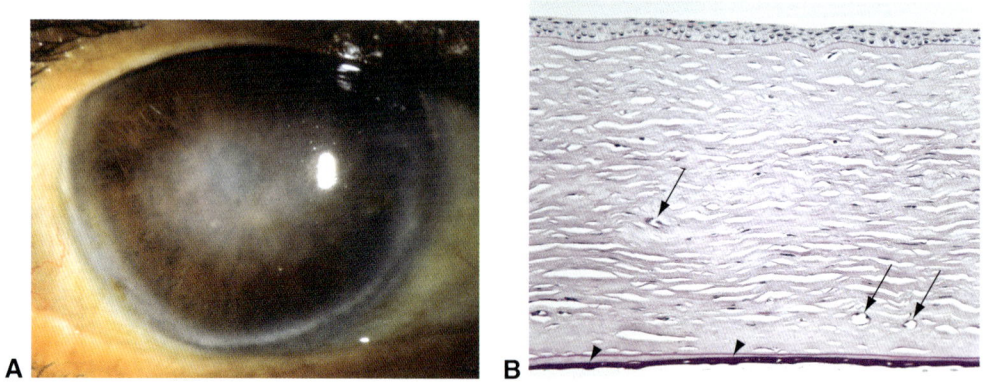

Figure 6-8 Interstitial keratitis of congenital syphilis. **A,** Clinical photograph depicting a stromal opacity, with intact overlying epithelium. **B,** PAS stain shows ghost vessels *(arrows)* in the midstroma and deep stroma, with surrounding fibrosis and a sparse chronic inflammatory cell infiltrate. Descemet membrane is multilaminated and demonstrates nodular excrescences *(arrowheads)*. Note the intact epithelium and Bowman layer. *(Part A courtesy of Anthony J. Lubniewski, MD; part B courtesy of Tatyana Milman, MD.)*

Although congenital syphilis represents the "classic" cause of IK, the most common etiologic agent of IK is HSV (see Fig 6-4). Other microorganisms that can cause IK include *Onchocerca volvulus, Mycobacterium tuberculosis, Mycobacterium leprae, Borrelia burgdorferi,* and Epstein-Barr virus. See also BCSC Section 8, *External Disease and Cornea.*

Noninfectious Keratitis

Corneal inflammation can also be a result of many noninfectious processes. For example, autoimmune diseases, especially rheumatoid arthritis and graft-vs-host disease, may be associated with sterile corneal ulceration and interstitial keratitis. Topical medication toxicity (eg, as occurs with overuse of topical anesthetics, nonsteroidal anti-inflammatory drugs [NSAIDs], or antiviral drugs) may also result in corneal melting. Histology varies depending on the etiology, but the unifying feature is absence of organisms. See also BCSC Section 8, *External Disease and Cornea.*

Degenerations, Depositions, and Ectasias

Corneal degenerations are secondary changes that occur in previously normal tissue. They are often associated with aging, are not inherited, and are not necessarily bilateral. See BCSC Section 8, *External Disease and Cornea,* for additional discussion.

Salzmann Nodular Degeneration

Salzmann nodular degeneration is a slowly progressive degenerative condition of the cornea. Often asymptomatic, it is characterized by the appearance of nodular gray-white to bluish, flat or raised opacities that vary in number and size and are located in the central or paracentral cornea (Fig 6-9A). Usually, the condition is bilateral and occurs in

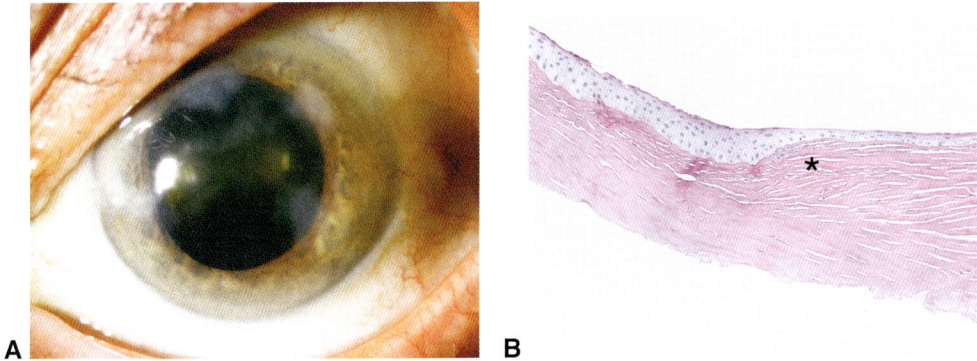

Figure 6-9 Salzmann nodular degeneration. **A,** Clinical photograph. Note the gray-white to bluish elevated superficial opacities. **B,** Histologic examination of a superficial keratectomy specimen (PAS stain) shows irregular epithelial thickness and loss of Bowman layer, as well as replacement of the latter with disorganized collagenous tissue *(asterisk). (Courtesy of George J. Harocopos, MD.)*

middle-aged and older individuals, with a female preponderance. It is typically associated with chronic ocular surface inflammation. Although the condition is often idiopathic, underlying causes include (from most to least common)

- meibomian gland dysfunction (MGD)
- exposure keratopathy
- conditions that lead to recurrent erosions
- dry eye/keratoconjunctivitis sicca
- contact lens wear (especially hard contact lenses)
- peripheral corneal vascularization
- pterygium
- actinic keratitis
- phlyctenular keratitis, vernal keratoconjunctivitis
- previous IK

Histologic examination reveals focal absence of Bowman layer with nodular, sclerotic subepithelial collagenous and/or fibrotic material (pannus). Sometimes there is focal thickening of the epithelial basement membrane (Fig 6-9B). The Bowman layer may be fragmented or absent.

Paranjpe V, Galor A, Monsalve P, Dubovy SR, Karp CL. Salzmann nodular degeneration: prevalence, impact, and management strategies. *Clin Ophthalmol.* 2019;13:1305–1314.

Calcific Band Keratopathy

Seen clinically as a band-shaped calcific plaque in the interpalpebral zone typically sparing the most peripheral clear cornea, calcific band keratopathy is characterized by the deposition of calcium at the level of Bowman layer and the anterior stroma. The calcium deposits appear as intensely basophilic (dark purple) granules in H&E sections; the presence of calcium can be further confirmed with the use of special stains such as alizarin red or von Kossa (Fig 6-10).

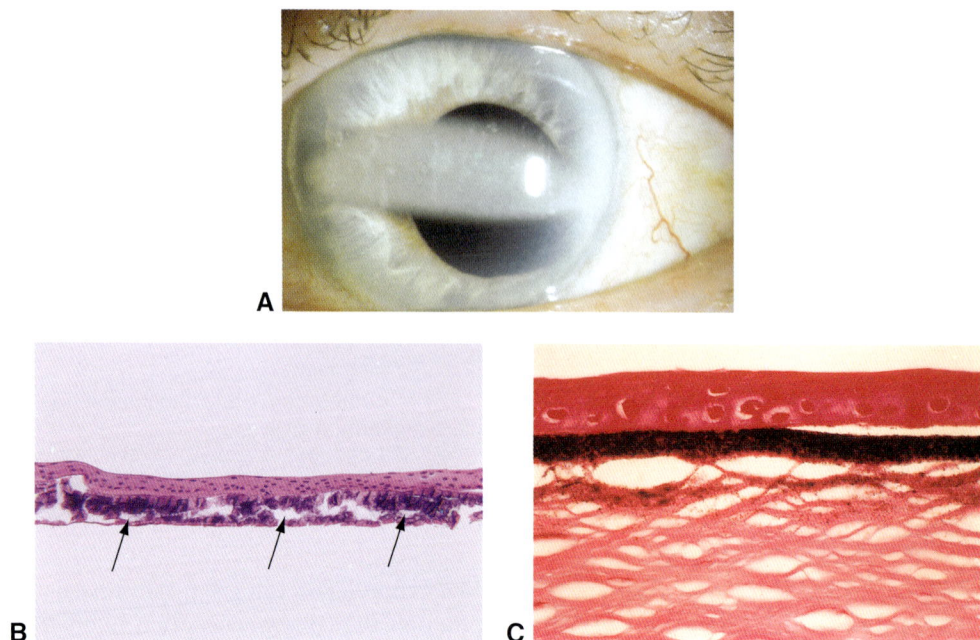

Figure 6-10 Calcific band keratopathy. **A,** Clinical photograph showing a white bandlike opacity extending from 3 o'clock to 9 o'clock, sparing the perilimbal cornea. **B,** The calcium is deposited at the level of Bowman layer *(arrows)*, appearing deeply basophilic *(dark purple)* on H&E stain. **C,** Calcium deposits appear black with von Kossa stain. *(Part A courtesy of Anthony J. Lubniewski, MD; part B courtesy of George J. Harocopos, MD; part C courtesy of Hans E. Grossniklaus, MD.)*

Band keratopathy may develop in chronically inflamed and/or traumatized eyes, following intraocular therapy (eg, intravitreal silicone oil), and, less commonly, in association with systemic hypercalcemic states. The exact pathophysiology is not well understood.

Actinic Keratopathy

Also known as *spheroidal degeneration, Labrador keratopathy,* or *climatic droplet keratopathy,* actinic keratopathy is characterized by aggregates of translucent, golden-brown spheroidal deposits in the interpalpebral superficial cornea (Fig 6-11A). The condition is generally bilateral and is more common in males. Smaller spheroidal deposits may mimic calcific band keratopathy; this phenomenon has been described as "actinic" band keratopathy.

The etiology is controversial, but cumulative evidence suggests that the deposits develop from ultraviolet (UV) radiation–induced alteration of preexisting structural connective tissue components or from the synthesis of abnormal extracellular material at the limbal conjunctiva. This abnormal material progressively diffuses into the superficial cornea, precipitates over a prolonged period, and may be further modified by UV light. Factors involved in the pathogenesis of actinic keratopathy include sun exposure and dry climate, as the condition is more prevalent in dry equatorial regions.

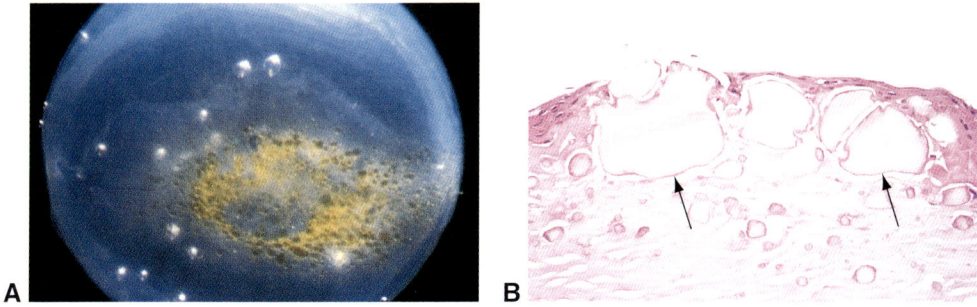

Figure 6-11 Actinic keratopathy (also called *spheroidal degeneration* or *climatic droplet keratopathy*). **A,** Gross appearance of a corneal button showing golden-brown superficial opacities. The air bubbles are artifacts. **B,** Histology shows irregular, pale, basophilic globules *(arrows)* extending from the epithelium into the superficial stroma. *(Courtesy of Hans E. Grossniklaus, MD.)*

Histologic examination reveals irregular, basophilic globules deep to the epithelium in the region of Bowman layer and the anterior stroma (Fig 6-11B). Analogous to the actinic degeneration of collagen in pingueculae and pterygia, the deposits stain black with special stains for elastin, such as Verhoeff–van Gieson.

Serra HM, Holopainen JM, Beuerman R, Kaarniranta K, Suarez MF, Urrets-Zavaliá JA. Climatic droplet keratopathy: an old disease in new clothes. *Acta Ophthalmol.* 2015;93(6):496–504.

Pinguecula and Pterygium

See Chapter 5 in this volume for discussion of these entities.

Pannus

Pannus—the growth of fibrovascular, fibroinflammatory, or fibrous tissue between the corneal epithelium and Bowman layer (Fig 6-12)—is frequently seen in cases of chronic corneal disease. Histologically, the term *inflammatory* is used when the Bowman layer is disrupted, because inflammatory conditions tend to destroy this layer. In contrast, *degenerative* is used when the Bowman layer remains intact under the fibrous or fibrovascular tissue.

Bullous Keratopathy

Bullous keratopathy can occur after cataract surgery (*pseudophakic* or *aphakic bullous keratopathy*) or after other forms of intraocular surgery. It may also occur in endothelial dystrophies such as Fuchs endothelial corneal dystrophy. Bullous keratopathy is a result of widespread endothelial cell loss or dysfunction. Corneal deturgescence cannot be maintained with insufficient endothelial cell function.

Clinically, bullous keratopathy is characterized initially by stromal edema and resulting folds in Descemet membrane, followed by intracellular epithelial edema (hydropic degeneration) and, ultimately, separation of the epithelium from the Bowman layer. Small separations called *microcysts* may coalesce to form large separations, known as *bullae*. In advanced cases of bullous keratopathy, secondary epithelial basement membrane changes, loss of stromal keratocytes, and pannus may occur (Fig 6-13).

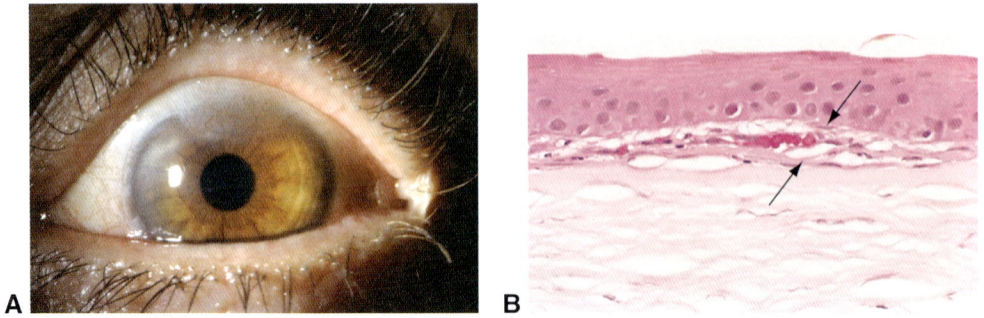

Figure 6-12   Corneal pannus. **A,** Clinical photograph of pannus in the superior cornea. **B,** Fibrovascular degenerative pannus *(area between arrows)* is interposed between the epithelium and Bowman layer. *(Part A courtesy of George J. Harocopos, MD.)*

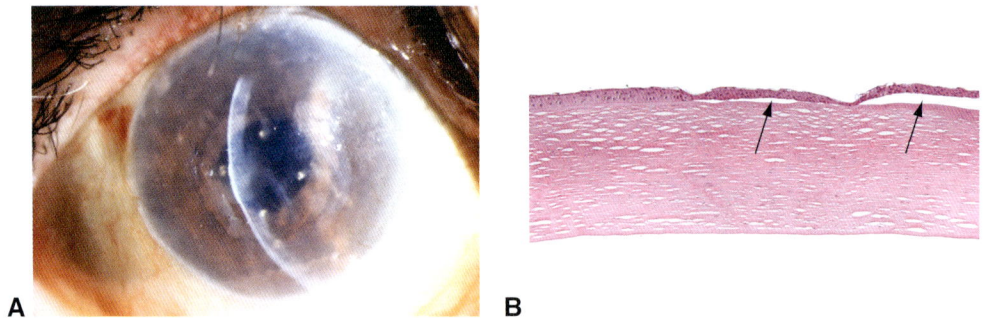

Figure 6-13   Pseudophakic bullous keratopathy. **A,** Clinical photograph showing severe bullous keratopathy associated with an iris clip anterior chamber lens implant. **B,** Corneal button from penetrating keratoplasty. Note the subepithelial bullae *(arrows)*. Also note stromal edema, characterized by focal absence of interlamellar clefts, and diffuse endothelial cell loss without thickening of Descemet membrane or guttae. *(Part A courtesy of Andrew J.W. Huang, MD; part B courtesy of George J. Harocopos, MD.)*

Corneal Graft Failure

Corneal graft failure typically results from significant loss of endothelial cells in grafted donor corneal tissue (Fig 6-14). It is one of the most common indications for PK or endothelial keratoplasty (EK). Graft failure after PK or EK may occur within a few weeks of surgery (primary graft failure), gradually over time, or following an acute rejection episode. Wound-related complications, such as *fibrous* or *epithelial ingrowth* or *downgrowth,* can also contribute to graft failure and are most common with PK grafts (see Fig 6-14E, F). The final common pathway is endothelial cell loss. When endothelial failure occurs, associated bullous keratopathy often develops. A delicate, fibrous retrocorneal membrane (fibrous downgrowth) may be seen, and there is a paucity or absence of endothelial cells. For various types of EK, additional important etiologies of graft failure include traumatic intracameral insertion of donor tissue, loss of adherence of the donor lenticule to the posterior stroma, and prolonged presence of the air bubble in the anterior chamber. See also BCSC Section 8, *External Disease and Cornea.*

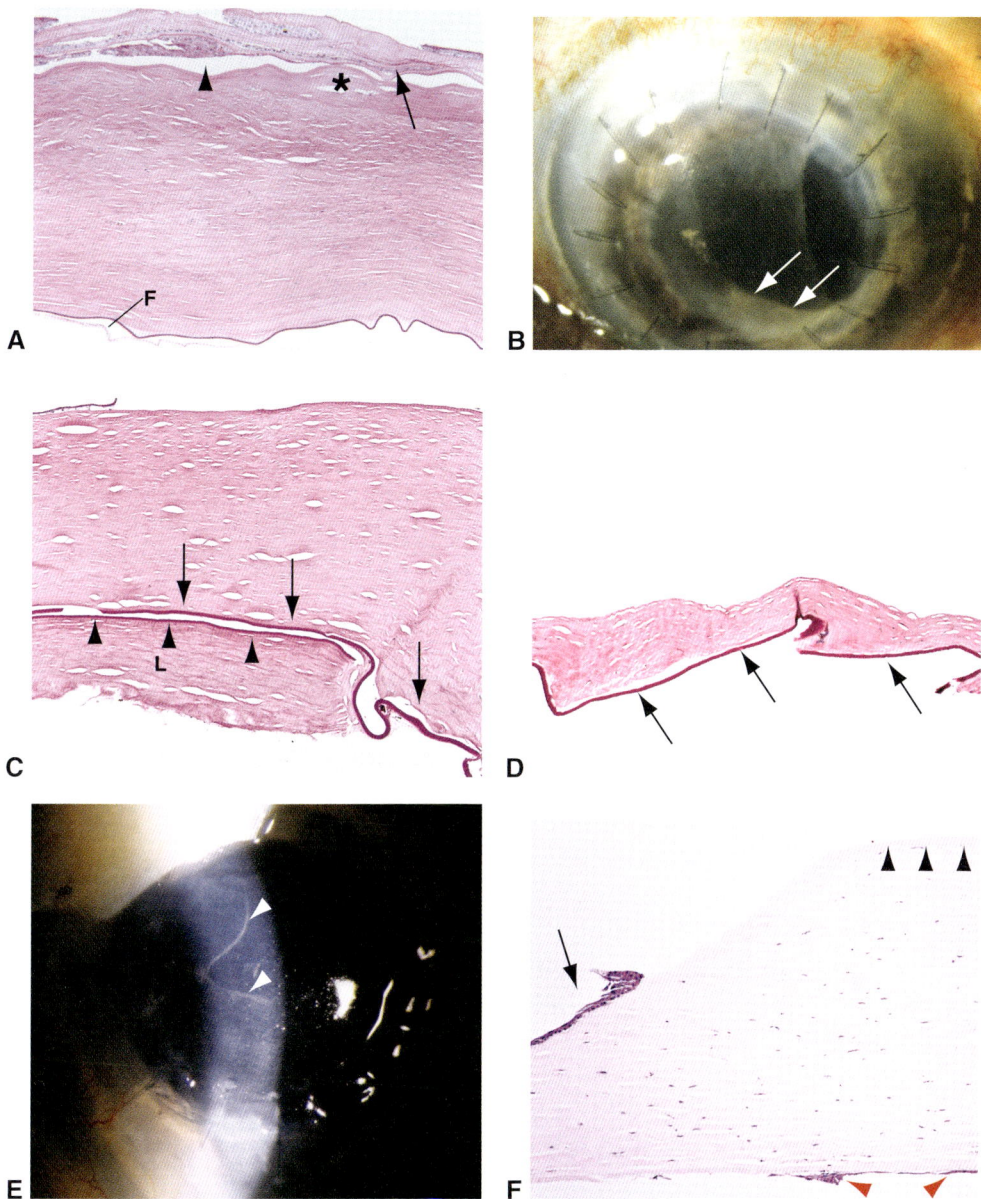

Figure 6-14 Corneal graft failure. **A,** PAS stain of a failed penetrating keratoplasty (PK) graft with diffuse endothelial cell loss; fibrous retrocorneal membrane (F); stromal edema with bullous keratopathy *(arrowhead)* and absence of stromal clefts; epithelial basement membrane thickening *(arrow);* and focal fibrous pannus *(asterisk).* **B,** Clinical photograph illustrating fibrous downgrowth *(arrows).* **C,** PAS stain of a failed graft following endothelial keratoplasty (EK). The donor lenticule is positioned upside down (L) with donor Descemet membrane *(arrowheads)* facing recipient Descemet membrane *(arrows).* Note the endothelial attenuation and marked stromal edema. **D,** PAS stain of a failed EK donor lenticule. Note the total absence of endothelium *(arrows).* **E,** Clinical photograph showing epithelial downgrowth *(arrowheads)* in a PK graft. **F,** Histology of a cornea from PK following failed EK shows full-thickness cornea with Bowman layer *(black arrowheads)* on the right and partial-thickness cornea on the left. The surface epithelium is discontinuous *(arrow).* A layer of squamous epithelium (epithelial ingrowth) *(red arrowheads)* replaces endothelial cells. *(Part A courtesy of George J. Harocopos, MD; parts B and F courtesy of Anthony J. Lubniewski, MD; parts C and E courtesy of Tatyana Milman, MD; part D courtesy of Hans E. Grossniklaus, MD.)*

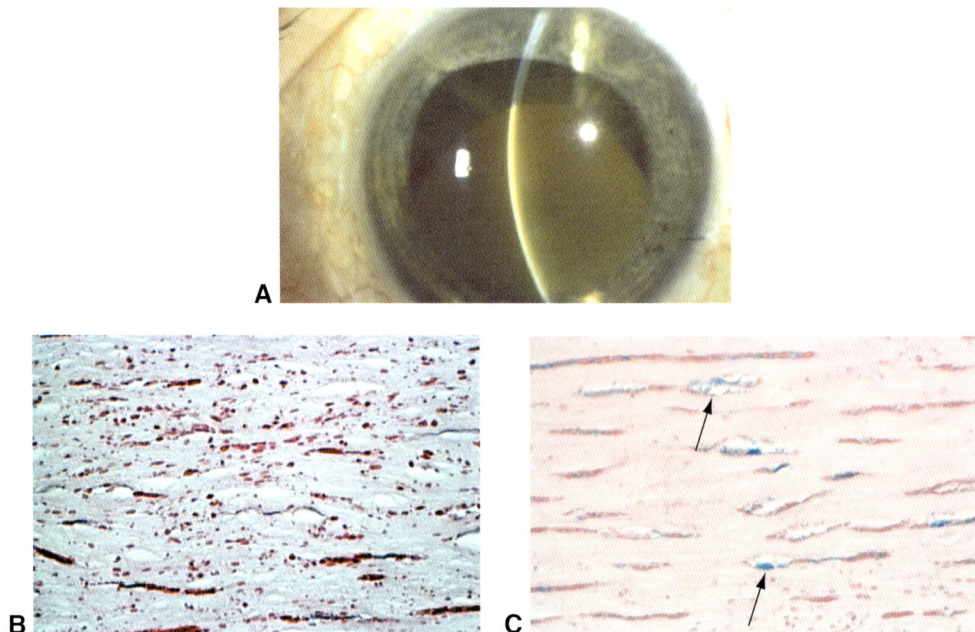

Figure 6-15 Corneal blood staining. **A,** Clinical photograph. Note the rust-colored opacity of the central cornea. **B,** Masson trichrome stain. The red particles represent erythrocytic debris and hemoglobin in the corneal stroma. **C,** An iron stain (blue staining) demonstrates hemosiderin *(arrows)* within stromal keratocytes. *(Part A courtesy of Anthony J. Lubniewski, MD; parts B and C courtesy of Hans E. Grossniklaus, MD.)*

Corneal Pigment Deposits

Various types of pigment and pigmented chemical compounds may deposit in corneal tissue, resulting in focal or diffuse opacities. Pigments that deposit in the corneal epithelium include melanin, alkapton (brown color, seen in alkaptonuria), iron, and amiodarone. Amiodarone can result in a clockwise whorl-like pattern of golden-brown or gray deposits in the inferior interpalpebral portion of the cornea, referred to as *cornea verticillate. Blood staining* of the cornea (Fig 6-15A) may complicate hyphema when intraocular pressure (IOP) is very high for a long duration; however, if the endothelium is compromised, blood staining can occur even at normal or low IOP. Histologically, red blood cells and their breakdown products (hemoglobin and hemosiderin) are observed in the corneal stroma (Fig 6-15B). The hemosiderin is found in the cytoplasm of keratocytes and may be demonstrated with iron stains such as Prussian blue (Fig 6-15C).

Ectatic Disorders

Keratoectasias (keratoconus, keratoglobus, and pellucid marginal degeneration) are predominantly sporadic, typically bilateral noninflammatory disorders that share a unifying feature: stromal thinning. See also BCSC Section 8, *External Disease and Cornea.*

Keratoconus

Keratoconus, which is typically diagnosed during adolescence or young adulthood, is characterized by inferior or inferotemporal corneal stromal ectasia (Fig 6-16A). Although it is frequently sporadic, familial inheritance and association with other ocular and systemic conditions, including atopy, Down syndrome, and Ehlers-Danlos syndrome, have been described. The basic pathophysiologic change is loss of stromal structural integrity, leading to keratoectasia, or stretching and thinning of the corneal stroma. The alteration

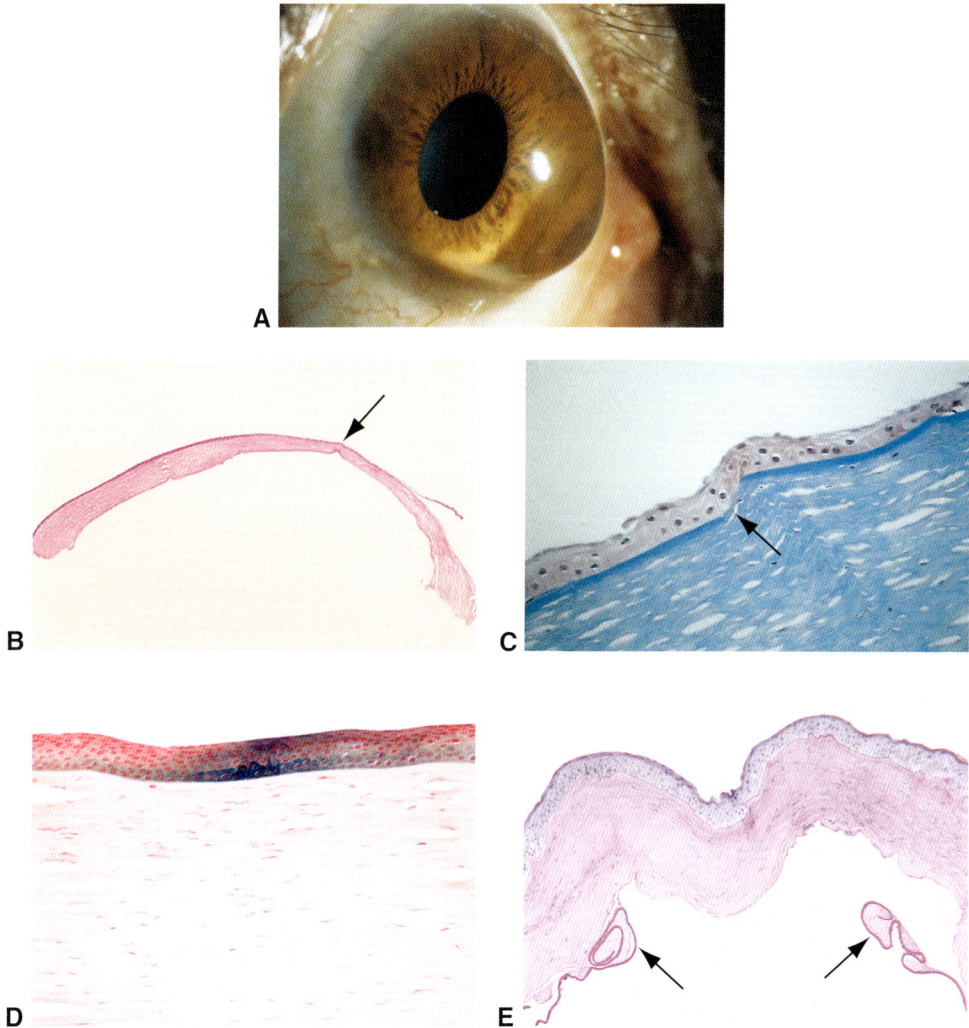

Figure 6-16 Keratoconus. **A,** Clinical photograph showing inferior conical deformity of the cornea. **B,** Low-magnification photomicrograph showing apical stromal thinning *(arrow)*. **C,** Masson trichrome stain demonstrating focal disruption of Bowman layer *(arrow)*. **D,** Prussian blue stain demonstrating focal intraepithelial iron deposition (Fleischer ring). **E,** In a patient with prior hydrops, PAS stain highlights the rupture of Descemet membrane, with rolled edges on either side *(arrows)*. *(Part A courtesy of Sander Dubovy, MD; part C courtesy of Hans E. Grossniklaus, MD; part D courtesy of Tatyana Milman, MD; part E courtesy of George J. Harocopos, MD.)*

in the normal corneal contour produces irregular astigmatism, occasionally requiring deep anterior lamellar keratoplasty (DALK). Advanced cases with significant apical scarring are managed with PK.

Histologic findings in keratoconus include central stromal thinning and small focal discontinuities in the Bowman layer. Apical anterior stromal fibrosis is often present (Fig 6-16B, C). Iron deposition in the epithelium at the base of the cone *(Fleischer ring)* can sometimes be demonstrated with Prussian blue stain (Fig 6-16D). In patients with a history of *corneal hydrops,* a focal break in Descemet membrane may be seen (Fig 6-16E).

In 2016, the US Food and Drug Administration (FDA) approved collagen crosslinking using UVA light and riboflavin (vitamin B_2) to slow or arrest the progression of the ectasia in keratoconus. There are no human studies describing the histologic and cellular changes following the procedure.

Pellucid marginal degeneration

Pellucid marginal corneal degeneration (PMCD) is a rare, bilateral, noninflammatory, ectatic peripheral corneal disorder, usually involving the inferior portion of the cornea; the band of thinning is separated from the limbus by a zone of normal corneal thickness. The cornea protrudes above the thinned area, resulting in high irregular astigmatism. Histologic examination demonstrates that the epithelium of the thinned region is intact, with microscopic disruptions in the Bowman layer similar to those seen in keratoconus. The pathogenesis of PMCD is poorly understood.

Dystrophies

Dystrophies of the cornea are primary, bilateral disorders with an underlying genetic cause. The International Committee for Classification of Corneal Dystrophies (IC3D) categorizes the major corneal dystrophies by the corneal layer (ie, epithelial, stromal, or endothelial) most involved and by the identified genetic alterations, when they are known. Thus, the classification system divides major corneal dystrophies into 4 groups:

- epithelial and subepithelial dystrophies
- epithelial–stromal *TGFB1* dystrophies
- stromal dystrophies
- endothelial dystrophies

The dystrophies are described according to a template consisting of clinical, pathologic, and genetic information (see BCSC Section 8, *External Disease and Cornea*). Although traditional pathologic methods continue to play an important role in the diagnosis of corneal dystrophies, clinicians increasingly rely on ancillary clinical diagnostic modalities, such as confocal microscopy and OCT, because treatment selection depends on the layers and structures involved. Molecular genetic studies are becoming more important in elucidating the pathogenetic mechanisms of corneal dystrophies, for example, the various dystrophies that are now known to be due to a mutation in the transforming growth factor β–induced gene *(TGFBI).* Such studies have also shown that various corneal dystrophy phenotypes may be caused by mutations in the same gene. Many of these genetic tests are commercially available and can be performed on peripheral blood.

The following subsections cover only the most common corneal dystrophies; see BCSC Section 8, *External Disease and Cornea,* for additional discussion.

Han KE, Choi SI, Kim TI, et al. Pathogenesis and treatments of *TGFBI* corneal dystrophies. *Prog Retin Eye Res.* 2016;50:67–88.

Seibelmann S, Scholz P, Sonnenschein S, et al. Anterior segment optical coherence tomography for the diagnosis of corneal dystrophies according to the IC3D classification. *Surv Ophthalmol.* 2018;63(3):355–380.

Weiss JS, Møller HU, Aldave AJ, et al. IC3D classification of corneal dystrophies—edition 2. *Cornea.* 2015;34(2):117–159.

Epithelial and Subepithelial Dystrophies

Epithelial basement membrane dystrophy

Also called *map-dot-fingerprint dystrophy,* epithelial basement membrane dystrophy (EBMD) is characterized by clinically observed patterns resembling maps, dots, and fingerprints in the superficial cornea. Regional thickening of the epithelial basement membrane with deposition of intraepithelial basal laminar material results in large, slightly gray outlines that look like a continent on a map. Intraepithelial pseudocysts containing degenerated epithelial debris appear as dots. Riblike intraepithelial extensions of basal laminar material give rise to patterns resembling fingerprints (Fig 6-17). EBMD results in focally impaired adhesion of the epithelial basement membrane to Bowman layer. As a result, patients may experience recurrent epithelial erosions. Management includes superficial keratectomy and phototherapeutic keratectomy and is described in BCSC Section 8, *External Disease and Cornea.*

Epithelial–Stromal *TGFBI* Dystrophies

A mutation in the *TGFBI* gene, located at 5q31, results in the most common corneal dystrophies that involve both epithelium and stroma. *TGFBI* encodes *keratoepithelin,* a protein elaborated predominantly by the corneal epithelium. Thus, these dystrophies arise in the epithelium, and the stroma is involved secondarily in their pathogenesis.

Reis-Bücklers corneal dystrophy

Reis-Bücklers corneal dystrophy (RBCD; formerly known as *corneal dystrophy of Bowman layer type I,* among other names) is an autosomal dominant disorder characterized by confluent irregular, coarse, and angulated geographic-like opacities with varying densities at the level of Bowman layer and the superficial stroma (Fig 6-18A). OCT demonstrates a homogeneous, confluent layer of hyperreflective deposits, often with a serrated anterior border, at the level of Bowman layer and the anterior stroma. Histologically, the Bowman layer is replaced by material comprising a multilayered pannus, which stains intensely red with Masson trichrome stain (Fig 6-18B) and immunoreacts with anti-*TGFBI* antibodies. The overlying epithelium is irregular in thickness. Ultrastructural studies show crystalloids that stain deeply black with osmium tetroxide, resembling those in granular corneal dystrophy.

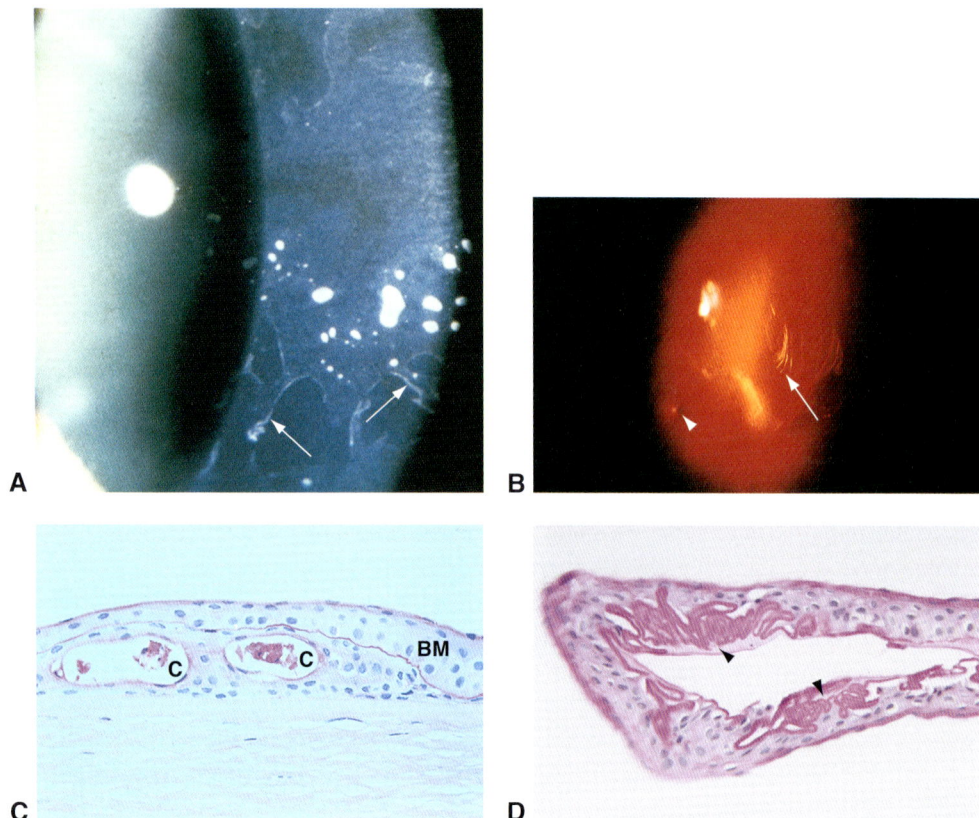

Figure 6-17 Epithelial basement membrane dystrophy (EBMD, also called *map-dot-fingerprint dystrophy*). **A,** Clinical photograph showing fine, lacy opacities *(arrows)*. **B,** Retroillumination demonstrating wavy lines *(arrow)* and dotlike lesions *(arrowhead)*. **C,** The changes in primary EBMD are essentially identical to those observed in the epithelium in cases of chronic corneal edema secondary to endothelial decompensation. Note the intraepithelial basement membrane (BM) highlighted with PAS stain and the degenerating epithelial cells trapped within cystoid spaces (C). **D,** When surgical treatment is required for EBMD, removal of abnormal epithelium (superficial keratectomy) may be performed, as in this case. PAS stain highlights irregular, wavy thickening *(arrowheads)* of the epithelial basement membrane. *(Part A courtesy of Andrew J.W. Huang, MD; part D courtesy of George J. Harocopos, MD.)*

Thiel-Behnke corneal dystrophy

Thiel-Behnke corneal dystrophy (TBCD; formerly known as *corneal dystrophy of Bowman layer type II,* among other names) manifests clinically as solitary flecks or irregularly shaped, scattered opacities at the level of Bowman layer that progress to symmetric subepithelial honeycomb opacities. OCT demonstrates prominent hyperreflective material at the level of Bowman layer that extends into the epithelium in a characteristic sawtooth pattern. Histologic evaluation shows diffuse replacement of Bowman layer by fibrous pannus and the sawtooth pattern observed with OCT (Fig 6-19). Ultrastructurally, the abnormal material in TBCD is composed of curly collagen fibers that are approximately 10 nm in diameter and distinctly different from the deposits in RBCD.

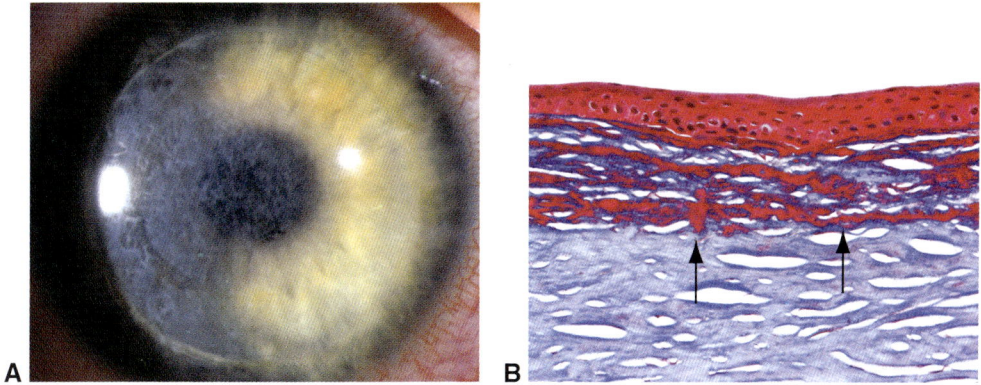

Figure 6-18 Reis-Bücklers corneal dystrophy. **A,** Clinical photograph shows coarse opacities resembling a geographic map in the superficial cornea. Note the circumferential linear scar in the peripheral cornea associated with a lamellar graft, in this case of recurrent corneal dystrophy. **B,** Masson trichrome stain demonstrates diffuse loss of Bowman layer, superficial stromal fibrosis, and numerous red deposits *(arrows)*. *(Part A courtesy of Brandon Ayres, MD; part B courtesy of Tatyana Milman, MD.)*

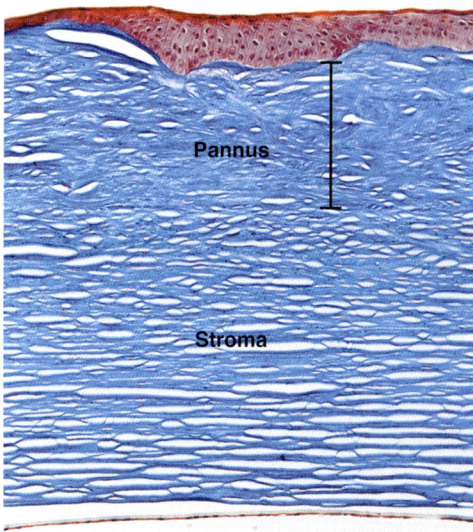

Figure 6-19 Thiel-Behnke corneal dystrophy. Masson trichrome stain demonstrates diffuse replacement of Bowman layer by a thick fibrous pannus *(bracket)*. The overlying epithelium exhibits a sawtooth configuration. The underlying stroma appears to be uninvolved. *(Courtesy of Tero Kivelä, MD.)*

Lattice corneal dystrophy type 1

Classic lattice corneal dystrophy (LCD), or *LCD type 1 (LCD1),* is an autosomal dominant stromal dystrophy characterized by branching, refractile lines in the central corneal stroma, as well as intervening stromal haze in the later stages of disease (Fig 6-20A). Histologic examination reveals poorly demarcated, fusiform amyloid deposits, most conspicuously in the anterior stroma and Bowman layer (Fig 6-20B). These deposits stain red orange with Congo red on standard light microscopy and exhibit apple-green birefringence (dichroism, ie, 2 different colors depending on lighting conditions) under polarized light (Fig 6-20C, D).

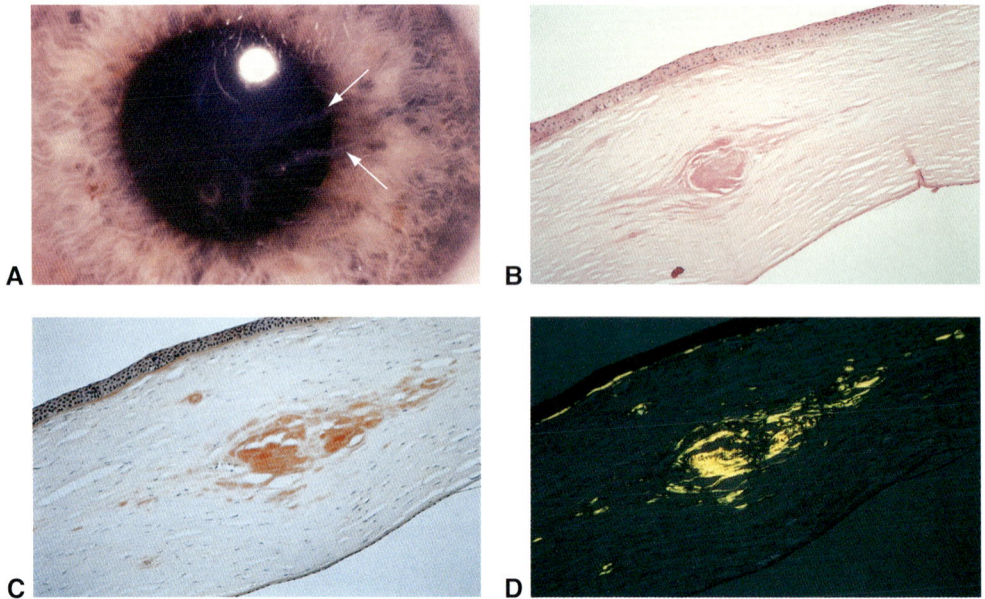

Figure 6-20 Lattice corneal dystrophy type 1. **A,** Clinical photograph. Note the fine lattice lines *(arrows)*. **B,** H&E stain shows scattered fusiform, eosinophilic deposits in the anterior and mid-stroma. **C,** Congo red stain (red orange) demonstrates that the fusiform deposits are amyloid. **D,** With Congo red stain, under polarized light, amyloid deposits exhibit apple-green birefringence (dichroism). *(Parts B–D courtesy of Hans E. Grossniklaus, MD.)*

Granular corneal dystrophy type 1

Granular corneal dystrophy type 1 (GCD1) is an autosomal dominant disorder character-ized by sharply demarcated (granular) central corneal stromal deposits separated by clear intervening stroma (Fig 6-21A). Histologically, irregularly shaped, well-circumscribed, crumblike deposits of hyaline material, which stain bright red with Masson trichrome, are visible in the stroma (Fig 6-21B, C).

Granular corneal dystrophy type 2

Formerly known as *Avellino dystrophy,* GCD type 2 (GCD2) demonstrates clinical, histo-logic, and ultrastructural features of both GCD1 and LCD1 (Fig 6-22).

Stromal Dystrophies

Macular corneal dystrophy

Macular corneal dystrophy (MCD), an autosomal recessive corneal stromal dystrophy, is caused by mutations in the carbohydrate sulfotransferase 6 gene *(CHST6),* located at 16q22. This dystrophy is characterized by diffuse stromal haze that extends from limbus to limbus and is associated with poorly demarcated focal opacities (macules) (Fig 6-23A). Histologically, H&E staining shows subtle eosinophilic stromal deposits. Alcian blue and colloidal iron stains highlight nonsulfated glycosaminoglycan deposits, which accumu-late intracellularly in the stromal keratocytes and endothelium and extracellularly in the

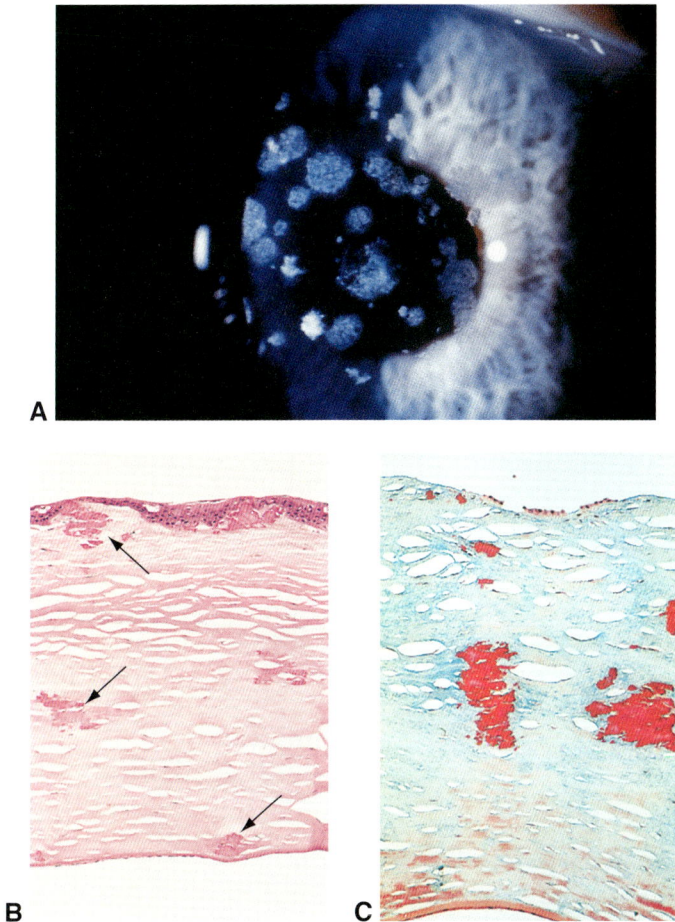

Figure 6-21 Granular corneal dystrophy type 1. **A,** Clinical photograph. Note the well-demarcated stromal opacities with clear intervening stroma. **B,** H&E stain. Note the eosinophilic deposits *(arrows)* at all levels of the corneal stroma. **C,** Masson trichrome stain. The stromal collagen stains blue, and the granular hyaline deposits stain brilliant red.

stroma (Fig 6-23B, C). Pathologic changes in the endothelium are frequently accompanied by guttae in the Descemet membrane (Fig 6-23D). See Table 6-1 for a histologic comparison of LCD1, GCD1, GCD2, and MCD.

Aggarwal S, Peck T, Golen J, Karcioglu ZA. Macular corneal dystrophy. *Surv Ophthalmol.* 2018; 63(5):609–717.

Descemet Membrane and Endothelial Dystrophies

Fuchs endothelial corneal dystrophy

Although Fuchs endothelial corneal dystrophy (FECD) can be inherited in an autosomal dominant fashion, the mode of inheritance is unknown in most cases. FECD is one of the leading causes of bullous keratopathy (discussed earlier), characterized in its early stage by

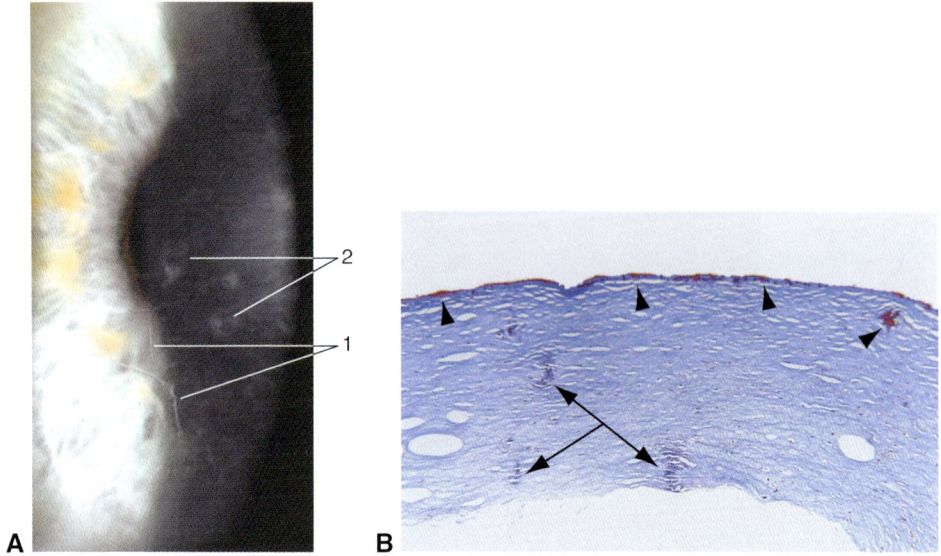

Figure 6-22 Granular corneal dystrophy type 2 (formerly known as *Avellino dystrophy*). **A,** Clinical photograph shows both lattice lines (1) and granular deposits (2). **B,** Trichrome stain of deep anterior lamellar keratoplasty (DALK) button highlights hyaline deposits at the level of Bowman layer and the anterior stroma *(arrowheads)*. Other deposits at various levels of the stroma stain a darker blue than the stromal background *(triple arrow)*; Congo red stain (not shown) confirmed that these deposits were amyloid. The large empty spaces in the posterior stroma were caused by pneumatic dissection. *(Part A modified with permission from Krachmer JH, Palay DA.* Cornea Atlas. *2nd ed. Mosby-Elsevier; 2006:163. Part B courtesy of George J. Harocopos, MD.)*

the presence of guttae along Descemet membrane, which when confluent have a "beaten metal" appearance (Fig 6-24A). In some cases, progressive endothelial cell loss occurs over time, ultimately resulting in visually significant corneal edema and bullous keratopathy, typically in middle-aged and older individuals. Endothelial cell loss and irregular thickening of Descemet membrane are the major histologic features of FECD. Histologically, the irregularly thickened Descemet membrane is studded with anvil-shaped or droplike guttae, which may protrude into the anterior chamber or may be buried within a new layer of basement membrane (Fig 6-24B, C). The epithelium demonstrates changes identical to those of bullous keratopathy from degenerative causes. Ultrastructural studies demonstrate the presence of new wide-spaced collagen, made of collagen type VIII, in the posterior banded layer of Descemet membrane and in the guttae. Treatment is surgical, with either PK or, more commonly, EK.

Congenital hereditary endothelial dystrophy
Congenital hereditary endothelial dystrophy (CHED) was traditionally classified as either an autosomal dominant (CHED1) or an autosomal recessive (CHED2) variant. This classification was recently revisited and modified, and the updated IC3D classification eliminates CHED1 as new evidence suggests that this entity be classified as part of the posterior polymorphous corneal dystrophy spectrum (see the following section). CHED2 is now known simply as *CHED*. A mutation in the *SLC4A11* gene, located at 20p13, has been implicated in this dystrophy.

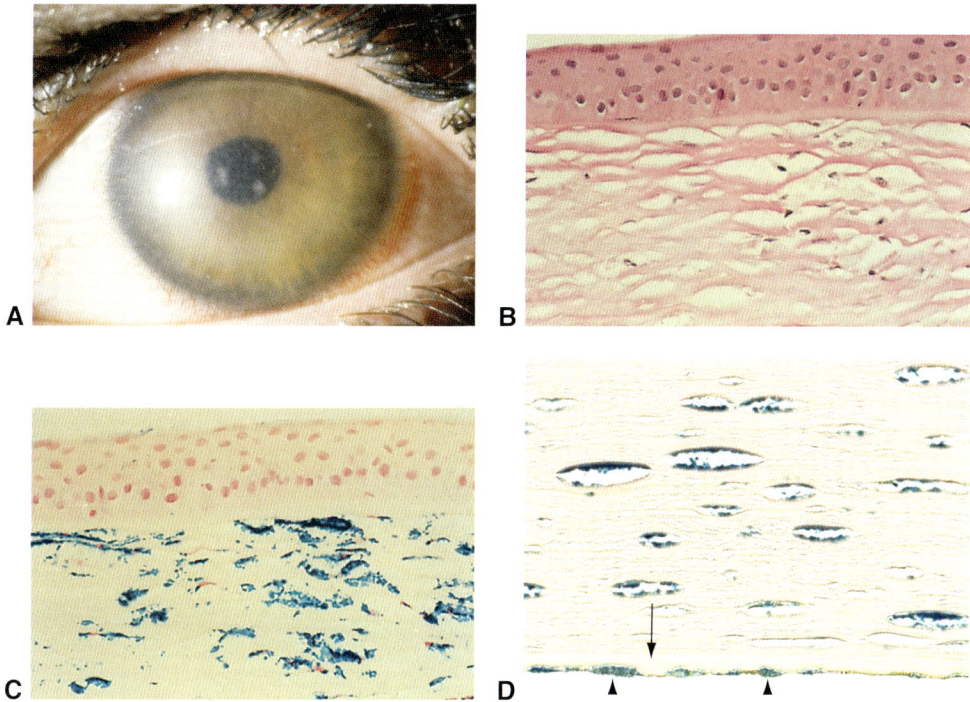

Figure 6-23 Macular corneal dystrophy. **A,** Clinical photograph showing a diffusely hazy cornea with focal opacities. **B,** H&E stain. Note the pale pink, fluffy material within the keratocytes and extracellularly in the stroma. **C,** Colloidal iron stain showing mucopolysaccharides (nonsulfated glycosaminoglycans) in the keratocytes and stroma. **D,** Colloidal iron stain highlighting muco-polysaccharides in the corneal endothelium *(arrowheads)*. Note the Descemet membrane excrescences, or guttae *(arrow)*. *(Part A courtesy of Sander Dubovy, MD; part D courtesy of Tatyana Milman, MD.)*

Table 6-1 Histologic Differentiation of Common Anterior Corneal Dystrophies

	Stains			
Dystrophy	Trichrome	Alcian Blue	Congo Red	Periodic Acid–Schiff
Granular, type 1	+ in deposits	–	–	–
Granular, type 2 (Avellino)	+ in deposits	–	+ (dichroism)	weakly + in deposits
Lattice, type 1	–	–	+ (dichroism)	weakly + in deposits
Macular	–	+ in deposits	–	weakly + in deposits
Reis-Bücklers	+ in deposits	–	–	–
Thiel-Behnke	–/+	–	–	–

Key: + = positive; – = negative.

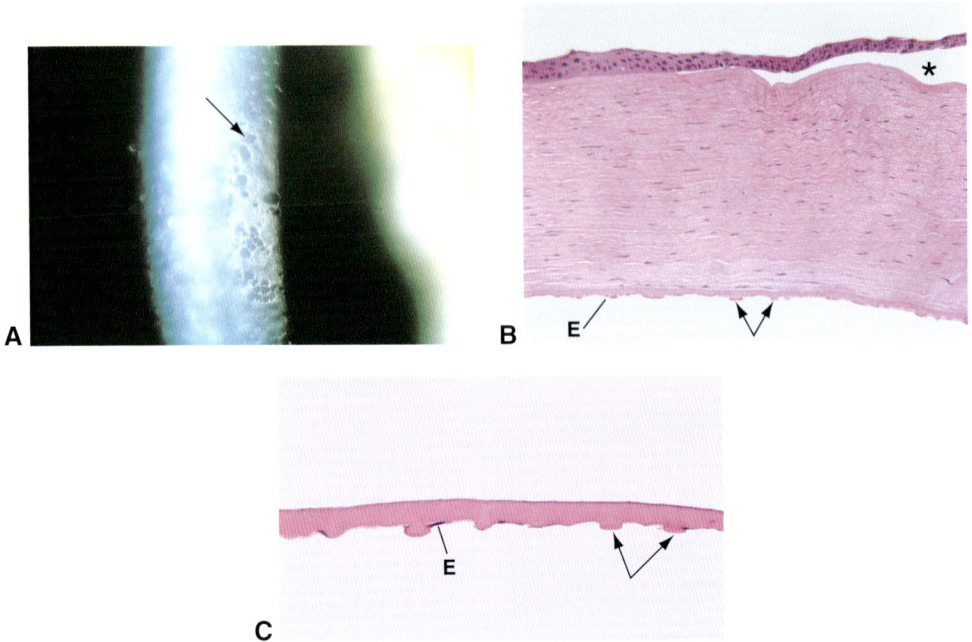

Figure 6-24 Fuchs endothelial corneal dystrophy. **A,** Slit-lamp illumination of the cornea shows the "beaten metal" appearance of Descemet membrane *(arrow).* **B,** Corneal button from PK shows endothelial cell loss, with only a few surviving endothelial cells (E). Numerous guttae are seen in Descemet membrane *(arrows).* The result of endothelial decompensation is bullous keratopathy. Note the diffuse stromal edema (loss of interlamellar clefts) and epithelial bulla *(asterisk).* **C,** Specimen from EK shows scant endothelial cells (E) and numerous guttae *(arrows). (Part A reproduced from* External Disease and Cornea: A Multimedia Collection. *San Francisco: American Academy of Ophthalmology; 2000. Parts B and C courtesy of George J. Harocopos, MD.)*

CHED presents early in life with diffuse or ground-glass, milky, and frequently asymmetric corneal clouding associated with marked corneal thickening (Fig 6-25A). The primary abnormality in CHED is thought to be a degeneration of endothelial cells during or after the fifth month of gestation. Histologically, the Descemet membrane is diffusely thickened and occasionally multilaminated. There is marked loss of endothelial cells (Fig 6-25B).

Posterior polymorphous corneal dystrophy

Posterior polymorphous corneal dystrophy (PPCD) is an autosomal dominant dystrophy that typically manifests early in life, frequently with asymmetric opacities of various shapes at the level of Descemet membrane, including nummular, vesicular (blisterlike), and "railroad track"–like lesions (Fig 6-26A). The condition can be progressive and can be associated with corneal edema, peripheral iridocorneal adhesions, and IOP elevation. Histologically, Descemet membrane is thickened and multilaminated with focal nodular and fusiform excrescences. Although the corneal endothelium is generally atrophic, overlapping or multilayered aggregates of endothelial cells with spindle morphology may be present focally (Fig 6-26B). These transformed endothelial cells demonstrate the

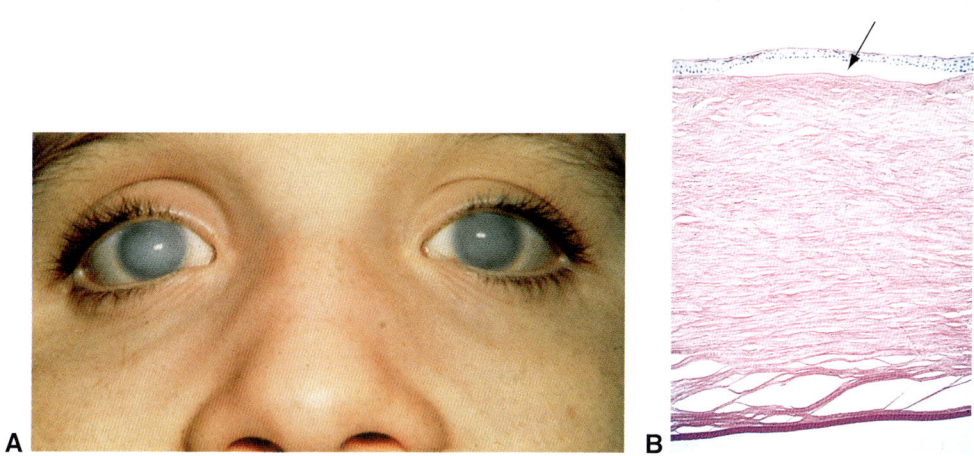

Figure 6-25 Congenital hereditary endothelial dystrophy. **A,** Clinical photograph showing bilateral diffuse, severe corneal clouding. **B,** PAS stain showing diffuse stromal edema with bullous keratopathy *(arrow).* The Descemet membrane is diffusely thickened, without guttae, and endothelial cells are absent. *(Courtesy of Hans E. Grossniklaus, MD.)*

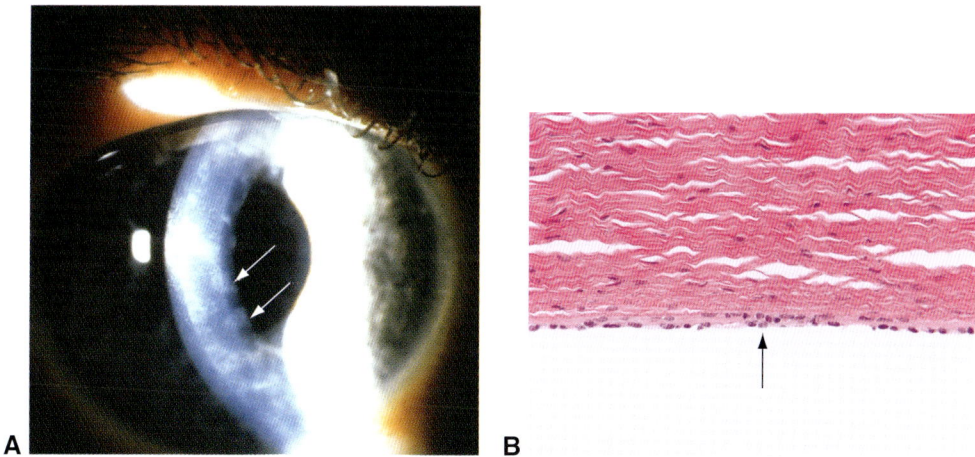

Figure 6-26 Posterior polymorphous corneal dystrophy. **A,** Clinical photograph showing nummular opacities *(arrows)* and linear opacities on the endothelial surface. **B,** Histology showing overlapping and multilayered aggregates of endothelial cells *(arrow).* *(Part A courtesy of Andrew J.W. Huang, MD; part B courtesy of George J. Harocopos, MD.)*

immunophenotypic and ultrastructural features of epithelial cells (ie, epithelialization of the endothelium) with aberrant expression of cytokeratins (CKs) such as CK19, CK5/6, and CK903.

Aldave AJ, Han J, Frausto RF. Genetics of the corneal endothelial dystrophies: an evidence-based review. *Clin Genet.* 2013;84(2):109–119.

Schmedt T, Silva MM, Ziael A, Jurkanas U. Molecular bases of corneal endothelial dystrophies. *Exp Eye Res.* 2012;95(1):24–34.

Neoplasia

Ocular surface squamous neoplasia, melanocytic neoplasms, and sebaceous carcinoma may extend from adjacent structures to involve the cornea. In rare cases, squamous neoplasia may arise primarily in the corneal epithelium. See Chapter 5 for more information on this topic.

CHAPTER **7**

Anterior Chamber
and Trabecular Meshwork

Highlights

- Gonioscopic landmarks of the anterior chamber angle correspond to histologically identifiable structures.
- The term *anterior segment dysgenesis* refers to a spectrum of developmental anomalies.
- Pseudoexfoliation syndrome is a systemic fibrillopathy, the features of which are manifested clinically and histologically in the eye.
- Pigment dispersion may be a primary process, or it may be secondary to inflammation or neoplasia.

Topography

The anterior chamber is bounded anteriorly by the corneal endothelium; posteriorly by the anterior surface of the iris, ciliary body, and pupillary portion of the lens; and peripherally by thc trabecular meshwork (Fig 7-1). The normal central depth of the anterior chamber is approximately 3.0–3.5 mm. The trabecular meshwork is derived predominantly from the neural crest.

The histologic features of the anterior chamber angle correlate with its gonioscopic landmarks (Fig 7-2). For example, the termination of Descemet membrane manifests gonioscopically as the Schwalbe line. The scleral spur, a triangular extension of the sclera that appears gonioscopically as a white band, can be identified histologically by tracing the outermost longitudinal ciliary muscle fibers to its insertion. Anterior to the scleral spur in an internal indentation of the sclera is the trabecular meshwork and Schlemm canal. On gonioscopy, the posterior trabecular meshwork appears more pigmented than the rest of the meshwork because of its increased thickness. The meshwork is lined with cells that appear flat and have slender spindle-shaped nuclei known as *trabeculocytes*. These cells function to phagocytose material from the aqueous humor and have contractile properties.

See Figures 2-13 and 2-23 in BCSC Section 2, *Fundamentals and Principles of Ophthalmology,* which includes additional images and discussion of the structure and physiology of the anterior chamber and trabecular meshwork.

117

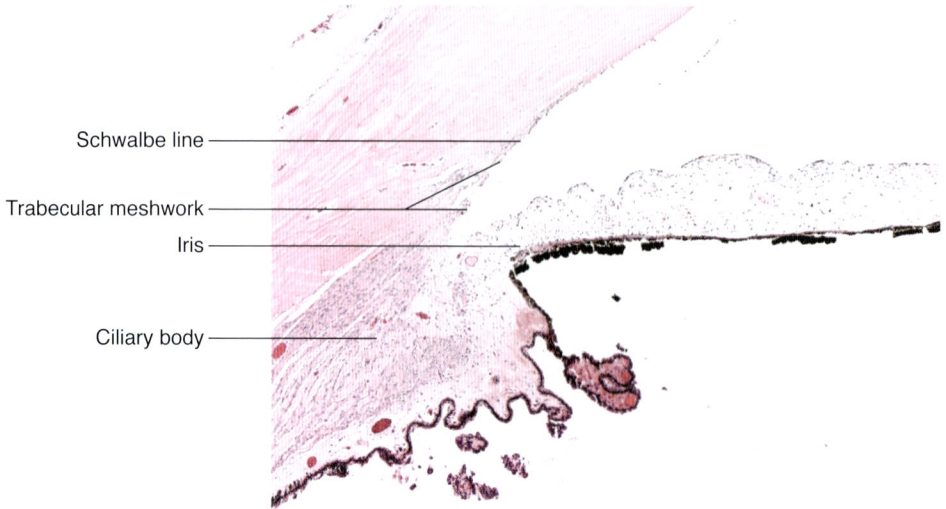

Figure 7-1 The normal anterior chamber angle, the site of drainage for the major portion of the aqueous humor flow, is defined by the anterior border of the iris, the pupillary zone of the anterior lens capsule, the face of the ciliary body, the internal surface of the trabecular meshwork, and the posterior surface of the cornea. *(Courtesy of Nasreen A. Syed, MD.)*

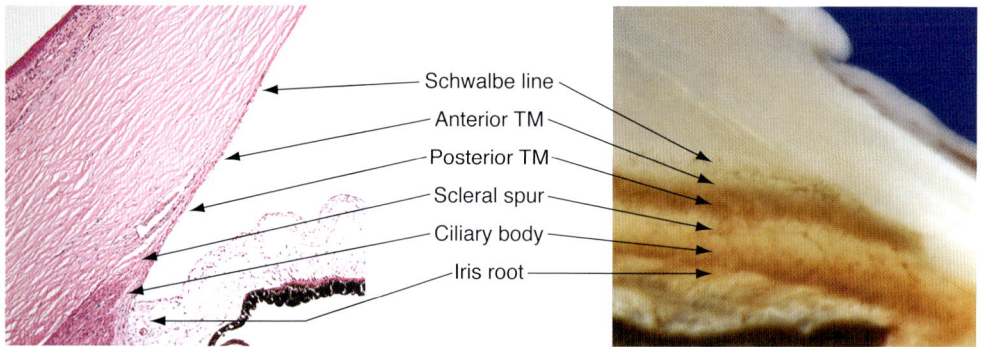

Figure 7-2 Gonioscopic landmarks of a normal anterior chamber angle with histologic correlation. TM = trabecular meshwork. *(Courtesy of Tatyana Milman, MD.)*

Abu-Hassan DW, Acott TS, Kelley MJ. The trabecular meshwork: a basic review of form and function. *J Ocul Biol.* 2014;2(1), https://www.avensonline.org/fulltextarticles/JOCB-2334 -2838-02-0017.html

Developmental Anomalies

See BCSC Section 10, *Glaucoma,* for additional discussion on the conditions described in the following sections.

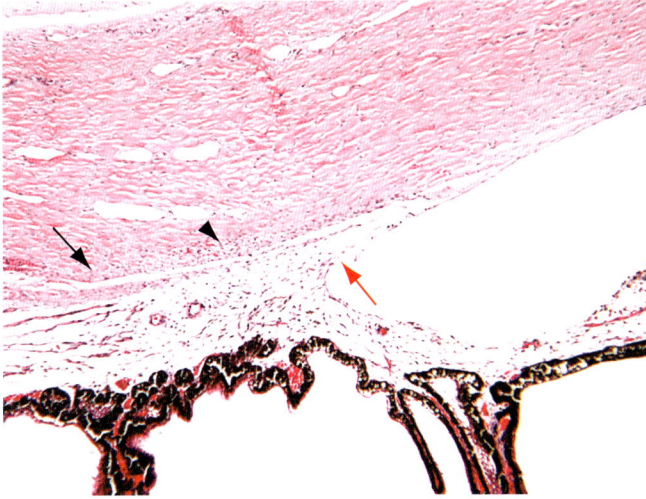

Figure 7-3 Congenital glaucoma. This histologic example of a "fetal" anterior chamber angle demonstrates the anterior insertion of the iris root *(red arrow),* the anteriorly displaced ciliary processes, and a poorly developed scleral spur *(black arrow)* and trabecular meshwork *(arrow-head). (Courtesy of Tatyana Milman, MD.)*

Primary Congenital Glaucoma

Primary congenital glaucoma (PCG), also referred to as *congenital* or *infantile glaucoma,* can be evident at birth or become evident within the first few years of life. The pathogenesis of PCG is likely related to arrested development of the anterior chamber angle structures. Histologically, the anterior chamber angle retains an "embryonic" or "fetal" conformation, characterized by the following:

- anterior insertion of the iris root
- mesenchymal tissue in the anterior chamber angle
- poorly developed scleral spur, allowing the ciliary muscle to insert directly into the trabecular meshwork (Fig 7-3)

See BCSC Section 6, *Pediatric Ophthalmology and Strabismus,* and Section 10, *Glaucoma,* for detailed discussion of PCG.

Anterior Segment Dysgenesis

The term *anterior segment dysgenesis* refers to a spectrum of developmental anomalies resulting from abnormalities of neural crest cell migration and differentiation during embryologic development (eg, Axenfeld-Rieger syndrome, Peters anomaly, posterior keratoconus, and iridoschisis). Maldevelopment of the anterior chamber angle is most prominent in *Axenfeld-Rieger syndrome,* an autosomal dominant disorder, which itself encompasses a spectrum of anomalies, ranging from isolated bilateral ocular defects to a fully manifested systemic disorder.

Ocular manifestations of Axenfeld-Rieger syndrome include posterior embryotoxon, iris strands attached to the Schwalbe line, iris hypoplasia and atrophy, corectopia and pseudopolycoria, a maldeveloped or "fetal" anterior chamber angle (discussed earlier),

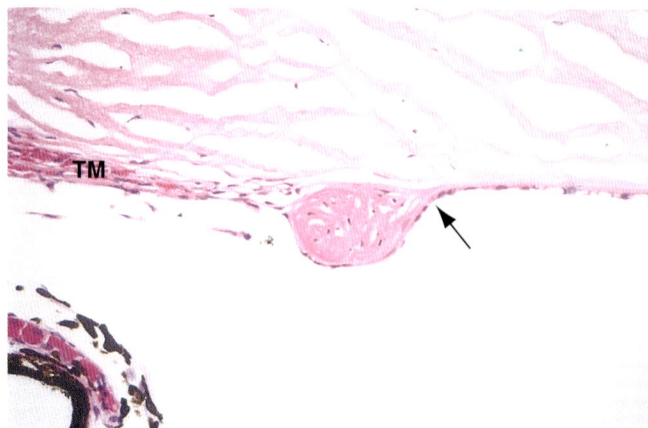

Figure 7-4 Posterior embryotoxon. Light micrograph shows a nodular, collagenous promi-
nence under the termination of Descemet membrane *(arrow)*. TM=trabecular meshwork.
(Courtesy of Hans E. Grossniklaus, MD.)

and glaucoma in 50% of the cases occurring in late childhood or adulthood (Figs 7-4,
7-5). Posterior embryotoxon is often described as a thickening of Descemet membrane at
its termination (Schwalbe line), but it is, in fact, a nodular thickening of the collagen just
under the terminal portion of Descemet membrane. See also BCSC Section 8, *External
Disease and Cornea.*

> Chang TC, Summers CG, Schimmenti LA, Grajewski AL. Axenfeld-Rieger syndrome: new
> perspectives. *Br J Ophthalmol.* 2012;96(3):318–322.

Inflammation

Inflammation in the anterior chamber and angle is typically secondary to inflammation
in adjacent structures (Fig 7-6). It may be infectious (eg, herpes virus) or noninfectious
(trauma, anterior uveitis). Inflammation in the angle structures can result in elevation of
intraocular pressure due to obstruction of aqueous outflow.

Degenerations

Iridocorneal Endothelial Syndrome

Iridocorneal endothelial (ICE) syndrome is a spectrum of acquired unilateral abnormalities of the corneal endothelium, anterior chamber angle, and iris. There are 3 recognized
clinical variants of ICE (when combined, the first letter of each variant also forms the
mnemonic *ICE*):

- iris nevus (Cogan-Reese) syndrome
- Chandler syndrome
- essential progressive iris atrophy

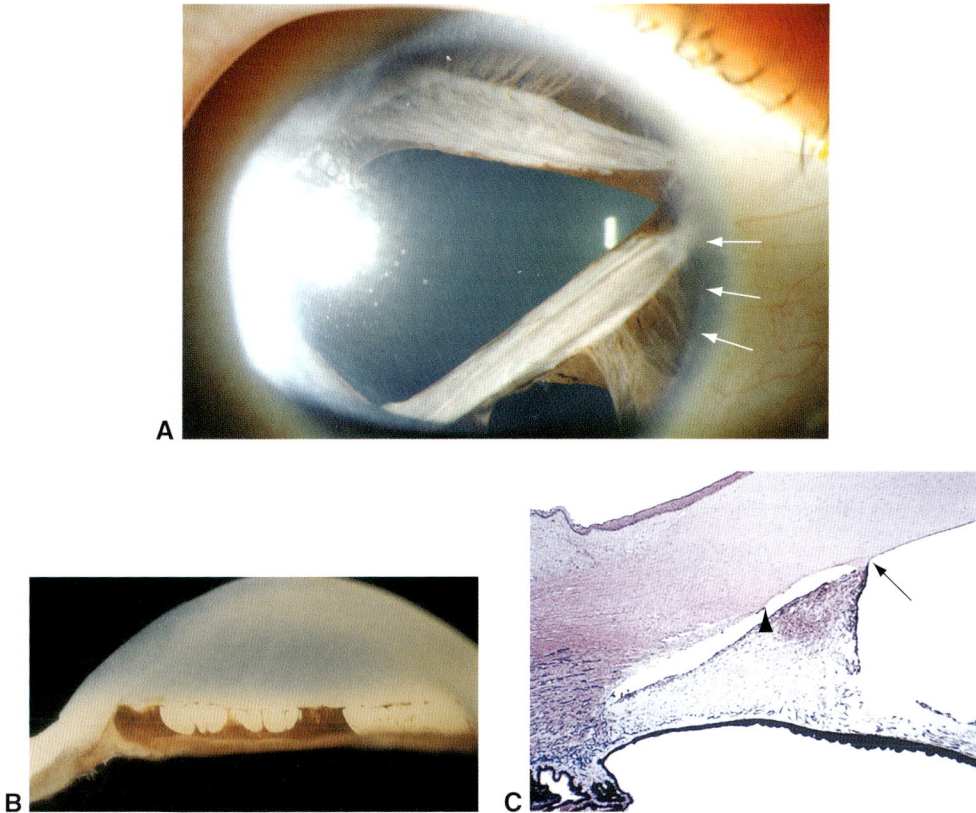

Figure 7-5 Axenfeld-Rieger syndrome. **A,** Clinical photograph of the anterior segment in a patient with Axenfeld-Rieger syndrome. Iris atrophy, pseudopolycoria, and iris strands in the periphery are present. Posterior embryotoxon can be seen laterally *(arrows)*. **B,** Gross photograph shows a prominent Schwalbe line and the anterior insertion of iris strands (Axenfeld anomaly). **C,** Light micrograph shows the anterior attachment of iris strands *(arrow)* to the Schwalbe line *(arrowhead)*. *(Part A courtesy of Wallace L.M. Alward, MD. Copyright University of Iowa. Part B courtesy of Robert Y. Foos, MD. Part C modified with permission from Yanoff M, Fine BS. Ocular Pathology: A Color Atlas. New York: Gower; 1988.)*

All forms of ICE syndrome, which typically affects young to middle-aged adults, have the following 2 features in common: epithelial-like metaplasia of the corneal endothelium and abnormal proliferation of the corneal endothelium. Abnormal endothelial cells migrate over the anterior chamber angle while laying down new basement membrane (Descemet membrane), leading to the formation of peripheral anterior synechiae (PAS) and subsequent secondary angle-closure glaucoma in approximately half of patients with this condition (Fig 7-7). See BCSC Section 8, *External Disease and Cornea,* and Section 10, *Glaucoma,* for further discussion.

Silva L, Najafi A, Suwan Y, Teekhasaenee C, Ritch R. The iridocorneal endothelial syndrome. *Surv Ophthalmol.* 2018;63(5):665–676.

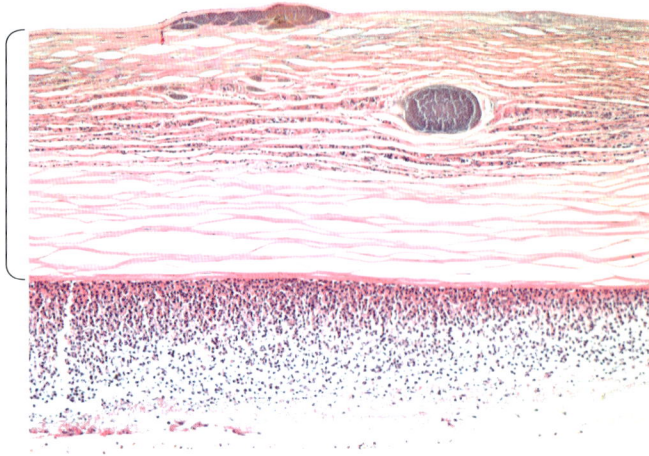

Figure 7-6 Collection of neutrophils and necrotic debris in the anterior chamber (hypopyon). The cornea *(bracket)* has a dense inflammatory infiltrate in the stroma, resulting in the hypopyon. Inflammation may result in the formation of peripheral anterior synechiae in the angle, leading to secondary angle-closure glaucoma. *(Courtesy of Steffen Heegaard, MD.)*

Secondary Glaucoma

Pseudoexfoliation syndrome

Pseudoexfoliation syndrome is a systemic condition characterized by the production and progressive accumulation of a fibrillar material in tissues throughout the anterior segment and in the connective tissue of various visceral organs (eg, lung, liver, kidney, and gallbladder) (Fig 7-8). These deposits help differentiate pseudoexfoliation syndrome from true exfoliation, in which infrared radiation induces splitting of the lens capsule. Pseudoexfoliation syndrome is usually identified in individuals older than 50 years.

Recent data suggest that the pathogenesis of pseudoexfoliation syndrome is a combination of excessive production and abnormal aggregation of elastic microfibril and extracellular matrix components (protein sink), as well as abnormal biomechanical properties of the elastic components of the trabecular meshwork and lamina cribrosa. Polymorphisms in the lysyl oxidase–like 1 gene, *LOXL1*, on chromosome 15 (15q24) are markers for pseudoexfoliation syndrome. Lysyl oxidase is a pivotal enzyme in extracellular matrix formation, catalyzing covalent crosslinking of collagen and elastin.

Pseudoexfoliative material is most apparent on the surface of the anterior segment structures, where it exhibits a positive periodic acid–Schiff reaction (PAS stain); presents as delicate, feathery or brushlike fibrils arranged perpendicular to the surfaces of the intraocular structures; and is easiest to identify on the anterior lens capsule (Fig 7-9A). Pseudoexfoliative material also accumulates in the trabecular meshwork and the wall of Schlemm canal, leading to increased intraocular pressure and secondary glaucoma. Associated degenerative changes in the iris pigment epithelium manifest histologically as a "sawtooth" configuration (Fig 7-9B). These degenerative changes lead to pigment aggregation in the anterior chamber angle. See also BCSC Section 10, *Glaucoma,* and Section 11, *Lens and Cataract.*

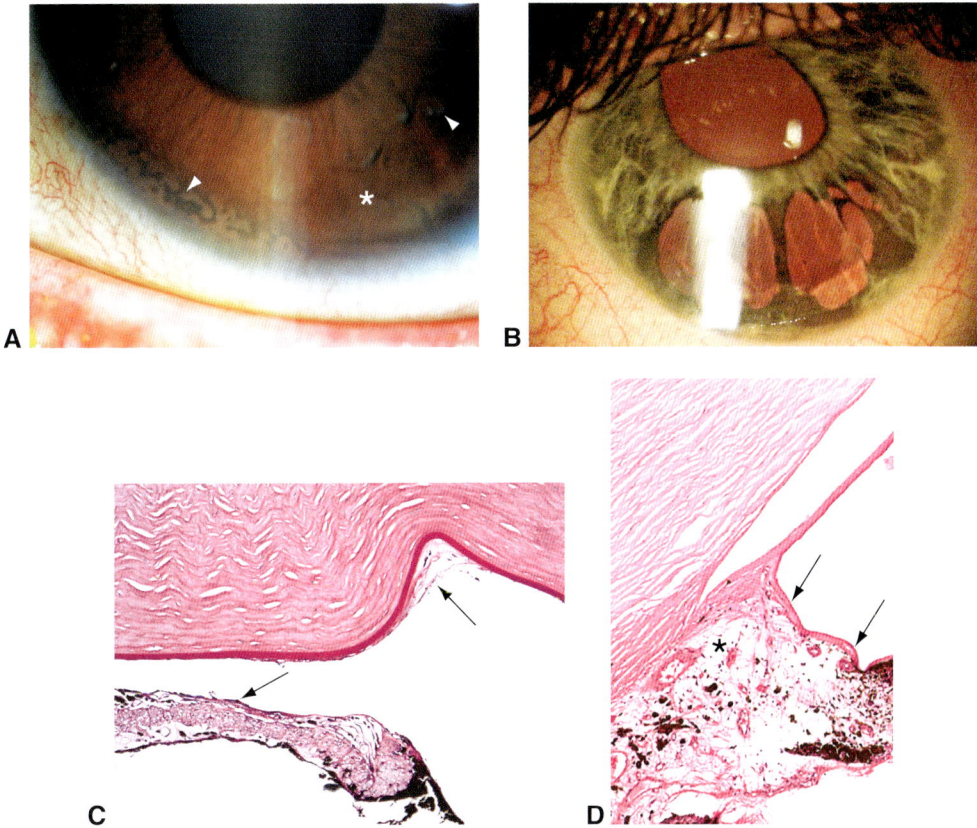

Figure 7-7 Iridocorneal endothelial (ICE) syndrome. **A,** Iris nevus syndrome. The normal anterior iris architecture is effaced by a membrane growing on the anterior iris surface *(asterisk)*. The membrane pinches off islands of normal iris stroma, resulting in a nodular, nevus-like appearance *(arrowheads)*. **B,** Essential iris atrophy. Atrophic holes in the iris and a narrow anterior chamber, consistent with peripheral anterior synechiae formation. **C,** A membrane composed of spindle cells lines the posterior surface of the cornea and the anterior surface of the atrophic iris *(arrows)*. Metaplastic endothelial cells deposit on the iris surface a thin basement membrane that exhibits positive periodic acid–Schiff staining and is analogous to Descemet membrane. **D,** Descemet membrane lines the anterior surface of the iris *(arrows)*. The iris is apposed to the cornea (peripheral anterior synechiae; *asterisk*). *(Part A courtesy of Paul A. Sidoti, MD; parts B and C courtesy of Tatyana Milman, MD.)*

Vazquez LE, Lee RK. Genomic and proteomic pathophysiology of pseudoexfoliation glaucoma. *Int Ophthalmol Clin.* 2014;54(4):1–13.

Phacolytic glaucoma

In phacolytic glaucoma, denatured lens protein leaks from a hypermature cataract through an intact but permeable lens capsule. The trabecular meshwork becomes occluded by the lens protein and by histiocytes that are engorged with phagocytosed proteinaceous, eosinophilic lens material (Fig 7-10).

Trauma

As detailed in the following discussion, blunt trauma may result in different types of secondary glaucoma.

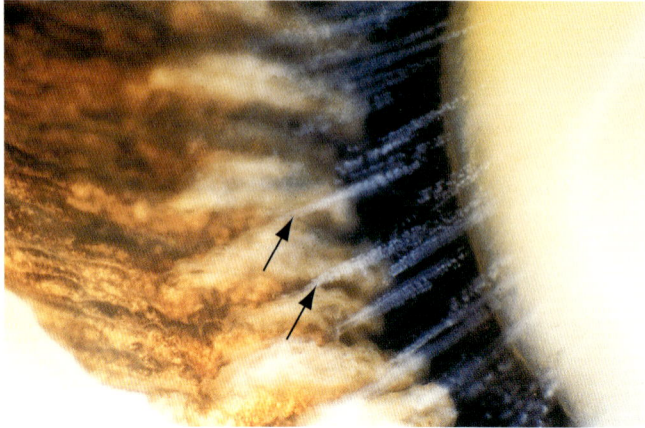

Figure 7-8 Gross photograph shows white fibrillar deposits on the lens zonular fibers *(arrows)* in pseudoexfoliation syndrome. *(Courtesy of Hans E. Grossniklaus, MD.)*

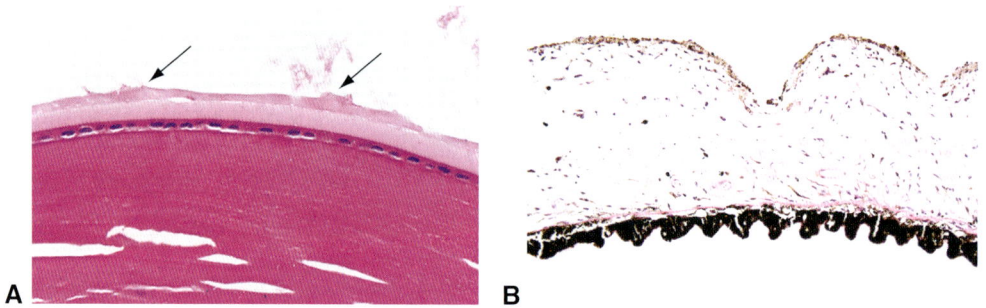

A **B**

Figure 7-9 Pseudoexfoliation syndrome. **A,** Abnormal material appears on the anterior lens capsule like iron filings on the edge of a magnet *(arrows).* **B,** The iris pigment epithelium demonstrates a "sawtooth" configuration, consistent with pseudoexfoliation. *(Part B courtesy of Tatyana Milman, MD.)*

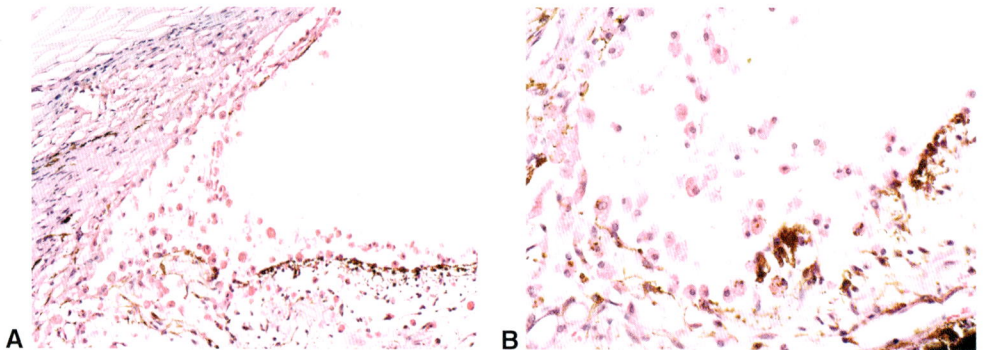

A **B**

Figure 7-10 Phacolytic glaucoma. **A,** Photomicrograph of histiocytes filled with degenerated lens cortical material in the angle. **B,** Higher magnification of the same image. *(Courtesy of Michele M. Bloomer, MD.)*

Hyphema (Fig 7-11), defined as blood in the anterior chamber, may lead to increased intraocular pressure, peripheral anterior synechiae, hemosiderosis bulbi, and, potentially, vision loss.

Following an intraocular hemorrhage, blood breakdown products may accumulate in the trabecular meshwork. The rigidity and spherical shape of hemolyzed erythrocytes (ghost cells) make it difficult for them to escape through the trabecular meshwork. The ghost cells obstruct the meshwork and block aqueous outflow, leading to ghost cell glaucoma (Fig 7-12), one type of secondary open-angle glaucoma. Ghost cell glaucoma often

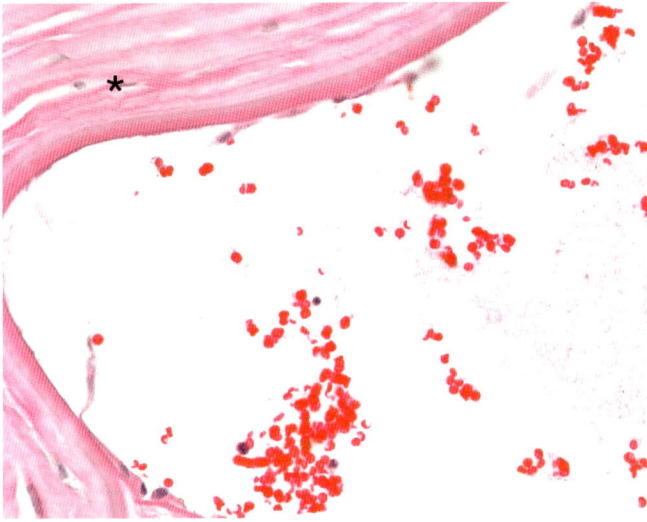

Figure 7-11   Erythrocytes in the anterior chamber (hyphema) posterior to the cornea *(asterisk)*. *(Courtesy of Steffen Heegaard, MD.)*

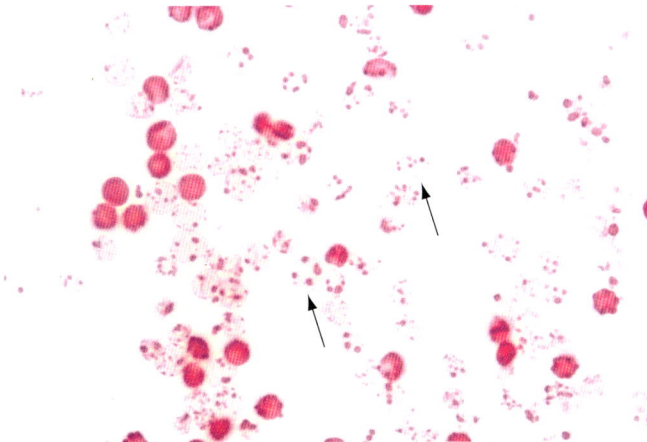

Figure 7-12   Aqueous aspirate demonstrates numerous ghost cells. The degenerating hemoglobin is present as small globules known as *Heinz bodies (arrows)* within the red blood cells. *(Courtesy of Nasreen A. Syed, MD.)*

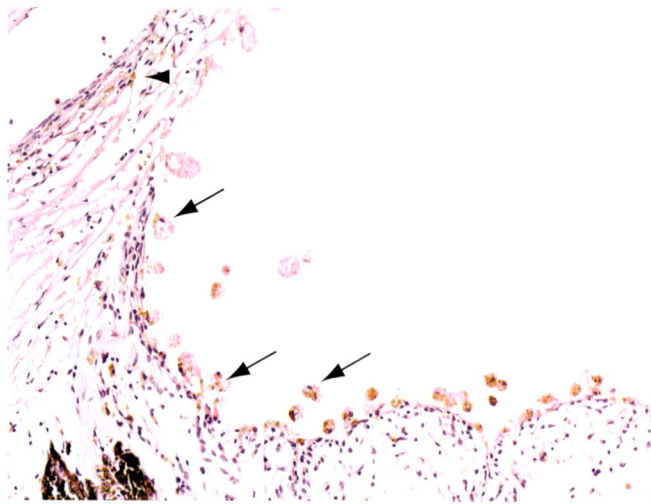

Figure 7-13 Hemolytic glaucoma. The anterior chamber angle contains histiocytes with erythrocyte debris and rust-colored intracytoplasmic hemosiderin *(arrows)*. Hemosiderin is also observed within the trabecular meshwork endothelium *(arrowhead)*. *(Courtesy of Michele M. Bloomer, MD.)*

follows a vitreous hemorrhage, in which blood cells may be retained for prolonged periods, allowing the hemoglobin in erythrocytes to denature.

In *hemolytic glaucoma,* another type of secondary open-angle glaucoma, histiocytes in the anterior chamber phagocytose erythrocytes and their breakdown products, and these hemoglobin-laden and hemosiderin-laden histiocytes block the trabecular outflow channels (Fig 7-13). The histiocytes may be a sign of trabecular obstruction rather than the actual cause of an obstruction.

In other cases of secondary open-angle glaucoma associated with chronic intraocular hemorrhage, histologic examinations have revealed hemosiderin within the trabeculocytes and within many ocular epithelial structures (see Fig 7-13). The hemosiderin likely releases intracellular iron, which results in intracellular toxicity, probably due to oxidative damage. This is the basis of intraocular dysfunction, including glaucoma, in both *siderosis bulbi* and *hemosiderosis bulbi.* The Prussian blue reaction can demonstrate iron deposition in hemosiderosis bulbi.

Blunt injury to the globe may be associated with *angle recession, cyclodialysis,* and *iridodialysis.* Progressive degenerative changes in the trabecular meshwork can contribute to the development of glaucoma after injury. See the section Pathologically Apparent Sequelae of Ocular Trauma in Chapter 4 for further discussion, including images.

Pigment dispersion associations

Pigment dispersion (of melanosomes) may be associated with a variety of other conditions in which pigment epithelium or uveal melanocytes are injured, such as uveitis and uveal melanoma. These conditions are characterized by the presence of pigment within the trabecular meshwork as well as in histiocytes littering the anterior chamber angle (Fig 7-14).

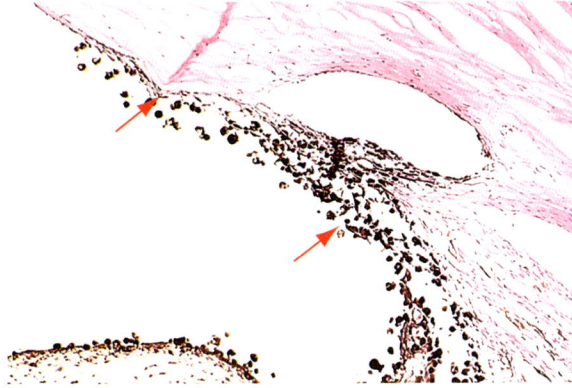

Figure 7-14 Melanomalytic glaucoma. The trabecular meshwork *(between arrows)* is obstructed by histiocytes that have ingested pigment from a necrotic intraocular melanoma.

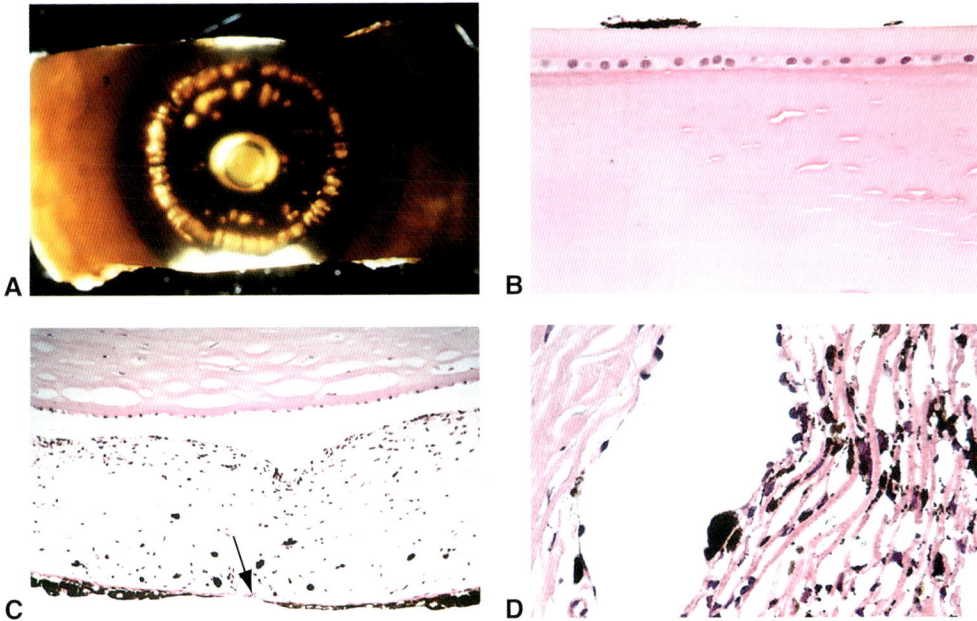

Figure 7-15 Pigment dispersion syndrome. **A,** Gross photograph demonstrating circumferential transillumination defects in the iris. **B,** Melanin is present on the anterior surface of the lens. **C,** Note the focal loss of iris pigment epithelium *(arrow)*. Chafing of the zonular fibers against the epithelium may release the pigment that is dispersed in this condition. **D,** Pigment accumulation in the trabecular meshwork.

Pigment dispersion syndrome can lead to a secondary open-angle glaucoma that is characterized by transillumination defects in the midperipheral iris in addition to pigment in the trabecular meshwork, the corneal endothelium *(Krukenberg spindle),* and other anterior segment structures, such as the lens capsule (Fig 7-15). The dispersed pigment is

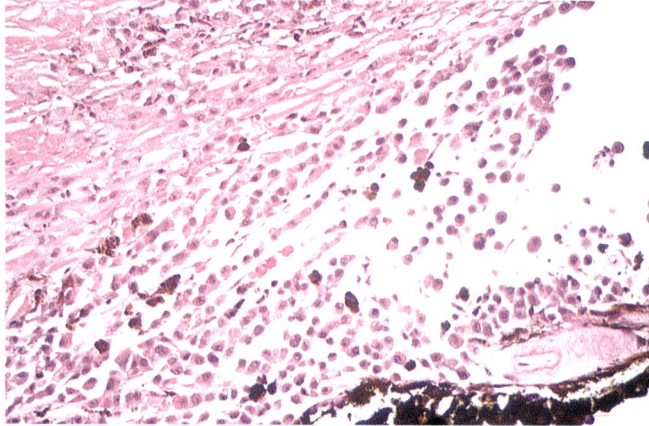

Figure 7-16 Photomicrograph shows melanoma cells filling the anterior chamber angle and obstructing the trabecular meshwork. The iris pigment epithelium is present in the lower right corner of the photomicrograph. *(Courtesy of Hans E. Grossniklaus, MD.)*

presumed to result from rubbing of the lens zonular fibers against the iris pigment epithelium. See also BCSC Section 10, *Glaucoma.*

Neoplasia

Primary tumors of the angle structures are not known to occur. Melanocytic nevi and melanomas that arise in the iris or extend to the iris from the ciliary body may invade or obstruct the trabecular meshwork (Fig 7-16). See also Chapter 17. In addition, pigment elaborated from melanomas and melanocytomas may be shed into the trabecular meshwork, leading to secondary glaucoma *(melanomalytic glaucoma)* (see Fig 7-14). Occasionally, epibulbar tumors such as conjunctival carcinoma can invade the eye through the limbus, resulting in trabecular outflow obstruction and glaucoma. See the section Neoplasia in Chapter 5 for further discussion.

CHAPTER 8

Sclera

Highlights

- The sclera is the tough, relatively avascular outer shell of the eye.
- Inflammation may occur in the sclera either focally or diffusely and is often granulomatous in nature.
- The sclera can thin for a variety of reasons, resulting in staphyloma formation.

Topography

The sclera is the white, nearly opaque portion of the outer wall of the eye that covers most of the eye's surface area. Anteriorly, it is continuous with the corneal stroma at the limbus. Posteriorly, the outer two-thirds of the sclera merge with the dural sheath of the optic nerve; the inner third continues as perforated sclera, known as the *lamina cribrosa,* through which the axonal fibers of the retinal ganglion cells pass and become the retrobulbar optic nerve (see Chapter 15, Fig 15-1). Histologically, the sclera is divided into 3 layers (from outermost inward): episclera, stroma, and lamina fusca (Fig 8-1). Embryologically, the sclera is derived predominantly from the neural crest. See BCSC Section 2, *Fundamentals and Principles of Ophthalmology,* for further discussion.

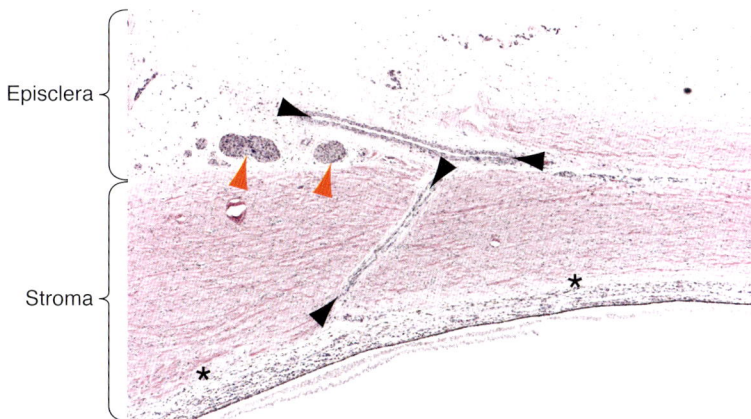

Figure 8-1 The 3 layers of the sclera—episclera, stroma, and lamina fusca *(asterisks).* Emissary structures, including ciliary arteries *(black arrowheads)* and nerves *(red arrowheads)* are shown entering and traversing normal sclera (hematoxylin-eosin stain). *(Courtesy of Nasreen A. Syed, MD.)*

129

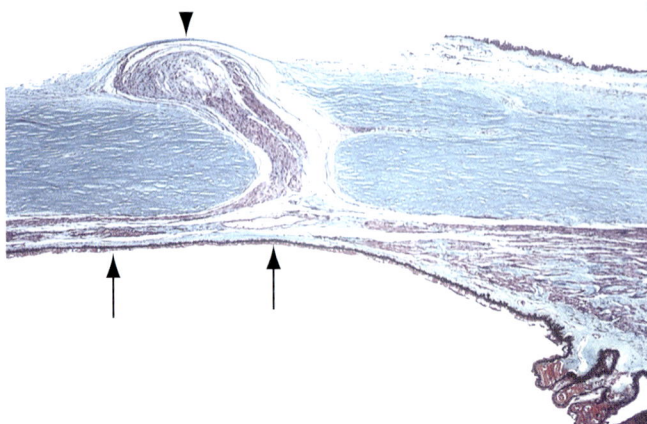

Figure 8-2   An emissary canal through the sclera with Axenfeld nerve loop *(arrowhead)*, which is overlying the pars plana *(arrows)* (trichrome stain). *(Courtesy of Harry H. Brown, MD.)*

The *episclera* is a thin layer of loose fibrovascular tissue that covers the outer surface of the scleral stroma. The bulk of the sclera is made up of the *stroma,* a layer of sparsely vascularized, dense type I collagen fibers. In comparison to the collagen lamellae of the corneal stroma, scleral collagen fibers are thicker and more variable in thickness and orientation, resulting in the opaque appearance of the sclera. Transmural *emissary canals* allow the passage of the ciliary arteries, vortex veins, and ciliary nerves through the scleral stroma (Fig 8-2; see also Fig 8-1). For additional discussion, see BCSC Section 2, *Fundamentals and Principles of Ophthalmology*, Chapter 2.

The *lamina fusca* is a delicate fibrovascular layer containing melanocytes that loosely binds the uveal tract to the sclera. Sclerouveal attachments are strongest surrounding the major emissary canals, at the anterior base of the ciliary body (scleral spur), and surrounding the optic nerve.

Developmental Anomalies

Choristoma

Epibulbar dermoids and other choristomatous lesions are discussed in Chapter 5.

Nanophthalmos

Nanophthalmos is a rare, usually bilateral, developmental disorder characterized by an eye with short axial length, a normal or slightly enlarged lens, thickened sclera, hyperopia, foveal changes, and a predisposition to uveal effusions and angle-closure glaucoma. The criteria for nanophthalmos differ in various studies, but in most, the size criterion is an axial length between 19 and 21 mm. For clinical purposes, 20.5 mm is often used as the cutoff. Nanophthalmos has a strong genetic basis, but sporadic cases (likely representing new mutations) occur.

Examination of tissue from nanophthalmic eyes has shown disarrangement, fraying, and splitting of scleral collagen fibrils. Abnormalities in the extracellular matrix glycosaminoglycans have also been described. These scleral changes may predispose the nanophthalmic eye to uveal effusion due to reduced protein permeability and impaired venous outflow through the vortex veins.

See BCSC Section 6, *Pediatric Ophthalmology and Strabismus,* and Section 10, *Glaucoma,* for additional discussion of nanophthalmos.

Carricondo PC, Andrade T, Prasov L, Ayres BM, Moroi SE. Nanophthalmos: a review of the clinical spectrum and genetics. *J Ophthalmol.* 2018 May 9;2018:2735465.

Fukuchi T, Sawada H, Seki M, Oyama T, Cho H, Abe H. Changes of scleral-sulfated proteoglycans in three cases of nanophthalmos. *Jpn J Ophthalmol.* 2009;53(2):171–175.

Microphthalmia

Microphthalmia refers to a smaller than average eye with associated developmental defects (eg, persistent fetal vasculature). Colobomas and scleral defects with cystic outpouchings of intraocular contents (microphthalmia with cyst) are also common, because of failure of the fetal fissure to close completely.

See BCSC Section 6, *Pediatric Ophthalmology and Strabismus,* and Section 7, *Oculofacial Plastic and Orbital Surgery,* for additional discussion of microphthalmia.

Inflammation

See BCSC Section 8, *External Disease and Cornea,* and Section 9, *Uveitis and Ocular Inflammation,* for in-depth discussion of episcleritis and scleritis, including pathogenesis, clinical presentation, laboratory evaluation, and management.

Episcleritis

Episcleritis is classified as simple or nodular. *Simple episcleritis* is a self-limited, often idiopathic condition. Histologic examination shows vascular congestion, stromal edema, and a chronic nongranulomatous perivascular inflammatory infiltrate that is composed primarily of lymphocytes.

Nodular episcleritis more often occurs in the setting of systemic inflammatory conditions such as rheumatoid arthritis. It is characterized by tender, elevated, mobile pink-red nodules on the anterior episclera. Histologically, the nodules are often composed of a granulomatous inflammatory infiltrate surrounding a focus of *necrobiosis* (collagen decay), similar to rheumatoid nodules in subcutaneous tissue.

Scleritis

Scleritis may be infectious or noninfectious. Infectious scleritis may be distinguished from noninfectious scleritis by appropriate laboratory testing; special stains may aid in identifying causative organisms (Fig 8-3).

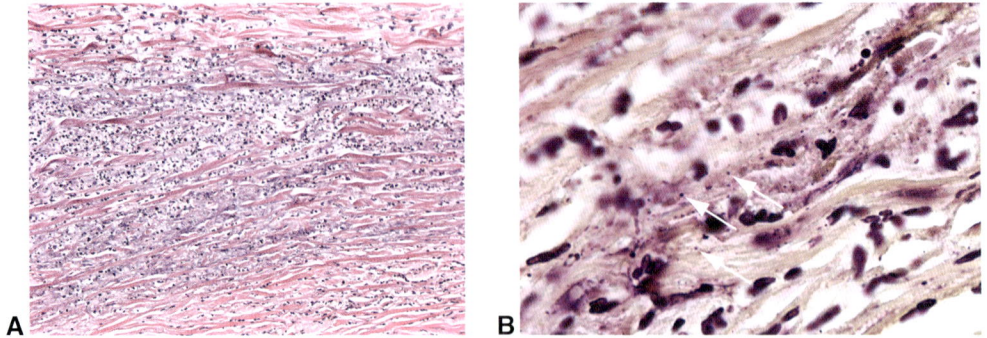

Figure 8-3 Infectious scleritis caused by bacteria. **A,** The sclera is infiltrated with numerous neutrophils, seen as blue dots between the scleral collagen lamellae. The purple areas represent necrobiosis of the sclera (hematoxylin-eosin stain). **B,** Tissue Gram stain illustrating the presence of scattered gram-positive cocci *(arrows)*. *(Courtesy of Nasreen A. Syed, MD.)*

Noninfectious scleritis is typically a painful ocular disease with potentially serious sequelae. Histologic examination of noninfectious scleritis reveals 2 main types: necrotizing and nonnecrotizing inflammation. Either type can occur anteriorly or posteriorly, but anterior scleritis is more common. *Necrotizing scleritis* may be nodular or diffuse (Figs 8-4, 8-5). Both forms demonstrate granulomatous inflammation within the sclera (Fig 8-6). Lymphocytes and plasma cells are usually present as well. Neutrophils may be present in some cases. Multiple foci may show different stages of evolution. In the course of healing, the necrotic stroma is resorbed, leaving a thinned scleral remnant that is prone to staphyloma formation (Fig 8-7). Severe ectasia of the scleral shell predisposes the sclera to herniation of uveal tissue through the defect (staphyloma). In *scleromalacia perforans,* the sclera undergoes focal progressive ectasia without clinical or histologic evidence of an inflammatory infiltrate. The ectasia can lead to scleral perforation requiring urgent medical and surgical intervention.

Nonnecrotizing scleritis is characterized by a perivascular lymphocytic and plasmacytic infiltrate, typically without a granulomatous inflammatory component. Vasculitis may be

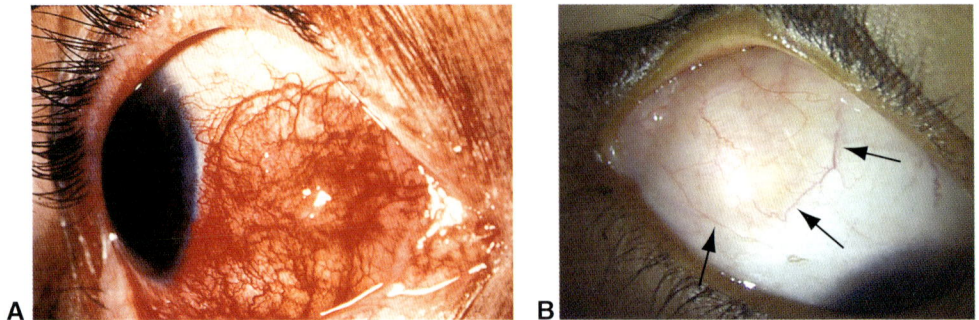

Figure 8-4 Nodular scleritis. **A,** An eye with sectoral nodular anterior scleritis with focal severe episcleral and scleral vascular congestion. **B,** Clinical photograph from a different patient following treatment. The nodule has a tan appearance *(arrows)*. *(Part A courtesy of Harry H. Brown, MD; part B courtesy of Nasreen A. Syed, MD.)*

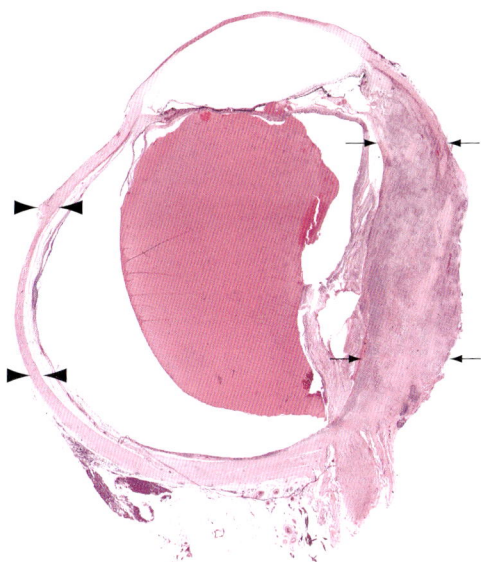

Figure 8-5 Diffuse anterior and posterior scleritis with marked thickening of the sclera *(arrows)* due to a dense inflammatory infiltrate. Compare the thickened sclera to normal sclera on the opposite side *(arrowheads).* *(Courtesy of Nasreen A. Syed, MD.)*

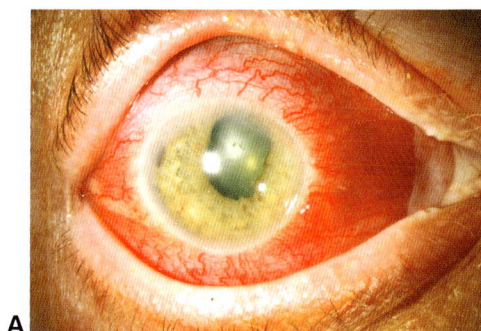

A

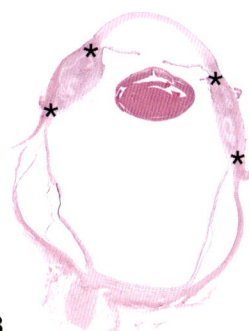

B

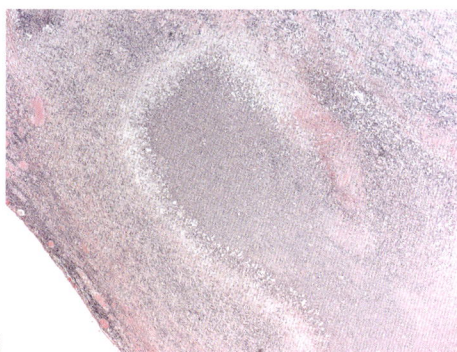

C

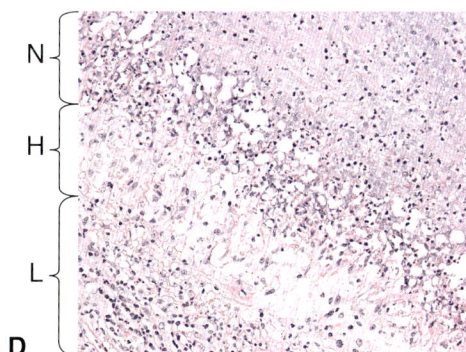

D

Figure 8-6 Necrotizing granulomatous anterior scleritis in a patient with rheumatoid arthritis. **A,** Clinical photograph of the anterior segment. **B,** Low-magnification photomicrograph illustrating the anterior location of the scleritis *(area between asterisks).* **C,** Medium-magnification photomicrograph showing the area of scleritis with central necrosis surrounded by a zonal inflammatory infiltrate. **D,** High-magnification photomicrograph of a zonal inflammatory infiltrate with central neutrophils and necrosis (N), a middle layer of epithelioid histiocytes (H), and an outer layer of lymphocytes (L). *(Courtesy of Nasreen A. Syed, MD.)*

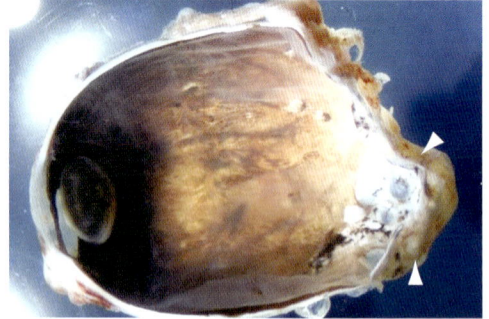

Figure 8-7 An eye with a posterior staphy-loma *(arrowheads)* as a sequela of scleritis. *(Courtesy of Hans E. Grossniklaus, MD.)*

present in the form of fibrinoid necrosis of the vessel walls. When treated, nonnecrotizing scleritis rarely leads to severe vision loss or enucleation.

Degenerations

Senile Calcific Plaque

Senile calcific plaques commonly occur in individuals older than 70 years. They appear as firm, flat, sharply circumscribed rectangular or ovoid gray scleral patches. The plaques, which appear bilaterally, are typically located anterior to the medial and lateral rectus muscle insertions in the interpalpebral fissure (Fig 8-8A). The etiology is unknown; various causes, such as scleral dehydration, actinic damage, and stress on scleral collagen exerted by rectus muscle insertions, have been proposed but not proven.

Histologic sections show that the calcium is present within the midportion of the scleral stroma. The plaque begins as a finely granular deposition but may progress to a confluent plaque involving both superficial and deep sclera (Fig 8-8B). Senile plaques may be high-lighted by special stains for calcium, such as von Kossa and alizarin red.

Scleral Staphyloma

Scleral staphylomas are scleral ectasias that are lined internally by uveal tissue. Staphylomas may develop at points of weakness in the scleral shell, either in inherently thin areas (such as posterior to the rectus muscle insertions; Fig 8-9) or in areas weakened by tissue destruction (as in scleritis; see Fig 8-7). In children, staphylomas may occur as a result of long-standing elevated intraocular pressure or axial myopia, owing to the relative distensibility of the sclera in young eyes. Thus, location and age at onset vary according to the underlying etiology. Histologic examination invariably reveals thinned sclera, with or without fibrosis and scar-ring, depending on the cause.

Melanoma-Associated Spongiform Scleropathy

The sclera may undergo degeneration at the base of a uveal melanoma. This change is typically not apparent clinically, but histologically, it appears as a feathery separation and

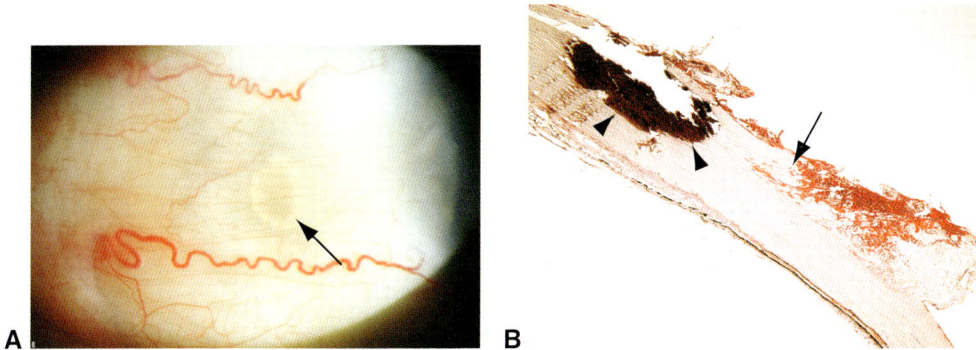

Figure 8-8 A calcific plaque of the sclera. **A,** Calcific plaques *(arrow)* are typically located just anterior to the insertion of the medial and lateral rectus muscles. **B,** Calcific deposits are noted in the sclera *(arrowheads)* anterior to the rectus muscle insertion *(arrow)* (von Kossa stain). *(Part A courtesy of Vinay A. Shah, MBBS; part B courtesy of Tatyana Milman, MD.)*

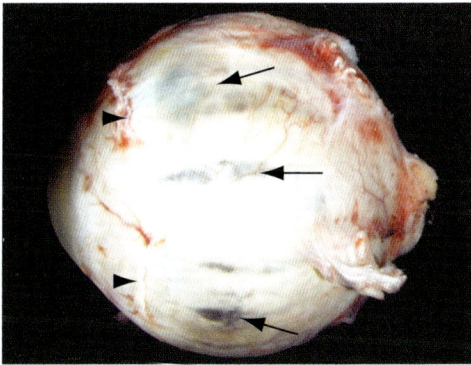

Figure 8-9 Scleral staphylomas. Several regions of scleral thinning *(arrows),* which appear blue because of the underlying uveal tissue, are present posterior to the rectus muscle insertions *(arrowheads)* and in the equatorial sclera. *(Courtesy of Nasreen A. Syed, MD.)*

fragmentation of the scleral collagen fibers. Studies have shown increased amounts of glycosaminoglycans in these areas. The change is postulated to result from activation of proteinases such as matrix metalloproteinase-2 in the sclera and may facilitate scleral extension of uveal melanoma.

Neoplasia

While neoplasms of the sclera can occur, they are exceedingly rare. Tumors originate predominantly in the conjunctiva or uveal tract with secondary scleral involvement.

CHAPTER **9**

Lens

Highlights

- Understanding the anatomical structure of the crystalline lens provides essential knowledge for performing cataract surgery as the structure(s) affected determines the techniques that the surgeon uses to achieve optimal outcomes for the patient.
- Developmental anomalies of the lens must be recognized early to prevent the development of amblyopia.
- Chronic postoperative endophthalmitis presents slowly because causative microorganisms are sequestered between the posterior capsule and the intraocular lens implant.
- Inflammation due to degeneration of the crystalline lens can cause various forms of glaucoma.

Topography

The crystalline lens is an avascular, elastic, disc-shaped biconvex structure located posterior to the iris and anterior to the vitreous body in the posterior chamber. In the adult eye, the lens measures approximately 9–10 mm in diameter equatorially and 5–6 mm anteroposteriorly (Fig 9-1). It is derived from surface ectoderm. See BCSC Section 11, *Lens and Cataract,* for in-depth discussion of the structure, embryology, and pathology of the lens.

Capsule

The capsule, which surrounds the lens, is a thick basement membrane elaborated by lens epithelial cells and composed partly of type IV collagen fibers (Fig 9-2). The lens capsule is thickest anteriorly (12–21 µm) and peripherally near the equator and thinnest posteriorly (2–9 µm) (Fig 9-3).

Epithelium

Embryologically, the lens epithelium is derived from the cells of the original lens vesicle that did not differentiate into primary lens fibers. The anterior or axial lens epithelium consists of a single layer of cuboidal cells. The basilar surface of the anterior epithelium is oriented toward the anterior lens capsule. The equatorial cells are mitotically active and appear more elongated as they differentiate into lens fibers. Epithelial cells are not typically observed posterior to the lens equator (see Fig 9-2).

137

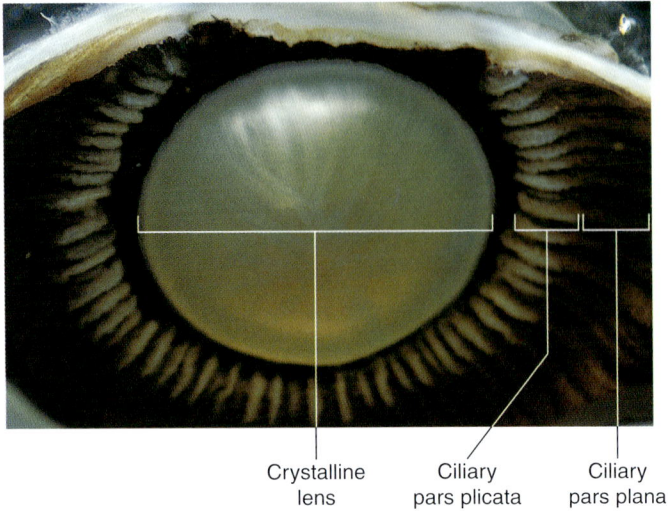

Crystalline   Ciliary   Ciliary
lens   pars plicata   pars plana

Figure 9-1 Posterior aspect of the crystalline lens, depicting its relationship to the peripheral iris and ciliary body. The zonular fibers are translucent and therefore are not visible. *(Courtesy of Hans E. Grossniklaus, MD.)*

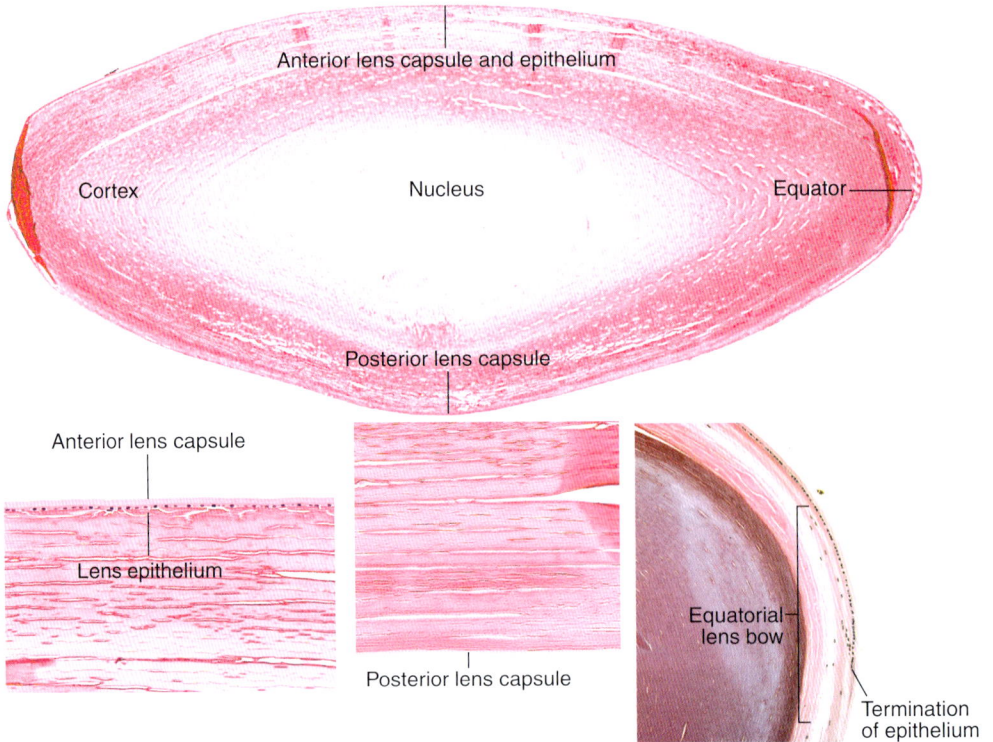

Anterior lens capsule and epithelium

Cortex   Nucleus   Equator

Posterior lens capsule

Anterior lens capsule

Lens epithelium

Equatorial
lens bow

Posterior lens capsule

Termination
of epithelium

Figure 9-2 Histologic appearance and structure of the adult lens. *(Courtesy of Tatyana Milman, MD, except for lower right image, courtesy of Nasreen A. Syed, MD.)*

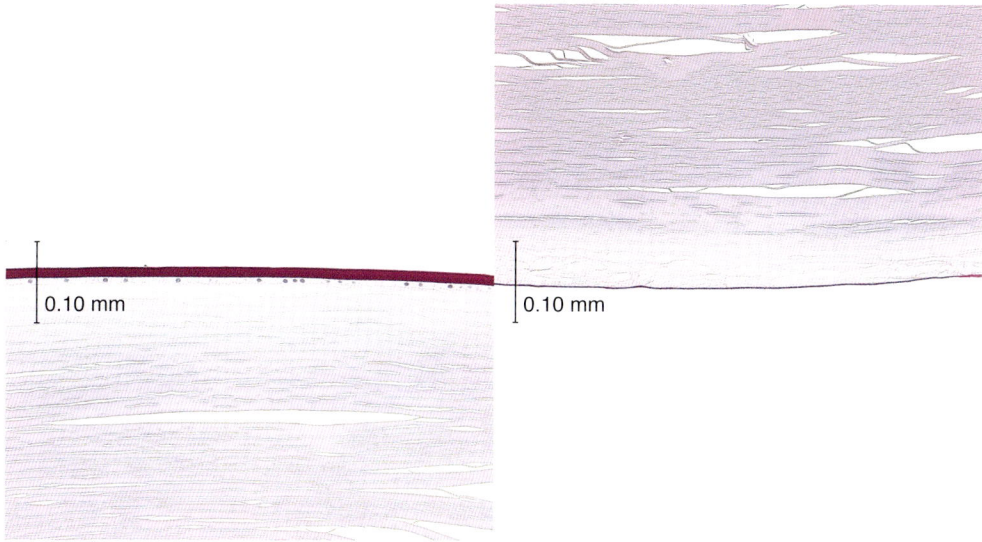

0.10 mm

0.10 mm

Figure 9-3 Lens capsule, periodic acid–Schiff (PAS) stain. Compare the thickness of the anterior capsule *(left)* with that of the posterior capsule *(right)*. Calibration bar = 0.01 mm. *(Courtesy of Nasreen A. Syed, MD.)*

Cortex and Nucleus

In the equatorial, or *bow,* region of the lens, the epithelial cells move centrally, elongate, produce crystalline proteins, lose organelles, and transform into lens fibers. As the lens epithelial cells differentiate, new fibers are continuously laid down over existing fibers, compacting them in a lamellar arrangement. Thus, the outermost fibers, derived from postnatally differentiated lens epithelial cells, are the most recently formed and make up the cortex of the lens, while older layers are located toward the center. The center of the lens contains the oldest fibers, the *embryonic and fetal lens nucleus.* Lens fibers are densely compacted in the nucleus. Clinically and histologically, the demarcation between the nucleus and cortex is not well defined (see Fig 9-2).

The overall shape of the lens changes over the first decade of life. With increasing age, the diameter of the lens nucleus and cortex increases from anterior to posterior.

Zonular Fibers

The lens is supported by the zonular fibers, which insert on both the anterior and the posterior lens capsule in the midperiphery (see Chapter 7, Fig 7-8). These fibers hold the lens in place through their attachments to the nonpigmented epithelium of the ciliary pars plana and the valleys of the pars plicata. The zonular fibers are composed of an elastic type of glycoprotein known as *fibrillin* and have an important role in molding the lens shape for accommodation.

See BCSC Section 2, *Fundamentals and Principles of Ophthalmology,* for more information on the structure and development of the crystalline lens.

Developmental Anomalies

Early recognition of developmental anomalies of the lens is important to prevent the development of amblyopia. See BCSC Section 6, *Pediatric Ophthalmology and Strabismus,* and Section 11, *Lens and Cataract,* for discussion of lens coloboma, ectopia lentis, and congenital cataract, as well as for additional information on the topics discussed in the following sections.

Congenital Aphakia

Congenital aphakia, a rare anomaly, can be divided into 2 forms: primary and secondary. In primary aphakia, the lens is absent histologically. The anomaly results from failed lens induction from the surface ectoderm during embryogenesis and is caused by homozygous mutations in the *FOXE3* gene. Primary aphakia is associated with severe ocular and systemic developmental anomalies. The histologic findings of secondary aphakia depend on the underlying etiology. In this form of congenital aphakia, the lens is developed but is resorbed or extruded before or during birth. Secondary aphakia is often associated with congenital infections such as rubella.

Anterior Lenticonus and Lentiglobus

The anterior surface of the lens can assume an abnormal shape, either conical *(lenticonus)* or spherical *(lentiglobus).* Clinically, these abnormalities can be seen in the red reflex, where, by retroillumination, they appear as an "oil droplet." Anterior lenticonus may be unilateral or bilateral.

Histologic examination reveals thinning of and small defects in the anterior lens capsule, a decrease in the number of anterior lens epithelial cells, and bulging of the anterior cortex. Electron microscopy demonstrates alterations in lens capsule collagen, and immunohistochemical analysis reveals abnormalities in type IV collagen.

Bilateral anterior lenticonus is usually associated with *Alport syndrome,* which is most often an X-linked disorder characterized by hemorrhagic nephritis, deafness, anterior polar cataract, and retinal flecks. Mutations in type IV collagen genes—specifically, *COL4A3, COL4A4,* and *COL4A5*—have been described in some forms of Alport syndrome.

Posterior Lenticonus and Lentiglobus

Posterior lenticonus (lentiglobus) is characterized by a conical (spherical in lentiglobus) deformity of the posterior surface of the lens (Fig 9-4). This condition usually occurs as a sporadic unilateral anomaly and is associated with congenital cataract. Other, rare ocular associations include microphthalmia, microcornea, persistent fetal vasculature, and uveal colobomas. Posterior lenticonus may also be a manifestation of Alport syndrome (see previous section) or *oculocerebrorenal syndrome (Lowe syndrome),* an X-linked disorder characterized by glaucoma, cognitive impairment, and infantile renal tubulopathy (Fanconi type) with resultant aminoaciduria, metabolic acidosis, proteinuria, rickets, and hypotonia. Histologically, the cataracts display focal, internally directed excrescences of the lens capsule. Oculocerebrorenal syndrome is due to mutations in the *OCRL* gene.

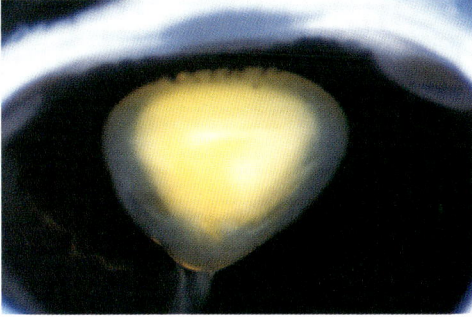

Figure 9-4 Macroscopic image showing posterior lenticonus. *(Courtesy of Hans E. Grossniklaus, MD.)*

Inflammation

Propionibacterium acnes Endophthalmitis

A chronic infectious endophthalmitis may develop following cataract surgery. Common causative organisms are *Propionibacterium acnes, Staphylococcus epidermidis,* and fungi. Chronic postoperative bacterial endophthalmitis is most commonly caused by *P acnes; P acnes* endophthalmitis often has a delayed presentation, usually between 2 months and 2 years following surgery. The organism, a gram-positive coccobacillus that is part of normal skin flora and grows best in anaerobic conditions, may sequester itself between a posterior chamber lens implant and the posterior capsule. In this relatively anaerobic environment, *P acnes* grows and forms colonies. Histologic examination of the lens capsule reveals sequestration of the bacteria within the capsule (Fig 9-5). See BCSC Section 9, *Uveitis and Ocular Inflammation,* Section 11, *Lens and Cataract,* and Section 12, *Retina and Vitreous,* for additional discussion of endophthalmitis.

Phacoantigenic Uveitis

Also known as *lens-induced granulomatous endophthalmitis* and previously called *phaco-anaphylactic endophthalmitis,* phacoantigenic uveitis is a type of lens-induced intraocular inflammation. It is thought to be precipitated by the deposition of antigen–antibody complexes in the lens (type III, Arthus-type reaction) following exposure of the immune system to lens antigens after the lens capsule has been violated. The inflammation may develop after accidental or surgical trauma to the lens.

Histologically, an eye with phacoantigenic uveitis shows a central nidus of degenerating lens material surrounded by concentric layers of inflammatory cells *(zonal granuloma).* Neutrophils are present in the innermost zone of inflammation. The intermediate zone consists primarily of epithelioid histiocytes and multinucleated giant cells. Lymphocytes and plasma cells are present in the outer zone. The inflammatory cells may be surrounded by fibrovascular connective tissue, depending on the duration of the inflammatory response (Fig 9-6). See also BCSC Section 9, *Uveitis and Ocular Inflammation.*

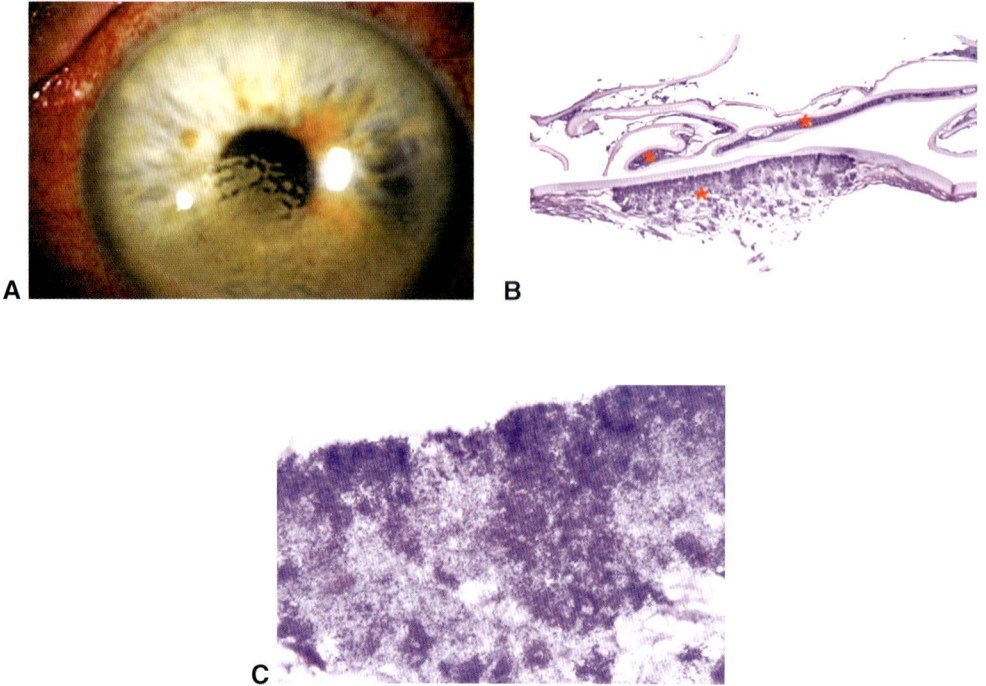

Figure 9-5 *Propionibacterium acnes* endophthalmitis. **A,** Slit-lamp photograph shows numerous keratic precipitates on the corneal endothelium. **B,** Giemsa stain shows large aggregates of coccobacilli within the capsular bag *(asterisks)*. **C,** Higher magnification of the numerous coccobacilli. *(Courtesy of Hans E. Grossniklaus, MD.)*

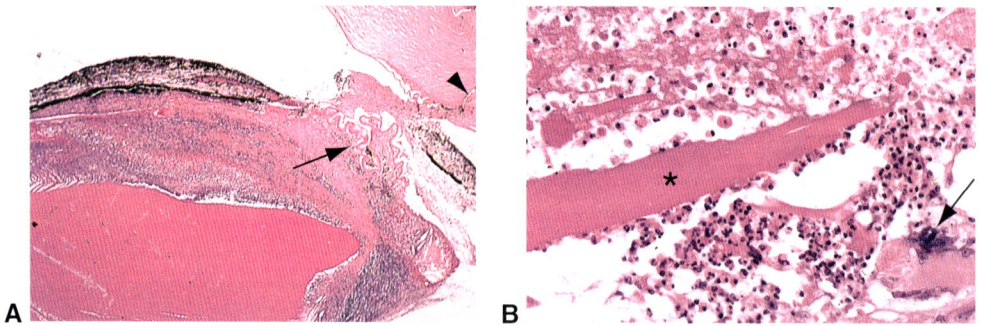

Figure 9-6 Phacoantigenic uveitis. **A,** A zonal inflammatory reaction surrounds the lens *(lower left)*. The torn capsule is visible in the pupillary region *(arrow)*. Note the corneal scar *(arrowhead)*, representing the site of ocular penetration. **B,** Acute and granulomatous inflammation, including giant cells *(arrow)*, surrounds inciting lens fibers *(asterisk)*.

Phacolytic Uveitis

Phacolytic uveitis is an inflammatory condition caused by leakage of lens protein from a hypermature or morgagnian cataract through a grossly intact lens capsule. The proteins are often engulfed by histiocytes. These protein-laden histiocytes may clog the trabecular meshwork or induce an inflammatory response in the angle, leading to a form of glaucoma called *phacolytic glaucoma*. See also BCSC Section 9, *Uveitis and Ocular Inflammation*, and Section 10, *Glaucoma*.

Degenerations

Cataract and Other Lens Abnormalities

Capsule

Mild thickening of the lens capsule can be associated with pathologic proliferation of lens epithelium or with chronic inflammation of the anterior segment. Elements with an affinity for basement membranes, such as copper or silver, can form pigmented deposits in the anterior lens capsule, conditions known as *chalcosis* and *argyrosis,* respectively.

Epithelium

The most common abnormality involving the lens epithelium may be *posterior subcapsular cataract* (Fig 9-7A; see also Fig 9-8A). Histologically, development of this cataract begins with epithelial disarray at the lens equator, followed by posterior migration of the lens epithelial cells along the posterior capsule. As the cells migrate posteriorly, they may enlarge significantly because of retention of lens protein in the cytoplasm. These swollen cells, referred to as *Wedl* (or *bladder*) *cells,* can cause significant visual impairment if they involve the axial portion of the lens (Fig 9-7B).

Inflammation, ischemia, or trauma can result in injury to the lens epithelium, stimulating epithelial metaplasia and the formation of *anterior subcapsular fibrous plaques* (Fig 9-8A). In this condition, the epithelial cells have undergone a metaplastic transformation into fibroblast-like cells that form a plaque just interior to the anterior capsule.

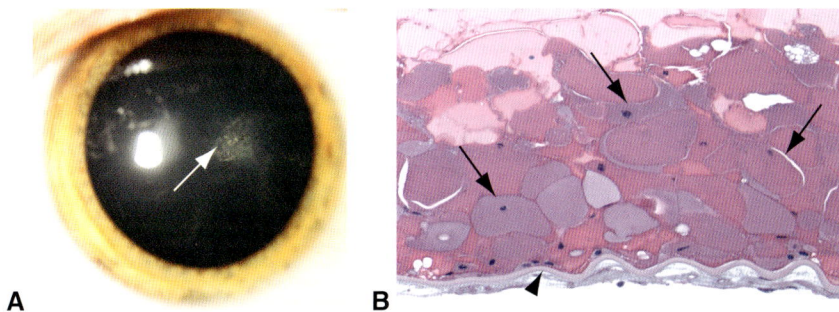

A   **B**

Figure 9-7   Posterior subcapsular cataract. **A,** Cataract *(arrow)* viewed at the slit lamp. **B,** Oval to round nucleated Wedl cells *(arrows)* and smaller lens epithelial cells line the posterior lens capsule *(arrowhead).* (Part A courtesy of Arlene V. Drack, MD; part B courtesy of Robert H. Rosa Jr, MD.)

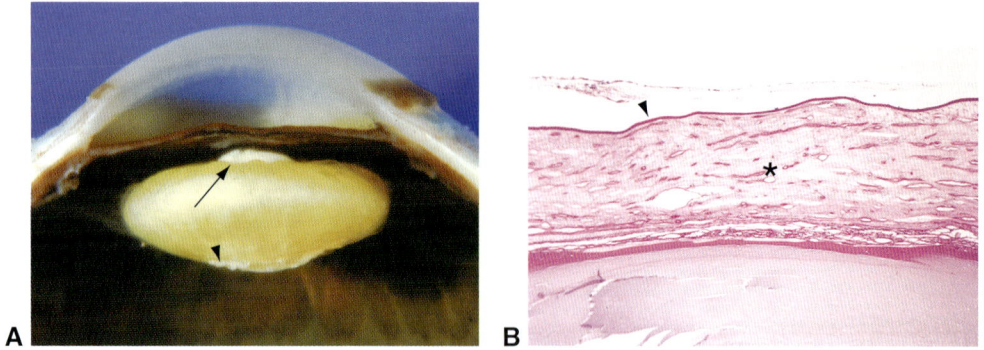

Figure 9-8 Anterior and posterior subcapsular cataracts. **A,** Gross photograph shows white anterior *(arrow)* and posterior *(arrowhead)* subcapsular plaques located centrally. **B,** A fibrous plaque *(asterisk)* is present internal to the original lens capsule *(arrowhead). (Part A courtesy of Tatyana Milman, MD; part B courtesy of Hans E. Grossniklaus, MD.)*

Following resolution of the inciting stimulus, the lens epithelium may produce another capsule, thereby completely surrounding the fibrous plaque and creating what is called a *duplication cataract* (Fig 9-8B).

Disruption of the lens capsule often results in proliferation of lens epithelial cells. For example, following extracapsular cataract extraction, remaining epithelial cells can proliferate and cover the inner surface of the posterior lens capsule, resulting in clinically appreciable posterior capsule opacification. These accumulations of proliferating epithelial cells may form partially transparent globular masses, referred to as *Elschnig pearls* (Fig 9-9), which are histologically identical to Wedl cells. Sequestration of proliferating lens fibers in the equatorial region may create a doughnut-shaped remnant, known as a *Soemmering ring secondary cataract* (Fig 9-10).

Severe elevation of intraocular pressure can damage lens epithelial cells, leading to cell degeneration. Clinically, patches of white flecks *(glaukomflecken)* are observed beneath

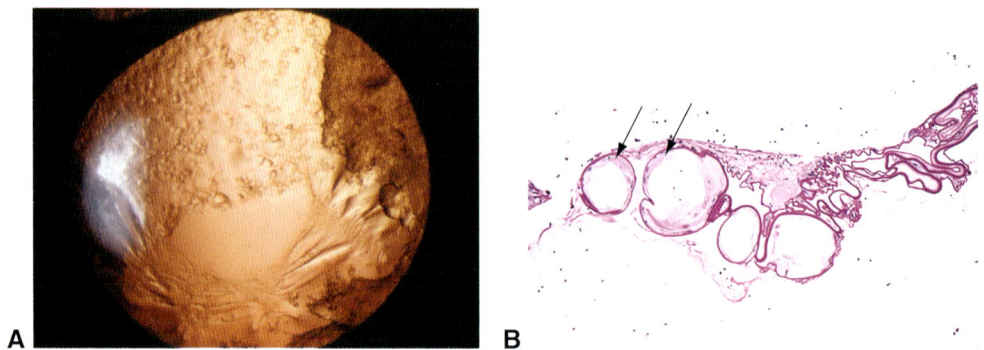

Figure 9-9 Elschnig pearls. **A,** Clinical appearance with slit-lamp retroillumination, demonstrating numerous cystic posterior capsule opacities behind the lens implant. **B,** Photomicrograph depicts proliferating lens epithelium *(arrows)* on remnants of the posterior capsule (PAS stain). *(Part A courtesy of Sander Dubovy, MD; part B courtesy of Nasreen A. Syed, MD.)*

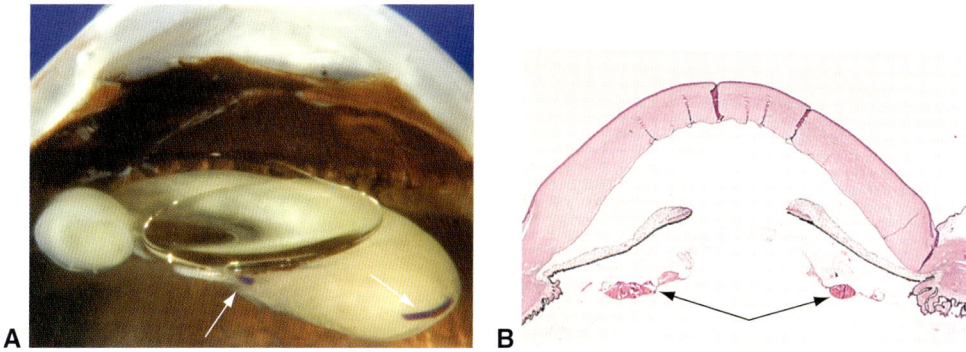

Figure 9-10 Soemmering ring secondary cataract. **A,** Doughnut-shaped white cataractous material is present in the equatorial region of the lens capsule and surrounds a lens haptic *(arrows)*. The lens optic and a second haptic are positioned in front of the lens capsular bag, in the sulcus. **B,** Photomicrograph shows accumulation of lens protein in the residual equatorial lens capsule *(arrows)*. *(Part A courtesy of Tatyana Milman, MD.)*

the anterior lens capsule. Histologic examination shows focal areas of necrotic lens epithelial cells, often with associated degenerated cortical material. See also BCSC Section 10, *Glaucoma.*

Retention of iron-containing metallic foreign bodies in the eye or long-standing intraocular hemorrhage may result in iron deposition in the lens epithelial cells from siderosis or hemosiderosis. The iron is toxic to the epithelial cells. The presence of iron within the epithelial cells can be demonstrated with Perls Prussian blue stain.

Cortex

Clinically, cortical degenerative changes fall into 2 broad categories: (1) generalized discolorations with loss of transparency; and (2) focal opacifications. Generalized loss of transparency cannot be reliably diagnosed histologically; the histologic stains used to colorize the lens tissue after it is processed prevent the assessment of lens clarity. The earliest sign of focal cortical degeneration is hydropic swelling of the lens fibers with decreased intensity of eosinophilic staining. Focal cortical opacities become more apparent when fiber degeneration is advanced enough to cause liquefactive change. Light microscopy shows the accumulation of eosinophilic globules (morgagnian globules) in slitlike spaces between the lens fibers (Fig 9-11; see also Fig 9-12C). As focal cortical lesions progress, these spaces become confluent and form globular collections of lens protein. Ultimately, the entire cortex can become liquefied, allowing the nucleus to sink inferiorly and the capsule to wrinkle; this condition is referred to as *morgagnian cataract* (Fig 9-12).

Nucleus

In the adult lens, the continual production of lens fibers subjects the nucleus to the stress of mechanical compression, which causes hardening of the lens nucleus. Aging is also associated with alterations in the chemical composition of the nuclear fibers that contribute to changes in color and refractive index. The pathogenesis of nuclear discoloration is poorly understood and probably involves more than one mechanism, including accumulation of

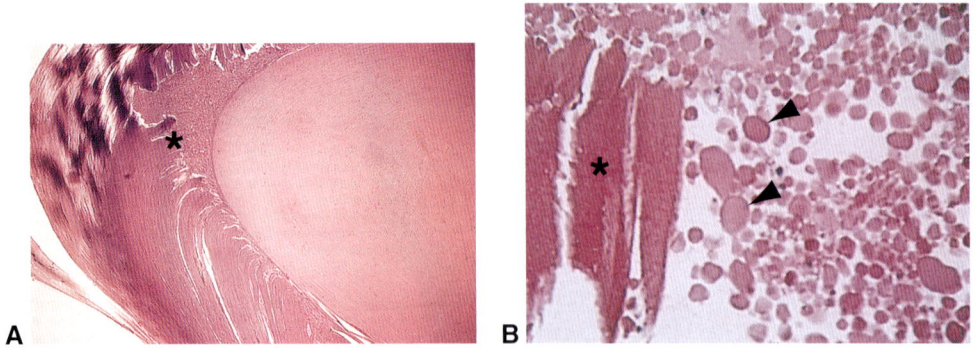

Figure 9-11 Cataract. **A,** Extensive cortical changes are present *(asterisk)*. **B,** Cortical degeneration. Lens cell fibers *(asterisk)* are swollen and fragmented. Note the morgagnian globules *(arrowheads)*. The lenticular fragments, which are opaque, increase osmotic pressure within the capsule. *(Courtesy of Hans E. Grossniklaus, MD.)*

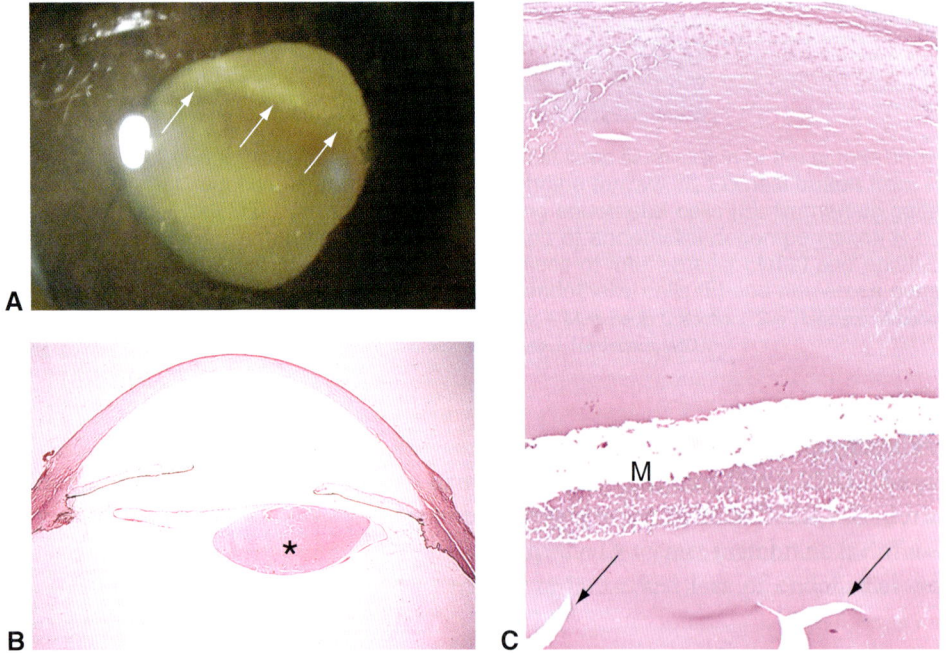

Figure 9-12 Morgagnian cataract. **A,** The brunescent nucleus has sunk inferiorly within the liquefied cortex. *Arrows* mark the superior edge of the nucleus. **B,** The lens cortex has liquefied, leaving the lens nucleus *(asterisk)* floating freely within the capsular bag. **C,** Artifactitious, sharply angulated clefts *(arrows)* are present in this nuclear sclerotic cataract. A zone of morgagnian globules (M) is visible. *(Part A courtesy of Bradford Tannen, MD; part B courtesy of Debra J. Shetlar, MD.)*

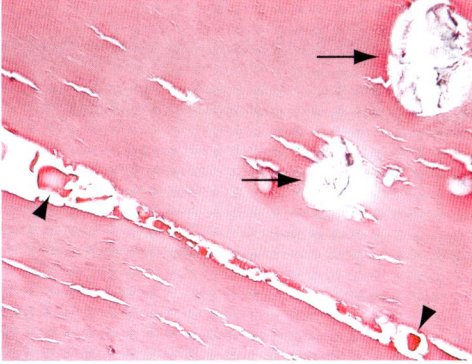

Figure 9-13 Crystalline deposits of calcium oxalate *(arrows)* are visible within the lens. Also apparent is a cortical cleft with morgagnian globules *(arrowheads)*. *(Courtesy of Tatyana Milman, MD.)*

urochrome pigment. Clinically, the lens nucleus may appear yellow, brunescent, or dark brown.

Nuclear cataracts are difficult to assess histologically because they take on a subtle homogeneous eosinophilic appearance. Clinically, the loss of laminations (artifactitious clefts) probably correlates better with nuclear firmness than it does with optical opacification (see Fig 9-12C). Occasionally, crystalline deposits, identified as calcium oxalate, may be observed within a nuclear cataract (Fig 9-13). These deposits are birefringent under polarized light. It is postulated that oxidative DNA damage to lens epithelial cells may contribute to age-related nuclear cataract.

Zonular fibers

Deposition of abnormal protein on the lens zonular fibers in *pseudoexfoliation syndrome* (also called *exfoliation syndrome*) can lead to degeneration of these fibers and their eventual dehiscence. See Chapter 7 in this volume for additional discussion of pseudoexfoliation syndrome. See also Chapter 5 in BCSC Section 11, *Lens and Cataract.*

Neoplasia and Associations With Systemic Disorders

There are no reported cases of neoplasms arising in the human lens. Premature opacification of the lens has been observed in many systemic disorders. See BCSC Section 11, *Lens and Cataract.*

Pathology in Intraocular Lenses

See BCSC Section 11, *Lens and Cataract,* for a discussion of this topic.

CHAPTER 10

Vitreous

Highlights

- A variety of developmental anomalies can occur in the vitreous. These range from Mittendorf dot and Bergmeister papilla to persistent fetal vasculature.
- Inflammation in the vitreous body can be a sign of potentially sight-threatening processes.
- Posterior vitreous detachment plays an important role in the development of many retinal conditions.
- Primary intraocular lymphoma generally presents as cells in the vitreous and may be a challenging diagnosis to make with routine cytology. This diagnosis usually requires special pathologic techniques, communication between the surgeon and pathologist regarding specimen handling, and a pathologist experienced with vitreous pathology.

Topography

The vitreous humor makes up most of the volume of the globe and is important in many diseases that affect the eye (Fig 10-1). The vitreous body is divided into 2 main topographic areas: the central, or core, vitreous; and the peripheral, or cortical, vitreous. See BCSC Section 2, *Fundamentals and Principles of Ophthalmology,* and Section 12, *Retina and Vitreous,* for discussion of the anatomy of the vitreous. The strength of vitreoretinal adhesion or attachment is important in the pathogenesis of retinal tears and detachment, macular hole formation, and vitreous hemorrhage from neovascularization.

The embryologic development of the vitreous is generally divided into 3 stages: primary, secondary, and tertiary (see Figure 4-11 in BCSC Section 2, *Fundamentals and Principles of Ophthalmology*). The *primary vitreous* consists of fibrillar material, mesenchymal cells, and vascular components (hyaloid artery, vasa hyaloidea propria, and tunica vasculosa lentis [see Fig 4-3 in BCSC Section 11, *Lens and Cataract*]). The *secondary vitreous* begins to form at approximately the ninth week of gestation and is destined to become the main portion of the vitreous in the postnatal and adult eye. The primary vitreous atrophies with formation of the secondary vitreous, leaving only a clear central zone through the vitreous (called the *hyaloid canal,* or *Cloquet canal*) and its anterior extension, the hyaloideocapsular ligament (also known as *ligament of Weiger*) (see Fig 10-1). The secondary vitreous is relatively acellular and completely avascular. It is composed of thin collagen fibrils and hyaluronic acid

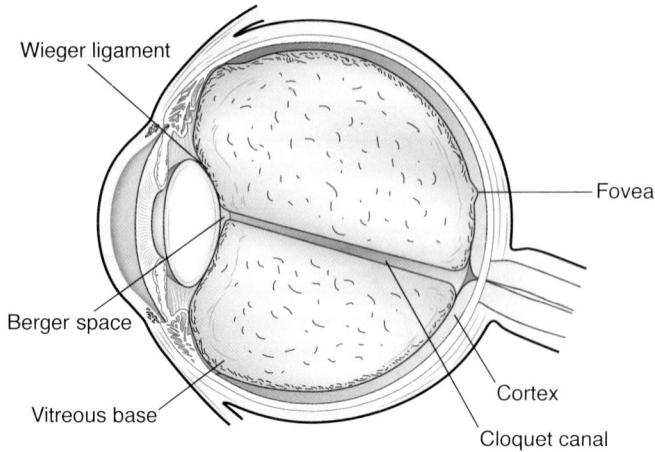

Figure 10-1 Schematic of the topography of the vitreous body demonstrating distribution of the collagen fibrils *(lines)* at the vitreous base, at the cortex, in the macular region, and at the optic nerve head. *(Illustration by Cyndie C. H. Wooley.)*

(hyaluronan), which is extremely hydrophilic. Although the vitreous cavity typically appears empty on routine histologic sections, the hyaluronic acid will stain with alcian blue. The rare cells present in the secondary vitreous are called *hyalocytes.* The lens zonular fibers (also referred to as the *zonule of Zinn*) represent the *tertiary vitreous.*

Developmental Anomalies

Persistent Fetal Vasculature

Persistent fetal vasculature (PFV; previously known as *persistent hyperplastic primary vitreous*) is characterized by the persistence of variable components of the primary vitreous and is most often unilateral. In most cases of clinically significant PFV, a fibrovascular plaque in the retrolental space extends laterally to involve the ciliary processes, which may be pulled toward the visual axis by traction from the fibrovascular tissue. The clinical and gross appearance of elongated ciliary processes results. The anterior fibrovascular plaque is generally contiguous posteriorly with a remnant of the hyaloid artery that may attach to the optic nerve head (optic disc) (Fig 10-2). Involvement of the posterior structures may be more extensive, with detachment of the peripapillary retina resulting from traction caused by preretinal membranes. The lens is often cataractous, and the posterior capsule may be discontinuous. Eyes affected by the more severe forms of PFV are often microphthalmic. See also Chapter 19 in this volume, BCSC Section 6, *Pediatric Ophthalmology and Strabismus,* and Section 12, *Retina and Vitreous.*

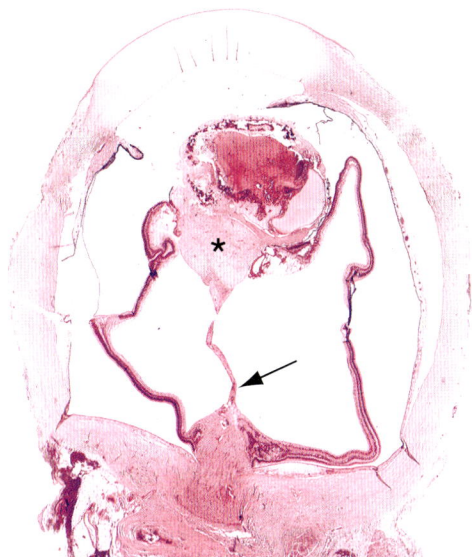

Figure 10-2 Persistent fetal vasculature. The photomicrograph shows a prominent anterior fibrovascular plaque adherent to the lens *(asterisk)*. The lens is distorted, and the peripheral retina is adherent to the plaque. The persistent remnant of the hyaloid artery is seen as a stalk traversing the vitreous cavity and attaching to the optic nerve head posteriorly *(arrow)*. *(Courtesy of Nasreen A. Syed, MD.)*

Bergmeister Papilla

The persistence of a small part of the posterior portion of the hyaloid artery is referred to as *Bergmeister papilla*. This anomaly generally takes the form of a veil-like structure or a fingerlike projection extending anteriorly from the surface of the optic nerve head (Fig 10-3). Retinal vessels may grow into a Bergmeister papilla and then return to the optic nerve head, creating prepapillary vascular loops (see Figure 17-9 in BCSC Section 12, *Retina and Vitreous*).

Mittendorf Dot

The hyaloid artery connects with the tunica vasculosa lentis just inferior and nasal to the center of the lens in utero. With regression of these vascular structures, a nodular mass of tissue may remain on the posterior lens capsule and appear as a focal posterior lens opacity at this site. This nodule is referred to as *Mittendorf dot* (see Figure 4-6 in BCSC Section 11, *Lens and Cataract*).

Vitreous Cysts

Vitreous cysts generally occur in eyes with no other pathologic findings, but they have been noted in retinitis pigmentosa and uveitis, as well as in eyes with remnants of the hyaloid system. These cysts may be clear, or they may be pigmented owing to the presence of pigment epithelium. Histologic studies have suggested the presence of hyaloid remnants in vitreous cysts. The exact origin of the cysts is not known.

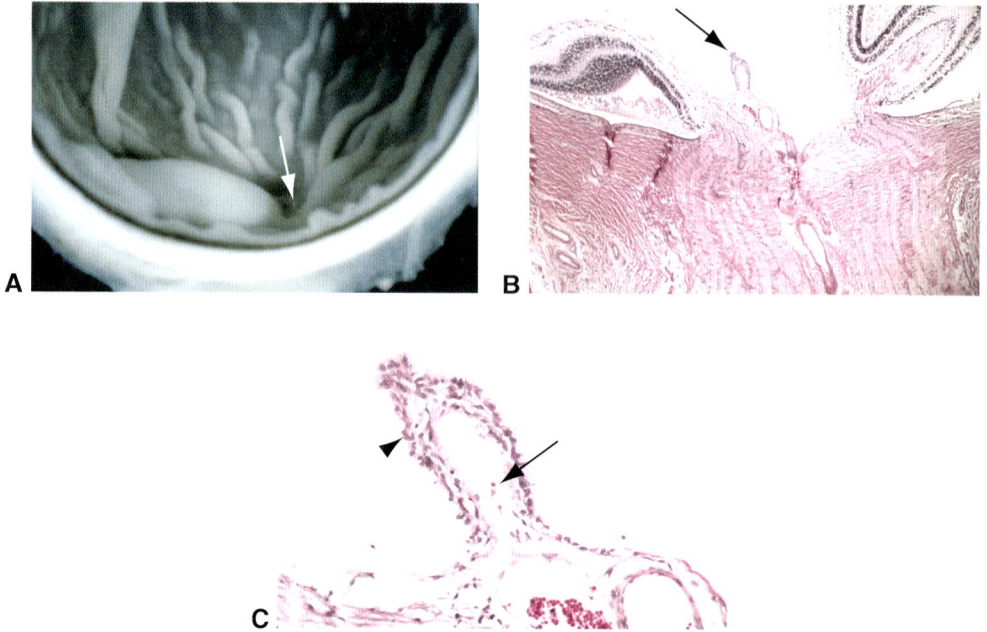

Figure 10-3 Bergmeister papilla. **A,** Gross photograph of an infant eye showing a fingerlike projection of whitish tissue *(arrow)* from the surface of the optic nerve head. **B,** Low-magnification photomicrograph of part **A** showing fibroglial tissue *(arrow)* projecting into the vitreous cavity from the optic nerve head. **C,** High-magnification photomicrograph of Bergmeister papilla demonstrating loose fibrous connective tissue with a small capillary *(arrow),* surrounded by a thin layer of fibrous astrocyte-like cells *(arrowhead). (Courtesy of Robert H. Rosa Jr, MD.)*

Inflammation

As a relatively acellular and completely avascular structure, the vitreous is generally not a primary site for the initiation of inflammatory disorders. It does become involved secondarily in inflammatory conditions of adjacent tissues, however. The term *vitritis* is used to denote the presence of benign or malignant white blood cells in the vitreous.

Vitreous inflammation associated with infectious agents, particularly bacteria and fungi, is clinically referred to as *infectious endophthalmitis.* Bacterial endophthalmitis and fungal endophthalmitis (Fig 10-4) are characterized by neutrophilic infiltration of the vitreous that leads to liquefaction of the vitreous, with subsequent posterior vitreous detachment. Fungal endophthalmitis may have a granulomatous component. Severe inflammation may be accompanied by formation of fibrocellular membranes, typically in the retrolental space; these may exert traction on the peripheral retina.

The vitreous infiltrate in noninfectious uveitis is typically composed of chronic inflammatory cells, including T and B lymphocytes and histiocytes (Fig 10-5). See also BCSC Section 9, *Uveitis and Ocular Inflammation.*

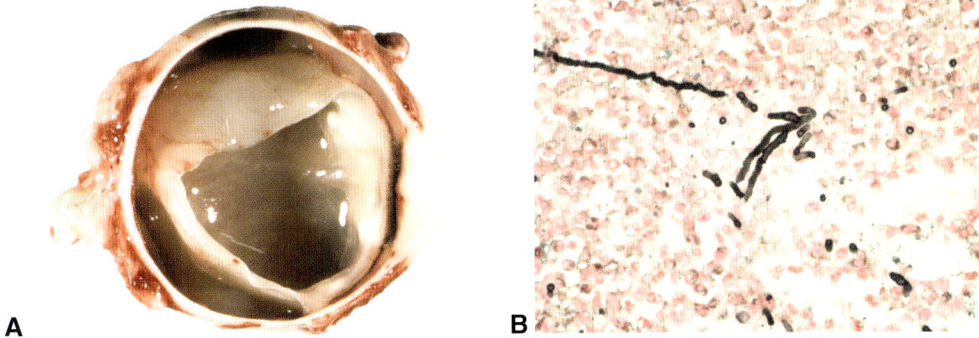

Figure 10-4 Endophthalmitis. **A,** Gross photograph showing opacification and infiltration of the vitreous by inflammatory cells as a result of fungal endophthalmitis. **B,** Photomicrograph showing fungal organisms and cellular infiltration of the vitreous in endophthalmitis. *(Courtesy of Steffen Heegaard, MD.)*

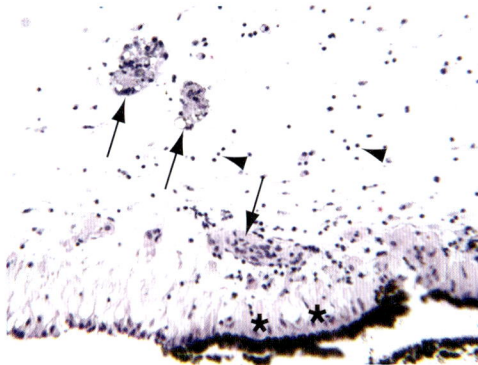

Figure 10-5 Noninfectious uveitis. Aggregates of epithelioid histiocytes *(arrows)* and scattered lymphocytes *(arrowheads)* in the vitreous base overlying the pigmented and nonpigmented ciliary epithelium *(asterisks)*. *(Courtesy of Tatyana Milman, MD.)*

Degenerations

Syneresis and Aging

Syneresis of the vitreous refers to liquefaction and collapse of the gel. Syneresis of the central vitreous is a nearly universal consequence of aging. It also occurs as a result of vitreous inflammation and hemorrhage and in the setting of significant axial myopia. The prominent lamellae and strands that develop in the aging eye and following inflammation or hemorrhage are the result of abnormally aggregated collagenous vitreous fibrils around syneretic pockets of hyaluronate (Fig 10-6). Syneresis is one of the contributing factors leading to vitreous detachment.

Posterior Vitreous Detachment

Posterior vitreous detachment (PVD) occurs when a dehiscence in the vitreous cortex allows fluid from a syneretic cavity to enter the potential subhyaloid space, causing the remaining

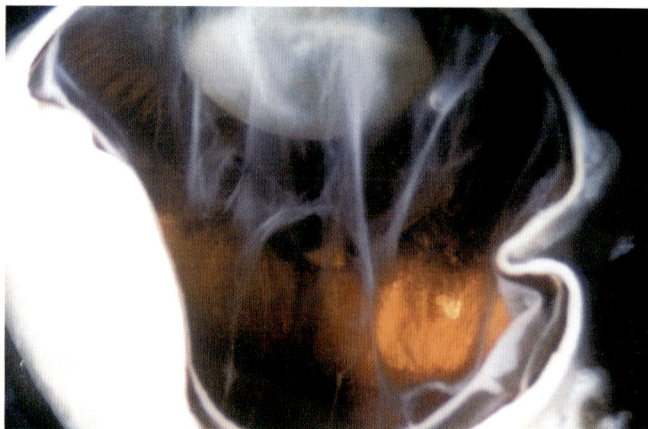

Figure 10-6 Gross photograph demonstrates vitreous condensations outlining syneretic cavities. *(Courtesy of Hans E. Grossniklaus, MD.)*

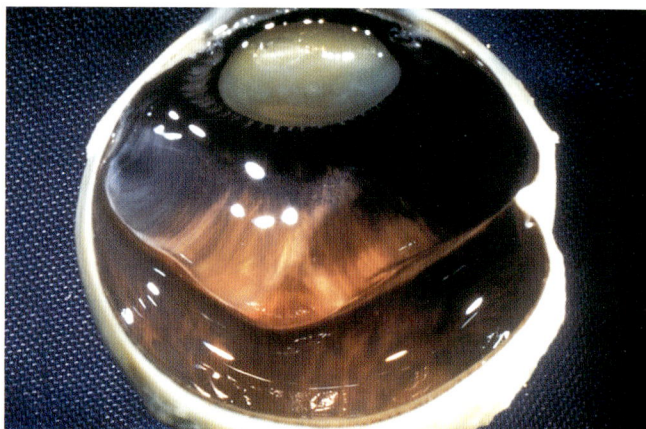

Figure 10-7 Gross photograph showing a posterior vitreous detachment. Retraction of the vitreous from the posterior retina is seen. *(Courtesy of Hans E. Grossniklaus, MD.)*

hyaloid face to be stripped from the internal limiting membrane (ILM) of the retina (Fig 10-7). As fluid drains out of the syneretic cavities under the newly formed posterior hyaloid, the vitreous body collapses anteriorly, remaining attached at its base. Vitreous detachment generally occurs rapidly over the course of a few hours to days. Occasionally, traction may occur on the peripheral retina, perifoveal macula, or retinal blood vessels as a PVD occurs.

An age-related weakening of the adherence of the cortical vitreous to the ILM also plays a role in PVDs. The prevalence of PVD in individuals aged 70 years and older has been reported as 50% or higher in clinical and pathologic studies. The incidence of PVD is increased in persons with intraocular inflammation, aphakia or pseudophakia, trauma, myopia, or vitreoretinal diseases. PVD is important in the pathogenesis of many conditions, including retinal tears and detachment, macular hole formation, and vitreous hemorrhage. See BCSC Section 12, *Retina and Vitreous,* for additional discussion of these conditions.

Retinal tears and potential sequelae

Retinal tears (breaks) are often the result of vitreous traction on the retina during or after a PVD or secondary to ocular trauma. Tears are most likely to occur at sites of greatest vitreoretinal adhesion, such as the vitreous base (Fig 10-8) or the margin of lattice degeneration. The vitreous base extends anteriorly from the ora serrata (approximately 2 mm) over the ciliary body, and posteriorly (about 4 mm) over the peripheral retina. Histologic examination of retinal tears reveals that the vitreous adheres to the retina along the flap of the tear. In the area of retina separated from the underlying retinal pigment epithelium (RPE), there is loss of photoreceptors.

Rhegmatogenous retinal detachment (RRD) occurs when vitreous traction and fluid currents resulting from eye movements combine to overcome the forces maintaining retinal adhesion to the RPE. With an RRD, cellular membranes may form on either surface (anterior or posterior) of the retina (Fig 10-9). Clinically, this process is referred to as *proliferative vitreoretinopathy (PVR)*. These membranes, which often have a contractile

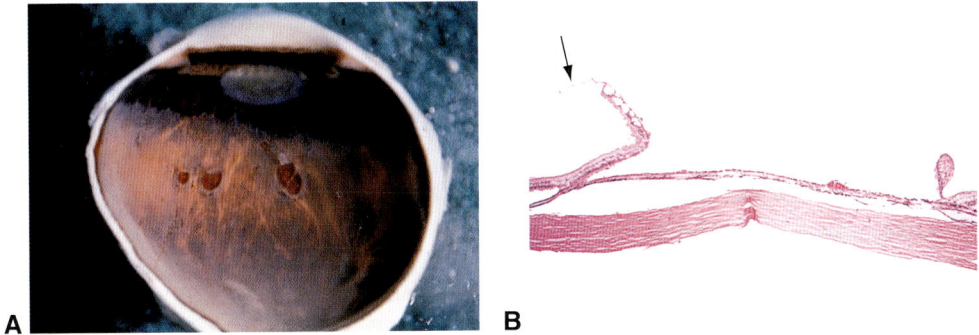

Figure 10-8 Peripheral retinal tears. **A,** The gross photograph shows several retinal tears at the vitreous base. **B,** The photomicrograph demonstrates condensed vitreous *(arrow)* attached to the anterior flap of the retinal tear. *(Courtesy of W. Richard Green, MD.)*

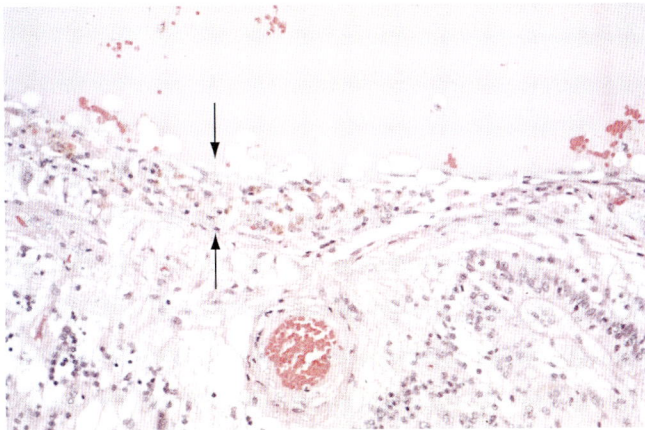

Figure 10-9 Preretinal membrane *(area between arrows)* on the surface of the retina, secondary to proliferative vitreoretinopathy. *(Courtesy of David J. Wilson, MD.)*

component, form as a result of proliferation of RPE cells and other cellular elements, including glial cells (Müller cells, fibrous astrocytes), histiocytes, fibroblasts, myofibroblasts, and possibly hyalocytes. The cell biology of PVR is complex and involves the interaction of various growth factors and integrins, as well as cellular proliferation. Studies have shown a significant association between clinical grades of PVR and the expression levels of specific cytokines and/or growth factors in the vitreous fluid.

Garweg JG, Tappeiner C, Halberstadt M. Pathophysiology of proliferative vitreoretinopathy in retinal detachment. *Surv Ophthalmol.* 2013;58(4):321–329.

Macular holes

Idiopathic macular holes most likely form as the result of degenerative changes in the vitreous. Optical coherence tomography (OCT) has greatly advanced our understanding of the anatomical features of full-thickness macular holes and early macular hole formation. The results of these studies are most consistent with a focal vitreomacular traction mechanism. Localized perifoveal vitreous detachment (an early stage of age-related PVD) appears to be the primary pathogenetic event in idiopathic macular hole formation (Fig 10-10). Detachment of the posterior hyaloid from the pericentral retina exerts anterior traction on the foveola and localizes the dynamic vitreous traction associated with ocular rotations into the perifoveolar region.

OCT has clarified the pathogenesis of macular holes, particularly the early stages: a foveal pseudocyst (stage 1A) is typically followed by disruption of the outer retina (stage 1B) before progressing to a full-thickness dehiscence (stage 2). Histologically, full-thickness macular holes are similar to holes in other locations. A full-thickness retinal defect with rounded tissue margins (stage 3) is accompanied by loss of the photoreceptor outer segments in adjacent retina, which is separated from the RPE by subretinal fluid (see Fig 10-10C). An epiretinal membrane composed of Müller cells, fibrous astrocytes, and myofibroblasts is often present on the surface of the retina adjacent to the macular hole. Cystoid macular edema in the parafoveal retina adjacent to the full-thickness macular hole is relatively common. Following surgical repair of macular holes, closer apposition of the remaining photoreceptors and variable glial scarring close the macular defect. See BCSC Section 12, *Retina and Vitreous,* for further discussion.

Smiddy WE, Flynn HW Jr. Pathogenesis of macular holes and therapeutic implications. *Am J Ophthalmol.* 2004;137(3):525–537.

Steel DHW, Lotery AJ. Idiopathic vitreomacular traction and macular hole: a comprehensive review of pathophysiology, diagnosis, and treatment. *Eye.* 2013;27(Suppl 1):S1–S21.

Hemorrhage

A constellation of pathologic features may develop in the vitreous following vitreous hemorrhage. After 3–10 days, red blood cell clots undergo fibrinolysis, and red blood cells may diffuse throughout the vitreous cavity. At this time, red blood cell breakdown may also occur. Denaturation of hemoglobin in the red blood cells produces ghost cells (see Chapter 7, Fig 7-12) and hemoglobin spherules. Obstruction of the trabecular meshwork by these cells may lead to *ghost cell glaucoma.* See also BCSC Section 10, *Glaucoma.*

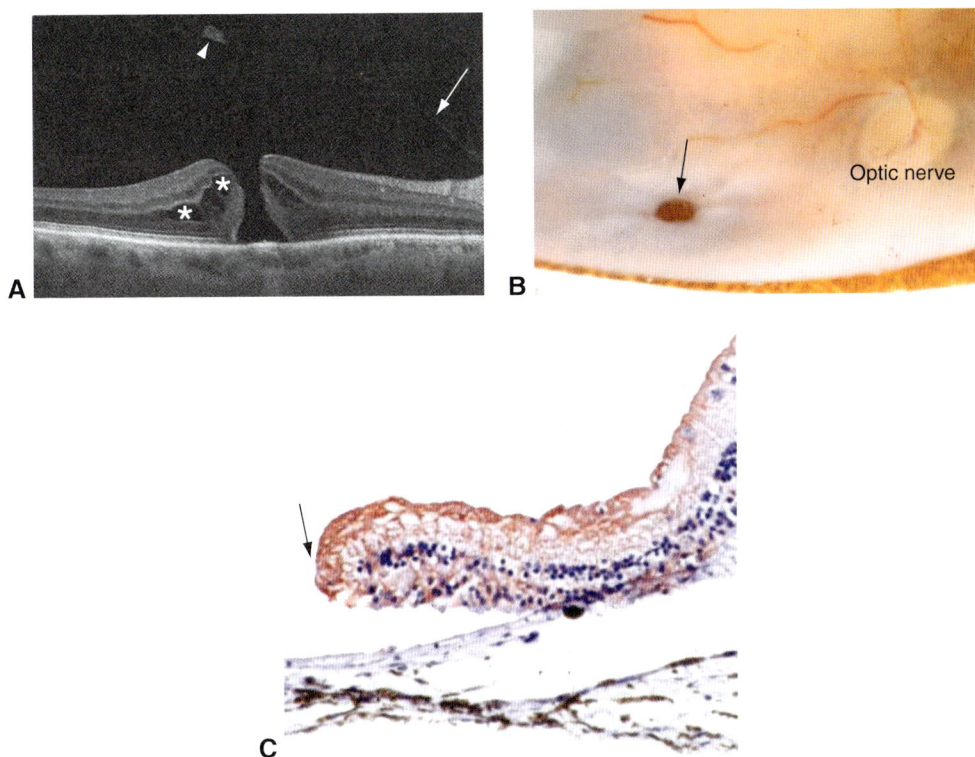

Figure 10-10 Macular holes. **A,** Spectral-domain optical coherence tomography (SD-OCT) image showing a stage 3 macular hole with full-thickness retinal defect, rounded margins, cystoid macular edema *(asterisks)*, and an operculum *(arrowhead)*. Note the posterior hyaloid face *(arrow)* tethered to the peripapillary retina near the optic nerve head. **B,** Gross photograph demonstrating a full-thickness macular hole *(arrow)*. **C,** Photomicrograph of the edge of a full-thickness macular hole showing a rounded gliotic margin *(arrow)* with positive brown staining for glial fibrillary acidic protein (GFAP), highlighting the Müller cells and fibrous astrocytes. *(Part A courtesy of Robert H. Rosa Jr, MD; parts B and C courtesy of Patricia Chévez-Barrios, MD.)*

The process of red blood cell dissolution attracts histiocytes, which phagocytose the degenerate red blood cells. Ferric iron (Fe^{3+}) is released during hemoglobin breakdown. This can occur intracellularly in histiocytes with iron storage as ferritin or hemosiderin, or extracellularly with iron binding to vitreous proteins such as lactoferrin and transferrin. In massive hemorrhages, cholesterol may deposit in the vitreous in the form of cholesterol crystals, which result from the breakdown of red blood cell membranes. Clinically, cholesterol appears as refractile crystals in the vitreous cavity (synchysis scintillans); the crystals are typically not attached to vitreous fibrils. Syneresis of the vitreous and PVD are common after vitreous hemorrhage.

Asteroid Hyalosis

Asteroid hyalosis is a condition with a dramatic clinical appearance (see Fig 17-12 in BCSC Section 12, *Retina and Vitreous*) but little clinical significance. Histologically, asteroid

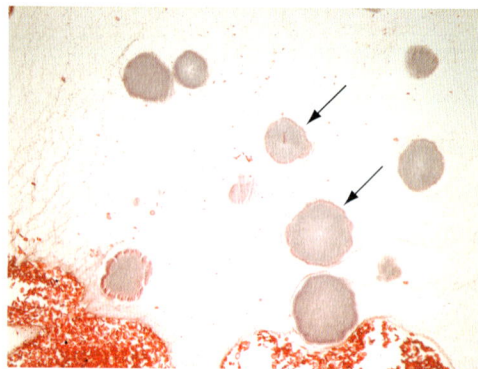

Figure 10-11 Asteroid bodies *(arrows)* and erythrocytic debris within the vitreous. *(Courtesy of Tatyana Milman, MD.)*

bodies are rounded structures measuring 10–100 nm, typically attached to vitreous fibrils (Fig 10-11). The bodies are basophilic with hematoxylin-eosin stain. They are usually positive with stains for calcium such as alizarin red and von Kossa. Occasionally, they will be surrounded by a foreign body giant cell reaction, but the condition is not generally associated with vitreous inflammation.

Studies have shown that asteroid bodies are composed of complex lipids and also have a component with structural and elemental similarity to hydroxyapatite, a calcium phosphate complex.

> Khoshnevis M, Rosen S, Sebag J. Asteroid hyalosis—a comprehensive review. *Surv Ophthalmol.* 2019;64(4):452–462.

Vitreous Amyloidosis

The term *amyloidosis* refers to a group of diseases that lead to extracellular deposition of amyloid. Amyloid is a group of proteins that have in common a characteristic ultrastructural appearance of nonbranching fibrils with variable length and a diameter of 7–10 nm. The proteins forming amyloid can form a tertiary structure known as a *β-pleated sheet,* which enables the proteins to bind Congo red stain and show birefringence under polarized light (Fig 10-12).

The type of amyloid protein that is deposited and the location of the deposition depend on the etiology of the underlying condition. Amyloid deposition can occur in the vitreous when the protein forming the amyloid is *transthyretin.* Multiple genetic mutations can result in various amino acid substitutions in the transthyretin protein and allow for a conformational change to a β-pleated sheet. The most common mutations were originally described in *familial amyloid polyneuropathy (FAP).* Systemic manifestations in patients with FAP include vitreous opacities and perivascular infiltrates (Fig 10-13), peripheral neuropathy, cardiomyopathy, and carpal tunnel syndrome. If amyloid protein is identified in the vitreous, referral to evaluate for systemic disease should be considered.

The mechanism by which the vitreous becomes involved is not known with certainty. Because amyloid deposits are found within the walls of retinal vessels and in the RPE and ciliary body, amyloid may gain access to the vitreous through these tissues. In addition,

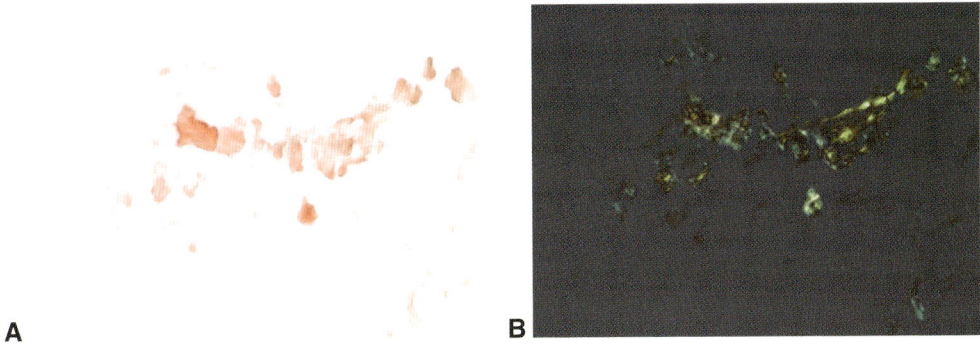

Figure 10-12 Amyloid of the vitreous. **A,** Congo red–stained material, aspirated from the vitreous, shows red-orange staining. **B,** Photomicrograph of the material shown in part **A** under polarized light; the material exhibits apple-green birefringence (dichroism). *(Courtesy of Nasreen A. Syed, MD.)*

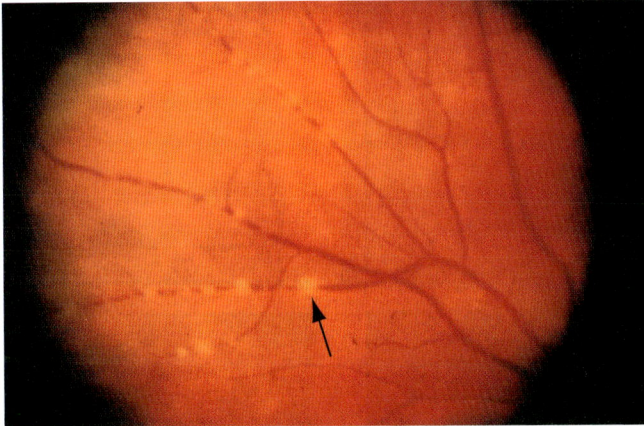

Figure 10-13 Perivascular sheathing of retinal vessels *(arrow)* associated with vitreous amyloidosis. *(Courtesy of Hans E. Grossniklaus, MD.)*

because transthyretin is a blood protein, it may gain access to the vitreous by crossing the blood–aqueous or blood–retina barrier.

Neoplasia

Intraocular Lymphoma

Primary neoplastic involvement of the vitreous is uncommon because of the relatively acellular nature of the vitreous. However, the vitreous can be the site of primary involvement in cases of large cell lymphoma, which has been referred to as *primary intraocular lymphoma (PIOL)* and *vitreoretinal lymphoma*. Immunohistochemical and molecular genetic studies have confirmed that this entity is typically a B-cell lymphoma; however, T-cell lymphomas may occur in rare instances.

Clinically, PIOL presents most commonly as a vitritis. Some patients have sub-RPE infiltrates with a characteristic speckled pigmentation overlying tumor detachments of the RPE (Fig 10-14). Evidence suggests that the lymphoma cells may be attracted to the RPE by B-cell chemokines and subsequently migrate from the sub-RPE space into the vitreous. In more than half of patients presenting with ocular findings, the central nervous system is or will become involved. Neuroimaging of the brain is essential in the workup of patients with PIOL (Fig 10-15). See Chapter 20 for more information on the clinical aspects of PIOL.

The diagnosis of PIOL can be challenging and relies primarily on cytologic analysis of vitreous and/or subretinal specimens. Cytologically, the vitreous infiltrate in PIOL is heterogeneous. The atypical cells are large lymphoid cells, frequently with a convoluted nuclear membrane and multiple, conspicuous nucleoli. An accompanying infiltrate of small

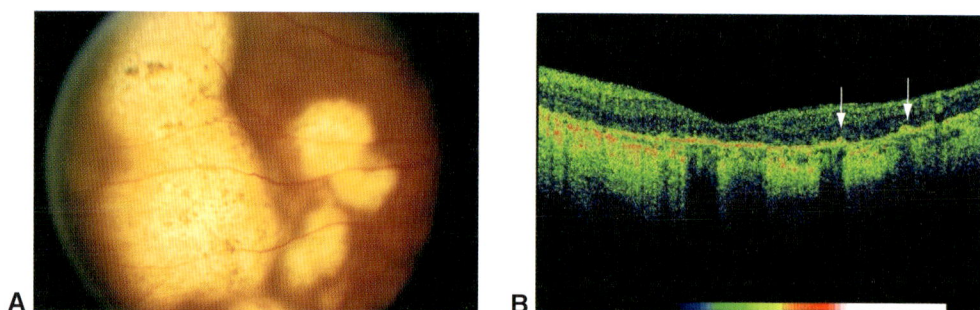

Figure 10-14 Sub-RPE infiltrates in a patient with primary intraocular lymphoma (PIOL). **A,** Note the characteristic speckled pigmentation over the tumor detachments of the RPE. **B,** OCT image shows disruption of the RPE cell layer and tumor cells on top of the RPE cells *(arrows)*. *(Part A courtesy of Robert H. Rosa Jr, MD; part B courtesy of Steffen Heegaard, MD.)*

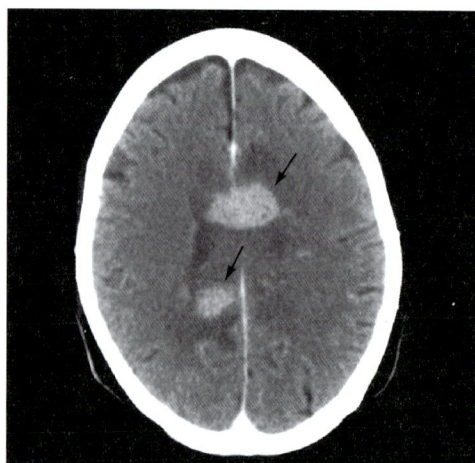

Figure 10-15 Axial computed tomography (CT) scan of the brain showing lymphomatous infiltrates *(arrows)*. *(Courtesy of Steffen Heegaard, MD.)*

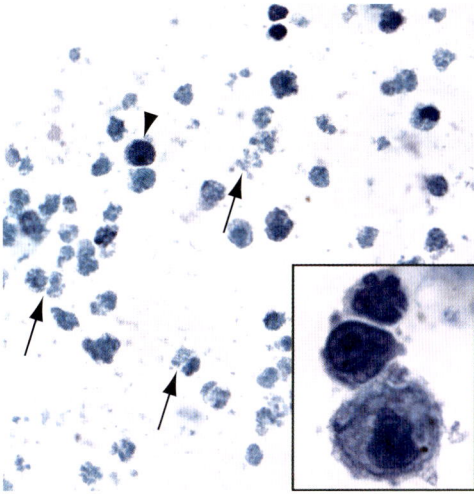

Figure 10-16 Cytologic appearance of PIOL (vitreoretinal lymphoma). Note the atypical cells with hyperchromatic nuclei, prominent nucleoli, and scant cytoplasm *(arrowhead)*. Numerous necrotic, smudgy cells *(arrows)* are present. *Inset:* Atypical lymphoid cells with irregular nuclear contours are shown. *(Courtesy of Robert H. Rosa Jr, MD.)*

lymphocytes is almost always present, and the normal cells may obscure the neoplastic cell population. These small round lymphocytes are mostly reactive T cells. Necrotic cells are usually present, and this feature is very suggestive of a diagnosis of intraocular lymphoma (Fig 10-16). Immunohistochemically, the viable tumor cells typically label with B-cell markers. Flow cytometry may be helpful in demonstrating a monoclonal population. Other laboratory tests that may be useful in the diagnosis of intraocular lymphoma include a panel of immunohistochemical markers (if the amount of tissue is sufficient) and molecular studies for lymphocyte gene rearrangement and translocation, as well as for *MYD88* mutations (found in 69% of cases of PIOL). An interleukin-10 to interleukin-6 ratio that is greater than 1.0 may be useful if this testing is available in the pathology laboratory.

The diagnosis of PIOL relies on good communication between the vitreoretinal surgeon and the pathologist prior to scheduling a biopsy. Each pathology laboratory has its own preferred methods for how a specimen is collected and submitted for pathologic analysis. Also, the amount of tissue in the specimen is usually small, which can be a limiting factor when a diagnosis is being made. To avoid performing multiple biopsies for a definitive diagnosis, the clinician should ensure that the pathologist is experienced with handling and diagnosing PIOL.

The subretinal/sub-RPE infiltrates are composed of neoplastic lymphoid cells. With or without treatment, the subretinal infiltrates may resolve, leaving a focal area of RPE atrophy. Optic nerve and retinal infiltration may also be present. Infiltrates in these locations tend to be perivascular and may lead to ischemic retinal or optic nerve damage. The choroid is typically free of lymphoma cells; however, a secondary reactive population of chronic inflammatory cells may be present in the choroid (Fig 10-17). In the setting of systemic lymphoma with ocular involvement, the choroid (rather than the vitreous, retina, or subretinal space) is usually the primary site of involvement. See Chapter 12 for more information on choroidal lymphoma.

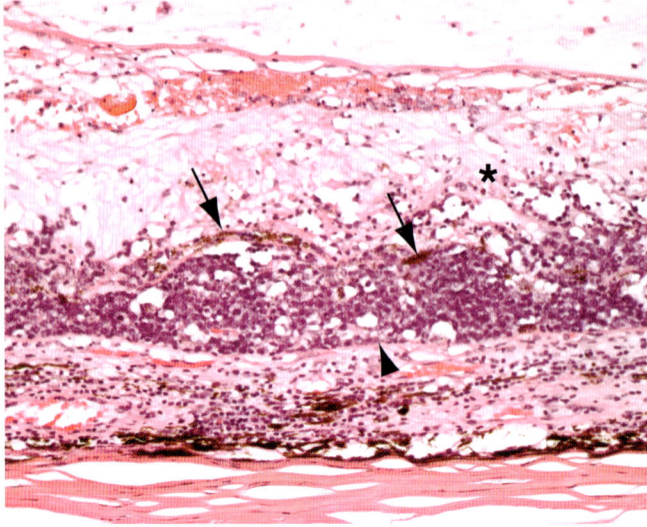

Figure 10-17 Histologic section through retina and choroid showing PIOL. Note the detachment of the RPE by tumor *(arrows)*, the overlying retinal gliosis *(asterisk)*, and the intact Bruch membrane *(arrowhead)*. Secondary chronic inflammation is present in the underlying choroid. *(Courtesy of Robert H. Rosa Jr, MD.)*

Chan CC, Rubenstein JL, Coupland SE, et al. Primary vitreoretinal lymphoma: a report from an International Primary Central Nervous System Lymphoma Collaborative Group symposium. *Oncologist.* 2011;16(11):1589–1599.

Coupland SE. Molecular pathology of lymphoma. *Eye (Lond).* 2013;27(2):180–189.

CHAPTER **11**

Retina and Retinal Pigment Epithelium

▶ *This chapter includes related videos. Go to www.aao.org/bcscvideo_section04 or scan the QR codes in the text to access this content.*

Highlights

- The neurosensory retina has 9 distinct histologic layers; the retinal pigment epithelium lines the outermost of these layers.
- There is a correlation between the clinical appearance and the histologic location of hemorrhage and other deposits in the retina.
- Two vascular sources supply the retina: the retinal circulation supplies the inner layers, and the choroidal circulation supplies the outer layers. Ischemic events involving either vascular source lead to atrophy and thinning of the corresponding retinal layers supplied.
- The retina heals with a fibroglial scar.
- In many cases of infantile abusive head trauma, histologic abnormalities can be identified in the retina.
- Retinoblastoma is the most common primary intraocular malignancy in children and has characteristic histologic features.

Topography

Two distinct layers form the inner lining of the posterior two-thirds of the globe:

- the neurosensory retina, which is a delicate, transparent layer derived from the inner layer of the optic cup
- the retinal pigment epithelium (RPE), which is a pigmented layer derived from the outer layer of the optic cup

The neurosensory retina is considered part of the central nervous system (CNS). It is continuous anteriorly with the nonpigmented ciliary epithelium, whereas the RPE is continuous with the pigmented ciliary epithelium. The RPE terminates posteriorly at the optic nerve head, along with the underlying Bruch membrane. The nuclear, photoreceptor, and synaptic layers of the neurosensory retina gradually taper at the optic nerve head, and

163

only the nerve fiber layer (NFL) continues to become the optic nerve, making a 90° turn posteriorly as it becomes the optic nerve head (optic disc). See BCSC Section 2, *Fundamentals and Principles of Ophthalmology,* and Section 12, *Retina and Vitreous,* for additional information on the anatomy of the retina and RPE.

Neurosensory Retina

The neurosensory retina has 9 distinct histologic layers (Fig 11-1). An additional layer, the middle limiting membrane (MLM), has been described, but it is not a distinct layer on routine histologic sections of the neurosensory retina. On optical coherence tomography (OCT), the photoreceptor inner segment layer appears as several layers because of its innate optical properties: the myoid zone (MZ), which is just external to the external limiting membrane; the ellipsoid zone (EZ), which is closest to the outer segments; and the interdigitation zone (IZ), which is between the outer segments and the RPE (Fig 11-2). The myoid zone contains ribosomes, endoplasmic reticulum, and Golgi bodies, whereas the ellipsoid zone is densely packed with mitochondria of the photoreceptors. In histologic cross sections of the neurosensory retina, the retinal fibers and synaptic processes are arranged perpendicular to the retinal surface, with the exception of the NFL, where

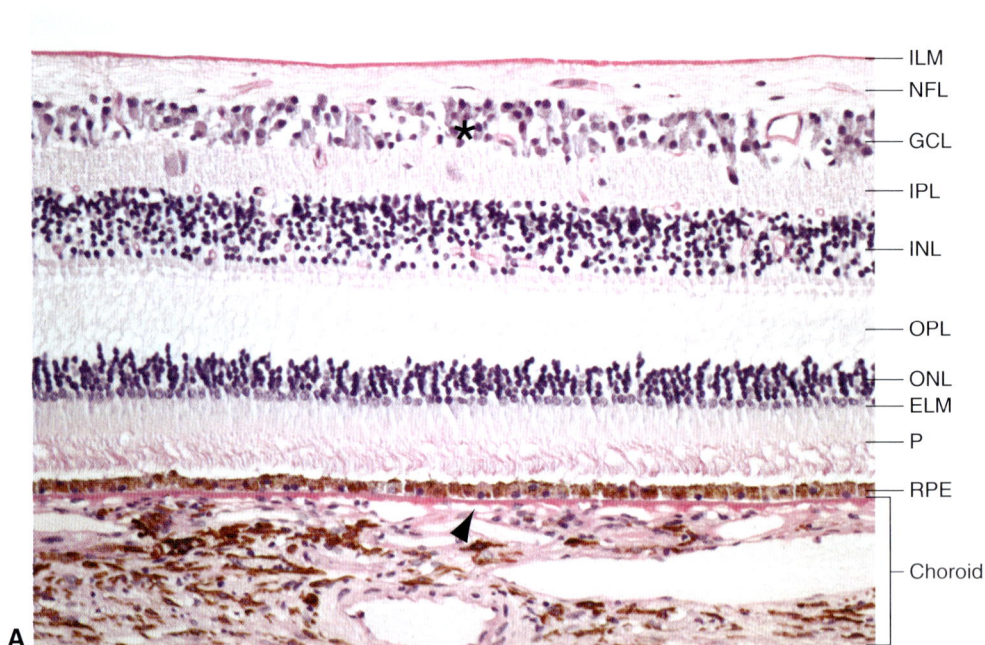

Figure 11-1 Photomicrographs illustrating retinal organization and how it differs depending on location. **A,** Macula, from vitreous *(top of photo)* to choroid *(bottom)*: ILM = internal limiting membrane; NFL = nerve fiber layer; GCL = ganglion cell layer *(asterisk)*; IPL = inner plexiform layer; INL = inner nuclear layer; OPL = outer plexiform layer; ONL = outer nuclear layer; ELM = external limiting membrane; P = photoreceptors (inner/outer segments) of rods and cones; RPE = retinal pigment epithelium; Bruch membrane *(arrowhead)*.

(Continued)

the axons run parallel to the retinal surface and converge at the optic nerve head. Consequently, deposits and hemorrhages in the deep retinal layers have a round appearance clinically as they displace the perpendicularly arranged fibers, whereas those in the NFL have a feathery or splinter-shaped appearance (Video 11-1).

> ▶ **VIDEO 11-1** Appearance of blood in various retinal layers.
> *Developed by Vivian Lee, MD.*
> Go to www.aao.org/bcscvideo_section04 to access all videos in Section 4.

The morphology of the retina varies depending on the region. For example, histologically, the *macula* is the area of the retina where the ganglion cell layer (GCL) is thicker than a single cell (see Fig 11-1A). Clinically, this area corresponds approximately with the area of the retina bounded by the inferior and superior major temporal vascular arcades. The center of the macula is further subdivided into the *fovea,* the central 1.5 mm of the macula, and the *foveola,* a small pit in the center of the fovea. The foveola contains only cone photoreceptor cells; ganglion cells, other nucleated cells (including Müller cells), and blood vessels are not present (see Fig 11-1E). The concentration of cones is greater in the macula than in the peripheral retina, and only cones are present in the fovea.

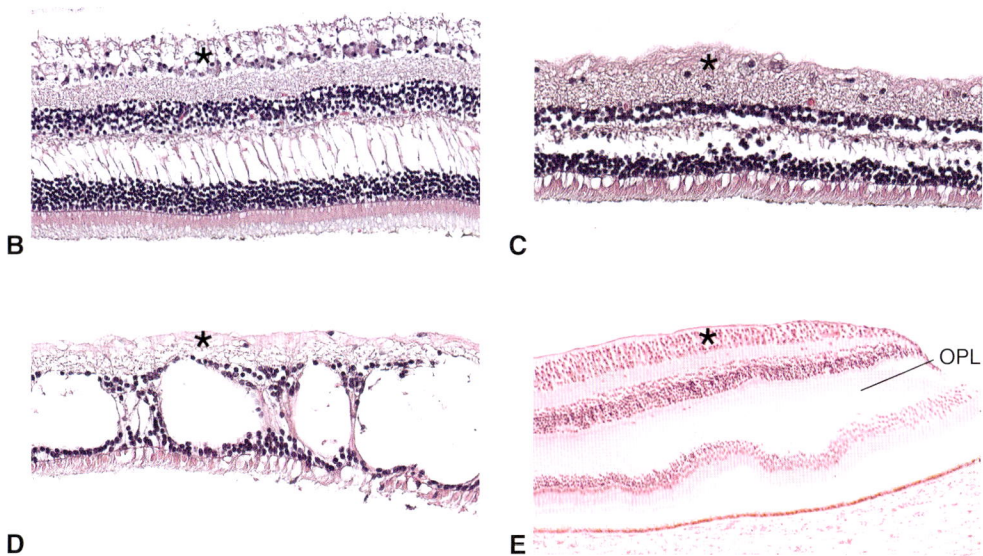

Figure 11-1 *(continued)* **B,** Retina peripheral to the major vascular arcades and posterior to the equator (near-peripheral retina). The *asterisk* denotes the GCL. **C,** Retina in the equatorial region. The *asterisk* denotes the GCL. **D,** Far-peripheral retina near the ora serrata. Note the reduced density of the GCL *(asterisk)* and overall thinning of the inner retinal layers. **E,** In the region of the foveola, the inner cellular layers taper off *(right side of photo),* with increased density of pigment in the RPE. The incident light falls directly on the photoreceptor outer segments, reducing the potential for distortion of light by overlying tissue elements. Note the multilayered GCL *(asterisk),* typical of the macula. The OPL fibers travel obliquely in the fovea (Henle fiber layer), and the photoreceptor layer in the fovea consists only of cones. *(Part A courtesy of Robert H. Rosa Jr, MD; parts B–D courtesy of Vivian Lee, MD; part E courtesy of Nasreen A. Syed, MD.)*

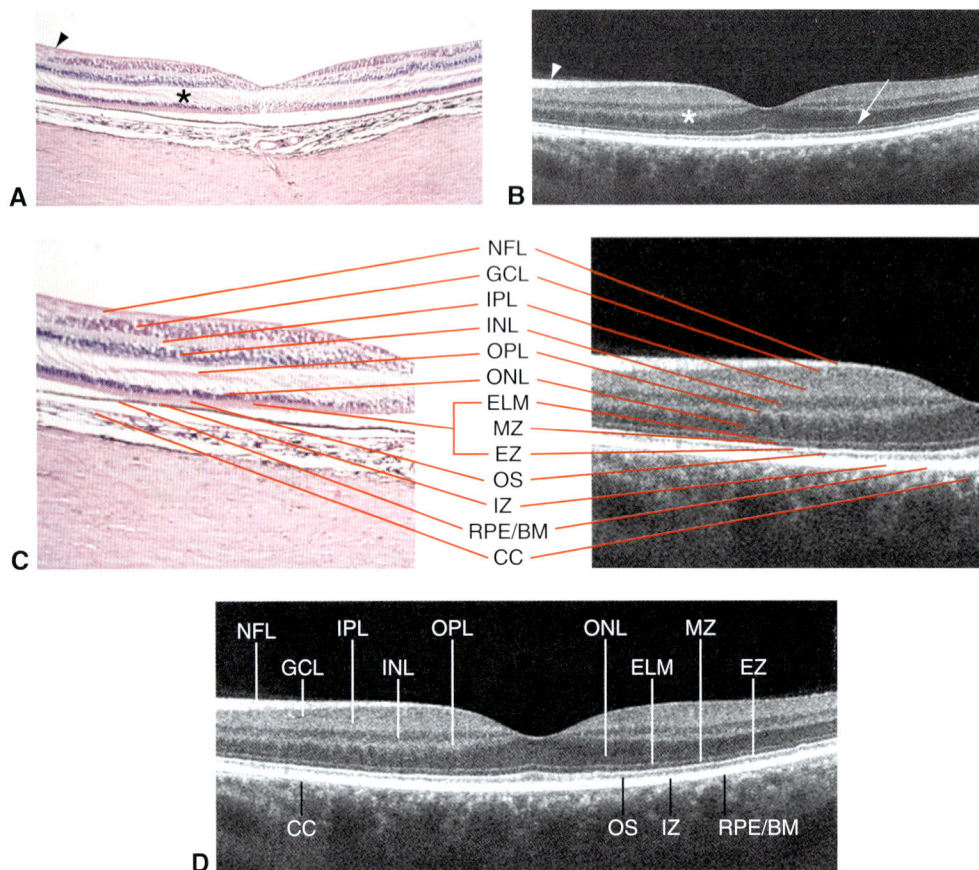

Figure 11-2 Macula. **A,** The normal macula is identified histologically by a thick, multilayered GCL and a central area of focal thinning, the foveola. Note the NFL *(arrowhead)* in the nasal macular region and the oblique orientation of Henle fiber layer (perifoveal OPL) *(asterisk).* Clinically, the macula lies between the inferior and superior temporal vascular arcades. **B,** Spectral-domain optical coherence tomography (SD-OCT) of the macula shows in vivo imaging with high-resolution details of the lamellar architecture of the retina. Note the NFL *(arrowhead)* in the nasal macular region, Henle fiber layer *(asterisk),* and the ELM *(arrow).* **C,** Higher magnification of the photomicrograph shown in part **A** and the SD-OCT image shown in part **B** illustrating the corresponding macular layers. **D,** SD-OCT image of the macula. NFL = nerve fiber layer; GCL = ganglion cell layer; IPL = inner plexiform layer; INL = inner nuclear layer; OPL = outer plexiform layer; ONL = outer nuclear layer; ELM = external limiting membrane; MZ = myoid zone; EZ = ellipsoid zone; OS = outer segments; IZ = interdigitation zone between outer segments and RPE; RPE/BM = retinal pigment epithelium/Bruch membrane; CC = choriocapillaris. *(Part B courtesy of Robert H. Rosa Jr, MD; parts C (right) and D adapted from Staurenghi G, Sadda S, Chakravarthy U, Spaide RF; International Nomenclature for Optical Coherence Tomography (IN-OCT) Panel. Proposed lexicon for anatomic landmarks in normal posterior segment spectral-domain optical coherence tomography: the IN-OCT consensus.* Ophthalmology. *2014;121(8):1572–1578.)*

In the outer plexiform layer (OPL) of the fovea (Henle fiber layer), nerve fibers run obliquely (Video 11-2; see also Figs 11-1E, 11-2A). This morphological feature results in the "flower petal" appearance of cystoid macular edema (CME) on fluorescein angiography

(FA), as well as the star-shaped configuration of hard exudates observed ophthalmoscopically in conditions that cause macular edema. Xanthophyll pigment gives the macula its yellow appearance clinically and grossly (macula lutea), but the xanthophyll dissolves during tissue processing and is not present in histologic sections. For more on the macula, see Table 1-1 in BCSC Section 12, *Retina and Vitreous*.

▶ **VIDEO 11-2** Foveal architecture and related pathologies.
Developed by Vivian Lee, MD.

Outside the macula, the GCL consists of a single layer of ganglion cells and astrocytes. The NFL progressively thins moving anteriorly toward the ora serrata from the optic nerve head. In addition, the most peripheral retina near the ora serrata may lack some of the 9 histologic neurosensory layers (see Fig 11-1B–D).

Two vascular sources supply the retina with some overlap (watershed zone) in the inner nuclear layer (INL). The *retinal blood vessels* supply the NFL, GCL, inner plexiform layer (IPL), and inner portion of the INL. The *choroidal vasculature*, specifically the *choriocapillaris*, which is derived from the posterior ciliary arteries, supplies the outer layers of the retina; these include the outer portion of the INL, OPL, outer nuclear layer, photoreceptors, and RPE. The venous network in these layers drains into the vortex veins.

Spaide RF, Curcio CA. Anatomical correlates to the bands seen in the outer retina by optical coherence tomography: literature review and model. *Retina.* 2011;31(8):1609–1619.

Retinal Pigment Epithelium

The RPE consists of a monolayer of hexagonal cells with apical microvilli. RPE cells appear cuboidal in cross section. The cytoplasm of RPE cells contains numerous melanosomes and lipofuscin. The RPE basement membrane forms the inner layer of Bruch membrane. In contrast to the retina, the RPE exhibits more subtle topographic variations. In the macula, the RPE is taller, narrower, and more heavily pigmented than in other regions, and it forms a regular hexagonal array. Anterior to the macula, RPE cells are shorter and larger in diameter. Variability in the diameter of RPE cells increases in the peripheral retina. The amount of cytoplasmic lipofuscin increases with age, particularly in the macula.

Developmental Anomalies

Albinism

The term *albinism* refers to the congenital absence or dilution of the pigment in the skin, eyes, or both. This condition results from genetic mutations that alter or prevent the biosynthesis of melanin. True albinism is divided into *oculocutaneous* and *ocular* forms. Clinically, this distinction is somewhat helpful; however, in reality, all cases of ocular albinism

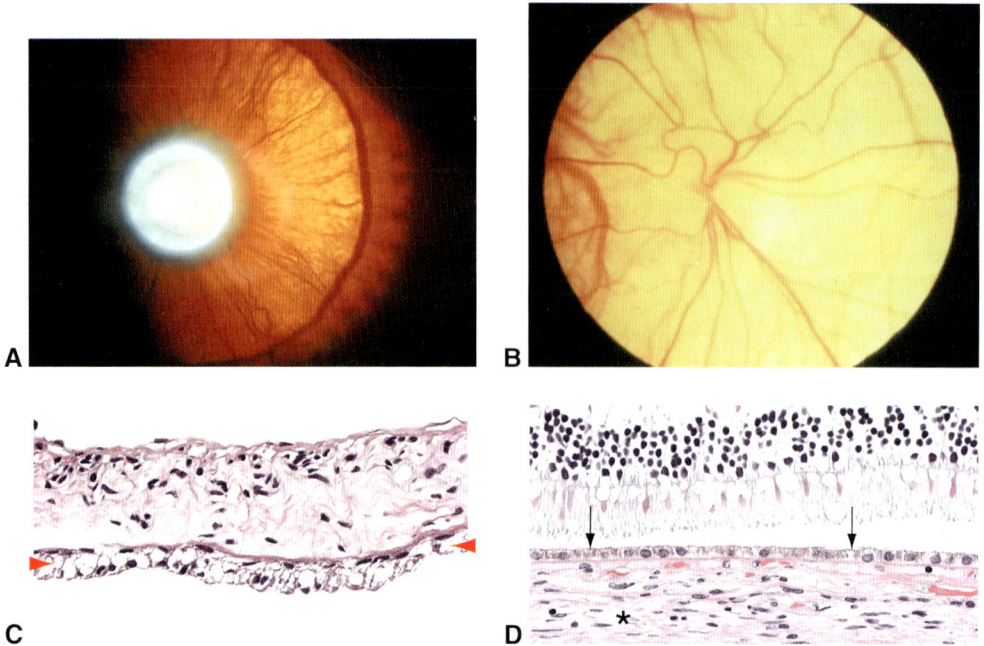

Figure 11-3   Albinism. **A,** Clinical appearance with total iris transillumination. **B,** Fundus photograph illustrating diffuse hypopigmentation. **C,** Photomicrograph illustrates lack of pigment in the iris pigment epithelium *(between arrowheads)*, allowing visualization of the nuclei. No appreciable pigmentation is present in the iris stroma. **D,** Photomicrograph showing the RPE and choroid in an albino eye. There is markedly reduced pigment in the RPE cells *(arrows)* and no appreciable pigmentation in the choroid *(asterisk)*. *(Parts A and B courtesy of Robert H. Rosa Jr, MD; parts C and D courtesy of Nasreen A. Syed, MD.)*

have some degree of cutaneous involvement. The 2 types of albinism do have a pathophysiologic difference: in oculocutaneous albinism, transmission is commonly autosomal recessive, and the amount of melanin in each melanosome is reduced; in ocular albinism, transmission is commonly X-linked recessive, and the number of melanosomes is reduced (Fig 11-3). See BCSC Section 6, *Pediatric Ophthalmology and Strabismus,* and Section 12, *Retina and Vitreous,* for further discussion of albinism.

Myelinated Nerve Fibers

Generally, the ganglion cell axonal fibers do not become myelinated until they pass through the lamina cribrosa. However, oligodendroglial cells in the NFL can occasionally produce a myelin sheath around nerve fibers in the retina. Although this type of myelination is usually contiguous with the optic nerve head, it may also occur in isolation, away from the optic nerve head. If large, it can produce a clinically significant scotoma. Myelinated nerve fibers have also been associated with myopia, amblyopia, strabismus, and nystagmus. See BCSC Section 6, *Pediatric Ophthalmology and Strabismus,* for additional discussion of myelinated nerve fibers.

Vascular Anomalies

Numerous developmental anomalies may be observed in the retinal vasculature, including Coats disease and hemangioblastoma. In Coats disease, exudative retinal detachment is due to leakage from abnormalities in the peripheral retina, which include telangiectatic vessels, aneurysms, and saccular dilatations of the retinal vessels (Fig 11-4). Histologically, retinal detachments secondary to Coats disease are characterized by "foamy" histiocytes and cholesterol crystals in the subretinal space (see Fig 11-4E).

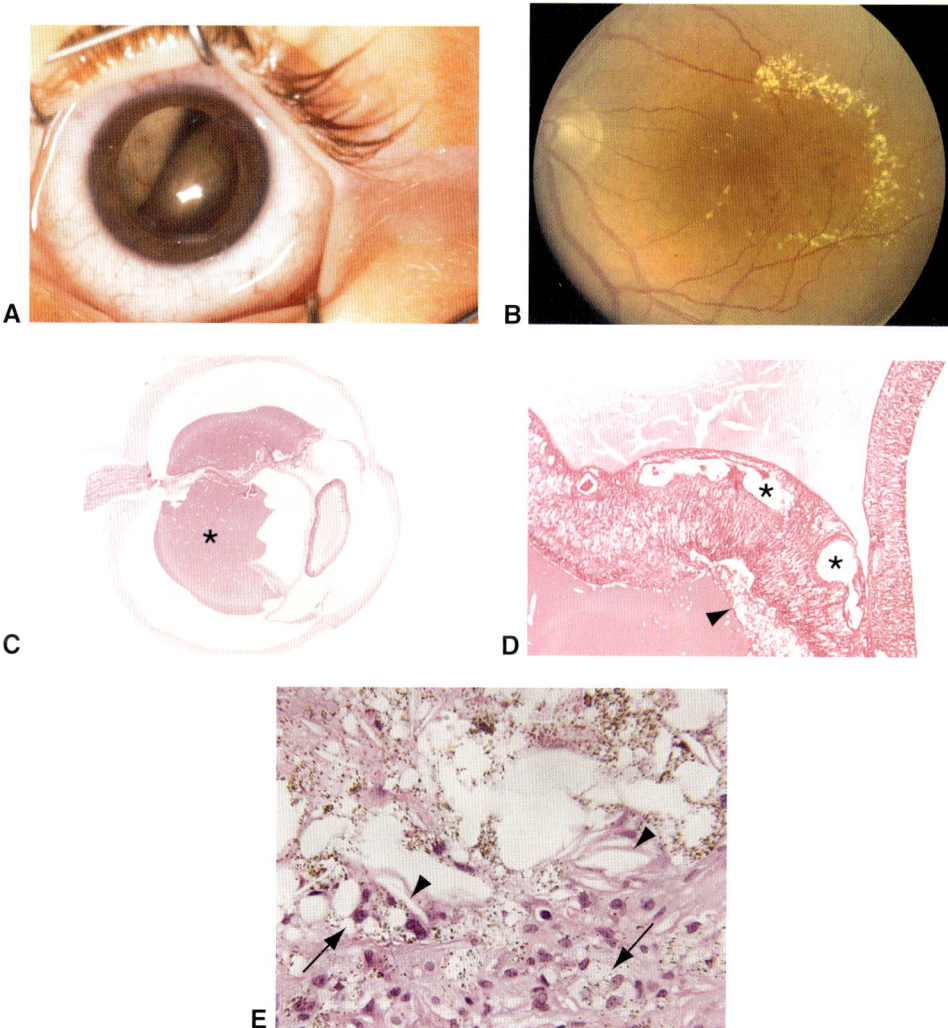

Figure 11-4 Coats disease. **A,** Leukocoria in a patient with Coats disease. **B,** Fundus photograph demonstrating multiple retinal macroaneurysms and lipid exudate. **C,** Total exudative retinal detachment in Coats disease with dense subretinal proteinaceous fluid *(asterisk)*. **D,** Telangiectatic retinal vessels *(asterisks)* and "foamy" histiocytes *(arrowhead)* typical of Coats disease. **E,** High-magnification of subretinal exudate showing lipid-laden and pigment-laden histiocytes *(arrows)* and cholesterol clefts *(arrowheads)*. *(Parts A, C, and D courtesy of Hans E. Grossniklaus, MD; part B courtesy of Benjamin J. Kim, MD; part E courtesy of George J. Harocopos, MD.)*

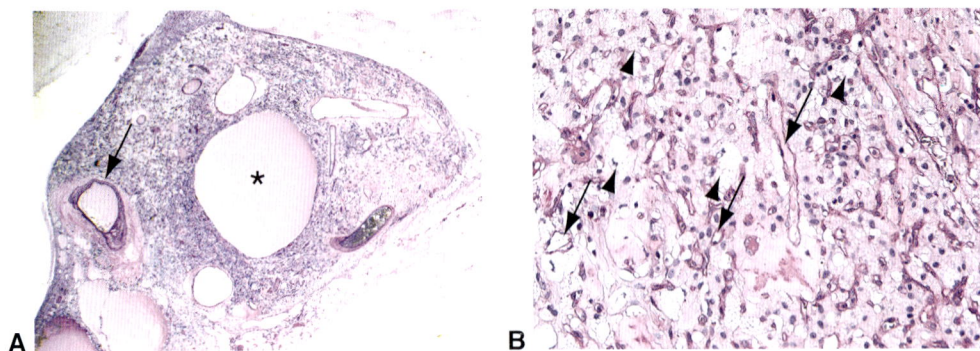

Figure 11-5 Retinal capillary hemangioblastoma in von Hippel–Lindau syndrome. **A,** Low-magnification photomicrograph showing a retinal tumor with a thick-walled feeder vessel *(arrow)* and a cystic area filled with proteinaceous material *(asterisk)*. Note the prominent blood vessels and area of dense cellularity composed of stromal cells (periodic acid–Schiff [PAS] stain). **B,** Higher magnification showing the numerous small, capillary-like vascular channels *(arrows)*. The vacuolated, foamy stromal cells *(arrowheads)* are the tumor cells that have the *VHL* gene mutation. *(Courtesy of Robert H. Rosa Jr, MD.)*

Retinal capillary hemangioblastoma is a vascular tumor that is often seen in patients with von Hippel–Lindau (VHL) syndrome (see Chapter 18). These tumors are composed of many abnormal, capillary-like, fenestrated channels surrounded by vacuolated, foamy stromal cells and reactive glial cells (Fig 11-5). Histologically, retinal and optic nerve hemangioblastomas are similar to hemangioblastomas of the CNS. Loss of heterozygosity of the *VHL* gene has been clearly identified in the vacuolated stromal cells but not in the vascular endothelial or reactive glial cells of retinal and optic nerve hemangioblastomas. Thus, the vacuolated, foamy stromal cells are the actual neoplastic cells of the retinal hemangioblastomas.

See BCSC Section 12, *Retina and Vitreous*, for further discussion of these vascular anomalies and their clinical features.

Congenital Hypertrophy of the RPE

Congenital hypertrophy of the RPE (CHRPE) is a relatively common congenital lesion. It is characterized clinically as a flat, heavily pigmented circumscribed lesion that varies in diameter (Chapter 17, Fig 17-11). Frequently, with age, central depigmentation may occur in these lesions (lacunae). Histologically, CHRPE is characterized by enlarged RPE cells with densely packed and larger-than-normal melanin granules (Fig 11-6). This benign condition can generally be distinguished from choroidal nevus and melanoma on the basis of ophthalmoscopic features. In rare instances, adenoma and adenocarcinoma of the RPE may develop in CHRPE.

RPE lesions mimicking CHRPE may be present in *Gardner syndrome,* a subtype of familial adenomatous intestinal polyposis. Histologic study of the RPE changes in Gardner syndrome reveals that they are more consistent with hyperplasia (increase in the number of cells) of the RPE than with hypertrophy. The RPE changes are probably more

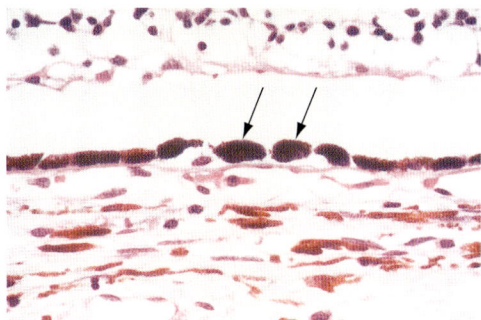

Figure 11-6 In congenital hypertrophy of the RPE (CHRPE), the RPE cells are larger than normal and contain more densely packed melanin granules *(arrows)* (hematoxylin-eosin [H&E] stain). For clinical images of CHRPE, see Chapter 17, Figure 17-11. *(Courtesy of Hans E. Grossniklaus, MD.)*

appropriately termed *hamartomas,* consistent with the loss of regulatory control of cell growth that results in other soft-tissue lesions in this syndrome. A mutation in the *APC* gene, which is linked to Gardner syndrome, confers an increased lifetime risk of developing colon polyps, benign tumors, and cancer.

Inflammation

Infectious Etiologies

Bacterial infection

See the discussion of endophthalmitis in Chapter 10 in this volume and in BCSC Section 9, *Uveitis and Ocular Inflammation.*

Viral infection

Multiple viruses may cause retinal infections, including rubella virus, measles virus, human immunodeficiency virus (HIV), herpes simplex virus (HSV), varicella-zoster virus (VZV), and cytomegalovirus (CMV). Two of the most frequent clinical presentations of retinal viral infection, acute retinal necrosis (ARN) and CMV retinitis, are discussed here.

Acute retinal necrosis is a rapidly progressive, necrotizing retinitis caused by infection with HSV types 1 and 2, VZV, or in rare instances, CMV. ARN can occur in healthy or immunocompromised individuals. Histologic findings include robust inflammation in the vitreous and anterior chamber with prominent obliterative retinal vasculitis and retinal necrosis (Fig 11-7). Inflammatory cells include neutrophils, lymphocytes, plasma cells, and epithelioid histiocytes. Electron microscopy has shown viral inclusions in retinal cells. Polymerase chain reaction analysis of aqueous or vitreous samples is the most sensitive and most rapid method for identifying the presence of virus, reducing the need for viral culture, intraocular antibody analysis, immunohistochemistry, or other diagnostic techniques.

CMV retinitis is an opportunistic infection that occurs in immunosuppressed patients (Fig 11-8). Histologically, it is characterized by retinal necrosis that heals with a thin fibroglial scar. Acute lesions show enlarged neurons (20–30 μm) that contain large eosinophilic intranuclear and/or intracytoplasmic inclusion bodies (see Fig 11-8C, D). At the cellular level, CMV may infect vascular endothelial cells, retinal neurons, the RPE, and

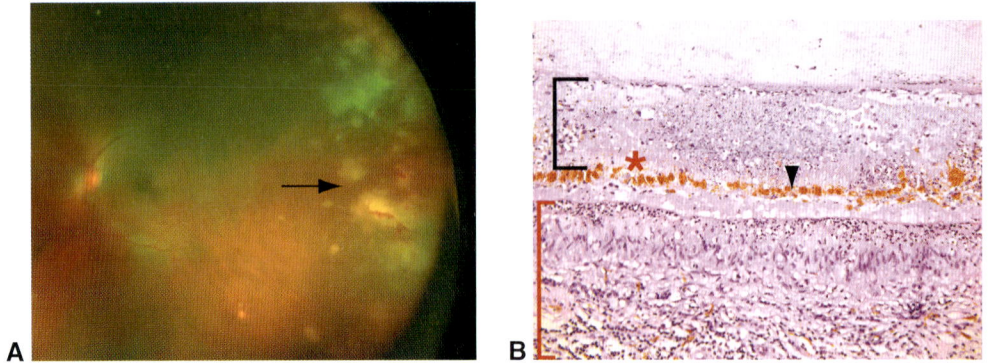

Figure 11-7 Acute retinal necrosis (ARN). **A,** Wide-field fundus photograph reveals areas of retinal necrosis manifesting as white areas and hemorrhage *(arrow)* in the periphery. The hazy appearance is due to vitritis. **B,** Photomicrograph from a different patient reveals full-thickness necrosis of the retina *(black bracket),* identified by remaining photoreceptor outer segments *(asterisk)* and RPE cells *(arrowhead).* Acute and chronic granulomatous inflammation is present below Bruch membrane *(red bracket).* Neutrophils, epithelioid histiocytes, lymphocytes, and plasma cells are present with a zonal arrangement from top to bottom. *(Part A courtesy of Benjamin J. Kim, MD; part B courtesy of Vivian Lee, MD.)*

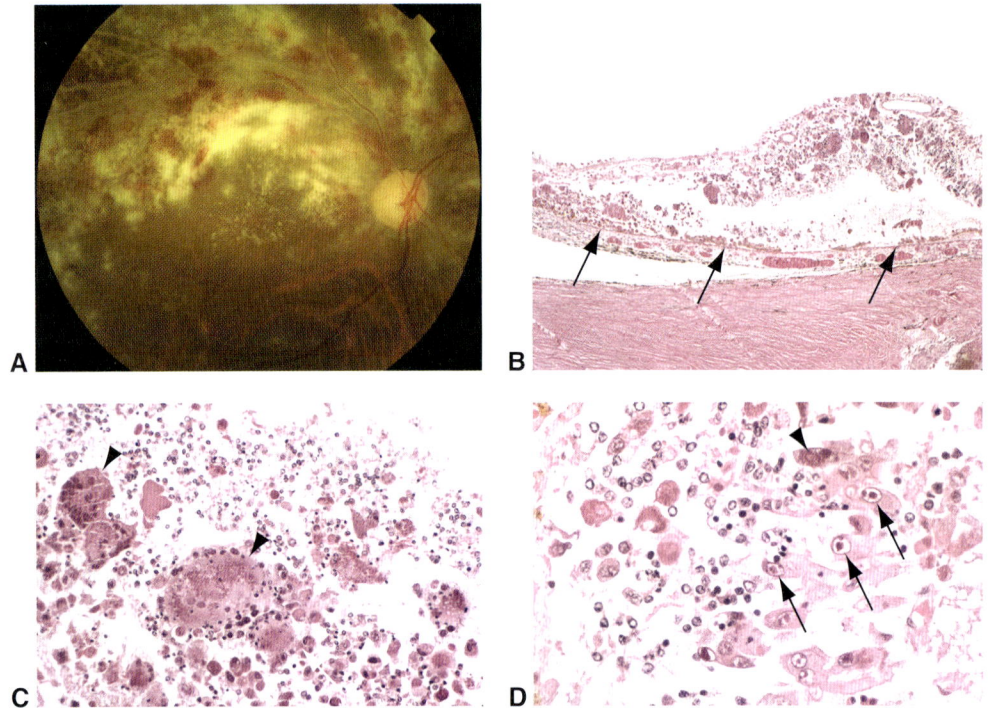

Figure 11-8 Cytomegalovirus (CMV) retinitis. **A,** Retinal hemorrhages and areas of opaque retina are present. Note the white vascular sheathing along the superotemporal arcade and hard exudates in the macular region. **B,** Histologically, full-thickness retinal necrosis is present. Note the loss of the normal lamellar architecture of the retina, including disruption of the RPE *(arrows).* **C,** Large syncytial cells infected with virus *(arrowheads)* are present in areas of necrosis, characteristic of CMV retinitis. **D,** Intranuclear "owl's eye" inclusions *(arrows)* and intracytoplasmic inclusion bodies *(arrowhead)* are present in CMV-infected cells. *(Courtesy of Robert H. Rosa Jr, MD.)*

histiocytes. Because of the immunocompromised status of the infected host, a prominent inflammatory infiltrate is typically not present.

Fungal infection

Fungal infections of the retina are uncommon, occurring most often in immunosuppressed patients and in patients with fungemia (eg, from parenteral nutrition or intravenous drug use). These infections usually begin as single or multiple small foci in the choroid or retina (Fig 11-9). The most common causative fungi are *Candida* species, particularly *C albicans.* Less common agents include *Aspergillus* species and *Cryptococcus neoformans.*

Histologically, fungal infections are characterized by necrotizing granulomatous inflammation. A central zone of necrosis is typically surrounded by the granulomatous inflammation with an outer layer of lymphocytes. Although histologic examination may reveal the causative agent, a culture and/or molecular studies are required for definitive identification of the organism. With treatment, these lesions heal with a fibroglial scar.

Protozoal infection

Toxoplasmic retinochoroiditis (also called *toxoplasmic chorioretinitis, ocular toxoplasmosis*) is the most common infectious retinitis. It may be due to reactivation of a congenitally acquired infection or to an acquired *Toxoplasma* infection in healthy or immunocompromised

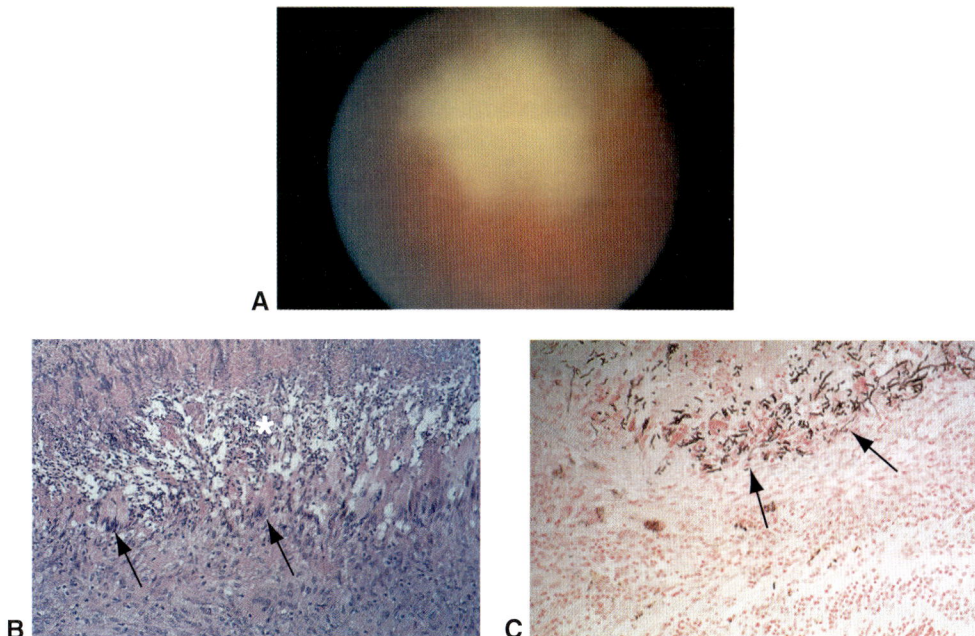

A

B

C

Figure 11-9   Fungal chorioretinitis. **A,** Clinical appearance of vitreous, retinal, and choroidal infiltrates in a patient with fungal chorioretinitis. The vitreous cells give the photograph a hazy appearance. **B,** Granulomatous infiltration surrounding a central area of necrosis *(asterisk)*. Frequent multinucleated giant cells are present *(arrows)*. **C,** Grocott-Gomori methenamine–silver nitrate stain of the section parallel to that shown in part **B** demonstrating numerous fungal hyphae, which stain black *(arrows)*. *(Courtesy of David J. Wilson, MD.)*

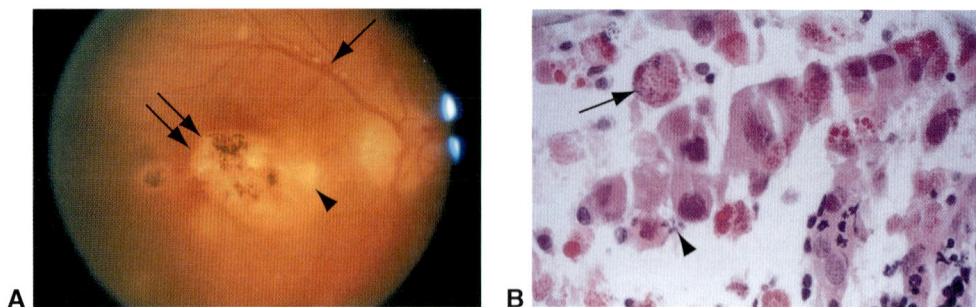

Figure 11-10 Toxoplasmic retinochoroiditis. **A,** Fundus photograph showing chorioretinal scars rimmed with pigment *(double arrow)*, typical of prior infection with *Toxoplasma* species. Active retinitis *(arrowhead)* and perivascular sheathing *(arrow)* are present. **B,** Cysts *(arrow)* and extracellular organisms (tachyzoites, *arrowhead*) in active toxoplasmic retinochoroiditis. *(Courtesy of Hans E. Grossniklaus, MD.)*

individuals. In patients with reactivated disease, toxoplasmic retinochoroiditis typically presents as a posterior uveitis or panuveitis with marked vitritis and focal retinochoroiditis adjacent to a pigmented chorioretinal scar. The absence of a preexisting chorioretinal scar suggests newly acquired disease.

Microscopic examination of active toxoplasmic retinochoroiditis reveals necrosis of the retina, a prominent infiltrate of neutrophils and lymphocytes, and *Toxoplasma* organisms in the form of tissue cysts and tachyzoites (Fig 11-10). There is generally a prominent lymphocytic infiltrate in the vitreous and the anterior segment and granulomatous inflammation in the inner choroid. Healing brings resolution of the inflammatory cell infiltrate with encystment of the organisms in the retina adjacent to the atrophic chorioretinal scar. See also BCSC Section 9, *Uveitis and Ocular Inflammation,* and Section 12, *Retina and Vitreous.*

Noninfectious Etiologies

Noninfectious inflammation of the retina may be acute with an infiltrate of neutrophils, chronic with an infiltrate of lymphocytes and plasma cells, or granulomatous with the presence of epithelioid histiocytes and/or multinucleated giant cells in the inflammatory infiltrate. Noninfectious inflammatory conditions, including autoimmune conditions involving the retina, are discussed in more detail in BCSC Section 9, *Uveitis and Ocular Inflammation,* and Section 12, *Retina and Vitreous.*

Degenerations

The clinical features of various retinal degenerations are discussed in BCSC Section 12, *Retina and Vitreous.*

Typical and Reticular Peripheral Cystoid Degeneration and Retinoschisis

In *typical peripheral cystoid degeneration (TPCD),* which is a universal finding in the eyes of individuals older than 20 years, cystoid spaces develop in the OPL of the retina. In

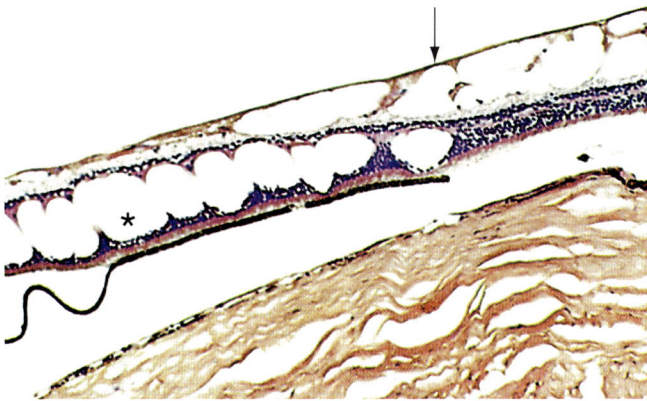

Figure 11-11 Typical peripheral cystoid degeneration (TPCD) consisting of cystoid spaces in the outer plexiform layer *(asterisk)*. The anterior eye is toward the left side of the photograph. Reticular peripheral cystoid degeneration (RPCD) is posterior to the TPCD *(arrow)* in the nerve fiber layer. Coalescence of these cystoid spaces results in retinoschisis.

reticular peripheral cystoid degeneration (RPCD), which is less common than TPCD, cystoid spaces develop in the NFL, posterior to areas of TPCD (Fig 11-11). Coalescence of the cystoid spaces of TPCD forms *typical degenerative retinoschisis,* usually in the inferotemporal region. In *reticular degenerative retinoschisis,* the retinal layers split in the NFL.

Lattice Degeneration

Although lattice degeneration (Fig 11-12) may be a familial condition, it is found in up to 10% of the general population. Retinal detachment develops in only a small number of individuals with lattice degeneration; on the other hand, lattice degeneration is seen in up to 40% of all patients with rhegmatogenous detachments.

The most important histologic features of lattice degeneration are

- discontinuity of the internal limiting membrane (ILM) of the retina
- an overlying pocket of liquefied vitreous
- focal sclerosis of retinal vessels, which remain physiologically patent
- condensation and adherence of vitreous at the margins of the lesion
- variable degrees of atrophy of the inner layers of the retina

Radial perivascular lattice degeneration has the same histologic features as typical lattice degeneration, but it occurs more posteriorly along the course of retinal vessels.

Although atrophic holes often develop in the center of the lattice lesion, they are rarely the cause of retinal detachment because the vitreous is liquefied over the surface of the lattice, preventing vitreous traction. Instead, retinal detachment is generally the result of vitreous adhesion at the margins of lattice degeneration, leading to retinal tears in this location when vitreous detachment occurs. With time, other degenerative changes occur.

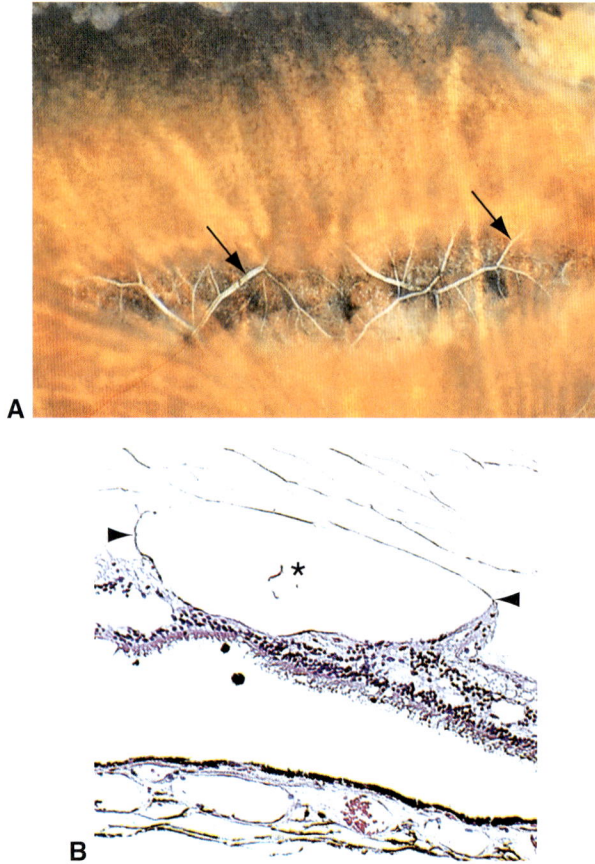

Figure 11-12   Retinal lattice degeneration. **A,** Lattice degeneration appears clinically as prominent sclerotic vessels *(arrows)* in a wicker or lattice pattern. **B,** The vitreous directly over the lattice degeneration is liquefied *(asterisk),* but formed vitreous remains adherent at the margins
(arrowheads) of the degenerated area. The internal limiting membrane is discontinuous, and
the inner retinal layers are atrophic.

Sequelae of Retinal Detachment

When any type of retinal detachment occurs, loss of the photoreceptor outer segments in
the region of the detachment is the earliest change identified. With time, if the detachment
is not repaired or does not resolve, other degenerative changes can be identified, including
loss of the photoreceptor cells, migration of Müller cells, and proliferation and migration
of RPE cells. RPE cells, when not in contact with the neurosensory retina, can undergo
metaplasia, becoming fibroblast-like cells or even osseous tissue. In addition, the RPE may
produce more basement membrane, focally leading to the formation of nodular and calcified drusen. Small cystic spaces develop in the detached retina over time, and in chronic
detachment, these cysts may coalesce into large macrocysts (Fig 11-13).

Paving-Stone Degeneration

Focal occlusion of the choriocapillaris can lead to loss of the outer retinal layers and RPE,
a condition known as *paving-stone* or *cobblestone degeneration.* This type of atrophy is

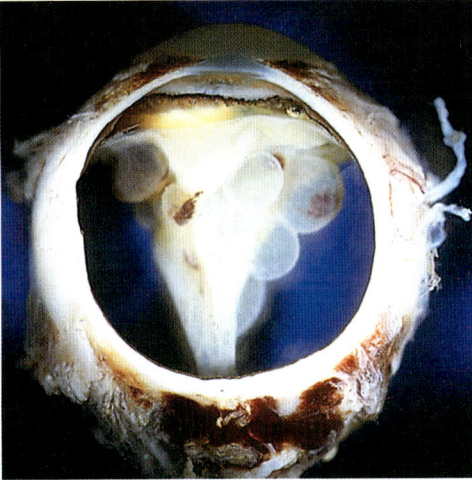

Figure 11-13 Long-standing total retinal detachment with macrocystic degeneration of the retina.

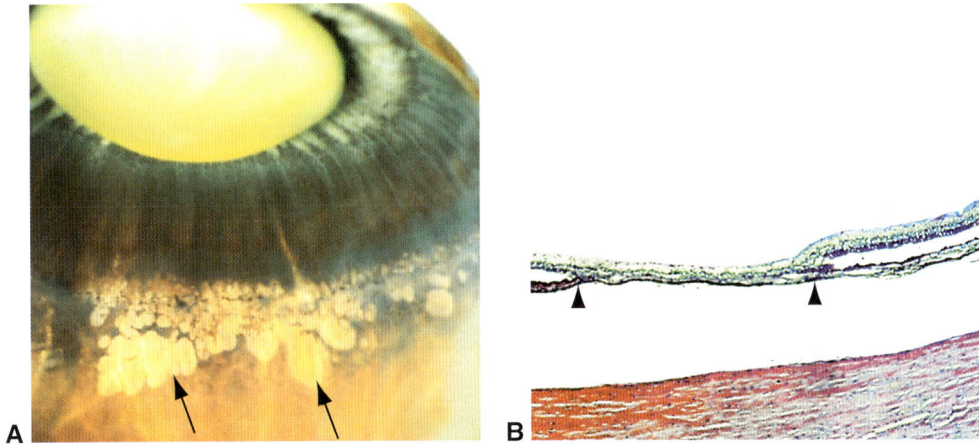

A   B

Figure 11-14 Paving-stone degeneration. **A,** Photograph shows the gross appearance of paving-stone degeneration: areas of depigmentation *(arrows)* in the peripheral retina near the ora serrata. **B,** Histologically, paving-stone degeneration shows atrophy of the outer retinal layers and adhesion of the remaining inner retinal elements to Bruch membrane. The sharp boundary *(arrowheads)* between the normal and the atrophic retina corresponds to the clinical appearance of paving-stone degeneration.

common in the retinal periphery in older individuals. The well-demarcated, flat, pale lesions seen clinically correspond to circumscribed areas of outer retinal and RPE atrophy and loss of the choriocapillaris, with adherence of the INL to Bruch membrane (Fig 11-14). Histologically, these findings are similar to those found in geographic atrophy in age-related macular degeneration.

Ischemia

Because of dual blood supplies to the retina, the histologic findings associated with ischemic vascular insults vary. In general, ischemia of the retinal vasculature produces

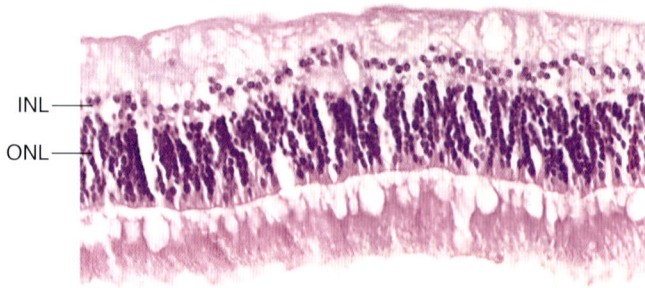

Figure 11-15 Inner ischemic retinal atrophy. The photoreceptor nuclei (outer nuclear layer; ONL) and the outer portion of the inner nuclear layer (INL) are normal in appearance. The inner portion of the INL is absent. There are no ganglion cells, and the nerve fiber layer is thin, appearing to merge with the inner plexiform layer. This pattern of ischemia corresponds to the supply of the retinal arteriolar circulation and may be seen after healing from retinal arterial and venous occlusions.

Figure 11-16 Outer ischemic retinal atrophy. Begin at the right edge of the photograph and trace the ganglion cell and inner nuclear layers *(red arrows toward the left)*. In this case, there is loss of the nuclei of the photoreceptor layer (outer nuclear layer) *(arrow)*, the photoreceptor inner and outer segments, and the RPE *(arrowhead)*. This is the pattern of outer retinal atrophy secondary to interruption in the choroidal blood supply. Compare with Figure 11-15.

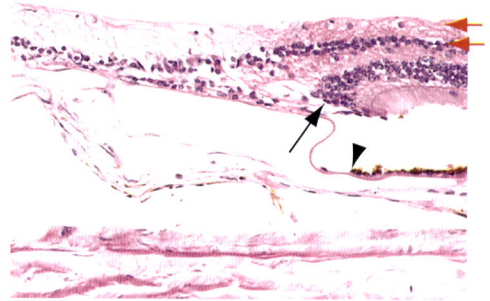

inner retinal atrophy, and choroidal ischemia produces outer retinal atrophy. Occlusion of the retinal vessels leads to *inner ischemic retinal atrophy* with atrophy of retinal ganglion cells and astrocytes, partial atrophy of the INL, and thinning of the NFL (Fig 11-15). Occlusion of the choroidal vessels leads to *outer ischemic retinal atrophy,* including loss of the photoreceptor segments and nuclei, loss of the OPL, and sometimes thinning of the INL (Fig 11-16).

Retinal ischemia can be caused by many conditions, including diabetes mellitus, retinal artery and vein occlusions, radiation retinopathy, retinopathy of prematurity, sickle cell retinopathy, vasculitis, and carotid occlusive disease (some of these diseases are discussed later in this chapter). Some of these entities result in focal retinal atrophy; others, in diffuse retinal atrophy. The development of optical coherence tomography angiography (OCTA), which depicts all capillary layers of the retina, may refine our understanding of vascular pathologies affecting this area. See BCSC Section 12, *Retina and Vitreous*, for further information on OCTA.

Nevertheless, certain histologic findings—both cellular and vascular responses—are common to all disorders that result in retinal ischemia.

Retinal changes

Cellular responses Neurons in the retina are highly active metabolically, requiring large amounts of oxygen for production of adenosine triphosphate (ATP) (see BCSC Section 2, *Fundamentals and Principles of Ophthalmology,* Part IV, Biochemistry and Metabolism). This makes them highly sensitive to interruption of their blood supply. With prolonged oxygen deprivation (>90 minutes in experimental studies), neuronal cell nuclei become pyknotic (ie, hyperchromatic and shrunken) and are subsequently phagocytosed by microglia. Microglia are involved in the phagocytosis of necrotic cells, as well as of extracellular material, such as lipid or blood, that accumulates in areas of ischemia in the CNS. Microglial cells are fairly resistant to ischemia.

Retinal neurons such as ganglion cells, photoreceptors, amacrine cells, horizontal cells, and bipolar cells have no capacity for regeneration after damage. In response to insult, the nerve fibers of the ganglion cells swell, appearing histologically as pseudo-cells, known as *cytoid bodies* (Fig 11-17). These localized accumulations of axoplasmic material are present in ischemic infarcts of the NFL. Cotton-wool spots are the clinical correlate of small infarctions in the NFL. They resolve over 4–12 weeks, leaving an area of inner ischemic retinal atrophy.

Like neurons, glial cells degenerate in areas of infarction. These cells may proliferate adjacent to focal areas of infarction as well as in ischemic areas without infarction, resulting in *gliosis,* a glial scar. The location and extent of atrophic retina resulting from ischemia depend on the size of the occluded vessel and on whether it is a retinal or a choroidal blood vessel.

Vascular responses One of the earliest manifestations of retinal ischemia is *edema,* which results from transudation across the damaged inner blood–retina barrier. Fluid and serum components accumulate in the extracellular space, and the fluid pockets are delimited by

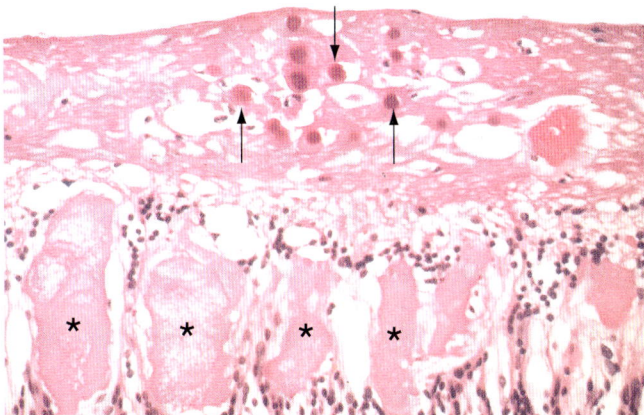

Figure 11-17 Cytoid bodies *(arrows)* within the nerve fiber layer that represent axoplasmic swelling of ganglion cell axons secondary to ischemia. The cystoid spaces *(asterisks)* in the deeper retina are filled with proteinaceous fluid and represent retinal exudation. *(Courtesy of W. Richard Green, MD.)*

the surrounding neurons and glial cells. In the perifoveal region, in the Henle fiber layer, this results in cystoid macular edema (CME) (Fig 11-18; see also BCSC Section 12, *Retina and Vitreous*, for additional images of CME). Lipid-rich exudate accumulation in the OPL of the macula produces a macular star configuration because of the orientation of the nerve fibers in this area (Fig 11-19A). Histologically, retinal exudates appear as sharply circumscribed eosinophilic spaces between the retinal fibers (Fig 11-19B).

Retinal hemorrhages may also develop as a result of ischemic damage to the inner blood–retina barrier. As with edema and exudates, the shape of the hemorrhage conforms to the surrounding retinal tissue. Consequently, hemorrhages in the NFL are flame-shaped, whereas those in the nuclear or inner plexiform layers are circular, or "dot-and-blot" (Fig 11-20). Subhyaloid hemorrhages have a boat-shaped configuration. White-centered hemorrhages *(Roth spots)* may be present in the retina in a number of conditions (see Fig 18-8 in BCSC Section 12, *Retina and Vitreous*). The white centers of these

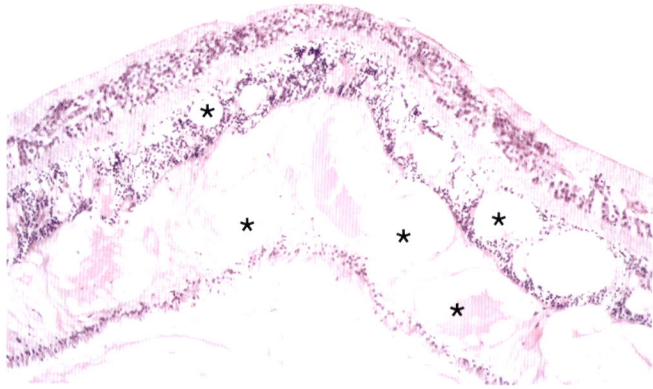

Figure 11-18   Cystoid macular edema. Cystoid spaces in the inner nuclear and outer plexiform layers *(asterisks)* of the macula. *(Courtesy of Nasreen A. Syed, MD.)*

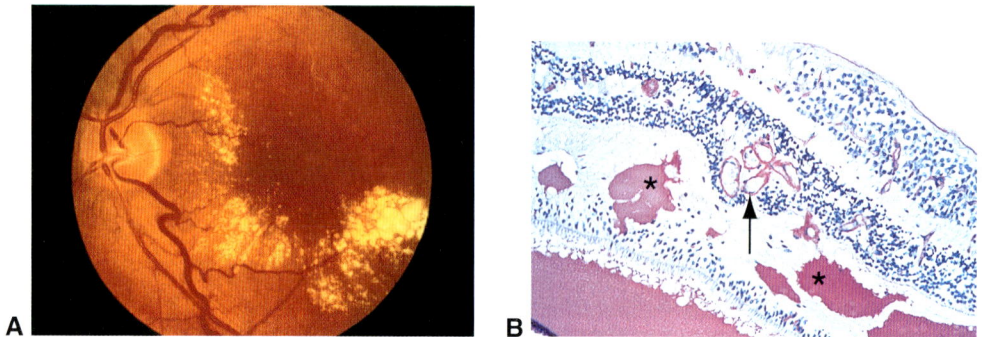

Figure 11-19   **A,** Clinical appearance of intraretinal lipid deposits, or hard exudates. **B,** PAS stain showing intraretinal exudates *(asterisks)* surrounding intraretinal microvascular abnormalities (IRMA) *(arrow)*. *(Part A courtesy of David J. Wilson, MD; part B courtesy of W. Richard Green, MD.)*

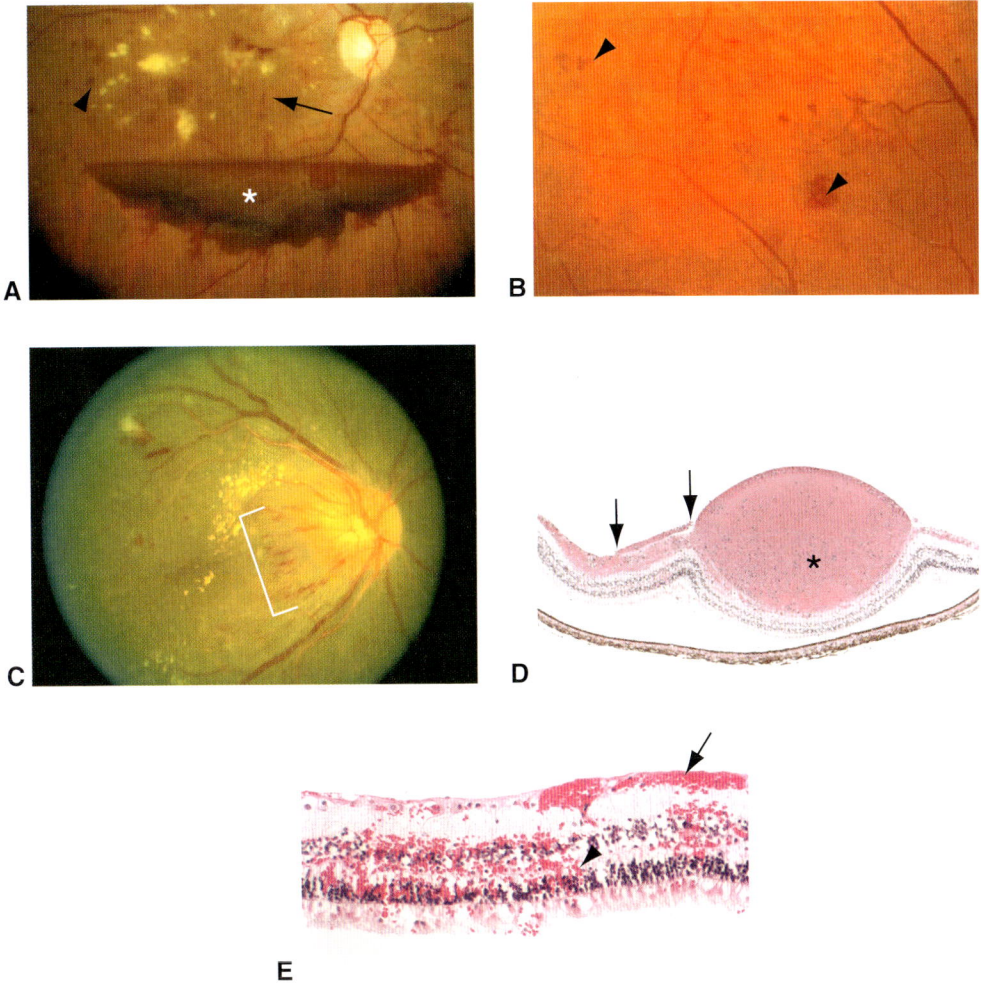

Figure 11-20 Retinal hemorrhage. **A,** Fundus photograph shows dot-and-blot *(arrowhead)* and flame-shaped *(arrow)* intraretinal hemorrhages and boat-shaped preretinal hemorrhage *(asterisk)* in proliferative diabetic retinopathy. **B,** Fundus photograph shows dot-and-blot intraretinal hemorrhages *(arrowheads)*. **C,** Fundus photograph shows multiple flame-shaped hemorrhages *(bracket)* in the retina surrounding the nerve. **D,** Histologically, preretinal hemorrhage may be just inside the internal limiting membrane (ILM) in the vitreous *(between arrows)* or just outside the ILM, creating a bullous hemorrhage in the innermost retina *(asterisk)*. **E,** Histologically, the dot-and-blot hemorrhage corresponds to blood in the middle layers (inner nuclear and outer plexiform layers) of the retina *(arrowhead)*, whereas flame-shaped hemorrhage corresponds to blood in the nerve fiber layer *(arrow)*. *(Parts A and E courtesy of Robert H. Rosa Jr, MD; part B courtesy of Benjamin J. Kim, MD; part D courtesy of Nasreen A. Syed, MD.)*

hemorrhages may contain multiple constituents, including aggregates of white blood cells, platelets and fibrin, microorganisms, or neoplastic cells, or they may be due to retinal light reflexes.

Chronic retinal ischemia leads to architectural changes in the retinal vessels. The capillary bed undergoes atrophy of the endothelial cells and pericytes and becomes acellular

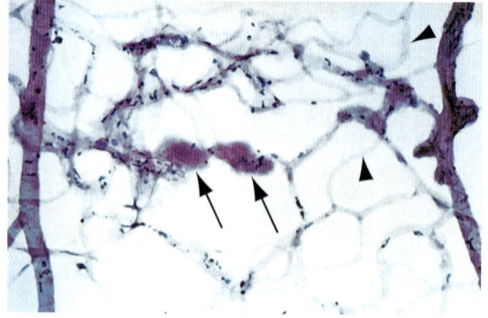

Figure 11-21 Trypsin digest preparation of the retina shows acellular capillaries *(arrowheads)* adjacent to IRMAs *(arrows)* (PAS stain). *(Courtesy of W. Richard Green, MD.)*

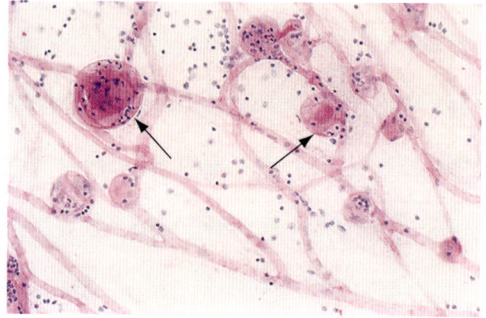

Figure 11-22 Retinal trypsin digest preparation (PAS stain) shows retinal microaneurysms in diabetic retinopathy *(arrows).*

in an area of vascular occlusion. Adjacent to acellular areas, irregular dilated vascular channels known as *intraretinal microvascular abnormalities (IRMAs)* (Fig 11-21) and microaneurysms often appear. *Microaneurysms* are fusiform or saccular outpouchings of the retinal capillaries and are best seen clinically with FA and histologically with trypsin digest flat mounts stained with periodic acid–Schiff (PAS) stain (Fig 11-22). The density of the endothelial cells that line IRMAs and microaneurysms frequently varies, with microaneurysms evolving from being thin-walled and hypercellular to being hyalinized and hypocellular.

In some cases of retinal ischemia, most commonly in diabetes mellitus and central retinal vein occlusion, neovascularization of the retina and the vitreous occurs. Retinal neovascularization arises from existing retinal blood vessels and penetrates the ILM, extending into the vitreous (Fig 11-23). Hemorrhage may develop from retinal neovascularization as the vitreous exerts traction on fragile new vessels.

Many of the vascular changes in retinal ischemia are mediated by vascular endothelial growth factor (VEGF), which is a potent stimulus of vascular permeability and angiogenesis. Biologic agents that inhibit VEGF (eg, bevacizumab, ranibizumab, and aflibercept) and intravitreally administered triamcinolone acetonide are used to treat various retinal diseases associated with macular edema and choroidal neovascularization. In studies that used these treatments for diabetic macular edema, retinal vein occlusion, and choroidal neovascularization, improvement in vision, mostly secondary to a decrease in macular edema and subretinal fluid, was shown (Fig 11-24). See BCSC Section 12, *Retina and Vitreous,* for more information on retinal neovascularization.

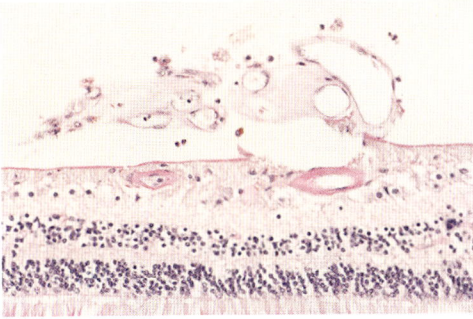

Figure 11-23 Retinal neovascularization. New blood vessels have broken through the internal limiting membrane into the vitreous (PAS stain).

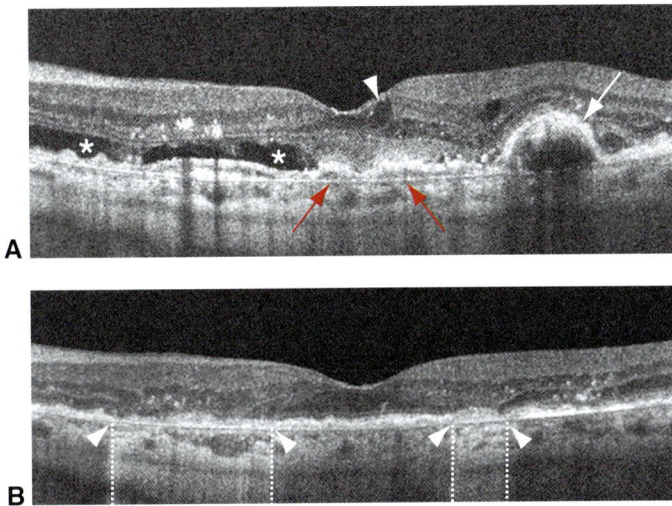

Figure 11-24 Cystoid macular edema (CME) before and after therapy with anti–vascular endothelial growth factor (anti-VEGF). **A,** SD-OCT shows mild CME *(arrowhead)*, subretinal fluid *(asterisks)*, and irregular elevation and detachment of the RPE *(white arrow)* secondary to neovascular age-related macular degeneration. Note the outer aspect of Bruch membrane *(red arrows)*. **B,** SD-OCT of the same retina after anti-VEGF therapy shows resolution of the CME and detachment of the RPE. Focal areas of geographic atrophy of the RPE with attenuation of the photoreceptor cell layer are more apparent *(between arrowheads)*. Note the hyperreflectivity *(between dashed lines)* in the choroid corresponding to the areas of geographic atrophy. *(Courtesy of Robert H. Rosa Jr, MD.)*

Specific ischemic retinal disorders

Central and branch retinal artery occlusions *Central retinal artery occlusion (CRAO)* results from localized arteriosclerotic changes, embolus, and in rare instances, vasculitis (as in giant cell arteritis). As the retina becomes ischemic, it swells and loses its transparency. This swelling is best seen clinically and histologically in the posterior pole, where the NFL and the GCL are thickest (Fig 11-25). Because the GCL and the NFL are thickest in the macula and absent in the fovea, a cherry-red spot can be appreciated clinically in the fovea, owing to the stark contrast between the normal color of the choroid and the surrounding

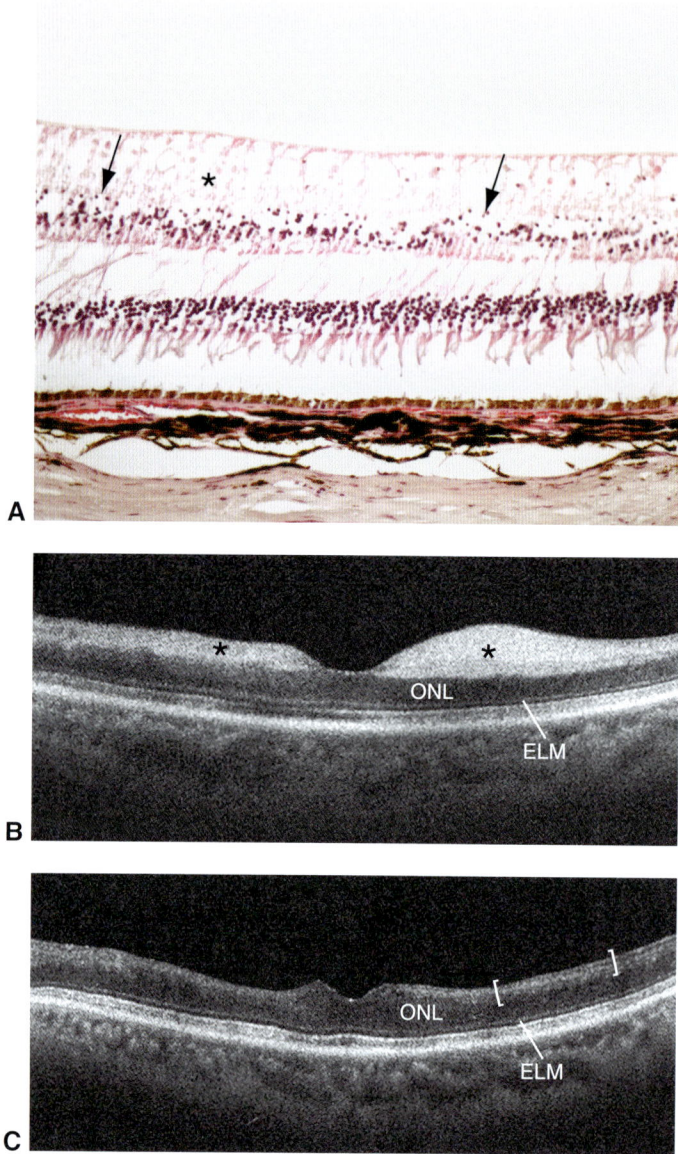

Figure 11-25 Central retinal artery occlusion (CRAO). **A,** Histologically, necrosis occurs in the inner retina *(asterisk),* corresponding to the retinal whitening observed on ophthalmoscopic examination. Note the pyknotic nuclei *(arrows)* in the inner aspect of the inner nuclear layer. **B,** SD-OCT reveals increased reflectivity in the area of retinal necrosis *(asterisks).* **C,** SD-OCT performed at a later date in the same patient as in part **B** reveals thinning of the inner retina *(in brackets)* with loss of the normal lamellar architecture up to the outer plexiform layer–outer nuclear layer junction. ELM = external limiting membrane; ONL = outer nuclear layer. *(Courtesy of Robert H. Rosa Jr, MD.)*

swollen white retina. When this sign is observed clinically, it suggests a CRAO. The retinal swelling eventually clears, leaving the classic histologic picture of inner ischemic retinal atrophy. After a CRAO, scarring and neovascularization are rare.

Branch retinal artery occlusion (BRAO) is usually the result of an embolus that lodges at the bifurcation of a retinal arteriole. As with CRAO, this embolic event may be the first or most important clue to a significant systemic disorder, such as carotid vascular disease (Hollenhorst plaques), cardiac valvular disease (calcific emboli), or cardiac thromboembolism (platelet-fibrin emboli). However, *Hollenhorst plaques,* which are cholesterol emboli within retinal arterioles, seldom occlude these vessels (see also BCSC Section 5, *Neuro-Ophthalmology*). In the acute phase, BRAO is characterized histologically by swelling of the inner retinal layers with early cell death. As the edema resolves, the classic picture of inner ischemic atrophy emerges in the distribution of the retina supplied by the occluded arteriole, with loss of cells in the NFL, GCL, IPL, and INL (see Fig 11-15). Arteriolar occlusions result in infarcts with subsequent complete atrophy of the affected layers.

American Academy of Ophthalmology Retina/Vitreous Panel. Preferred Practice Pattern Guidelines. *Retinal and Ophthalmic Artery Occlusions.* American Academy of Ophthalmology; 2016. www.aao.org/ppp

Central and branch retinal vein occlusions *Central retinal vein occlusion (CRVO)* is due to structural changes in the central retinal artery and lamina cribrosa that lead to compression of the central retinal vein. This compression creates turbulent flow in the vein and predisposes the patient to thrombosis. The pathophysiology of CRVO, which is similar to that of hemiretinal vein occlusion but different from that of branch retinal vein occlusion (see the following discussion), occurs in arteriosclerosis, hypertension, diabetes mellitus, and glaucoma.

CRVO occurs in 2 forms:

- milder, perfused type, with <10 disc areas of nonperfusion on FA
- more severe, nonperfused (ischemic) type, with >10 disc areas of nonperfusion on FA

Both forms of CRVO are recognized clinically by the presence of retinal hemorrhages in all 4 quadrants. Usually, prominent edema of the optic nerve head is noted, along with dilatation and tortuosity of the retinal veins, variable numbers of cotton-wool spots, and macular edema.

Histologically, acute ischemic CRVO is characterized by marked retinal edema, focal retinal necrosis, and extensive intraretinal hemorrhage. With long-standing CRVO, glial cells respond to the insult by replication and intracellular deposition of filaments *(gliosis).* The hemorrhage, disorganization of the retinal architecture, hemosiderosis, and gliosis seen in vein occlusions distinguish the final histologic picture from that of CRAO (Fig 11-26). After a CRVO, numerous microaneurysms develop in the retinal capillaries, and acellular capillary beds are present to a variable degree. With time, dilated collateral vessels develop at the optic nerve head. A significant amount of VEGF is often elaborated by oxygen-deprived retinal cells and endothelial cells, with resultant neovascularization of the iris and angle, and less often, the retina.

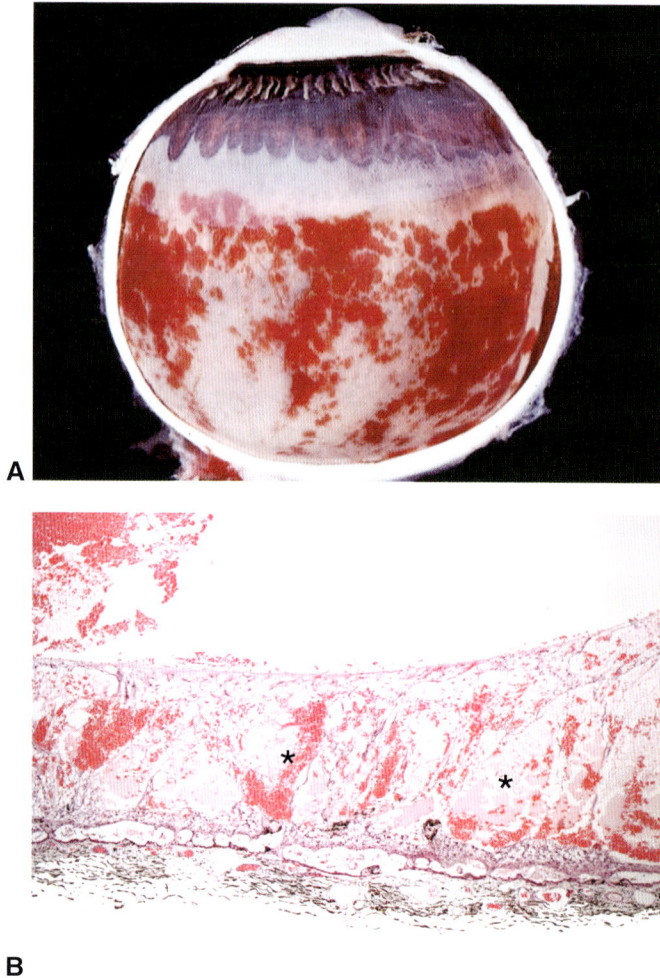

Figure 11-26 Central retinal vein occlusion (CRVO). **A,** Gross appearance of diffuse retinal hemorrhage after CRVO. **B,** Photomicrograph of a long-standing CRVO showing loss of the normal lamellar architecture of the retina, marked edema with cystoid spaces *(asterisks)* containing blood and proteinaceous exudate, and vitreous hemorrhage. *(Part B courtesy of Robert H. Rosa Jr, MD.)*

In *branch retinal vein occlusion (BRVO)*, occlusion of a tributary retinal vein occurs at the site of an arteriovenous crossing. At the crossing of a branch retinal artery and vein, the 2 vessels share a common adventitial sheath. With arteriovascular changes in the arteriole, the retinal venule may become compressed, leading to turbulent flow and thrombosis similar to that causing CRVO. Systemic arteriosclerosis and hypertension are risk factors for developing BRVO. BRVO leads to sectoral retinal hemorrhages and cotton-wool spots; however, because it does not always result in total inner retinal ischemia, neovascularization is unlikely unless the ischemia is extensive (>5 disc diameters). Findings in eyes with permanent vision loss from BRVO include CME, retinal nonperfusion, macular edema with hard lipid exudates, late pigmentary changes in the macula, subretinal fibrosis, and epiretinal membrane formation.

The histologic picture of BRVO resembles that of CRVO, but the changes are localized to the retinal area in the distribution of the occluded vein. Inner ischemic retinal atrophy is a characteristic late histologic finding in both retinal arterial and venous occlusions (see Fig 11-15). Numerous microaneurysms and dilated collateral vessels may be present. Acellular retinal capillaries are present to a variable degree, correlating with retinal capillary nonperfusion on retinal angiography.

See BCSC Section 12, *Retina and Vitreous,* for additional discussion of BRVO and CRVO.

Baseline and early natural history report: the Central Vein Occlusion Study. *Arch Ophthalmol.* 1993;111(8):1087–1095.

Natural history and clinical management of central retinal vein occlusion. The Central Vein Occlusion Study Group. *Arch Ophthalmol.* 1997;115(4):486–491.

Diabetic retinopathy

Diabetic retinopathy is one of the most common causes of new blindness in the United States and remains the leading cause among 20- to 60-year-olds. Early in the course of diabetic retinopathy, certain physiologic abnormalities occur:

- impaired autoregulation of the retinal vasculature
- alterations in retinal blood flow
- breakdown of the blood–retina barrier

Histologically, the primary changes occur in the retinal microcirculation and include

- thickening of the retinal capillary basement membrane
- selective loss of capillary pericytes
- microaneurysm formation
- retinal capillary closure (histologically recognized as acellular capillary beds)

Dilated intraretinal telangiectatic vessels, or IRMAs, may develop (see Figs 11-19, 11-21), and neovascularization may follow (see Fig 11-23). Intraretinal edema, hemorrhages, exudates, and microinfarcts of the NFL may develop secondary to primary retinal vascular changes. Acutely, microinfarcts of the NFL (see Fig 11-17) manifest as cotton-wool spots. Subsequently, focal inner ischemic atrophy appears (see Fig 11-15).

Laser photocoagulation, used in the treatment of diabetic retinopathy, results in focal destruction of the retina and RPE and occlusion of the choriocapillaris (Fig 11-27). These burns heal by proliferation of the underlying RPE and glial scarring, forming a chorioretinal adhesion.

Diabetic choroidopathy

In patients with diabetes mellitus, alterations to the choroid are common in addition to retinal findings. Risk factors for diabetic choroidopathy include diabetic retinopathy, poor diabetic control, and the diabetic treatment regimen. Histologic studies have shown loss of the choriocapillaris, tortuous blood vessels, microaneurysms, drusenoid deposits on the Bruch membrane, and choroidal neovascularization. Most of these findings occur at or anterior to the equator.

Lutty GA. Diabetic choroidopathy. *Vision Res.* 2017;39:161–167.

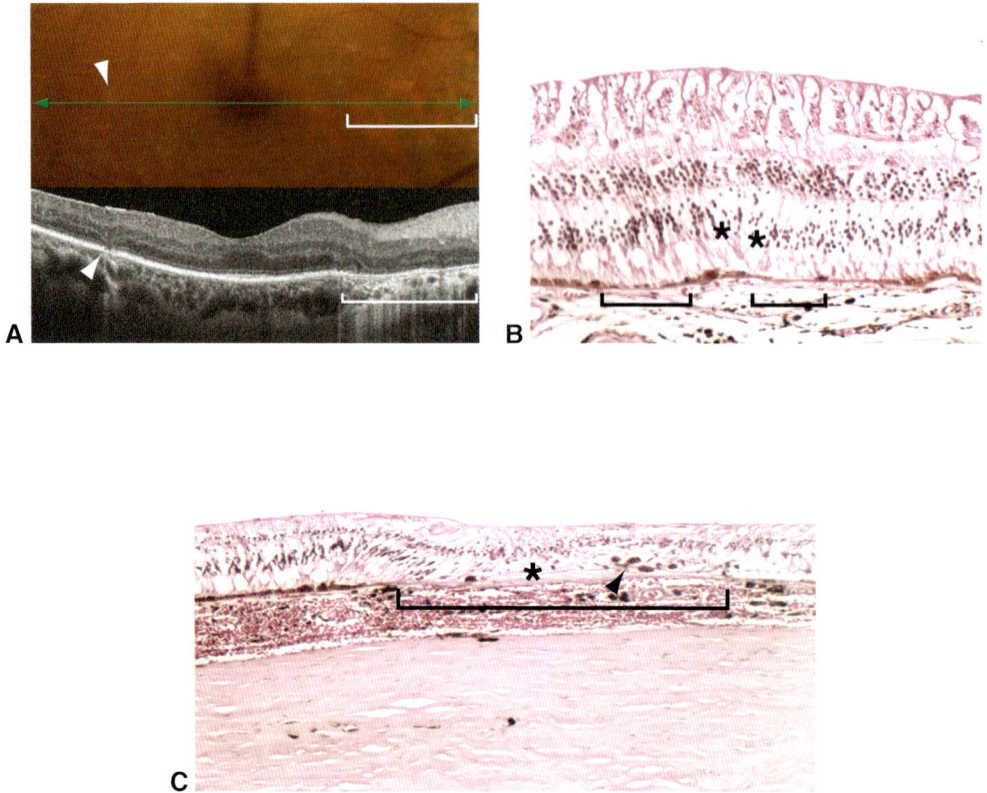

Figure 11-27 Laser photocoagulation scars. **A,** Clinical photograph *(upper panel)* and SD-OCT *(lower panel)* show a focal laser scar *(arrowheads)* and area of peripapillary atrophy *(brackets)*. The *double-headed arrow (upper panel)* indicates the meridian of the SD-OCT scan through the macula *(lower panel)*. In the *lower panel*, note the disruption of the outer plexiform layer, outer nuclear layer, ellipsoid zone, and RPE in the region of the focal laser scar *(bracket)*. **B,** In light applications of laser photocoagulation, focal disruption and attenuation of the outer nuclear layer *(asterisks)*, inner/outer segments, and RPE *(brackets)* may occur. **C,** In more intense laser applications, loss of the photoreceptor cell layer and RPE and obliteration of the choriocapillaris *(bracket)* may occur. Note the thin subretinal fibrosis *(asterisk)* in the laser scar. Variable RPE hypertrophy, hyperplasia, and migration into the retina *(arrowhead)*, as well as breaks in Bruch membrane, can occur. *(Courtesy of Robert H. Rosa Jr, MD.)*

Other intraocular changes in diabetes mellitus

In diabetes mellitus, prolonged hyperglycemia can result in many intraocular changes. The corneal epithelial basement membrane thickens and can result in inadequate adherence of the epithelium to the underlying Bowman layer. This change predisposes patients with diabetes mellitus to corneal abrasions and poor corneal epithelial healing. Lacy vacuolation of the iris pigment epithelium (Fig 11-28A) occurs in association with acute hyperglycemia. Histologically, the intraepithelial vacuoles contain glycogen, which is PAS-positive and diastase-sensitive. Thickening of the basement membrane of the pigmented ciliary epithelium (Fig 11-28B) is almost universally present in the eyes of patients with longstanding diabetes mellitus. The incidence of cataract formation is also increased.

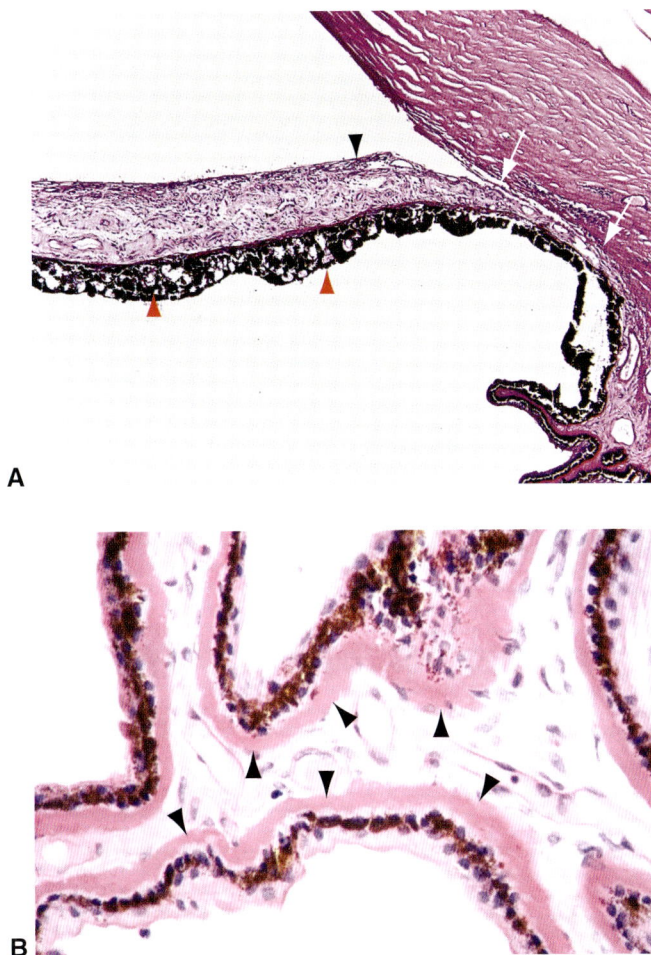

Figure 11-28 Histologic intraocular changes in diabetes mellitus. **A,** Photomicrograph (PAS stain) shows iris neovascularization *(black arrowhead)*, angle closure by peripheral anterior synechiae *(between white arrows)*, and lacy vacuolation of the iris pigment epithelium *(red arrowheads)*. **B,** High-magnification photomicrograph shows PAS-stained ciliary body with marked thickening of the basement membrane of the pigmented ciliary epithelium *(arrowheads)*. *(Part A courtesy of Tatyana Milman, MD; part B courtesy of Nasreen A. Syed, MD.)*

Abusive Head Trauma

Abusive head trauma (AHT) or nonaccidental trauma, previously referred to as *shaken baby syndrome*, is physical abuse that results in traumatic brain injury as well as injury to other structures in the head and neck in a young child. Victims are usually younger than 5 years and are most commonly younger than 24 months. Though not necessarily a degenerative process, AHT induces a variety of changes over time and therefore is included in this section.

In a young child, ocular findings in AHT often result from repetitive acceleration-deceleration forces applied to the head with or without direct head trauma. Injuries stem from the complex interactions of ocular and intracranial forces, as well as injuries to other parts of the body. In cases of suspected AHT, the ophthalmologist may provide critical clinical evidence by performing a thorough dilated fundus examination. On clinical examination, the most frequent ocular finding is retinal hemorrhage, present in up to 90% of cases. However, the absence of retinal hemorrhages does not entirely exclude a diagnosis of AHT. Circumferential perimacular folds are considered a specific finding of AHT, but they are not pathognomonic.

Because AHT is sometimes fatal, forensic examination of the eyes at autopsy is important. On gross examination of the globe, retinal hemorrhages may be dispersed throughout the fundus (Fig 11-29A). Subdural hemorrhage in the optic nerve sheath is also present (Fig 11-29B) and can be appreciated as a bluish discoloration of the optic nerve sheath.

Histologic findings in the eye may include

- hemorrhages involving any layer of the retina
- hemorrhagic retinal schisis cavities, usually between the ILM and the rest of the neurosensory retina
- retinal hemorrhages extending to the ora serrata
- subretinal hemorrhage
- subdural hemorrhage in the optic nerve
- subarachnoid, focal intradural and/or focal epidural hemorrhage of the optic nerve sheath
- perimacular circumferential retinal fold, often surrounding hemorrhagic macular retinoschisis cavity
- intrascleral hemorrhage adjacent to the optic nerve

As noted previously, no clinical or histopathologic findings are pathognomonic for AHT. Each case needs to be interpreted in the context of the clinical history and other clinical and pathologic findings. Whenever AHT is suspected, a physician is required by

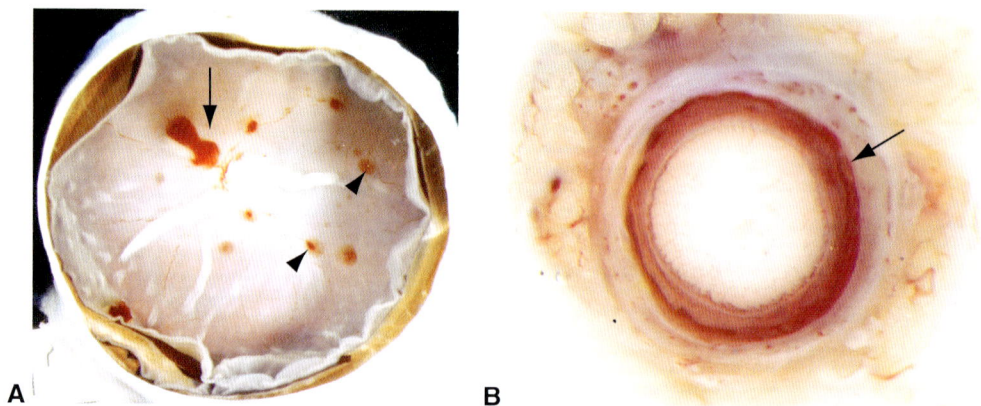

Figure 11-29 Abusive head trauma. **A,** Gross examination of the globe reveals multiple retinal hemorrhages *(arrowheads)*, including sub-internal limiting membrane hemorrhage *(arrow)* as a result of abusive head trauma. **B,** Cross section of the optic nerve reveals 360° of subdural hemorrhage *(arrow)*. *(Courtesy of Nasreen A. Syed, MD.)*

law in all US states and Canadian provinces to report the incident to a designated government agency. See BCSC Section 6, *Pediatric Ophthalmology and Strabismus,* for additional information on this topic.

Breazzano MP, Unkrich KH, Barker-Griffith AE. Clinicopathological findings in abusive head trauma: analysis of 110 infant autopsy eyes. *Am J Ophthalmol.* 2014;158(6):1146–1154.e2.

Age-Related Macular Degeneration

Age-related macular degeneration (AMD) is the leading cause of new blindness in adults in the United States. Although the etiology of AMD is poorly understood, evidence suggests that both genes and environmental factors are involved. Genome-wide and candidate association studies have identified risk loci for AMD and implicated certain genes, particularly *CFH* and *ARMS2*. Older age, tobacco use, positive family history, and cardiovascular disease increase the risk of AMD development. In addition, randomized clinical trials showing the benefit of antioxidant supplementation in AMD suggest that oxidative stress has a role in disease progression.

Several characteristic changes in the retina, RPE, Bruch membrane, and choroid occur in AMD. The first detectable pathologic change is the appearance of deposits between the basement membrane of the RPE and the elastic portion of Bruch membrane (basal linear deposits) and similar deposits between the plasma membrane and the basement membrane of the RPE (basal laminar deposits). Electron microscopy can distinguish between these types of deposits; in advanced cases, the deposits may become confluent and visible with light microscopy without being clinically apparent (Fig 11-30). This histologic appearance has been described clinically as *diffuse drusen.*

The first clinically detectable feature of AMD is the appearance of drusen. The clinical term *drusen* has been correlated pathologically to large, extracellular PAS-positive deposits between the RPE and Bruch membrane. Drusen may be transient in their clinical appearance. Clinical types of drusen with their histologic descriptions are listed in Table 11-1, and Figures 11-31, 11-32, and 11-33 depict some of these drusen.

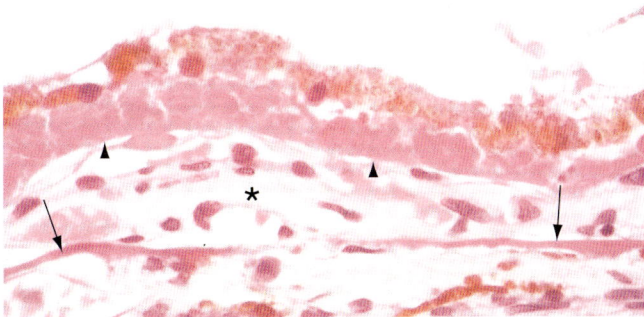

Figure 11-30 Diffuse drusen. Note the diffuse deposition of eosinophilic material *(arrowheads)* beneath the RPE. Choroidal neovascularization *(asterisk)* is present between the diffuse drusen and the elastic portion of Bruch membrane *(arrows)* (PAS stain). *(Courtesy of Hans E. Grossniklaus, MD.)*

Table 11-1 Clinical and Histologic Appearance of Drusen

Type of Drusen	Clinical Appearance	Histologic Appearance
Hard (nodular)	Discrete, yellowish, circumscribed, deep retinal lesions; sometimes have a glistening appearance	PAS-positive deposits composed of hyaline material between the RPE and Bruch membrane or on Bruch membrane (see Fig 11-31)
Soft	Yellow, somewhat amorphous lesions with poorly demarcated edges; usually >63 μm in size; may have appearance of fluid under RPE on optical coherence tomography	Focal areas of cleavage of the RPE and basal laminar or linear deposits from Bruch membrane that are composed of sub-RPE eosinophilic lipoproteinaceous material (see Fig 11-32)
Basal laminar or cuticular	Small, regular, diffuse nodular deposits that may be difficult to appreciate clinically	Linear deposits of eosinophilic material along the inner surface of Bruch membrane or within the basal portion of RPE cells
Calcific	Sharply demarcated, glistening, white-to-yellow refractile lesions	Nodular excrescences along the inner surface of Bruch membrane that are deep purple on H&E stain due to calcification
Reticular pseudodrusen	Ill-defined, whitish-yellow lesions in the deep retina with a reticular pattern; usually seen in the superior and temporal macula, with enhanced visibility when viewed with blue light, near-infrared imaging, or fundus autofluorescence	Accumulation of lipid-rich material in the subretinal space between photoreceptor inner/outer segments and RPE (see Fig 11-33)

H&E = hematoxylin-eosin; PAS = periodic acid–Schiff; RPE = retinal pigment epithelium.

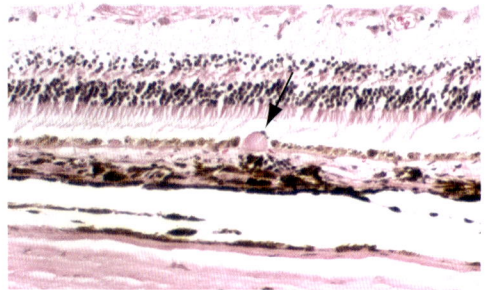

Figure 11-31 Photomicrograph illustrating a dome-shaped, nodular, hard druse *(arrow)* and attenuation of the overlying RPE. *(Courtesy of Robert H. Rosa Jr, MD.)*

Histochemical and molecular/biological analyses have demonstrated that the major constituents of human drusen include albumin, apolipoproteins, complement factors and related proteins, immunoglobulins, lipids, and β-amyloid. *Reticular pseudodrusen (RPD),* also known as *subretinal drusenoid deposits,* are extracellular material interposed between the photoreceptor inner/outer segments and the RPE that contain membranous debris, unesterified cholesterol, complement factors and related proteins, and apolipoproteins but lack opsins. RPD may be associated with progression to advanced AMD (geographic

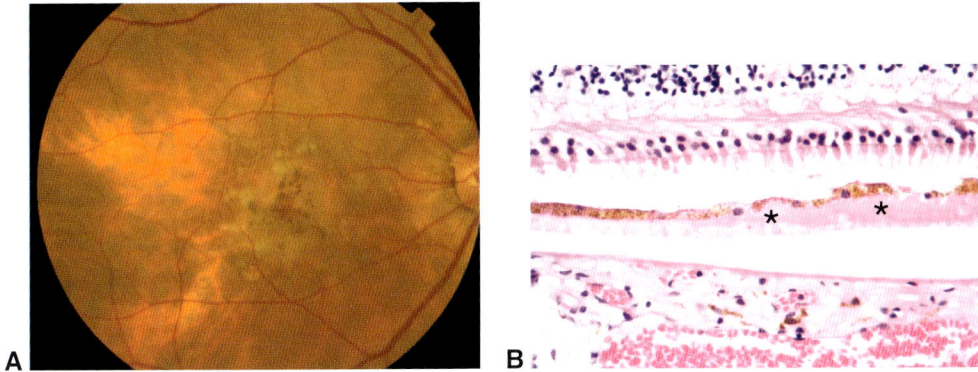

Figure 11-32 Confluent soft drusen. **A,** Clinical photograph of soft drusen. Note the pigment clumping overlying the confluent drusen in the central macula. **B,** Photomicrograph shows thick eosinophilic deposits *(asterisks)* between the RPE and Bruch membrane. The separation between the retina and RPE and the RPE and Bruch membrane is artifact. Note the marked attenuation of the photoreceptor cell nuclei in the outer nuclear layer and the loss of the outer segments over the confluent drusen. *(Part A courtesy of Robert H. Rosa Jr, MD; part B courtesy of Nasreen A. Syed, MD.)*

atrophy and choroidal neovascularization). Many eyes with clinically apparent drusen (especially soft drusen) are found to have basal laminar and/or basal linear deposits and diffuse drusen on histologic analysis.

Photoreceptor atrophy occurs to a variable degree in macular degeneration. This atrophy may be a primary abnormality of the photoreceptors or may be secondary to the underlying changes in the RPE, Bruch membrane, and/or choriocapillaris. In addition to photoreceptor atrophy, large zones of RPE atrophy may appear. When RPE atrophy occurs in the macular region, it is termed *geographic atrophy* (Fig 11-34). Drusen, photoreceptor atrophy, and RPE atrophy may all be present to varying degrees in *dry,* or *nonneovascular, AMD.* In addition, neovascular buds arising from the choriocapillaris are present in areas adjacent to the atrophic areas and in the peripheral choroid.

In eyes with choroidal neovascularization *(neovascular AMD;* also called *wet,* or *exudative, AMD),* fibrovascular tissue is present between the inner and outer layers of Bruch membrane, beneath the RPE, and/or in the subretinal space (Fig 11-35). Excised choroidal neovascular membranes (CNVMs) have demonstrated vascular channels, RPE, and various other components of the RPE–Bruch membrane complex, including photoreceptor outer segments, basal laminar and linear deposits, and inflammatory cells. CNVMs are classified as type 1, type 2, or type 3 depending on their pathologic and clinical features (see Fig 11-35C–E). *Type 1 CNVM* is characterized by neovascularization originating from the choriocapillaris that involves the Bruch membrane and the sub-RPE space (see Fig 11-35A, C). It is typically associated with basal laminar deposits and diffuse drusen. RPE atrophy and/or hyperplasia may overlie type 1 CNVM. *Type 2 CNVM* (see Fig 11-35B, D) occurs in the subretinal space and generally features only a small defect in the RPE. Type 1 CNVM is more characteristic of AMD, whereas type 2 is more characteristic of ocular histoplasmosis. *Type 3 CNVM* (see Fig 11-35E), previously referred to as *retinal angiomatous proliferation,* arises from the deep capillary plexus of the retina and grows toward the RPE.

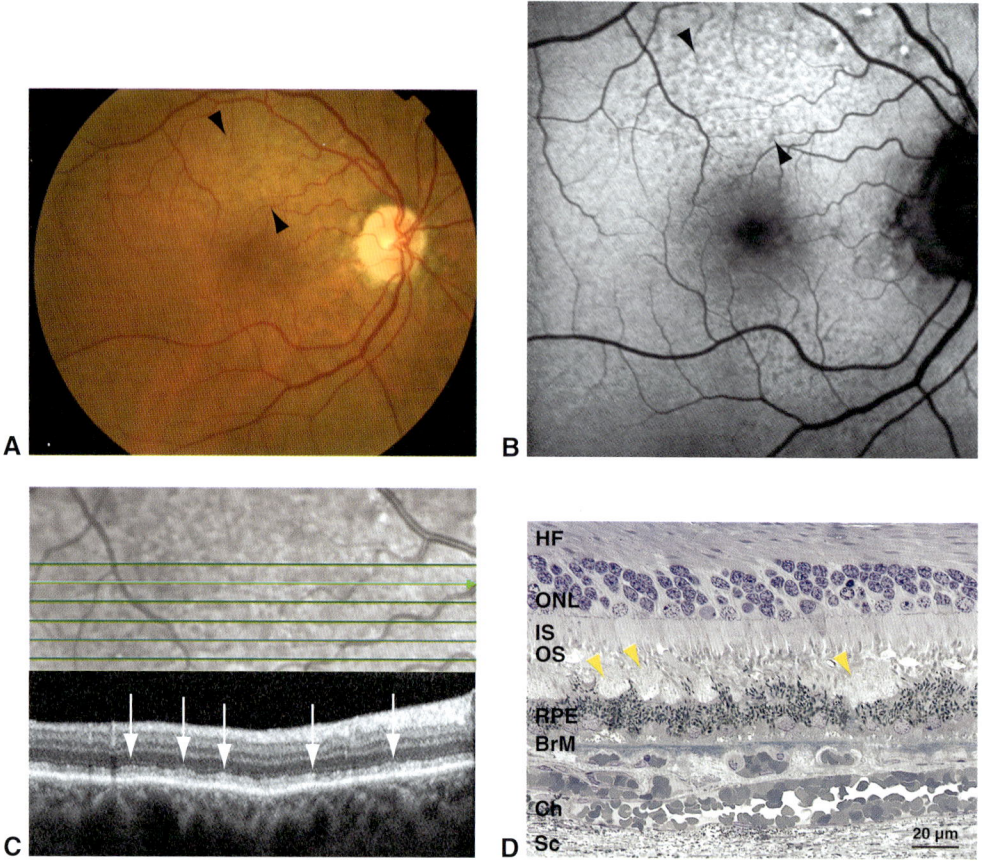

Figure 11-33 Reticular pseudodrusen. **A,** Color photograph shows the ill-defined, yellowish reticular pattern *(between arrowheads)* in the superior macula. **B,** Fundus autofluorescence (FAF) image shows the corresponding region *(between arrowheads)* with dotlike areas of decreased and increased FAF. **C,** Near-infrared image *(upper panel)* shows similar dotlike areas of decreased reflectance that, on SD-OCT *(lower panel)*, correspond to deposits *(arrows)* interposed between the photoreceptor outer segments and the RPE with focal disruption of the ellipsoid zone. **D,** Subretinal drusenoid deposits *(yellow arrowheads)* are the histologic correlate of reticular pseudodrusen. Note their location in the region of the outer segments. HF = Henle fiber layer; ONL = outer nuclear layer; IS = inner segment; OS = outer segment; RPE = retinal pigment epithelium; BrM = Bruch membrane; Ch = choroid; Sc = sclera. (Toluidine blue stain). *(Parts A–C courtesy of Robert H. Rosa Jr, MD; part D courtesy of Christine A. Curcio, PhD.)*

The choroidal and subretinal neovascular blood vessels leak fluid and may rupture easily, producing the exudative consequences of neovascular AMD, including macular edema, serous retinal detachment, and subretinal and intraretinal hemorrhages. VEGF inhibition with intravitreally administered anti-VEGF agents has been shown to reduce macular edema, slow progression of the neovascularization, and improve visual outcomes of patients with neovascular (wet) AMD. For further information, see BCSC Section 12, *Retina and Vitreous.*

Ratnapriya R, Chew EY. Age-related macular degeneration—clinical review and genetics update. *Clin Genet.* 2013;84(2):160–166.

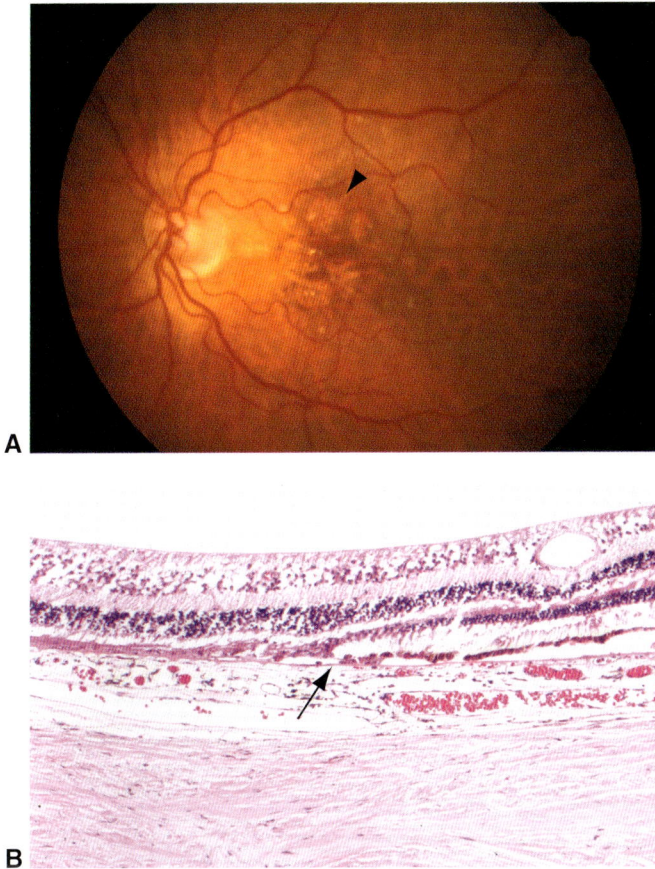

Figure 11-34 Geographic atrophy of the RPE. **A,** Fundus photograph shows focal geographic atrophy of the RPE *(arrowhead)* and drusen in nonneovascular age-related macular degeneration. **B,** Histologically, there is loss of the photoreceptor cell layer, RPE, and choriocapillaris *(left of arrow)* with an abrupt transition zone *(arrow)* to a more normal-appearing retina and RPE *(right of arrow).* Note the thick multicellular ganglion cell layer that identifies the macular region. *(Courtesy of Robert H. Rosa Jr, MD.)*

Seddon JM, McLeod DS, Bhutto IA, et al. Histopathological insights into choroidal vascular loss in clinically documented cases of age-related macular degeneration. *JAMA Ophthalmol.* 2016;154(11):1272–1280.

Polypoidal Choroidal Vasculopathy

Polypoidal choroidal vasculopathy, previously called *posterior uveal bleeding syndrome* and *multiple recurrent serosanguineous RPE detachments,* is a disorder in which dilated, thin-walled vascular channels (Figs 11-36, 11-37) are interposed between the RPE and the outer aspect of Bruch membrane. Associated choroidal neovascularization is often present in these lesions, as observed in several histologic specimens. See BCSC Section 12, *Retina and Vitreous,* for more information on this condition.

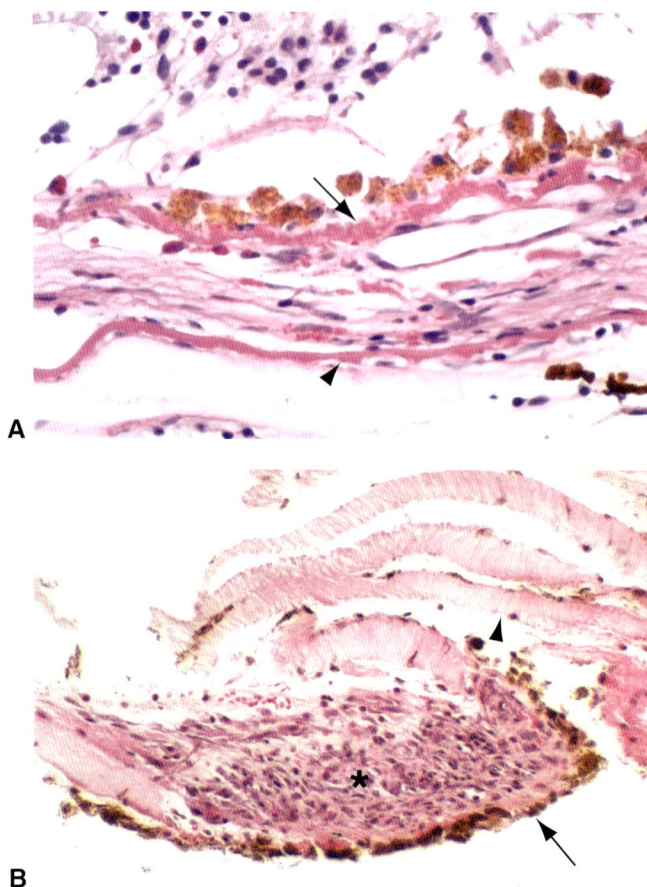

Figure 11-35 Choroidal neovascularization. **A,** Choroidal neovascular membranes (CNVMs) located between the inner *(arrow)* and outer *(arrowhead)* layers of Bruch membrane (sub-RPE; type 1 CNVM). Note the loss of overlying photoreceptor inner and outer segments, the RPE hyperplasia, and the PAS-positive basal laminar deposit *(arrow)*. **B,** Surgically excised CNVM (subretinal, type 2) composed of fibrovascular tissue *(asterisk)* that is lined externally by RPE *(arrow)* with adherent photoreceptor outer segments *(arrowhead)*.

(Continued)

Macular Dystrophies

See BCSC Section 12, *Retina and Vitreous,* for additional discussion of macular dystrophies.

Fundus flavimaculatus and Stargardt disease

Fundus flavimaculatus and Stargardt disease are thought to represent opposite ends of an inherited disease spectrum characterized by yellowish flecks at the RPE level, a generalized vermilion (reddish) fundus clinically, variable late RPE atrophy, dark choroid on FA, and gradually decreasing vision (Fig 11-38; see also Fig 13-11 in BCSC Section 12, *Retina and Vitreous*). The inheritance pattern is generally autosomal recessive, but

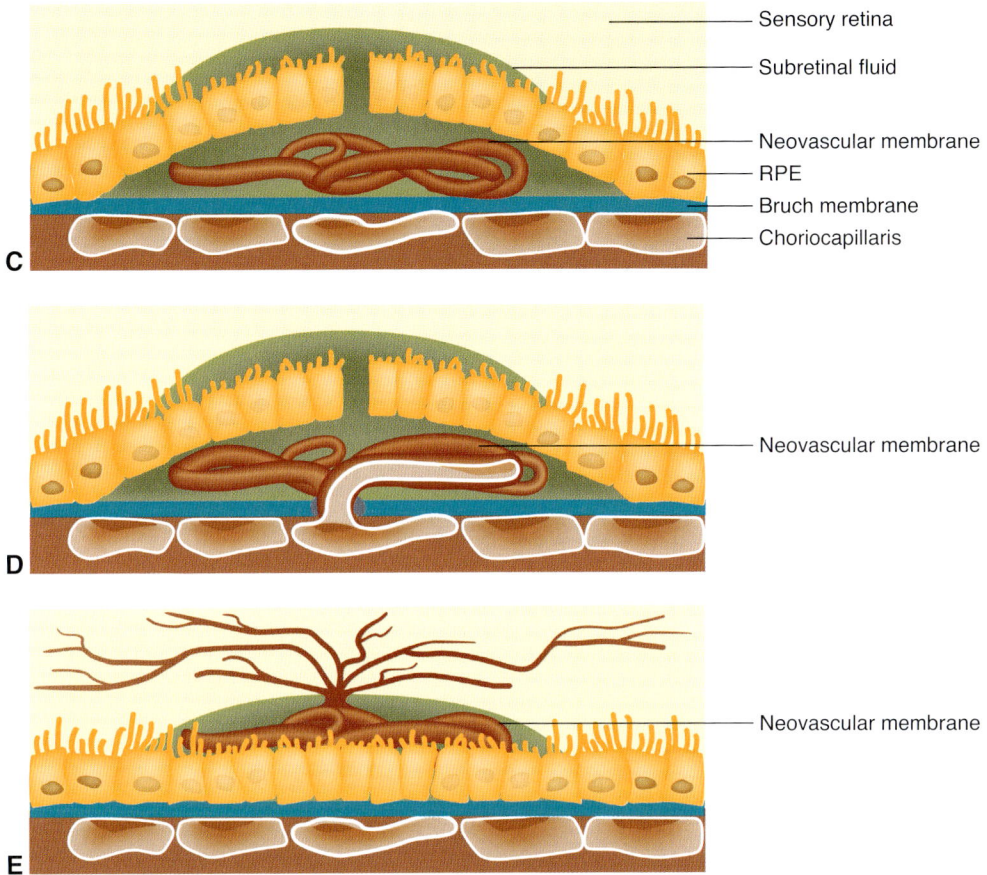

Figure 11-35 *(continued)* Schematic illustrations of CNVM types 1 **(C)**, 2 **(D)**, and 3 **(E)**. *(Parts A and B courtesy of Robert H. Rosa Jr, MD. Illustrations by Cyndie C. H. Wooley.)*

autosomal dominant forms have been reported. The most striking feature of Stargardt disease revealed by light and electron microscopy is the marked engorgement of RPE cells with lipofuscin-like, PAS-positive material and apical displacement of the normal RPE melanin granules (see Fig 11-38D; see also Fig 13-12 in BCSC Section 12, *Retina and Vitreous*).

Pattern dystrophies

The term *pattern dystrophies* refers to a heterogeneous group of inherited disorders characterized by varying patterns of pigment deposition in the macular RPE. The most common genetic mutation associated with the pattern dystrophies occurs in the *PRPH2 (peripherin 2)* gene. Recognized pattern dystrophies include butterfly-shaped pattern dystrophy (BPD), adult-onset foveomacular vitelliform dystrophy (AFMVD), reticular dystrophy, and fundus pulverulentus. BPD is characterized by an irregular, butterfly-shaped,

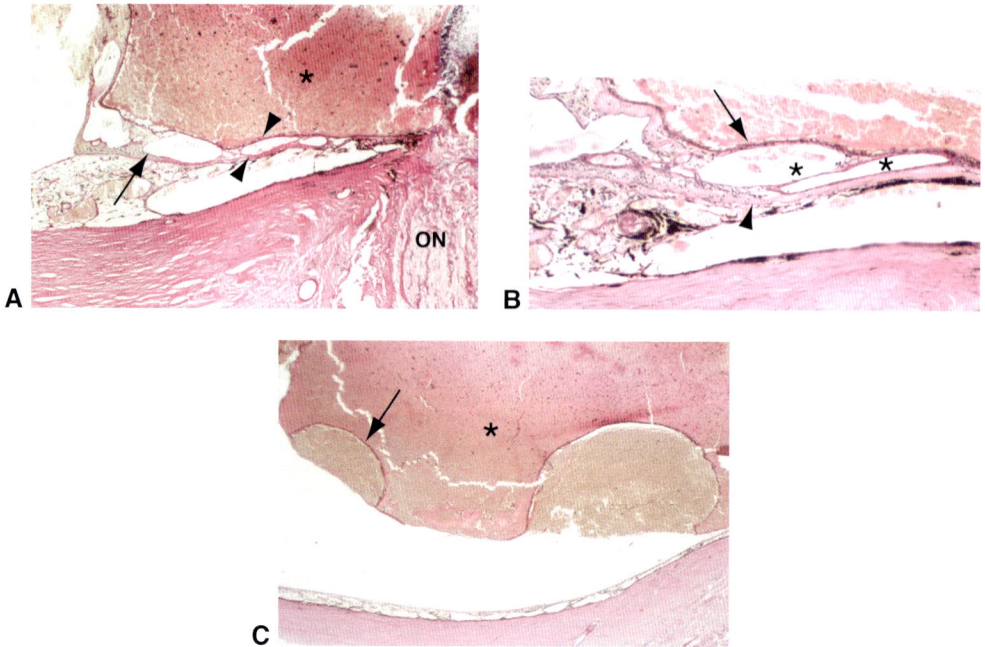

Figure 11-36 Polypoidal choroidal vasculopathy. **A,** Peripapillary dilated vascular channels *(arrow)* between the RPE and the outer aspect of Bruch membrane *(arrowheads)*. Note the dense subretinal hemorrhage *(asterisk)*. ON=optic nerve. **B,** Higher-magnification view of thin-walled vascular channels *(asterisks)* interposed between the RPE *(arrow)* and the Bruch membrane *(arrowhead)*. **C,** Hemorrhagic RPE detachments *(arrow)* and serosanguineous subretinal fluid *(asterisk)*. *(Courtesy of Robert H. Rosa Jr, MD.)*

depigmented lesion at the RPE level. AFMVD is characterized by slightly elevated, symmetric, round-to-oval yellow lesions at the RPE level; these lesions are typically smaller than the vitelliform lesion characteristic of Best disease (Fig 11-39).

Spectral-domain optical coherence tomography (SD-OCT) in patients with pattern dystrophy reveals elevation of the photoreceptor layer, with localization of the dystrophic material between the photoreceptors and RPE (see Fig 11-39C). Histologic studies reveal central loss of the RPE and photoreceptor cell layer with a moderate number of pigment-containing histiocytes (macrophages) in the subretinal space and outer neurosensory retina (see Fig 11-39D). The adjacent RPE is distended with lipofuscin (see Fig 11-39E). Basal laminar and linear deposits may be present throughout the macular region. The pathologic finding of pigment-containing cells with lipofuscin and drusenlike material in the subretinal space correlates with the vitelliform pattern seen clinically.

Diffuse Photoreceptor Dystrophies

Inherited dystrophies that affect the rods and cones are discussed in greater detail in BCSC Section 12, *Retina and Vitreous*. Only the most common photoreceptor dystrophy, retinitis pigmentosa (RP), is discussed here.

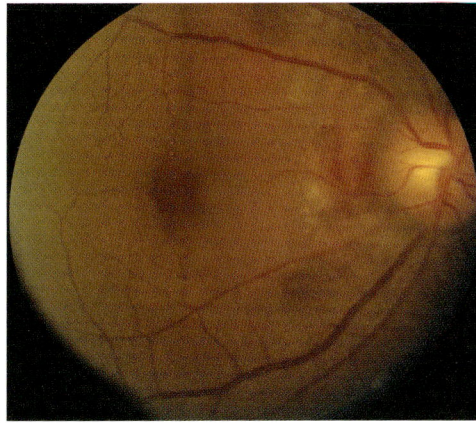

A

FA 1:00.06 30° ART + ICGA 1:00.03 30° ART [HS]

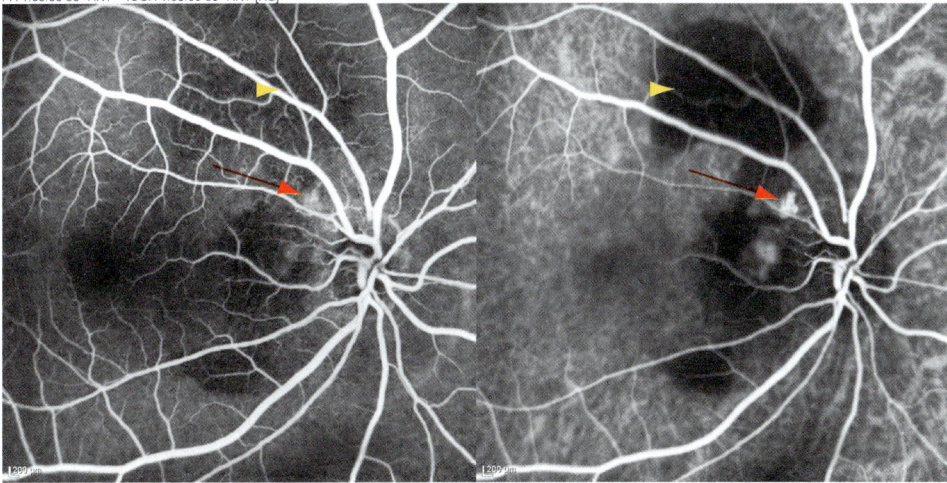

B

IR 30° ART + OCT 30° (8.5 mm) ART (20) Q: 28 [HR]

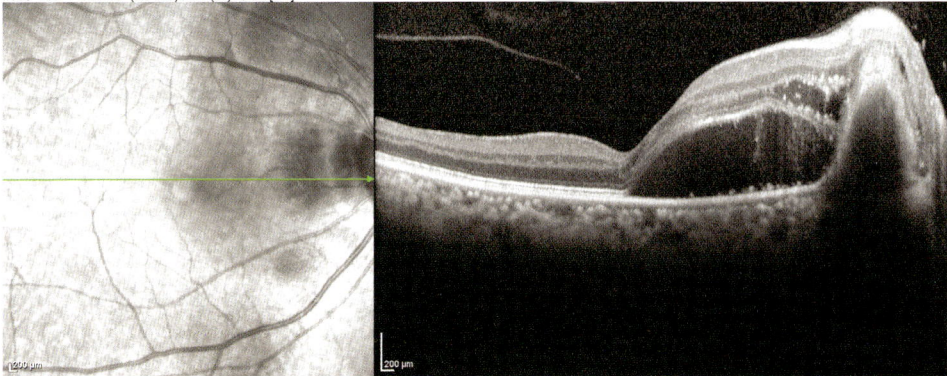

C

Figure 11-37 Polypoidal choroidal vasculopathy. **A,** Fundus photograph reveals elevated, red-orange, nodular subretinal lesions in the peripapillary area. **B,** Fluorescein angiogram (60 seconds) on the left shows mildly hyperfluorescent polypoidal lesions *(arrow),* which are best seen on the indocyanine green (ICG) angiogram on the right *(arrow).* Hypofluorescent areas on the fluorescein angiogram *(arrowhead)* and ICG angiogram *(arrowhead)* are due to hemorrhage. **C,** OCT from the same patient shows an elevated sub-RPE lesion in the peripapillary region with associated intraretinal and subretinal fluid. *(Courtesy of Robert M. Carroll, MD.)*

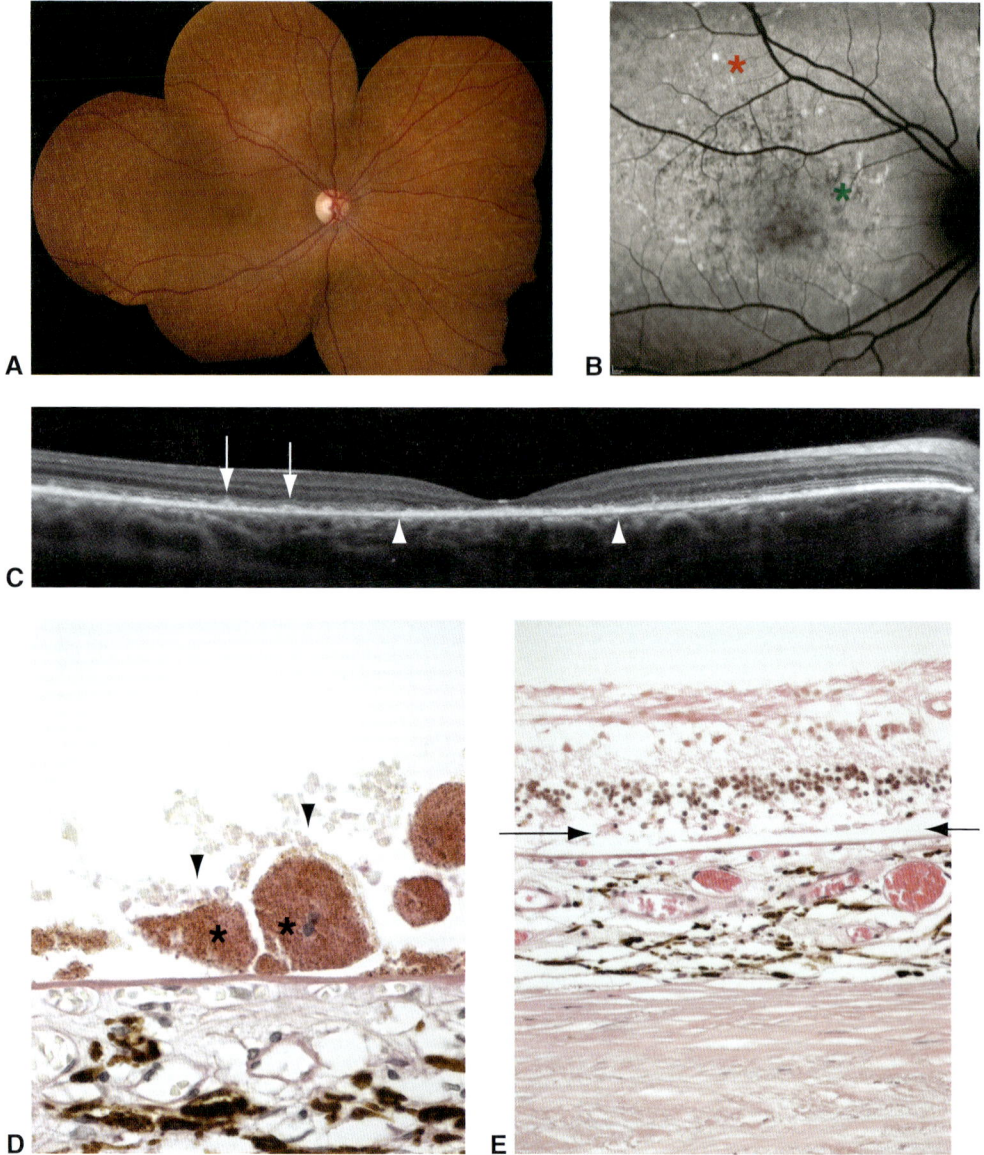

Figure 11-38 Stargardt disease. **A,** Fundus photograph shows diffuse retinal flecks. **B,** FAF imaging reveals increased autofluorescence corresponding to the retinal flecks *(red asterisk)* and decreased autofluorescence corresponding to areas of RPE atrophy *(green asterisk).* **C,** SD-OCT image shows hyperreflectivity at the level of the RPE (corresponding histologically with enlarged RPE cells with increased lipofuscin content) *(arrows),* markedly thinned retina in the foveal region, and focal attenuation or loss of the photoreceptor cell layer in areas corresponding to RPE atrophy *(area between arrowheads).* **D,** Photomicrograph of a PAS-stained section demonstrates hypertrophic RPE cells *(arrowheads)* with numerous PAS-positive cytoplasmic granules containing lipofuscin *(asterisks).* This histologic finding corresponds to the retinal flecks seen clinically. **E,** In advanced stages of Stargardt disease, geographic RPE atrophy with loss of the photoreceptor cell layer *(between arrows)* may be noted. *(Parts A–C courtesy of Tomas S. Aleman, MD; parts D and E courtesy of Sander Dubovy, MD.)*

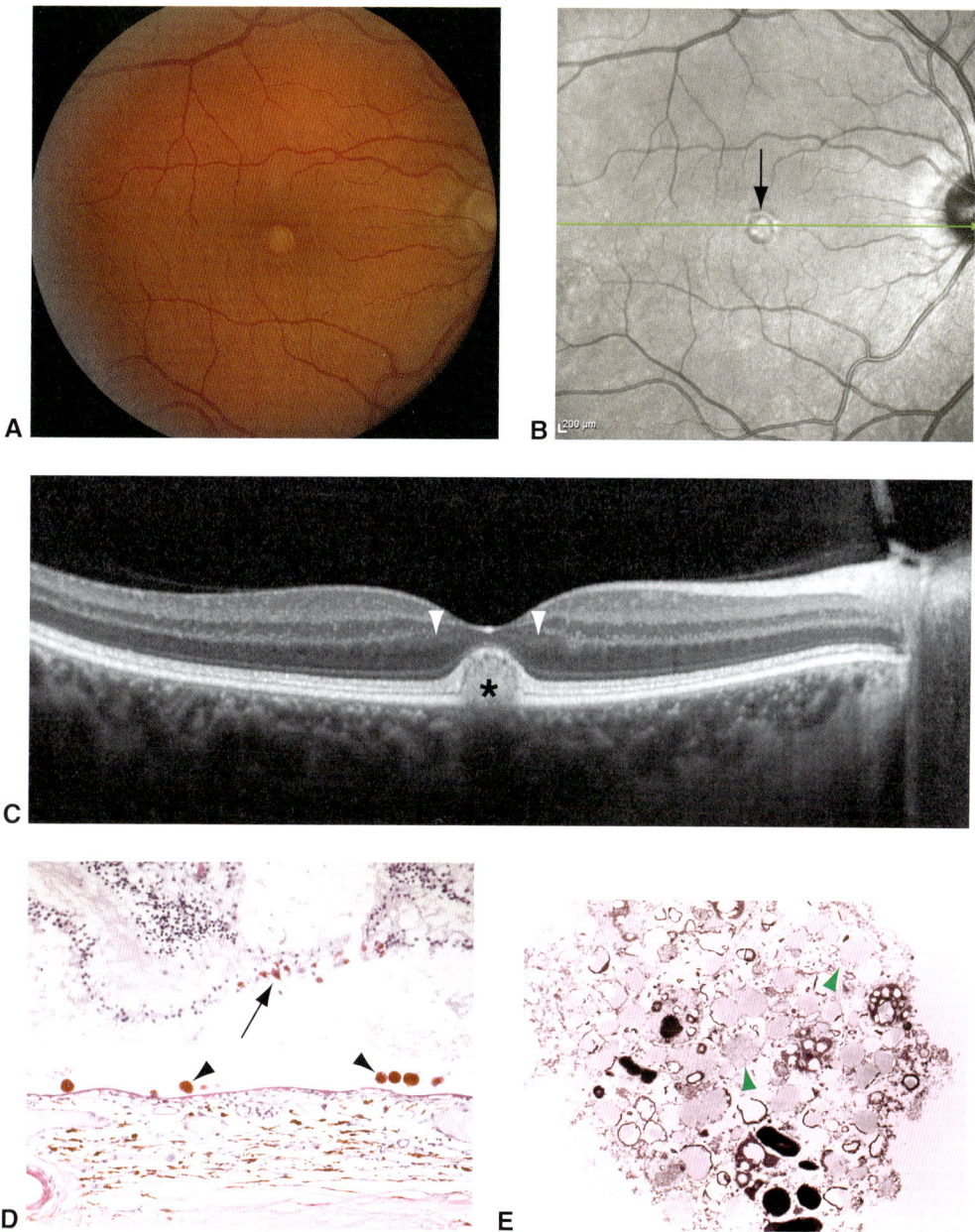

Figure 11-39 Adult-onset foveomacular vitelliform dystrophy. **A,** Fundus photograph shows a yellowish, egg yolk–like lesion with focal pigment clumping and mottling in the central macula. **B,** Near-infrared FAF image from the same patient shown in part **A** reveals increased autofluorescence corresponding to the vitelliform lesion *(arrow)*. **C,** SD-OCT (same patient as in parts **A** and **B**) reveals subfoveal hyperreflective material *(asterisk)*. Note the irregular RPE elevation *(between arrowheads)*. **D,** Histologic findings include pigment-containing cells in the subretinal space *(arrowheads)* and outer neurosensory retina *(arrow)*. **E,** Electron microscopy shows pigment-containing cells filled with lipofuscin *(arrowheads)*. *(Parts A–C courtesy of Tomas S. Aleman, MD; parts D and E courtesy of Sander Dubovy, MD.)*

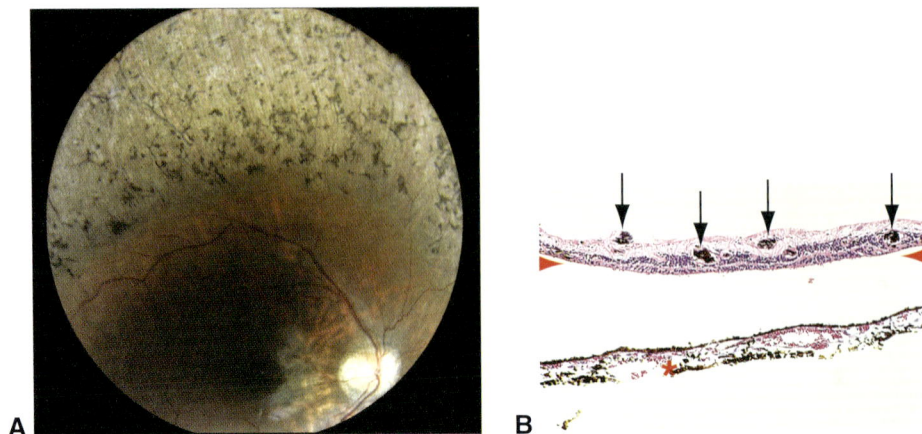

Figure 11-40 Retinitis pigmentosa. **A,** Fundus photograph shows pallor of the optic nerve, retinal arteriolar narrowing, focal depigmentation, and bone-spicule pigmentation in the peripheral fundus. **B,** Histologically, marked photoreceptor cell loss *(between red arrowheads)* and RPE migration into the retina in a perivascular distribution *(black arrows)* are apparent and correspond to the bone-spicule–like pattern seen clinically. The retina is artifactitiously detached from the underlying RPE and choroid *(asterisk)*. *(Part A courtesy of Tomas S. Aleman, MD.)*

RP refers to a group of inherited retinal diseases characterized by RPE and photoreceptor dysfunction and degeneration, resulting in progressive visual field loss. The genetics of RP are complex: it can be sporadic, autosomal dominant, autosomal recessive, or X-linked. Mutations in the rhodopsin gene *(RHO)* are the most common cause of autosomal dominant RP.

The term *retinitis pigmentosa* is a misnomer because clear evidence of inflammation is lacking. Ophthalmoscopic findings include pigment arranged in a bone-spicule–like configuration around the retinal arterioles, arteriolar narrowing, and optic nerve head atrophy (Fig 11-40A). The disease is characterized primarily by the loss of rod photoreceptor cells via apoptosis. Cones are seldom directly affected; however, they degenerate secondary to the loss of rods. Microscopically, loss of photoreceptor cells is seen, as well as RPE migration into the neurosensory retina around retinal vessels (Fig 11-40B). The arterioles, though narrowed clinically, show no histologic abnormality initially. Later, thickening and hyalinization of the vessel walls develop. The optic nerve may show diffuse or sectoral atrophy, with gliosis as a late change.

Neoplasia

The tumors discussed in this chapter arise from tissue derived from the inner layer of the optic cup.

Retinoblastoma

Retinoblastoma is the most common primary intraocular malignancy in childhood, occurring in 1 in 14,000–20,000 live births. Chapter 19 discusses the clinical aspects of retinoblastoma. Retinoblastoma is also discussed in BCSC Section 6, *Pediatric Ophthalmology and Strabismus.*

Pathogenesis

Although retinoblastoma was once thought to be of glial origin (eg, lesions clinically simulating retinoblastoma were formerly called *pseudogliomas*), the tumor's neuroblastic origin from the nucleated layers of the retina has been well established. In immunohistochemical studies, tumor cells stain positively for neuron-specific enolase, retinal S-antigen, and rhodopsin. Tumor cells also secrete an extracellular substance known as *interphotoreceptor retinoid-binding protein (IRBP),* which is produced by normal photoreceptors. Retinoblastoma cells grown in culture have expressed red and green photopigments, as well as cone cell α-subunits of transducin. These findings further support the hypothesis that retinoblastoma may be a neoplasm of cone cell lineage. However, immunohistochemical and molecular studies cast some doubt on a single-cell progenitor for retinoblastoma. The presence of small amounts of glial tissue within retinoblastomas suggests that resident glial cells may undergo reactive proliferation or become trapped within the tumor.

Retinoblastoma develops when both copies of the retinoblastoma gene *(RB1)* become nonfunctional, either by a deletion error or by mutation. *RB1* is located on the long arm of chromosome 13 and encodes for retinoblastoma protein, pRB, which functions as a tumor suppressor. Thus, loss of the gene does not actively cause tumorigenesis but rather leads to loss of tumor suppression, resulting in the development of retinoblastoma (and other tumors, such as osteosarcoma).

A single normal gene copy is sufficient to suppress the development of retinoblastoma. However, when 1 abnormal gene is present, if a mutation in the remaining normal gene occurs during retinal differentiation, loss of tumor suppression occurs and retinoblastoma is likely to develop.

Recently, *MYCN* oncogene amplification was demonstrated in a minority (approximately 3%) of retinoblastomas that lacked *RB1* gene mutations. This type of retinoblastoma is associated with very early age (ie, median age of 4.5 months) at diagnosis and unilateral occurrence, as well as more aggressive growth compared to retinoblastoma with *RB1* mutations.

Rushlow DE, Mol BM, Kennett JY, et al. Characterisation of retinoblastomas without *RB1* mutations: genomic, gene expression, and clinical studies. *Lancet Oncol.* 2013;14(4): 327–334.

Histologic features

On hematoxylin-eosin stain, retinoblastoma is histologically distinguished by 3 predominant colors, appreciated best at low magnification: blue, representing the retinoblastoma tumor cells; pink, representing areas of necrosis; and purple, representing areas of calcification. Commonly referred to as a *small blue cell tumor*, retinoblastoma consists of cells with round or oval nuclei that are approximately twice the size of a lymphocyte. The nuclei are hyperchromatic and surrounded by a scant amount of cytoplasm. The cells are generally tightly packed, and the nuclei can be indented by adjacent cells (nuclear molding). Mitotic activity is usually high, although frequent apoptotic cells may complicate identification of mitoses. As the tumor expands into the vitreous or subretinal space, retinoblastoma cells surround blood vessels for sustenance, creating a characteristic pattern referred to as *pseudorosettes* (ie, viable tumor cells surrounding a blood vessel) (Fig 11-41). However, they frequently outgrow their blood supply, and regions of ischemic necrosis begin 90–120 μm from the central vessel. Associated with the necrosis are foci of calcification. DNA released from degenerate cells sometimes accumulates in the walls of tumor blood vessels (Fig 11-42) or within vessels in other ocular tissues, such as the iris. Neovascularization of the iris, sometimes resulting in angle closure, may occur in the setting of retinoblastoma (Fig 11-43).

Small clumps of cells shed from the tumor may remain viable in the vitreous (vitreous seeds) and subretinal space without a blood supply and may eventually develop into focal tumor implants throughout the eye. It may be difficult to determine histologically whether multiple intraocular foci of the tumor represent multiple primary tumors, implying a systemic *RB1* mutation, or tumor implants due to intraocular seeding.

Various forms of differentiation may occur in retinoblastomas. The formation of highly organized *Flexner-Wintersteiner rosettes* is a characteristic of retinoblastoma that occurs only rarely in other neuroblastic tumors and represents cellular differentiation toward retinal tissue. These rosettes comprise a single row of columnar cells with eosinophilic cytoplasm and peripherally situated nuclei arranged radially (Fig 11-44A). The cells surround a central lumen lined by a refractile membranous structure that corresponds to the external limiting membrane of the retina. A rosette without features of retinal differentiation, known as a *Homer Wright rosette,* is also found in retinoblastomas as well as in other neuroblastic tumors, such as neuroblastomas and medulloblastomas. Unlike the Flexner-Wintersteiner rosette, the Homer Wright rosette lacks a central lumen and is filled with a tangle of eosinophilic cytoplasmic processes (Fig 11-44B).

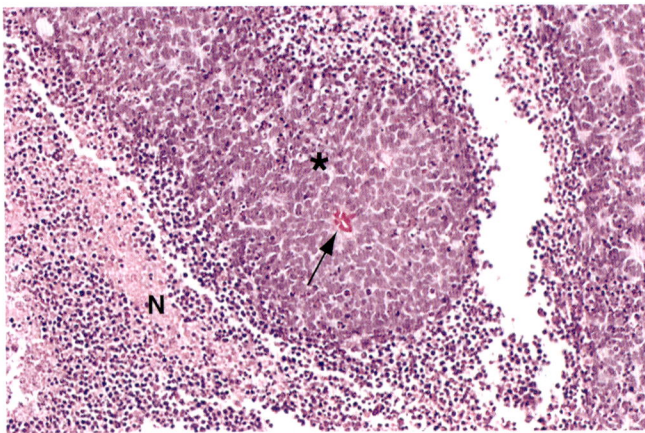

Figure 11-41 Retinoblastoma. Note the viable tumor cells *(asterisk)* surrounding a blood vessel *(arrow)* and the alternating zones of necrosis (N). This histologic arrangement is referred to as a *pseudorosette.*

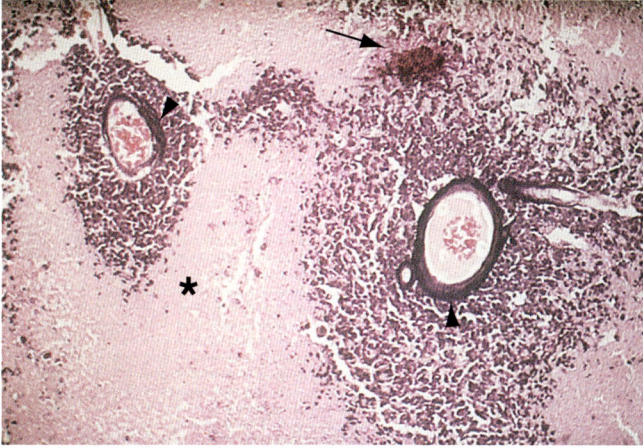

Figure 11-42 Retinoblastoma. Zones of viable tumor (usually surrounding blood vessels) alternate with zones of tumor necrosis *(asterisk)*. Calcification *(arrow)* occurs in the necrotic areas. The basophilic material surrounding and within the blood vessel walls *(arrowheads)* is DNA, liberated from degenerating tumor cells.

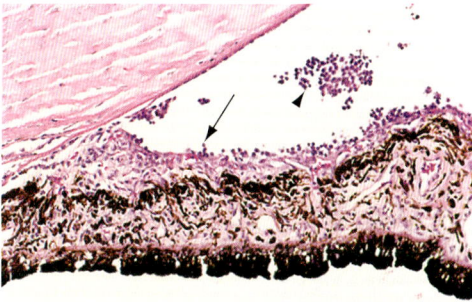

Figure 11-43 Retinoblastoma, anterior segment of the globe. Note the thick neovascular membrane *(arrow)* on the iris surface extending into the angle, resulting in angle closure. Free-floating tumor cells *(arrowhead)* are present in the anterior chamber.

Evidence of photoreceptor differentiation has also been documented for a form of differentiation known as a *fleurette*. Fleurettes, which resemble a bouquet of flowers, are curvilinear clusters of cells composed of rod and cone inner segments that are often attached to abortive outer segments (Fig 11-44C). A fleurette expresses a greater degree of retinal differentiation than a Flexner-Wintersteiner rosette. Nevertheless, in a typical retinoblastoma, undifferentiated tumor cells greatly outnumber fleurettes and Flexner-Wintersteiner rosettes, and differentiation is not an important prognostic indicator.

Tumors secondary to *MYCN* amplification demonstrate distinct histologic features such as undifferentiated cells with prominent and multiple nucleoli, necrosis, apoptosis, little calcification, and absence of Flexner-Wintersteiner rosettes and nuclear molding (Fig 11-45). Despite aggressive growth and poor differentiation, these tumors appear unlikely to spread systemically.

Tumor progression

Histologic features of retinoblastoma that are associated with higher risk of metastasis and poorer survival include

- optic nerve invasion (laminar, retrolaminar, or surgical cut end of the nerve)
- massive choroidal invasion
- direct extraocular extension
- anterior chamber involvement

The most common route for retinoblastoma to extend out of the eye is through the optic nerve. Direct infiltration of the optic nerve can lead to extension into the brain (Fig 11-46). Cells that spread into the leptomeninges can gain access to the cerebrospinal fluid, with the potential for seeding throughout the CNS. Therefore, invasion of the optic nerve is a poor prognostic indicator.

Massive choroidal invasion (Fig 11-47) is defined as an invasive focus of a tumor with a diameter (in any dimension) of at least 3 mm and the tumor reaching at least the inner

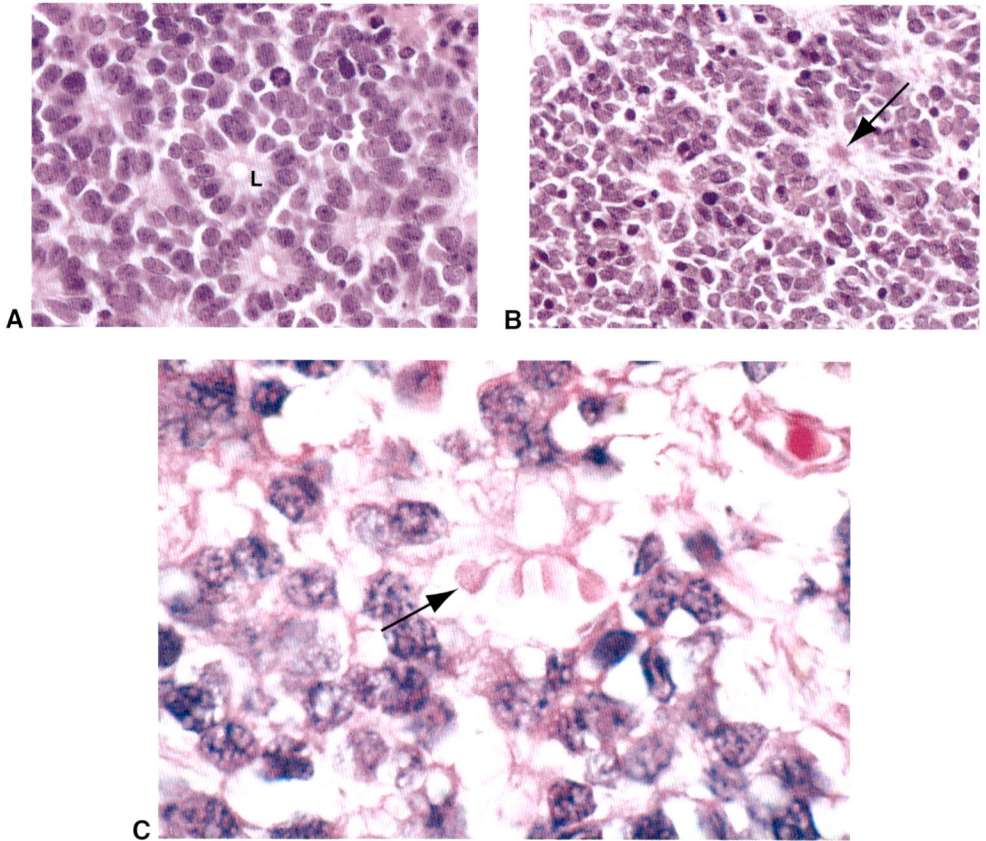

Figure 11-44 Retinoblastoma differentiation *(rosettes).* **A,** Flexner-Wintersteiner rosettes. Note the central lumen (L). **B,** Homer Wright rosettes. Note the neurofibrillary tangle *(arrow)* in the center of these structures. **C,** The fleurette *(arrow)* demonstrates bulbous extensions of retinoblastoma cells that represent differentiation toward photoreceptor inner segments.

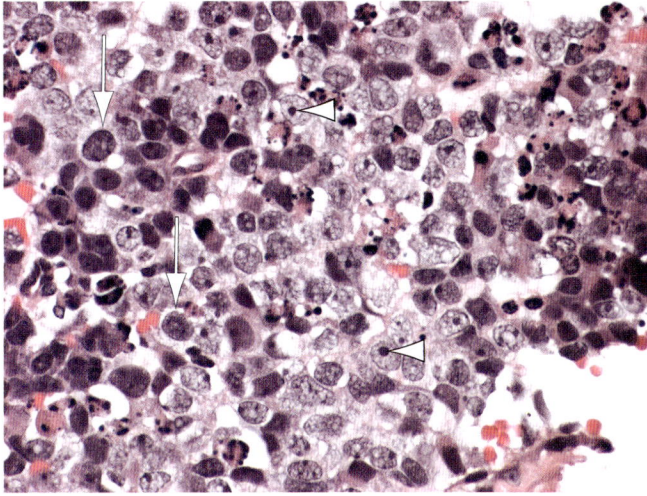

Figure 11-45 High-magnification photomicrograph of retinoblastoma cells with *MYCN* onco-gene amplification. Tumor cells are very poorly differentiated and highly pleomorphic. Nuclei are often hyperchromatic and enlarged *(arrows)* or have prominent nucleoli *(arrowheads)*. *(Courtesy of Nasreen A. Syed, MD.)*

fibers of the scleral tissue. Massive choroidal invasion is a poor prognostic factor that is thought to be related to hematogenous spread of tumor via the highly vascular choroid. See Chapter 19 for a discussion of prognosis. Choroidal involvement that is less than 3 mm in any dimension and does not reach the sclera is termed *focal choroidal invasion*. Focal choroidal invasion is not associated with a worse prognosis in retinoblastoma.

Sastre X, Chantada GL, Doz F, et al; International Retinoblastoma Staging Working Group. Proceedings of the consensus meetings from the International Retinoblastoma Staging Working Group on the pathology guidelines for the examination of enucleated eyes and evaluation of prognostic risk factors in retinoblastoma. *Arch Pathol Lab Med.* 2009;133(8):1199–1202.

Retinocytoma

Retinocytoma is a rare, highly differentiated retinoblastic tumor. The pathogenesis of this variant is the subject of debate. Some authors contend that the tumor is a fully differentiated form of retinoblastoma, whereas others argue that it is the benign counterpart of retinoblastoma. Retinocytoma is characterized histologically by numerous fleurettes admixed with individual cells that demonstrate varying degrees of photoreceptor differentiation (Fig 11-48). Retinocytoma differs from retinoblastoma in the following ways:

- retinocytoma cells have more cytoplasm and more evenly dispersed nuclear chromatin
- mitoses are not observed in retinocytomas
- although calcification may be identified in retinocytomas, necrosis is usually absent

Retinocytoma should be distinguished from the spontaneous regression of retinoblastoma that is the end result of coagulative necrosis. See the discussion in Chapter 19.

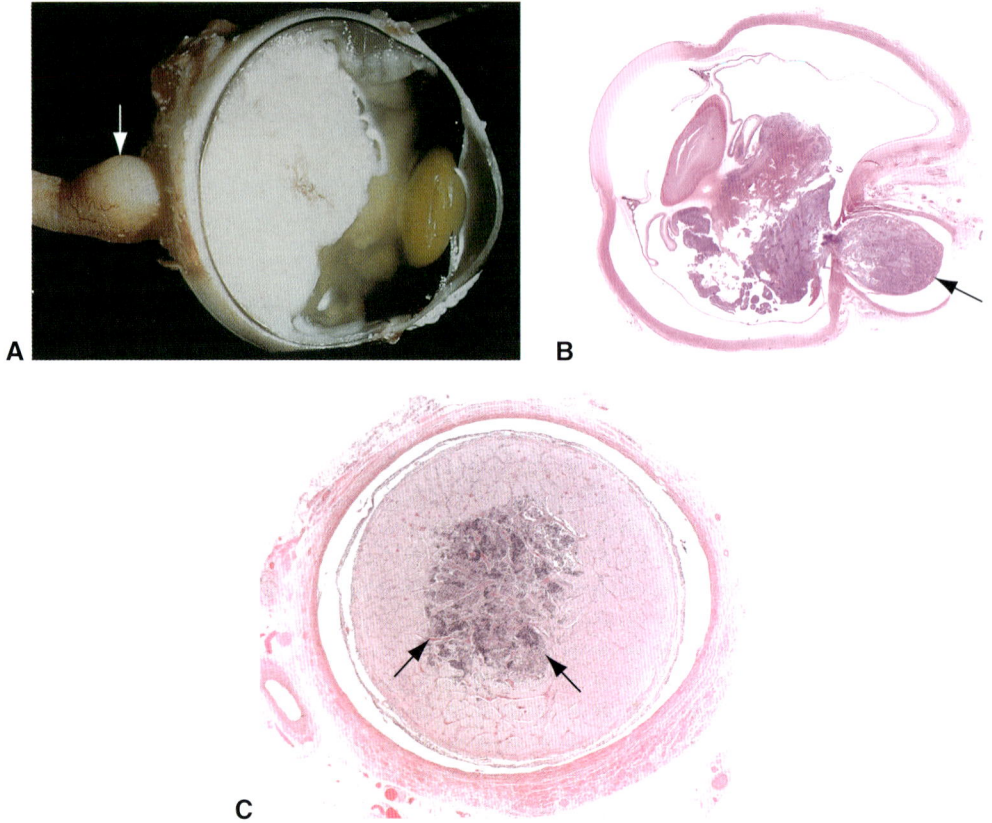

Figure 11-46 Retinoblastoma optic nerve invasion. **A,** Gross examination of the globe reveals a large intraocular tumor in the posterior segment with bulbous enlargement of the optic nerve *(arrow)* caused by direct extension. **B,** Retinoblastoma has invaded the optic nerve and has extended posterior to the lamina cribrosa to the margin of surgical resection *(arrow).* **C,** Cross section through the optic nerve shows tumor *(arrows)* present at the surgical cut end (surgical margin). This finding portends a poor prognosis. *(Parts B and C courtesy of Nasreen A. Syed, MD.)*

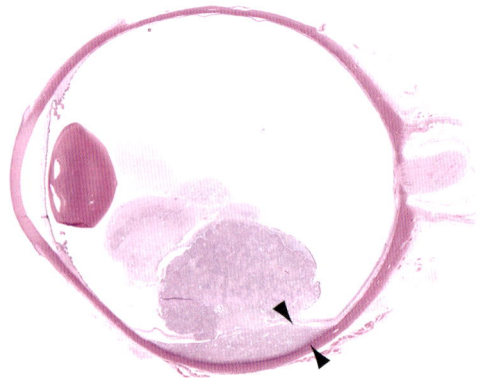

Figure 11-47 Retinoblastoma with the high-risk histologic feature of massive choroidal invasion *(between arrowheads).* Massive choroidal invasion is defined as an invasive focus of tumor with a diameter (in any dimension) of at least 3 mm and a choroidal focus of tumor that reaches at least the inner fibers of the scleral tissue. *(Courtesy of Nasreen A. Syed, MD.)*

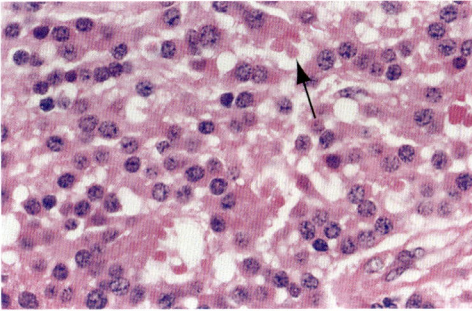

Figure 11-48 Retinocytoma. Note the significant degree of photoreceptor differentiation with apparent stubby inner segments *(arrow)*.

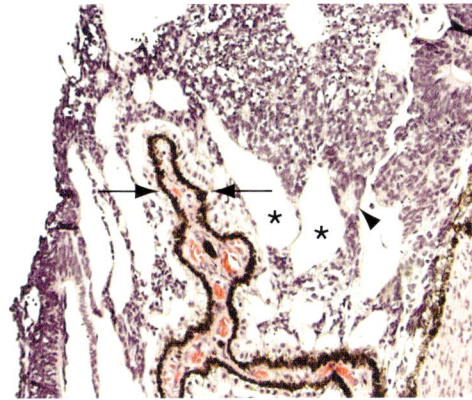

Figure 11-49 Medulloepithelioma. Photomicrograph shows a ciliary process *(between arrows)* surrounded by ribbons, cords, and small sheets of blue tumor cells with pockets of vitreous *(asterisks)* and occasional Flexner-Wintersteiner rosettes *(arrowhead)*. *(Courtesy of George J. Harocopos, MD.)*

Medulloepithelioma

Medulloepithelioma is a neuroepithelial tumor arising from primitive medullary epithelium (ie, the inner layer of the optic cup). This tumor usually arises from the ciliary epithelium but has been documented in the retina and optic nerve in rare instances. In the ciliary body, medulloepithelioma may appear clinically as a lightly pigmented or white cystic mass with erosion into the anterior chamber and iris root (see Chapter 19, Fig 19-15). Within the tumor, undifferentiated round-to-oval cells with little cytoplasm are organized into ribbon-like structures that have a distinct cellular polarity (Fig 11-49). Cell nuclei are stratified in 3–5 layers, and the entire structure is lined on one side by a thin basement membrane. One surface secretes a mucinous substance, rich in hyaluronic acid, that resembles vitreous. Stratified sheets of cells are capable of forming mucinous cysts that are clinically characteristic. Homer Wright and Flexner-Wintersteiner rosettes may also be present.

Medulloepitheliomas that contain solid masses of neuroblastic cells indistinguishable from retinoblastomas are more difficult to classify. Heteroplastic tissue, such as cartilage or smooth muscle, may be found in medulloepitheliomas. This variant of the tumor, composed of cells from 2 different embryonic germ layers, is referred to as *teratoid medulloepithelioma.* Medulloepitheliomas that have substantial numbers of undifferentiated cells with high mitotic rates and demonstrate tissue invasion are considered malignant; however, patients treated with enucleation have high survival rates, and "malignant"

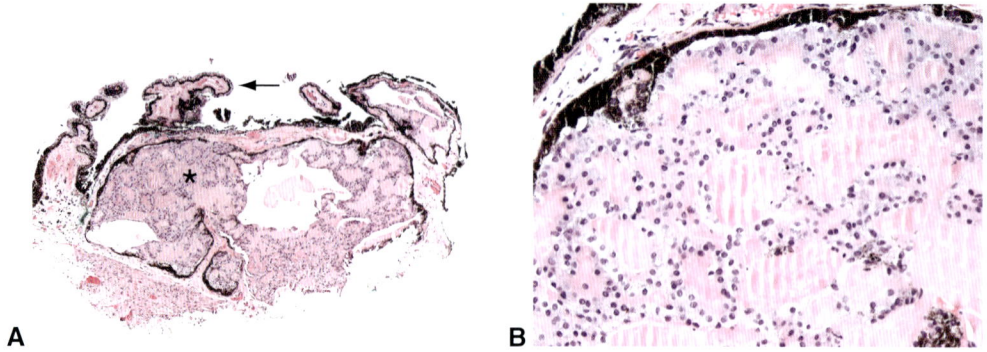

A **B**

Figure 11-50   **A,** Low-magnification photomicrograph of Fuchs adenoma *(asterisk)* arising from the nonpigmented ciliary body epithelium *(arrow)*. Note the pigmented layer of the ciliary body epithelium surrounding the tumor. **B,** High magnification reveals interweaving trabeculae of bland nonpigmented ciliary epithelial cells surrounding eosinophilic hyaline material. *(Courtesy of Nasreen A. Syed, MD.)*

medulloepithelioma typically follows a relatively benign course if the tumor remains confined to the eye.

In rare cases, ciliary body medulloepithelioma presents in association with pleuropulmonary blastoma as part of a familial tumor syndrome. In these cases, tumors are typically secondary to a germline mutation in the *DICER1* gene.

Schultz KA, Yang J, Doros L, et al. *DICER1*-pleuropulmonary blastoma familial tumor predisposition syndrome: a unique constellation of neoplastic conditions. *Pathol Case Rev.* 2014;19(2):90–100.

Fuchs Adenoma

Fuchs adenoma, derived from the inner layer of the optic cup, is an acquired, age-related benign tumor of the nonpigmented ciliary epithelium. It often goes undetected clinically unless it reaches significant size but is often identified on autopsy examination of eyes of older adults. It occasionally may be associated with sectoral cataract and may mimic other iris or ciliary body neoplasms. Histologically, Fuchs adenoma consists of hyperplastic nonpigmented ciliary epithelium arranged in sheets and tubules (Fig 11-50), with alternating areas of PAS-positive basement membrane material.

Shields JA, Eagle RC Jr, Ferguson K, Shields CL. Tumors of the nonpigmented epithelium of the ciliary body: the Lorenz E. Zimmerman tribute lecture. *Retina.* 2015;35(5):957–965.

Combined Hamartoma of the Retina and RPE

A combined hamartoma of the retina and RPE is not a true neoplasm but may present as a tumorous growth in the eye. It is characterized clinically by a slightly elevated, variably pigmented mass that involves the RPE, peripapillary retina, optic nerve, and overlying vitreous (see Chapter 17, Fig 17-14C). Frequently, a preretinal membrane that distorts the tumor's inner surface is present. The lesion is often diagnosed in childhood, supporting

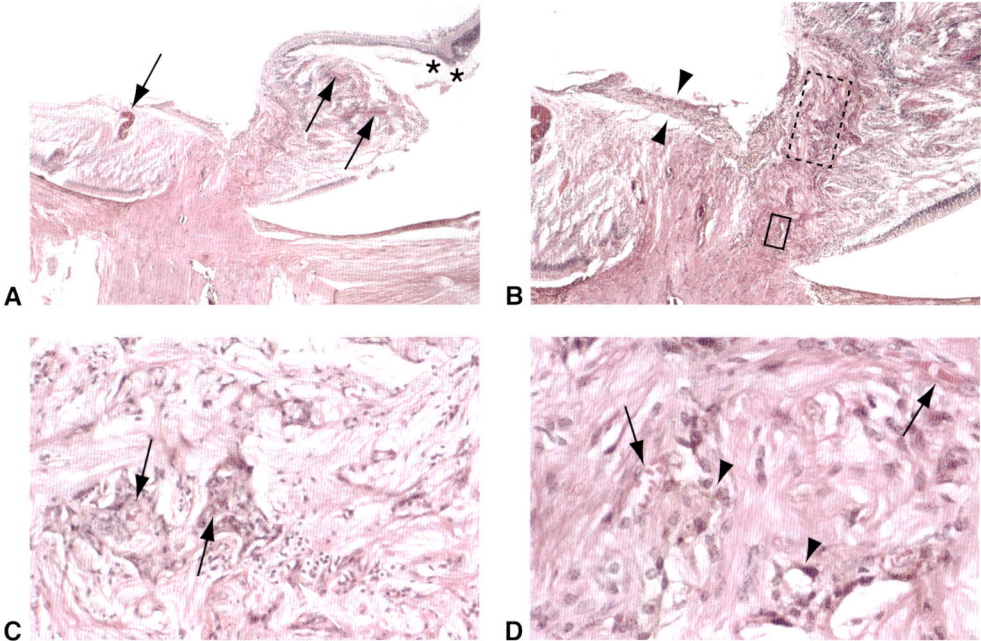

Figure 11-51 Combined hamartoma of the retina and RPE. **A,** Low-magnification photomicrograph showing thickening of the peripapillary retina, increased vascularity with variably sized blood vessels *(arrows)*, and cystic change in the outer plexiform layer *(asterisks)*. **B,** Thickening of the optic nerve head and peripapillary retina with a fibroglial membrane on the optic nerve surface *(between arrowheads)*. Box with dashed line is shown at higher magnification in part **C.** Smaller box is shown at higher magnification in part **D. C,** Hyperplastic RPE surrounding small blood vessels *(arrows)* in the peripapillary nerve fiber layer. **D,** Small-caliber vascular channels *(arrows)* and hyperplastic RPE *(arrowheads)* in the optic nerve head. *(Courtesy of Robert H. Rosa Jr, MD.)*

a probable hamartomatous origin. However, the vascular changes can be primary, with secondary changes in the adjacent RPE.

Histologically, the tumor is characterized by increased thickness of the optic nerve head and peripapillary retina, with an increased number of blood vessels (Fig 11-51). The RPE is hyperplastic and frequently migrates into the retina in a perivascular distribution. Vitreous condensation and fibroglial proliferation may be present on the surface of the tumor.

Adenomas and Adenocarcinomas of the RPE

Neoplasia of the RPE is rare. Histologically, *adenomas* in this layer typically retain characteristics of RPE cells, including basement membranes, cell junctions, and microvilli. *Adenocarcinomas* are distinguished from adenomas by greater anaplasia, mitotic activity, and invasion of the choroid or retina. Adenoma and adenocarcinoma of the RPE may arise from CHRPE. No metastases have been documented in patients with RPE adenocarcinomas. Adenomas and adenocarcinomas may also arise from the ciliary epithelium. See also Chapter 17.

CHAPTER 12

Uveal Tract

Highlights

- Dalen-Fuchs nodules may be seen in some cases of sympathetic ophthalmia and are located between the retinal pigment epithelium and Bruch membrane.
- The uveal tract is the most common site of ocular involvement in sarcoidosis, a nonnecrotizing granulomatous condition.
- Tumor cell type, tumor size, extraocular extension, and tumor location, including ciliary body involvement, are prognostic factors in posterior uveal melanoma.
- Metastatic tumors to the uvea constitute the most common intraocular tumors in adults.

Topography

The *iris, ciliary body,* and *choroid* constitute the uveal tract (also called *uvea*), a distinct, highly vascular layer in the eye (Fig 12-1). The constituents of the uveal tract

- have a layer of associated neuroepithelium
- are highly vascular with blood supply from the anterior and/or posterior ciliary arteries
- have a high concentration of dendritic melanocytes

The uveal tract is embryologically derived from mesoderm and neural crest cells. The neuroepithelium is derived from the optic cup. Firm attachments between the uveal tract and the sclera exist at only 3 sites: the scleral spur, the exit points of the vortex veins, and the optic nerve.

Iris

The iris is located in front of the crystalline lens. It separates the anterior segment of the eye into 2 compartments, the anterior chamber (between the cornea and iris) and the posterior chamber (between the iris and the lens/zonular fibers), and forms a circular aperture (pupil) that controls the amount of light transmitted into the eye. The iris comprises 4 layers:

- anterior border layer
- stroma
- muscular layer
- iris pigment epithelium (consisting of 2 layers: anterior and posterior)

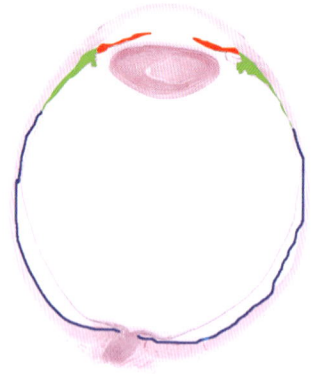

Figure 12-1 Uveal topography. The uveal tract consists of the iris *(red)*, ciliary body *(green)*, and choroid *(blue)*. *(Courtesy of Nasreen A. Syed, MD.)*

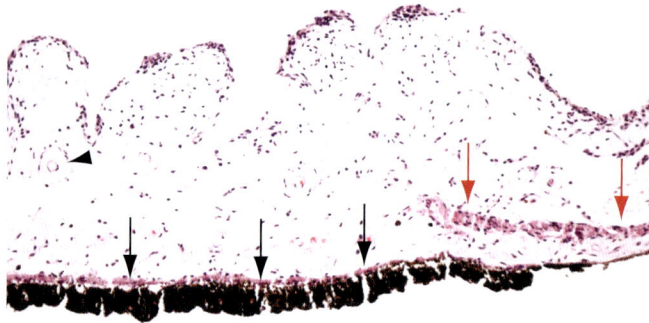

Figure 12-2 Histologic appearance of a normal iris: the anterior border layer is thrown into numerous crypts and folds. The sphincter muscle *(red arrows)* is present at the pupillary border, and the dilator muscle *(black arrows)* lies just anterior to the posterior pigment epithelium. Normal iris vessels demonstrate a thick collagen cuff *(arrowhead)*. *(Courtesy of Nasreen A. Syed, MD.)*

The *anterior border layer* represents a condensation of iris stroma, particularly melanocytes, and is coarsely ribbed with numerous crypts (Fig 12-2).

The *stroma* contains blood vessels, nerves, melanocytes, fibrocytes, and 2 types of clump cells containing pigment: histiocytes containing phagocytosed pigment (type I, or clump cells of Koganei) and variants of neuroepithelial cells (type II). The vessels within the stroma are surrounded by a thick cuff of collagen.

The *muscular layer* is made up of the dilator muscle and the sphincter muscle. Both muscles are composed of smooth muscle cells and are under autonomic control. The dilator muscle is a flat, radially arranged muscle that extends from the peripupillary region to the iris root. This muscle is integrated with the anterior layer of pigment epithelium. The sphincter muscle is a thicker muscle present just around the pupil in a radial arrangement.

The posterior iris surface is lined with a double layer of cuboidal epithelium (anterior and posterior layers of the pigment epithelium) arranged in an apex-to-apex configuration. The cytoplasm of these epithelial cells is packed with melanin granules. The number of melanin granules in the epithelium does not vary with iris color; rather, iris color is

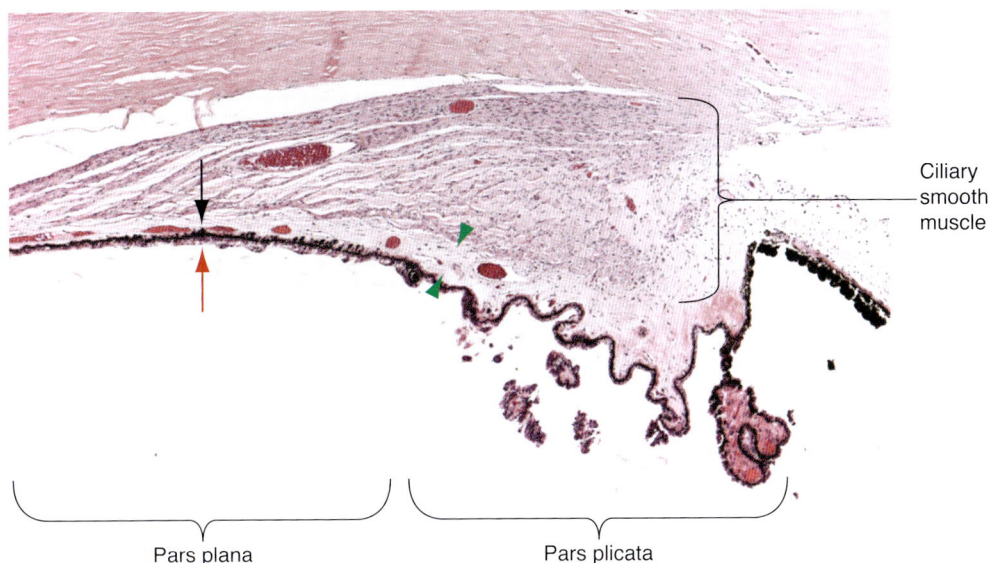

Figure 12-3 Normal ciliary body. The inner face of the ciliary body is lined with a double layer of epithelium: an inner, nonpigmented layer *(red arrow)* and an outer, pigmented layer *(black arrow)*. Note the fibrovascular connective tissue interposed between the pigmented ciliary epithelium and the ciliary muscle fibers *(between green arrowheads)*. *(Courtesy of Nasreen A. Syed, MD.)*

determined by the number of melanin granules and their size within the melanocytes of the anterior border layer.

Ciliary Body

The ciliary body is a ring-shaped structure approximately 6–7 mm wide that extends from the base of the iris and becomes continuous with the choroid at the ora serrata. The ciliary body is subdivided into 2 parts: the anterior *pars plicata,* which includes the ciliary processes, and the more posterior *pars plana.* The zonular fibers of the lens attach to the ciliary body in the valleys of the ciliary processes and along the pars plana. The inner portion of the ciliary body is lined by a double layer of epithelial cells: the inner, nonpigmented layer and the outer, pigmented layer (Fig 12-3).

Composed of smooth muscle fibers, the ciliary muscle comprises 3 layers of fibers: the outermost *longitudinal* layer, the middle *radial* layer, and the innermost *circular* layer. These individual muscle layers function as a unit during accommodation. Histologically, the layers are difficult to distinguish, and the muscle appears wedge-shaped in cross section.

Choroid

The choroid is the pigmented vascular tissue that forms the middle coat of the posterior part of the eye. It extends from the ora serrata anteriorly to the optic nerve posteriorly and consists of 3 principal layers:

- lamina fusca—outermost, pigmented layer with fine attachments to the sclera

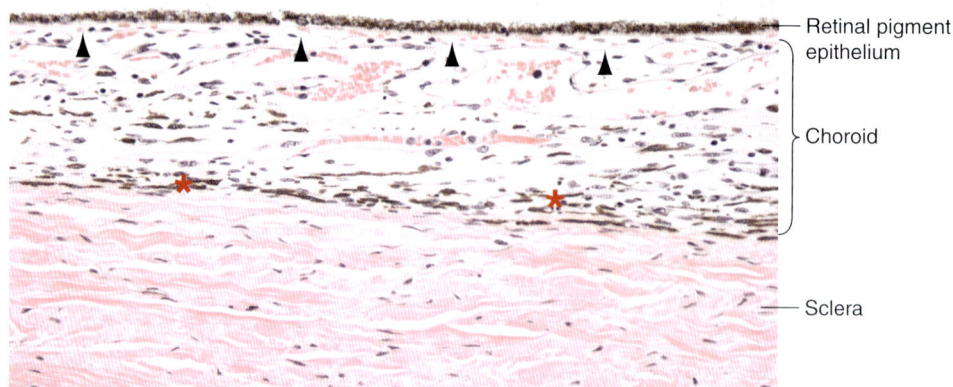

Figure 12-4 Normal choroid. The choroid is a vascular, pigmented structure located between the retinal pigment epithelium (RPE) and the sclera. The layer closest to the RPE is composed of capillaries and is known as the *choriocapillaris (arrowheads)*. The lamina fusca is also shown *(asterisks)* (hematoxylin-eosin [H&E] stain). *(Courtesy of Nasreen A. Syed, MD.)*

- stroma—central layer of loose fibrovascular connective tissue with arterioles originating from the short posterior ciliary arteries and veins draining to the vortex veins
- choriocapillaris—innermost layer containing thin-walled capillaries that are contiguous with Bruch membrane

The choriocapillaris is the blood supply for the retinal pigment epithelium (RPE) and the outer retinal layers (Fig 12-4). In addition to blood vessels, the choroid contains melanocytes, fibrocytes, nerves (eg, long posterior ciliary nerve), and various inflammatory cells. See BCSC Section 2, *Fundamentals and Principles of Ophthalmology,* for more information on the uveal tract.

Developmental Anomalies

See BCSC Section 2, *Fundamentals and Principles of Ophthalmology,* and Section 6, *Pediatric Ophthalmology and Strabismus,* for discussion of various developmental ocular anomalies, including aniridia and coloboma.

Aniridia

True aniridia, or complete absence of the iris, is rare. Most cases of aniridia are incomplete, with a narrow peripheral rim of rudimentary iris tissue present (Fig 12-5). Aniridia is usually bilateral, though sometimes asymmetric. Histologically, the rudimentary iris consists of underdeveloped ectodermal/mesodermal neural crest elements. The angle is often incompletely developed, and peripheral anterior synechiae that have an overgrowth

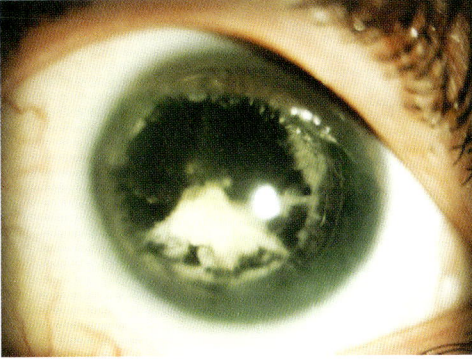

Figure 12-5 Aniridia, with a rudimentary iris present (visible near the limbus in this photograph). Cataract is also present. *(Courtesy of Daniella Bach-Holm, MD.)*

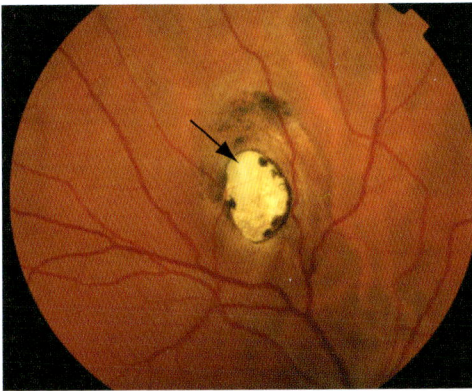

Figure 12-6 Choroidal coloboma. Note the RPE hyperplasia at the margin of the colobomatous defect and the fibroglial tissue within the coloboma *(arrow)*. *(Courtesy of Adela Castaño, COA, and Robert H. Rosa Jr, MD.)*

of corneal endothelium are often present, most likely accounting for the high incidence of glaucoma associated with aniridia. Other ocular findings in aniridia include cataract, corneal pannus, and foveal hypoplasia.

Both autosomal dominant and sporadic inheritance patterns have been described. An association between sporadic aniridia and Wilms tumor has been linked to 11p13 deletions and to mutations in the *PAX6* gene, located in the same region of chromosome 11. Microcephaly, cognitive impairment, and genitourinary abnormalities have also been associated with aniridia.

Hingorani M, Hanson I, van Heyningen V. Aniridia. *Eur J Hum Genet.* 2012;20(10): 1011–1017.

Coloboma

Coloboma, a partial or complete absence of normal tissue, may affect the iris, ciliary body, or choroid or all 3 structures (Fig 12-6). Colobomas are often a result of incomplete closure of the fetal fissure in the optic cup. Histologically, choroidal colobomas appear as an area nearly devoid of both retinal and choroidal tissue. A thin layer of glial tissue (intercalary membrane) may be the only tissue overlying the sclera.

Inflammation (Uveitis)

See BCSC Section 9, *Uveitis and Ocular Inflammation,* for in-depth discussion of the conditions described in the following sections and the immunologic processes involved.

Infectious Uveitis

Infectious processes in the uveal tract may be restricted to that layer of the eye or may be part of a generalized inflammatory process affecting multiple or all coats of the eye. If the eye is the primary source of the infection (eg, as in posttraumatic bacterial infection), that infection is termed *exogenous.* If, however, the infection originates elsewhere in the body (eg, a ruptured diverticulum) and subsequently spreads hematogenously to involve the uveal tract, the infection is referred to as *endogenous.* A wide variety of organisms can cause infections of the uveal tract, including bacteria, fungi, viruses, and protozoa.

Histologic examination often shows a mix of acute and chronic inflammatory cells within the choroid, ciliary body, or iris stroma. In cases of infection with viral, fungal, or protozoal (eg, toxoplasmosis) agents, epithelioid histiocytes are typically present (granulomatous inflammation). If infection is suspected, special stains for microorganisms may be helpful (Fig 12-7).

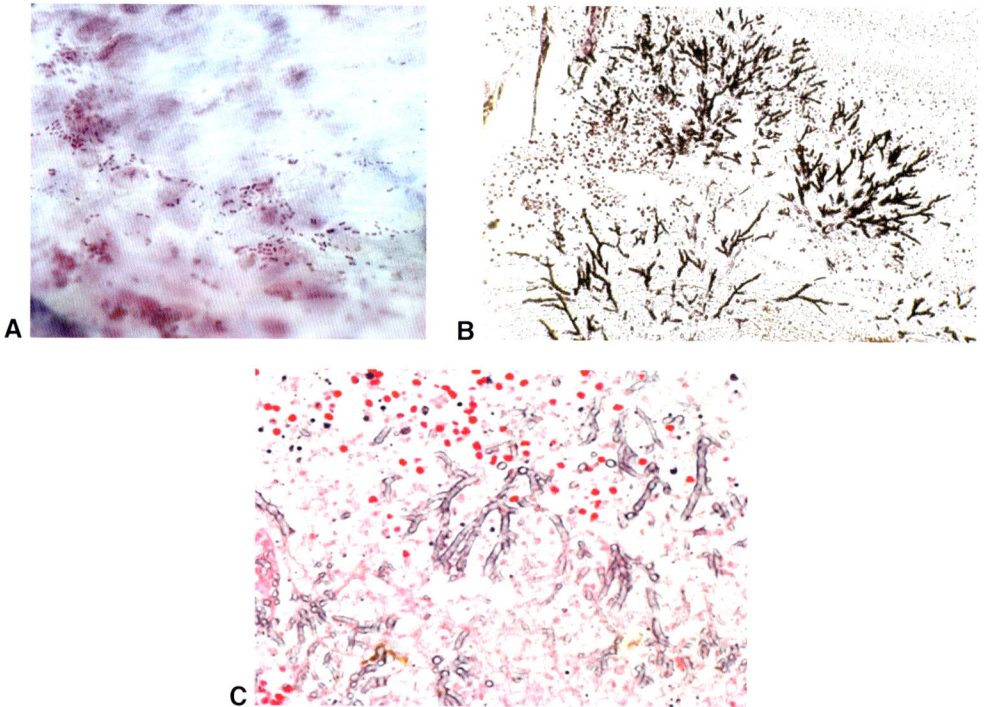

Figure 12-7 Infectious uveitis, with the infectious organisms demonstrated with special stains. **A,** Gram-positive bacilli seen on Gram stain. **B,** Filamentous fungi seen with Gomori methenamine silver (GMS) stain. **C,** Filamentous fungi on periodic acid–Schiff (PAS) stain. *(Courtesy of Steffen Heegaard, MD.)*

See Chapter 2, Table 2-2, which presents histochemical stains commonly used in ophthalmic pathology.

Noninfectious Uveitis

Noninfectious uveitis can be divided into nonspecific and specific forms. Most uveitides are nonspecific with no etiologic causes found and likely represent localized autoimmune disease. Several types of specific uveitis are discussed in the following sections.

Sympathetic ophthalmia

Sympathetic ophthalmia is a rare bilateral granulomatous panuveitis that occurs after accidental or surgical injury to one eye (the *exciting*, or *inciting, eye*), followed by a latent period of weeks to years before development of uveitis in the uninjured globe (the *sympathizing eye*).

Sympathetic ophthalmia is a clinical diagnosis. The histologic findings are not pathognomonic. Furthermore, immunomodulatory therapy may modify these findings. Histologically, a diffuse granulomatous inflammatory reaction occurs within the uveal tract and is composed of lymphocytes and epithelioid histiocytes containing phagocytosed melanin (Figs 12-8, 12-9). Plasma cells are usually scant, suggesting a cell-mediated response. Classically, in the early stages of the disease, the choriocapillaris is spared. Varying degrees of inflammation may be present in the anterior chamber, such as clusters of histiocytes deposited on the corneal endothelium *(mutton-fat keratic precipitates)*. *Dalen-Fuchs nodules,* which are accumulations of epithelioid histiocytes and lymphocytes between the RPE and Bruch membrane, may be seen in some cases (see Fig 12-9). As these nodules may also be present in other diseases, such as Vogt-Koyanagi-Harada syndrome, they are not pathognomonic of sympathetic ophthalmia.

See BCSC Section 7, *Oculofacial Plastic and Orbital Surgery,* for additional discussion.

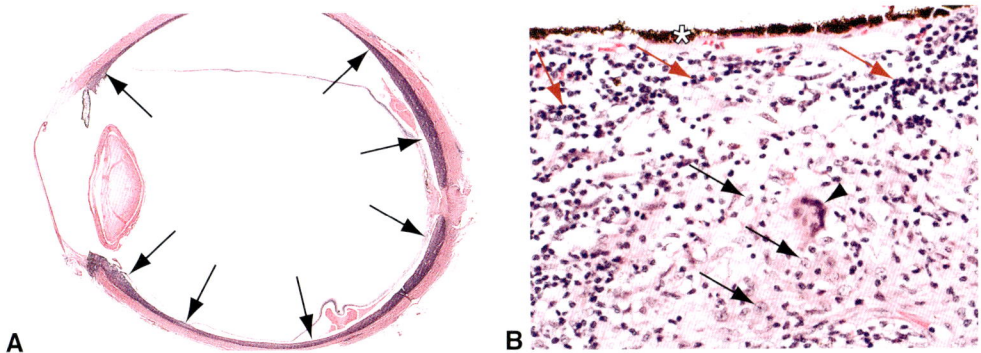

Figure 12-8 Sympathetic ophthalmia. **A,** Diffuse infiltration of the uveal tract by chronic inflammatory cells, seen as a purple layer beneath the retina *(arrows).* **B,** Higher magnification of the RPE *(asterisk)* and choroid shows a multinucleated giant cell *(arrowhead),* epithelioid histiocytes *(black arrows),* and lymphocytes *(red arrows).* Note the relative sparing of the choriocapillaris, beneath the RPE. *(Part A courtesy of Hans E. Grossniklaus, MD; part B courtesy of Michele Bloomer, MD.)*

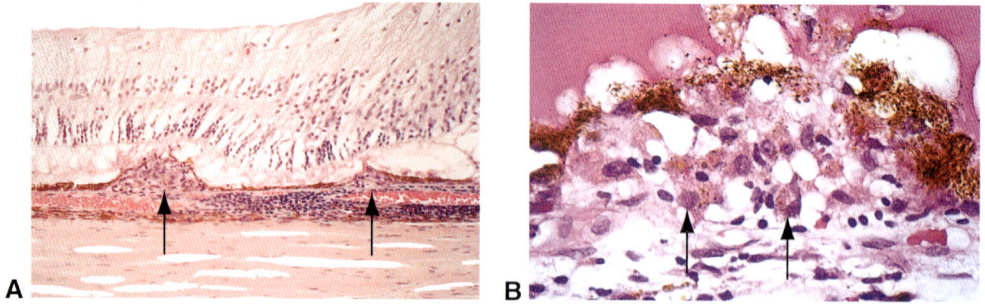

Figure 12-9 Dalen-Fuchs nodules in sympathetic ophthalmia. **A,** Focal aggregates of inflammatory cells are present between the RPE and Bruch membrane *(arrows).* **B,** Higher magnification demonstrates epithelioid histiocytes containing cytoplasmic pigment *(arrows)* within the nodules (H&E stain). *(Courtesy of Hans E. Grossniklaus, MD.)*

Vogt-Koyanagi-Harada syndrome

Vogt-Koyanagi-Harada (VKH) syndrome is a rare cause of posterior or diffuse uveitis and may have both ocular and systemic manifestations. The syndrome occurs more commonly in patients with Asian or Native American ancestry and usually affects individuals between 30 and 50 years of age.

The chronic, diffuse granulomatous uveitis of VKH resembles the uveitis seen in sympathetic ophthalmia. However, in VKH, the entire choroid, including the choriocapillaris, is typically involved by the inflammatory reaction. The granulomatous inflammation may extend into the retina. Because the disease is one of exacerbation and remission, chorioretinal scarring and RPE hyperplasia and/or atrophy may also occur.

Sarcoidosis

Sarcoidosis is an inflammatory disorder (or group of disorders) that can affect nearly all systems of the body. The disease is characterized by granulomatous inflammation, specifically, the formation of granulomas, in various organs and tissues. The uveal tract is the most common site of ocular involvement. Anteriorly, inflammatory nodules of the iris may develop, either at the pupillary margin *(Koeppe nodules)* or elsewhere in the iris stroma *(Busacca nodules)*. In the posterior segment, chorioretinitis (Fig 12-10A, B), periphlebitis, and chorioretinal nodules may be present. Periphlebitis may appear clinically as inflammatory lesions, referred to as *candlewax drippings* (perivenous exudates). Inflammatory cell infiltration may cause the optic nerve head to become swollen.

Histologically, the classic sarcoid nodule is a nonnecrotizing (noncaseating) granuloma. These granulomas are collections of epithelioid histiocytes, sometimes accompanied by multinucleated giant cells, surrounded by a cuff of lymphocytes (Fig 12-10C). In the uveal tract, the inflammatory infiltrate may show a more diffuse distribution of lymphocytes and epithelioid histiocytes (granulomatous inflammation). Multinucleated giant cells may contain *asteroid bodies* (star-shaped, acidophilic inclusion bodies) and/or *Schaumann bodies* (spherical, basophilic, calcified inclusion bodies) in their

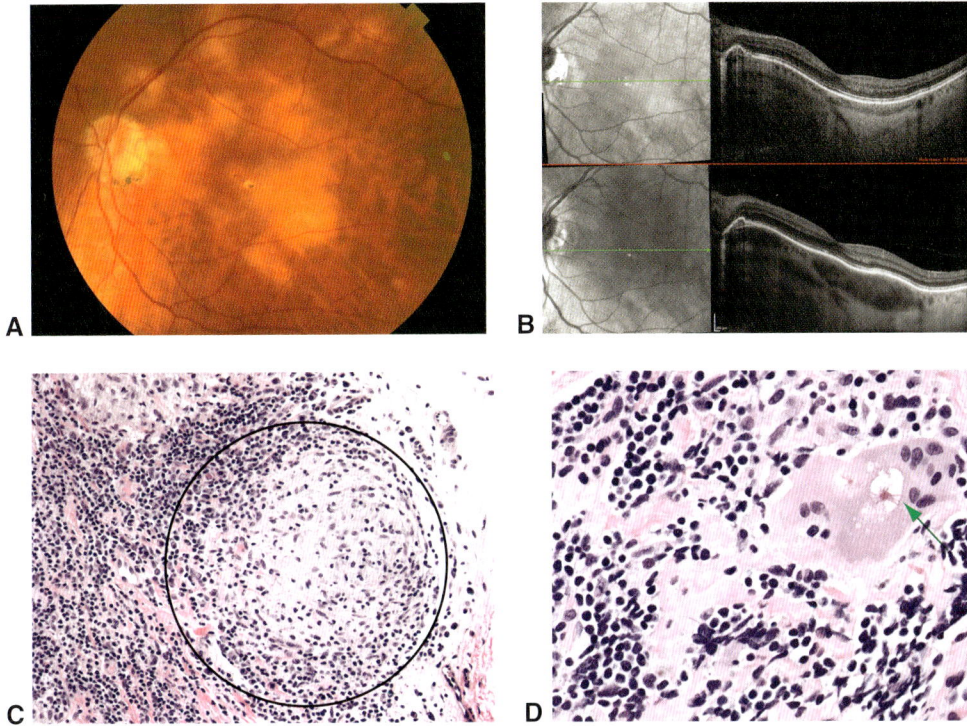

Figure 12-10 Sarcoidosis. **A,** Chorioretinitis in the fundus. **B,** Optical coherence tomography of the unaffected eye *(top)* and the eye with chorioretinitis *(bottom)* demonstrating thickening of the choroid in the eye with inflammation. **C,** Biopsy of a sarcoid nodule showing epithelioid histiocytes and lymphocytes (chronic granulomatous inflammation) arranged as a nonnecrotizing granuloma *(circle)*. **D,** High-magnification photomicrograph of a sarcoid nodule demonstrating an asteroid body *(arrow)* within a multinucleated giant cell. *(Parts A and B courtesy of H. Josefine Fuchs, MD; parts C and D courtesy of Nasreen A. Syed, MD.)*

cytoplasm (Fig 12-10D). Neither asteroid nor Schaumann bodies are pathognomonic for sarcoidosis.

Behçet disease

Behçet disease is an occlusive systemic vasculitis that can cause nongranulomatous, necrotizing inflammation in the uveal tract. See BCSC Section 9, *Uveitis and Ocular Inflammation,* for further discussion of this disease.

Juvenile xanthogranuloma

Juvenile xanthogranuloma is an uncommon inflammatory condition that occurs in children. The skin and uvea are commonly affected. In the uveal tract, lesions may present as a solid mass, mimicking a neoplastic process. The characteristic histologic features of the lesions include lipid-laden histiocytes, Touton giant cells, lymphocytes, and occasional eosinophils (Fig 12-11). The lesions are often vascularized, and the blood vessels tend to be fragile, resulting in intralesional hemorrhage. Iris lesions in juvenile xanthogranuloma may cause a spontaneous hyphema.

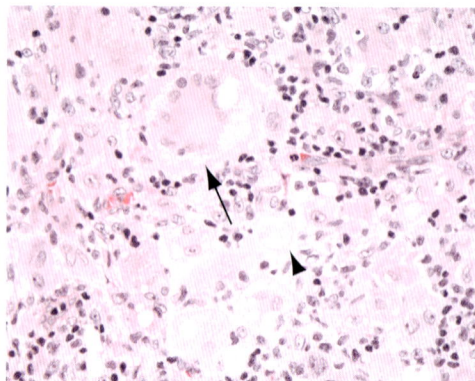

Figure 12-11 Juvenile xanthogranuloma. Touton giant cells *(arrow)* with a ring of nuclei, inner eosinophilic cytoplasm, and outer vacuolated or foamy cytoplasm; foamy histiocytes *(arrowhead);* and lymphocytes are admixed. *(Courtesy of Nasreen A. Syed, MD.)*

Degenerations

Rubeosis Iridis

Rubeosis iridis, or neovascularization of the iris (Fig 12-12; see also Chapter 11, Fig 11-28), is commonly found in surgically enucleated blind eyes. It is often due to severe inflammation or production of vascular endothelial growth factor in the eye. Rubeosis iridis may be associated with a wide variety of conditions (see BCSC Section 10, *Glaucoma,* Table 10-2).

Histologically, the new vessels tend to lack supporting tissue and do not possess the thick collagenous cuff that encircles normal iris vessels. The new vessels grow on the anterior surface of the iris, eventually forming a fibrovascular membrane, and may extend into the anterior chamber angle. The neovascular membrane has a myofibroblastic component, which contracts and eventually leads to angle closure due to formation of peripheral anterior synechiae. Neovascularization of the angle often results in *neovascular glaucoma,* a secondary form of angle-closure glaucoma. Membrane contraction may also lead to *ectropion uveae,* an anterior displacement or dragging of the posterior iris pigment epithelial layer onto the anterior iris surface at the pupillary border. The anterior surface of the iris often becomes flattened. In advanced cases, atrophy of the dilator muscle, attenuation of the pigment epithelium, and stromal fibrosis may occur (see Fig 12-12).

Hyalinization of the Ciliary Body

With age, the ciliary processes become hyalinized and fibrosed, losing stromal cellularity; occasionally, dystrophic calcification develops. The thin, delicate processes become blunted and attenuated, and the stroma becomes more eosinophilic (Fig 12-13). This process is a normal age-related change to the ciliary body and is not considered pathologic, although it does contribute functionally to the development of presbyopia.

Choroidal Neovascularization

Choroidal neovascularization is discussed at length in Chapter 11 and in BCSC Section 12, *Retina and Vitreous.*

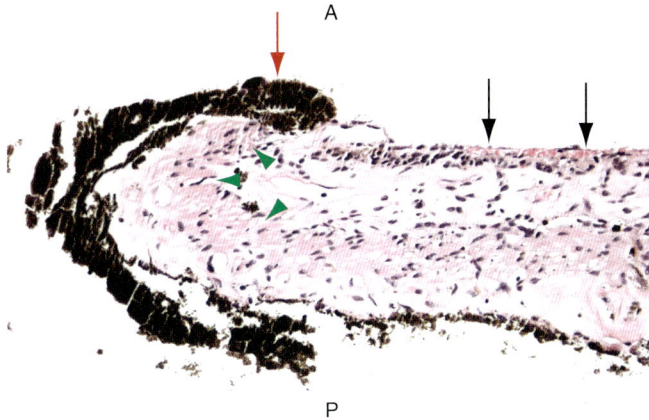

Figure 12-12 Iris neovascularization (rubeosis iridis). Tiny blood vessels sprout from existing iris vasculature, typically on the surface of the iris *(black arrows)*. Note the flat anterior surface of the iris (A = anterior; P = posterior). The contractile component of the neovascular membrane may result in dragging of the iris pigment epithelium *(red arrow)* and sphincter muscle *(green arrowheads)* anteriorly at the pupillary margin, in turn resulting in ectropion uveae. *(Courtesy of Nasreen A. Syed, MD.)*

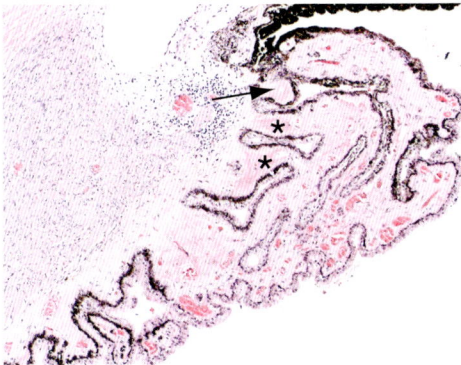

Figure 12-13 Age-related changes in the ciliary body include sclerotic vessels *(arrow)* and hyalinization *(asterisks)*. *(Courtesy of Michele Bloomer, MD.)*

Neoplasia

Uveal neoplasms are also discussed in detail in Chapters 17, 18, and 20. The discussion of uveal neoplasms in this chapter focuses primarily on histology.

Iris

Nevus

An *iris nevus* is a localized proliferation of melanocytic cells that generally appears as a darkly pigmented lesion of the iris stroma with minimal distortion of the iris architecture (see Chapter 17, Fig 17-1).

Figure 12-14 Iris nevus. Spindle-shaped nevus cells *(arrows)* form a plaque on the surface of the iris and extend downward into the iris stroma just anterior to the pigmented epithelium *(asterisk). (Courtesy of Michele Bloomer, MD.)*

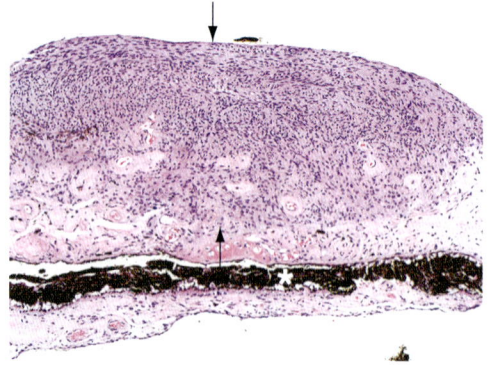

An iris nevus appears histologically as a combination of, or an accumulation of, any of the following:

- branching dendritic nevus cells
- spindle nevus cells
- epithelioid nevus cells (least common)

All of these cell types usually contain melanin granules in the cytoplasm. The nuclei of these cells are typically oblong or ovoid with a bland appearance and indistinct nucleoli. Less commonly, epithelioid nevus cells may be observed. A variety of growth patterns and cytologic appearances are possible, but cellular atypia and significant mitotic activity are not present. The nevus cells aggregate within the stroma and sometimes also appear as a plaque on the surface of the iris (Fig 12-14). Occasionally, nevus cells may extend into the adjacent angle structures.

Melanoma

Melanomas arising in the iris tend to follow a relatively nonaggressive clinical course, in contrast to posterior (ciliochoroidal) melanomas. Most iris melanomas develop in the inferior sectors of the iris (see Chapter 17, Fig 17-3). The lesions can be quite vascularized and may occasionally cause spontaneous hyphema.

Iris melanomas can be composed of spindle melanoma cells, epithelioid melanoma cells, or a combination of these. Histologically, spindle cells possess plump, spindle-shaped nuclei that have a coarse, granular appearance and prominent nucleoli. These cells are the equivalent of spindle-B cells in posterior uveal melanoma (see the "Melanoma" section under Choroid and Ciliary Body). Epithelioid cells are polyhedral, with large, round nuclei that have a clumped chromatin pattern and prominent eosinophilic nucleoli. Both types of cells tend to have a high nuclear-to-cytoplasmic ratio. The cytoplasm of melanoma cells can range from amelanotic to heavily pigmented.

Typically, iris melanomas grow as a solid mass in the stroma, sometimes covered by a surface plaque. Occasionally, the tumor demonstrates satellite lesions or a diffuse growth pattern and replaces normal iris stroma (Fig 12-15). In some cases, iris melanoma may be seen arising from a nevus on histology. The modified Callender classification for posterior melanomas (see "Melanoma" section under Choroid and Ciliary Body) is not applicable to iris melanomas in terms of prognostic significance. Iris melanomas are classified by a

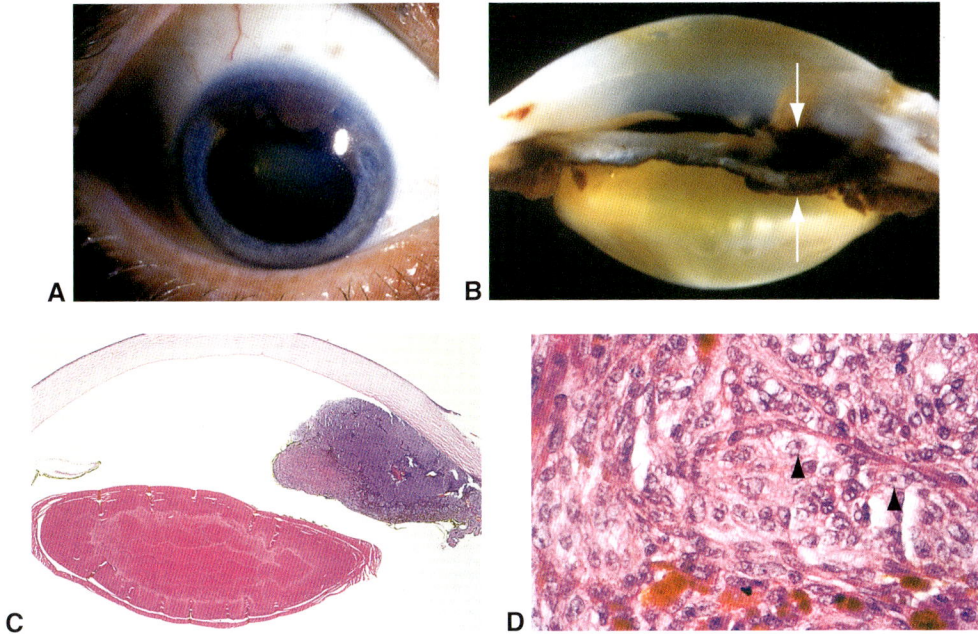

Figure 12-15 Iris melanoma. **A,** Clinical photograph. The pigmented tumor is seen between the 10:30 and 2:00 clock-hours. **B,** Gross appearance of a pigmented iris mass *(between arrows).* **C,** Low magnification shows the melanoma completely replacing the normal iris stroma, extending into the anterior chamber, touching the posterior cornea, and occluding the angle. **D,** Histologic examination shows numerous plump epithelioid melanoma cells containing prominent nucleoli *(arrowheads).* *(Courtesy of Hans E. Grossniklaus, MD.)*

separate staging system, one based on infiltration of adjacent structures and the presence or absence of coexisting glaucoma. In some cases, distinguishing between iris nevus and melanoma histologically can be challenging and requires the expertise of an experienced ophthalmic pathologist.

Although iris melanomas may grow in a locally aggressive fashion, they rarely metastasize. One exception occurs when melanomas grow to diffusely involve the entire iris stroma. This diffuse form of melanoma may invade the anterior chamber angle and extend posteriorly to involve the ciliary body.

Kivelä T, Simpson ER, Grossniklaus HE, et al. Uveal melanoma. In: Amin MB, Edge SB, Greene FL, eds. *AJCC Cancer Staging Manual.* 8th ed. Springer; 2017:805–817.

Choroid and Ciliary Body

Nevus

Most uveal nevi (>90%) develop in the choroid (see Chapter 17, Fig 17-4). Choroidal nevi may be composed of 4 types of nevus cells:

- plump polyhedral nevus cells: Abundant cytoplasm is filled with pigment and has a small round to oval nucleus with bland appearance.

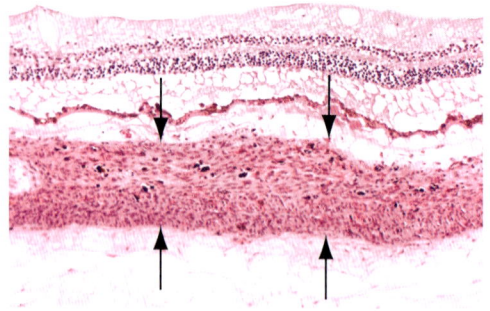

Figure 12-16 Spindle-cell choroidal nevus *(between arrows)* is composed of slender spindle-shaped cells with thin, homogeneously staining nuclei. *(Courtesy of Nasreen A. Syed, MD.)*

- slender spindle nevus cells (Fig 12-16): The cytoplasm contains scant pigment and a small, dark, elongated nucleus.
- plump fusiform dendritic nevus cells: Morphology is intermediate between that of plump polyhedral and slender spindle.
- balloon cells: Abundant, foamy cytoplasm lacks pigment and has a bland nucleus.

Depending on the size and location of the nevus, it may exert nonspecific effects on adjacent ocular tissues. The associated choriocapillaris may become compressed or obliterated, and drusen may form along Bruch membrane overlying the nevus. In rare cases, a choroidal nevus may be associated with localized serous detachments of the overlying RPE or neurosensory retina; in addition, secondary choroidal neovascularization may occur.

Most choroidal nevi remain stationary over long periods of observation. However, the presence of nevus cells contiguous with a choroidal melanoma on histologic examination provides evidence that melanomas may arise from choroidal nevi.

Melanocytoma

Uveal melanocytoma (magnocellular nevus) is a specific type of uveal nevus that warrants separate consideration. These benign jet-black lesions can occur anywhere in the uveal tract but appear most commonly in the peripapillary region (see Chapter 15, Fig 15-12B).

Histologically, a melanocytoma is composed of large polyhedral cells with small round to oval nuclei and abundant cytoplasm. Because the nevus cells are so heavily pigmented, it is usually necessary to apply melanin bleaching techniques to sections to accurately study the cytologic features (see Chapter 15, Fig 15-12D). Areas of cystic degeneration or necrosis may be observed in these nevi. In rare cases, melanocytoma can give rise to melanoma.

Melanoma

The most common primary intraocular malignancy in adults is melanoma arising from the ciliary body and/or choroid. When this type of tumor grows to a significant size, it may extend beyond its site of origin (ie, from the choroid to the ciliary body and vice versa). Ciliary body and choroidal melanomas exhibit overlapping clinical features with similar prognostic implications and may be referred to collectively as *posterior uveal melanomas.*

Histologically, posterior uveal melanomas are composed of spindle cells and/or epithelioid melanoma cells (Figs 12-17, 12-18, 12-19). Less commonly, balloon cells similar

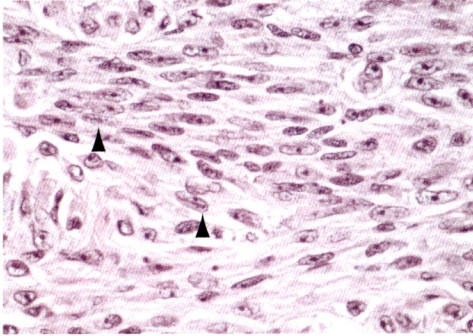

Figure 12-17 Posterior uveal melanoma. Spindle-A melanoma cells have slender, elongated nuclei with small nucleoli. A central stripe may be present down the long axis of the nucleus *(arrowheads)* (H&E stain). *(Courtesy of Nasreen A. Syed, MD.)*

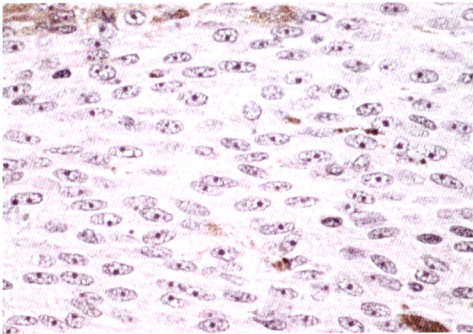

Figure 12-18 Posterior uveal melanoma. In spindle-B melanoma cells, coarse, granular chromatin and plump, large nuclei are seen. Nucleoli are prominent. Mitoses may be present, though not in large numbers. Tumors composed of a mix of spindle-A and spindle-B melanoma cells are designated *spindle cell melanomas.* *(Courtesy of Nasreen A. Syed, MD.)*

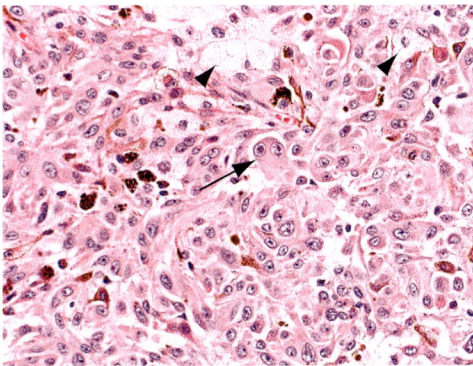

Figure 12-19 Posterior uveal melanoma. Epithelioid melanoma cells resemble epithelium because of their abundant eosinophilic cytoplasm and enlarged round to oval nuclei. They often lack cohesiveness and demonstrate marked pleomorphism, including the formation of multinucleated tumor cells *(arrow).* Their nuclei have a conspicuous nuclear membrane, very coarse chromatin, and large nucleoli. Note the balloon cells *(arrowheads)* with abundant foamy cytoplasm. *(Courtesy of Michele Bloomer, MD.)*

to those seen in choroidal nevi may be present. *Spindle cell melanoma* consists primarily of spindle-B melanoma cells (see Fig 12-18). It may also contain spindle-A cells (see Fig 12-17); however, a tumor consisting entirely of spindle-A cells is considered a nevus.

The cytoplasmic melanin content in melanoma cells can vary considerably. The mitotic rate in posterior uveal melanomas tends to be quite low, and mitotic counts by the pathologist typically require 40 high-power fields. These tumors may exhibit variable amounts of necrosis.

Choroidal melanomas typically start as dome-shaped lesions and, as they grow and break through Bruch membrane, they acquire a mushroom or collar-button shape (Fig 12-20). Tumors may involve both the choroid and the ciliary body in some cases

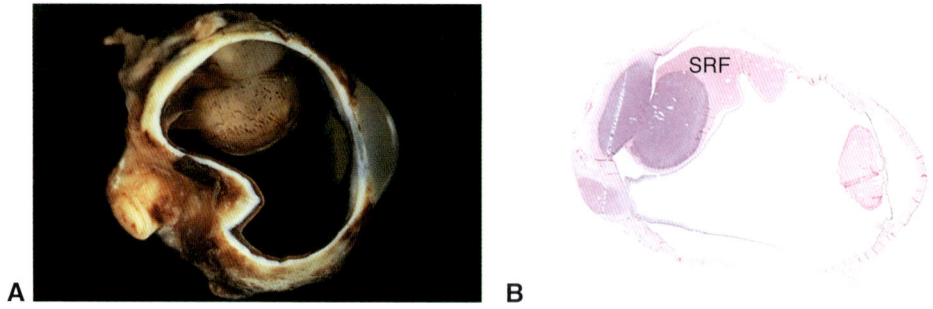

Figure 12-20 Choroidal melanoma with rupture through Bruch membrane. **A,** Gross appearance of a mushroom-shaped mass. The mushroom shape is a direct result of rupture through Bruch membrane. **B,** Microscopic appearance. Note the subretinal fluid (SRF) adjacent to the tumor.

Figure 12-21 Some choroidal melanomas grow in a diffuse placoid fashion, replacing normal choroid, without achieving significant height *(arrows)*. Note the eosinophilic protein-aceous fluid *(asterisks)* interposed between the retina and the tumor, corresponding to the exudative retinal detachment overlying the tumor.

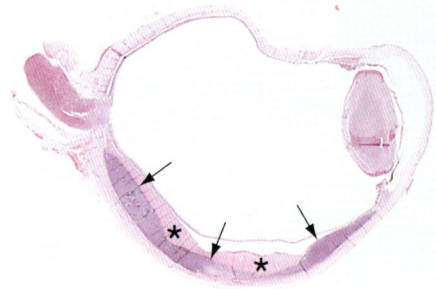

Figure 12-22 Ciliary body ring melanoma. By definition, a ring melanoma *(asterisks)* follows the major arterial circle of the iris at the iris root circumferentially around the eye.

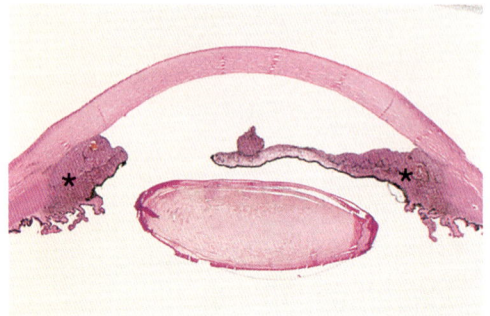

(ciliochoroidal melanoma), and it may be difficult to determine where the lesion originated. Less commonly, choroidal lesions grow in a diffuse pattern, replacing normal choroid without achieving significant height (Fig 12-21). In the ciliary body, tumors usually grow in a fashion similar to that of their choroidal counterparts. Likewise, there is a ciliary equivalent of the diffuse pattern seen in the choroid, known as a *ring melanoma,* in which the tumor extends for the entire circumference of the ciliary body (Fig 12-22).

Choroidal melanomas may cause serous detachments of the overlying and adjacent retina, with subsequent degenerative changes in the outer segments of the photoreceptors (see Figs 12-20B, 12-21). Melanoma may extend through the scleral emissary canals to gain access to the episcleral surface and the orbit (extrascleral tumor extension) (Fig 12-23). Less commonly, melanoma may directly invade the underlying sclera or overlying retina (Fig 12-24). Direct invasion of the anterior chamber or mechanical blockage of the chamber due to anterior iris displacement may lead to secondary glaucoma (Fig 12-25). In addition, tumor necrosis may lead to the dispersion of melanin in the anterior chamber and angle. The trabecular meshwork becomes obstructed by histiocytes that have ingested this pigment, causing a type of secondary glaucoma called *melanomalytic glaucoma* (see Chapter 7, Fig 7-14).

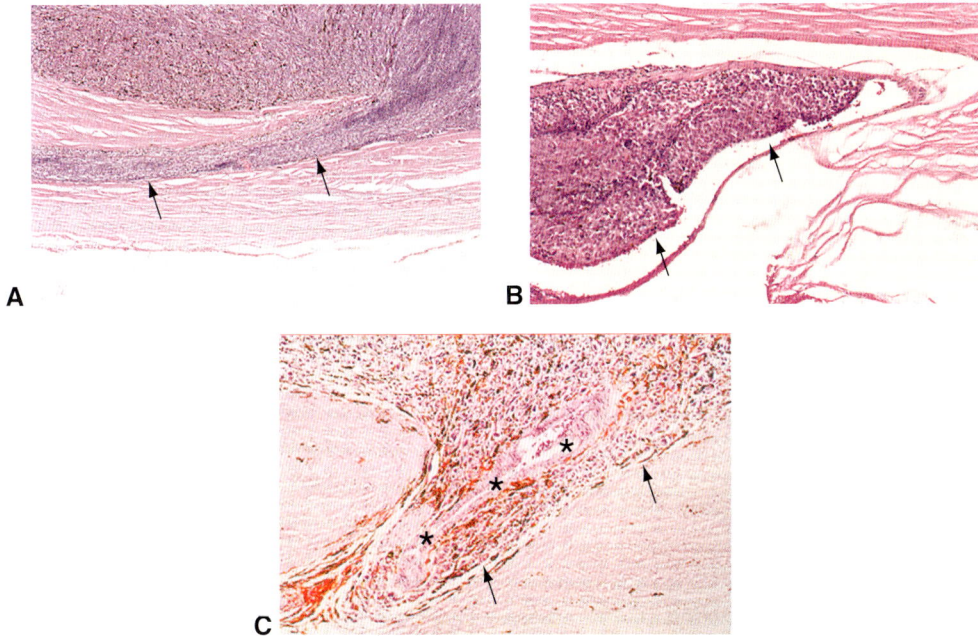

Figure 12-23 Invasion of scleral emissary canals by posterior melanoma. **A,** Note the melanoma cells tracking along an emissary canal within the sclera *(arrows).* **B,** Melanoma is found within the vortex vein *(arrows).* **C,** Melanoma *(arrows)* can spread by tracking along the outer sheaths of posterior ciliary vessels *(asterisks)* and nerves.

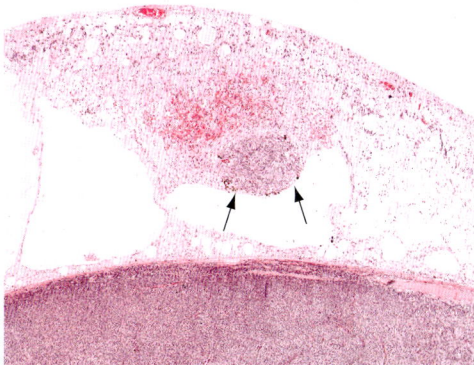

Figure 12-24 Invasion of the neurosensory retina by melanoma *(arrows).* Note the atrophy of overlying outer retina, cystoid edema, and intraretinal hemorrhage. *(Courtesy of Nasreen A. Syed, MD.)*

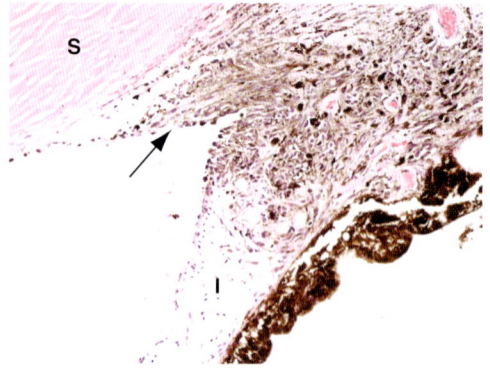

Figure 12-25 Ciliary body melanoma invading the iris root and angle. Pigmented melanoma cells from a ciliary body melanoma extend anteriorly into the trabecular meshwork *(arrow).* I = iris; S = sclera. *(Courtesy of Michele Bloomer, MD.)*

Histologic prognostic factors Several factors that can be identified via pathologic examination have been significantly correlated with survival in patients with posterior uveal melanoma. The most important histologic variables statistically associated with patient survival are

- tumor cell type (modified Callender classification)
- size of tumor in contact with the sclera (greatest basal dimension of tumor)
- direct extraocular extension
- tumor location (eg, ciliary body)
- complexity of extravascular matrix patterns and high microvascular density

Posterior uveal melanomas are classified by cell type via the modified Callender classification:

- spindle cell melanoma: >90% spindle cells
- epithelioid melanoma: >90% epithelioid cells
- mixed-cell type: mixture of spindle and epithelioid cells

Cell type, defined with the modified Callender classification, has one of the highest associations with survival. Spindle cell melanoma has the best prognosis; epithelioid melanoma, the worst. Melanomas of mixed-cell type have an intermediate prognosis. Some authors have suggested that, in mixed-cell melanoma, survival following enucleation decreases with increasing proportions of epithelioid cells. In rare cases, a melanoma undergoes extensive necrosis, which precludes classification. The prognosis for completely necrotic melanomas is the same as that for mixed-cell melanomas.

The modified Callender classification has some disadvantages. First, there is continuing controversy about the minimum number of epithelioid cells needed for a melanoma to be classified as mixed-cell type. Second, tumor classification can vary between pathologists, even with experienced ophthalmic pathologists, because the cytologic features of melanoma represent a continuous spectrum.

Tumor size is a factor that is also strongly associated with patient survival. In general, larger tumors are associated with poor survival. Many studies use greatest basal dimension and greatest tumor thickness to classify tumors based on size. These measurements can be obtained clinically for many tumors with the use of ultrasonography. Methodical measurements of tumor size are obtained on pathologic examination of tumors that are treated with enucleation. In studies of uveal melanomas that have been enucleated, 10 mm is often used as the cutoff for stratification by size to evaluate prognosis. Most studies have demonstrated that tumor size is an independent risk factor for patient survival and that the larger the tumor, the worse the survival rate. The American Joint Committee on Cancer (AJCC) staging system, commonly used for staging uveal melanoma, stratifies tumor size into 4 categories; these are described in Chapter 17.

Extrascleral extension of tumor is another factor that correlates with prognosis for survival. Extrascleral extension may be classified as macroscopic (ie, extension that can be detected clinically or by ultrasonography and, for enucleated eyes, seen on gross examination) or as microscopic (extension seen only under the microscope in enucleated specimens). The AJCC staging system categorizes extrascleral extension as present or not present; if extension is present, the largest diameter of the extrascleral component is categorized as 5 mm or less, or as greater than 5 mm in greatest dimension. In general, extrascleral extension, particularly macroscopic extension, is associated with less favorable survival.

Yet another prognostic factor that correlates with survival is the location of posterior uveal melanoma. Tumors with a scleral base 1 mm or less from the optic disc (juxtapapillary) have a less favorable prognosis. Posterior uveal melanomas with any ciliary body involvement are also associated with a worse prognosis.

Intrinsic tumor extravascular matrix patterns have prognostic significance. This is a feature that is difficult to assess without histologic evaluation. Tumors demonstrating more-complex extravascular matrix patterns, such as closed loops or networks (3 or more back-to-back loops), are associated with a higher rate of subsequent metastases (Fig 12-26).

Many other histologic factors have some association with survival and/or rate of metastasis. The *mean diameter of the 10 largest melanoma cell nucleoli (MLN)* correlates well with mortality after enucleation. However, because of the time-intensive nature of

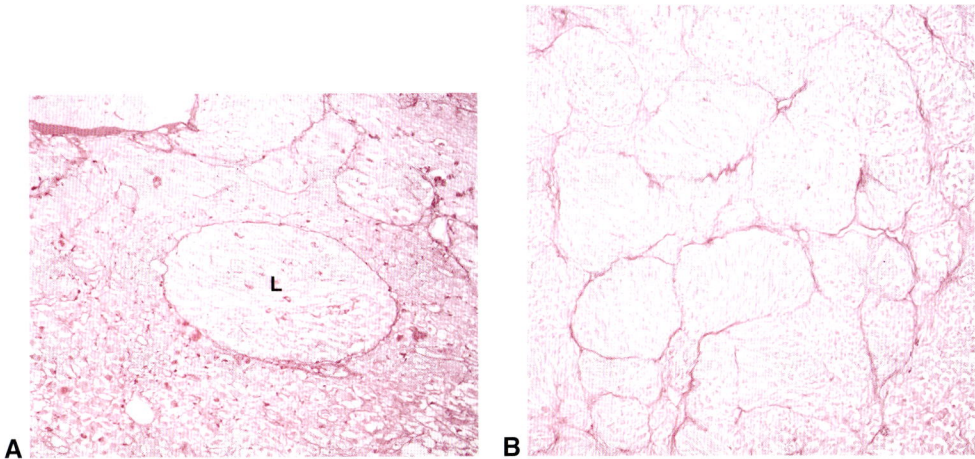

A   **B**

Figure 12-26 Complex extravascular matrix patterns in uveal melanoma (PAS stain). **A,** Closed loop (L). **B,** Network (3 or more back-to-back loops). *(Courtesy of Nasreen A. Syed, MD.)*

calculating this particular variable, it is not often included in pathology reports. High microvascular density is associated with an increased rate of subsequent metastases; this association is as strong as, if not stronger than, that of MLN and extravascular matrix patterns, and is relevant given that the mode of metastasis is overwhelmingly hematogenous. The presence of a large number of tumor-infiltrating lymphocytes and/or histiocytes is associated with a higher metastatic rate as well. It is important to note that invasion through Bruch membrane is not associated with a decrease in survival rates.

Metastases almost invariably result from the hematogenous spread of melanoma to the liver; in more than 95% of tumor-related deaths there is liver involvement. In as many as one-third of tumor-related deaths, the liver is the sole site of metastasis.

Some types of posterior uveal melanomas exhibit biological behavior that cannot be predicted according to the criteria just discussed. Survival rates of patients with diffuse ciliary body melanomas (ring melanoma) are particularly poor. These relatively flat tumors, which are almost always of mixed-cell type, may grow circumferentially without becoming significantly elevated. Diffuse choroidal melanomas have a similarly poor prognosis.

Cytogenetic studies of posterior uveal melanoma have shown that mutually exclusive mutations in *GNAQ* and *GNA11* are an initiating event in the development of uveal melanomas and nevi from melanocytes. Approximately half of uveal melanomas demonstrate monosomy of chromosome 3; a smaller proportion shows gain or loss of a chromosome in chromosomes 1, 6, or 8. Tumors with monosomy 3, especially when associated with gains in 8q, are associated with increased mortality.

Molecular analysis of posterior uveal melanomas by gene expression profiling provides a prognostic classification of uveal melanoma. The analysis, which requires a small amount of fresh or paraffin-embedded tissue, classifies these tumors as follows: class 1A (low metastatic potential), class 1B (intermediate metastatic potential), or class 2 (high metastatic potential). Gene expression profiling analyzes the status of several genes within the tumor. One of these genes is *BAP1* (BRCA1-associated protein-1). Mutations leading to inactivation of this gene within the tumor are associated with a higher rate of metastasis. Expression of mRNA by the *PRAME* gene in tumors may also be associated with rate of metastasis, but this needs to be validated in further studies. Identification of the genetic alterations in uveal melanoma is important not only for prognostication but also in the development of potential targeted therapies for posterior uveal melanoma.

See Chapter 17 for further discussion of posterior uveal melanomas.

Coupland SE, Lake SL, Zeschnigk M, Damato BE. Molecular pathology of uveal melanoma. *Eye (Lond).* 2013;27(2):230–242.

Field MG, Durante MA, Anbunathan H, et al. Punctuated evolution of canonical genomic aberrations in uveal melanoma. *Nat Commun.* 2018;9(1):116.

Metastatic Tumors

Metastatic tumors to the uveal tract are the most common intraocular tumors in adults when eyes have been examined in large autopsy series. When these lesions are identified clinically, they most often involve the choroid, but metastatic disease can affect any part of the uvea. Unlike primary uveal melanoma, uveal metastatic lesions are often multiple

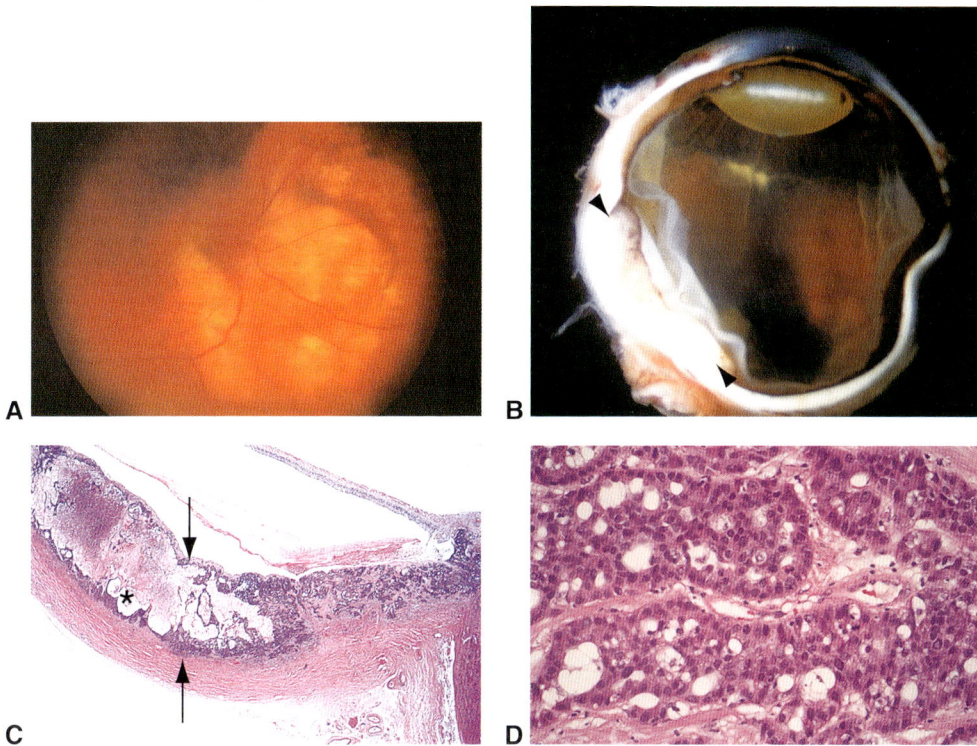

Figure 12-27 Choroidal metastasis. **A,** Clinical appearance of a metastatic lesion from a primary lung tumor. **B,** Gross appearance of the same lesion shown in part **A** *(between arrowheads)*. **C,** Choroidal metastasis from lung adenocarcinoma; histology shows adenocarcinoma *(between arrows)* with mucin production *(asterisk)*. Note the overlying exudative retinal detachment. **D,** Higher magnification depicts a well-differentiated adenocarcinoma with a distinct glandular morphology. *(Courtesy of Hans E. Grossniklaus, MD.)*

and may be bilateral. They are typically flat, nonpigmented lesions, but rare cases of collar-button or mushroom-shaped lesions have been reported. The most common primary tumors metastasizing to the eye are breast carcinoma in women and lung carcinoma in men (Fig 12-27), although tumors from many different primary sites have been reported. Histologically, metastatic tumors may recapitulate the appearance of the primary lesion, or they may appear less differentiated. Special histochemical stains and a panel of immunohistochemical stains can be helpful in diagnosing metastatic lesions, determining the origin of the primary tumor, and, in some cases, guiding therapy for that tumor. The importance of a careful clinical history cannot be overemphasized. See Chapter 20 for further discussion of metastatic tumors.

Other Uveal Tumors

Hemangioma

Hemangiomas of the choroid occur in 2 specific forms: circumscribed (ie, localized) and diffuse. *Circumscribed* choroidal hemangioma typically occurs in patients without

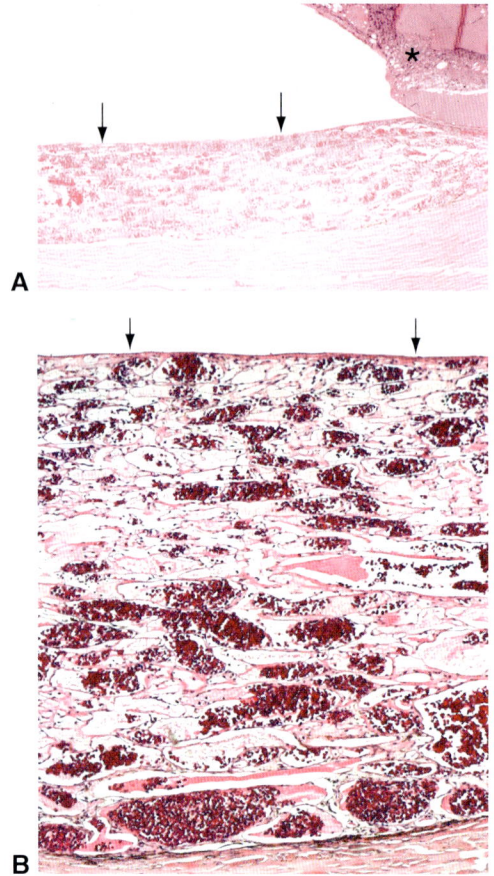

Figure 12-28 Choroidal hemangioma with a large number of thin-walled, variably sized vessels within the choroid. **A,** Low-magnification view shows exudative retinal detachment overlying the lesion *(asterisk)*. *Arrows* designate Bruch membrane. **B,** Higher-magnification photomicrograph from a different patient showing the numerous choroidal blood vessels; *arrows* designate Bruch membrane. *(Part A courtesy of Nasreen A. Syed, MD; part B courtesy of Steffen Heegaard, MD.)*

systemic disorders. *Diffuse* choroidal hemangioma is generally seen in patients with Sturge-Weber syndrome (encephalofacial angiomatosis).

Histologically, both forms show collections of variably sized vessels within the choroid (Fig 12-28). The lesions may appear as predominantly capillary hemangiomas, cavernous hemangiomas, or a mix of the two. There may be compressed melanocytes, hyperplastic RPE, and fibrous tissue proliferation in the adjacent and overlying choroid. See Chapter 18 (particularly Figs 18-1, 18-2) in this volume for detailed discussion of choroidal hemangiomas. See also BCSC Section 12, *Retina and Vitreous.*

Choroidal osteoma

Choroidal osteomas are benign bony tumors that typically arise from the juxtapapillary choroid. They are seen in adolescent and young adult patients and are more common in females. The characteristic lesion appears yellow to orange and has well-defined margins (see Chapter 17, Fig 17-12D). These tumors may affect vision in the involved eye and may lead to development of choroidal neovascularization. The tumor is located in the

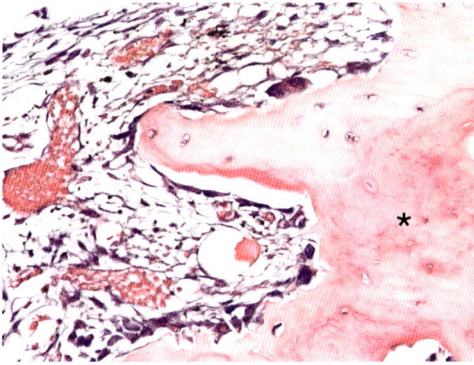

Figure 12-29 Choroidal osteoma. This choristomatous lesion is composed of compact bone *(asterisk)* and intratrabecular connective tissue. *(Courtesy of Steffen Heegaard, MD.)*

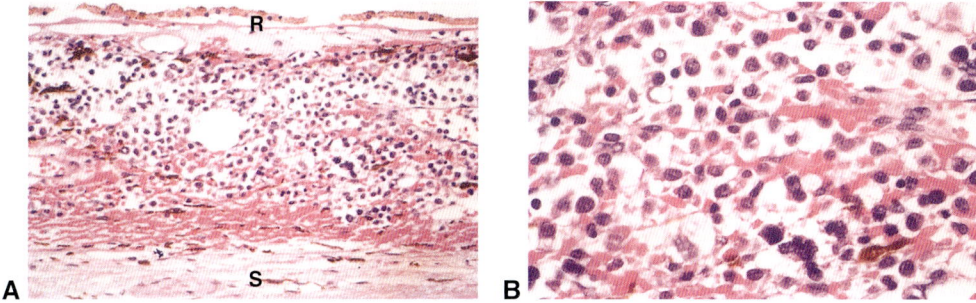

Figure 12-30 Choroidal lymphoma. **A,** Diffuse infiltration of the choroid by lymphoma (blue cells). R = RPE; S = sclera. **B,** Higher magnification demonstrates atypical pleomorphic lymphocytes. *(Courtesy of Hans E. Grossniklaus, MD.)*

peripapillary choroid and, histologically, is composed of compact bone (Fig 12-29). The intratrabecular spaces are filled with loose connective tissue that contains large and small blood vessels, vacuolated mesenchymal cells, and scattered mast cells. The bony trabeculae contain osteocytes, cement lines, and occasional osteoclasts.

Lymphoid proliferation

The choroid may be the site of lymphoid proliferation, either as a primary ocular process or in association with systemic lymphoproliferative disease.

Primary choroidal lymphomas (previously known as *uveal lymphoid hyperplasia* or *uveal lymphoid infiltration*) are mostly low-grade, B-cell tumors similar to extranodal marginal zone B-cell lymphomas occurring elsewhere in the body. High-grade choroidal lymphomas (Fig 12-30) are usually secondary to systemic disease or are an extension of vitreoretinal lymphoma. The classification of lymphoproliferative lesions is further discussed in Chapter 14.

Sagoo MS, Mehta H, Swampillai AJ, et al. Primary intraocular lymphoma. *Surv Ophthalmol.* 2014;59(5):503–516.

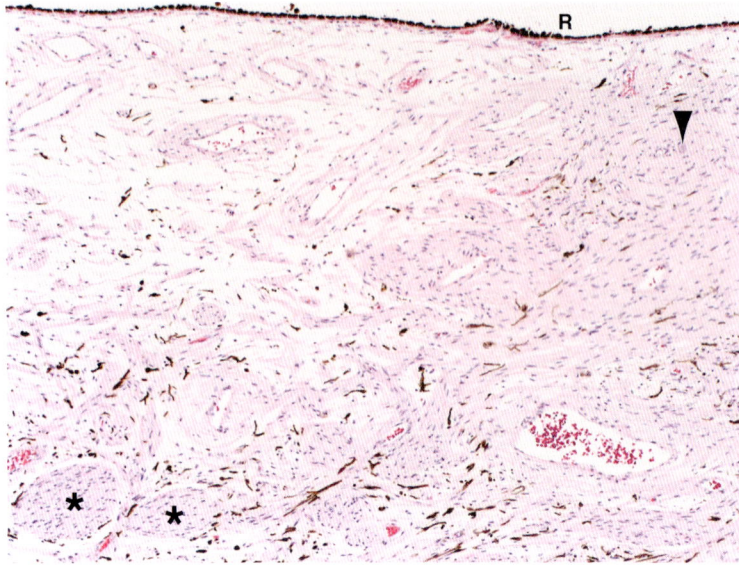

Figure 12-31 Choroidal neurofibromatosis. The choroid is diffusely infiltrated by spindle-shaped cells with slender, wavy nuclei; occasional neurons *(arrowhead);* and enlarged choroidal nerves *(asterisks).* R = RPE. *(Courtesy of Michele Bloomer, MD.)*

Neural sheath tumors

Neurilemomas (schwannomas) and neurofibromas are rare in the uveal tract. Multiple neurofibromas may occur in the ciliary body, iris, and choroid in patients with neurofibromatosis 1 (Fig 12-31). For more information on these tumors, see Chapter 14.

Leiomyoma

Neoplasms arising from the smooth muscle of the ciliary body have been reported in rare instances. They typically occur in young adult females. When leiomyoma occurs, it may be confused clinically with amelanotic melanoma or neurofibroma. Histologically, leiomyoma is identical to leiomyoma of the uterus (uterine fibroid) and consists of a proliferation of tightly packed, slender spindle cells lacking pigment. Immunohistochemical stains may be useful in diagnosing leiomyomas because these tumors express smooth muscle–related antigens. They also may express hormonal receptors such as progesterone and androgen receptor. Under light microscopy and transmission electron microscopy, leiomyoma sometimes exhibits both myogenic and neurogenic differentiation. In such cases, the tumor is called *mesectodermal leiomyoma.*

CHAPTER 13

Eyelids

Highlights

- The eyelid contains a number of distinct structures that can give rise to various types of pathologic conditions.
- Benign neoplasms of the eyelid are common in both children and adults.
- Malignant eyelid neoplasms increase in incidence with age. Basal cell carcinoma is the most common of these neoplasms.
- Sebaceous carcinoma frequently propagates along the eyelids and ocular surface via pagetoid and in situ spread.
- Eyelid nevi are common, and they evolve and proliferate with age.

Topography

The eyelids extend from the eyebrow superiorly to the cheek inferiorly and can be divided into orbital and tarsal components. At the level of the tarsus, the eyelid consists of 4 main histologic layers, from anterior to posterior (Fig 13-1):

- skin
- orbicularis oculi muscle
- tarsus
- palpebral conjunctiva

There is a surgical plane of dissection into the eyelid that is accessed through an incision starting at the gray line, an isolated slip of orbicularis muscle known as the *Riolan*

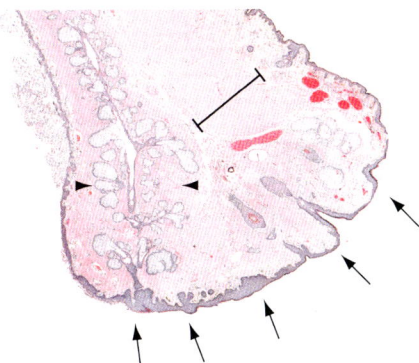

Figure 13-1 Cross section of a normal eyelid. Proceeding from left (posterior) to right (anterior) are the palpebral conjunctiva; the tarsus, containing the meibomian glands *(between arrowheads);* the orbicularis oculi muscle *(bracket);* and the dermis, underlying the epidermis. *Arrows* indicate the eyelid margin. *(Courtesy of Heather Potter, MD.)*

237

muscle. This dissection plane functionally separates the eyelid into anterior and posterior lamellae. See also BCSC Section 7, *Oculofacial Plastic and Orbital Surgery.*

The skin of the eyelids is thinner than that of most other body sites. The surface epidermis consists of keratinized stratified squamous epithelium, which contains melano-cytes and antigen-presenting Langerhans cells. Deep to the epidermis is the dermis (stromal tissue), which is composed of loose collagenous connective tissue and contains the following:

- cilia, or eyelashes, and associated sebaceous glands (of Zeis; specialized pilosebaceous units)
- apocrine sweat glands (of Moll)
- eccrine sweat glands
- pilosebaceous units (vellus hairs)

Eyelid glands secrete their products in various ways. Sebaceous glands are holocrine glands, meaning that their secretion contains entire secreting cells. The secretion from apocrine sweat glands contains the apical part of the secreting cells (decapitation secretion). Eccrine sweat glands and lacrimal glands secrete sweat and tears, respectively, without loss of any part of the secreting cells.

Two muscles elevate the upper eyelid: the *levator palpebrae superioris* (a skeletal muscle), of which only the aponeurotic portion is present in the eyelid, and the *Müller muscle* (a smooth muscle). The *orbicularis oculi* (a striated skeletal muscle), whose fibers are arranged circumferentially around the eye, closes the eyelid. The *tarsal plate*—a thick plaque of dense, collagenous connective tissue—contains the meibomian glands (specialized sebaceous glands). Also present near the upper border of the superior tarsal plate (and less so along the lower border of the inferior tarsal plate) are the accessory lacrimal glands of Wolfring; the accessory lacrimal glands of Krause are located in the conjunctival fornices. The *palpebral conjunctiva* adheres tightly to the posterior surface of the tarsus.

The following are some common dermatopathologic terms that also are applicable to eyelid pathology:

- *acanthosis:* increased thickness (hyperplasia) of the stratum malpighii (cellular layers of the epidermis)
- *hyperkeratosis:* increased thickness of the stratum corneum (keratin layer) of the epidermis
- *parakeratosis:* retention of nuclei within the stratum corneum
- *papillomatosis:* formation of fingerlike upward projections of epidermis surrounding fibrovascular cores
- *dyskeratosis:* premature keratinization of the individual cells within the stratum malpighii
- *acantholysis:* loss of cohesion (dissolution of intercellular bridges) between adjacent squamous epithelial cells

Developmental Anomalies

For additional discussion of the developmental anomalies covered in this chapter, see BCSC Section 7, *Oculofacial Plastic and Orbital Surgery.*

Distichiasis

Distichiasis is the aberrant formation of cilia within the tarsus, which causes them to exit the eyelid margin through the orifices of the meibomian glands and results in an extra row of eyelashes. The pathogenesis of distichiasis is thought to be an anomalous formation within the tarsus of a complete pilosebaceous unit rather than just the normal sebaceous (meibomian) gland. Histologically, hair follicles can be seen within the tarsal plate. The tarsus may be rudimentary, and the glands of Moll are often hypertrophic. See BCSC Section 6, *Pediatric Ophthalmology and Strabismus,* and Section 8, *External Disease and Cornea,* for additional discussion.

Phakomatous Choristoma

A rare developmental tumor, phakomatous choristoma (Zimmerman tumor) results from the aberrant retention of parts of the lens placode in the lower eyelid during embryologic development. As a result, lens epithelium proliferates within the inferonasal portion of the lower eyelid. The epithelial cells may undergo cytoplasmic enlargement, identical to the enlargement of "bladder" cells seen in posterior subcapsular cataract. Basement membrane material is produced, recapitulating the lens capsule (Fig 13-2); this material stains positively with periodic acid–Schiff (PAS) stain. The eyelid mass formed is usually present at birth and enlarges slowly. Complete excision is the usual treatment.

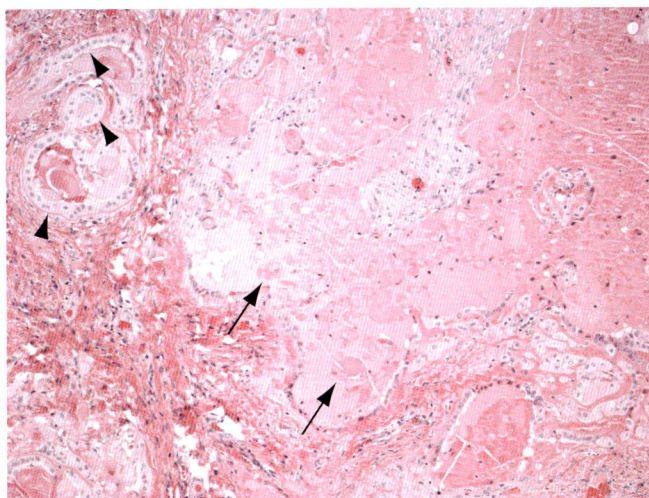

Figure 13-2 Phakomatous choristoma of the eyelid. The dermis displays a disorganized proliferation of lens epithelium *(arrowheads)* and occasional "bladder" cells *(arrows)* similar to those seen in posterior subcapsular cataract. Note the large amount of eosinophilic material, which represents lens crystalline proteins. *(Courtesy of Nasreen A. Syed, MD.)*

Dermoid Cyst

Dermoid cysts are not uncommon in the lateral portion of the upper eyelid and brow in young children. However, they are more traditionally regarded as orbital lesions and are therefore discussed in Chapter 14 of this volume.

Inflammation

Infectious Inflammatory Disorders

Depending on the causative agent, infectious organisms can cause disease that is localized (eg, hordeolum), multicentric (eg, papillomas), or diffuse (eg, cellulitis). Common routes of infection include primary inoculation through a bite or wound and direct spread from a contiguous site, such as an infected paranasal sinus. Infectious agents may be

- bacterial, such as *Staphylococcus aureus* in hordeolum and infectious blepharitis
- viral, such as poxvirus in molluscum contagiosum
- parasitic, such as *Demodex folliculorum*

Bacterial infections

Hordeolum A hordeolum (also called a *stye*) is an acute, generally self-limited primary inflammatory process typically involving the glands of Zeis and, less often, the meibomian glands. A small abscess, or focal collection of neutrophils and necrotic debris (ie, pus), forms at the site of infection, which is usually caused by *S aureus*. Lesions may drain spontaneously or require surgical management.

Cellulitis The diffuse spread of acute inflammatory cells through tissue planes is known as *cellulitis*. *Preseptal* cellulitis involves the tissues of the eyelid anterior to the orbital septum, which is the collagenous membrane connecting the nonmarginal borders of the tarsal plates to the bony orbital rim. Cellulitis is most often secondary to bacterial infection of the paranasal sinuses. Histologic examination reveals neutrophilic infiltration of the soft tissues, accompanied by interstitial edema and, occasionally, necrosis (Fig 13-3). See BCSC Section 7, *Oculofacial Plastic and Orbital Surgery,* for additional discussion.

Viral infections

Human papillomavirus may infect the skin of the eyelids, typically manifesting as *verruca vulgaris,* or *wart.* Clinically, verruca vulgaris is usually an elevated lesion with fine papillary projections. Histologically, the lesions exhibit a papillary growth pattern and demonstrate parakeratosis, hyperkeratosis, and acanthosis (Fig 13-4A). Infected epidermal cells may show cytoplasmic clearing (koilocytosis) (Fig 13-4B). A mixed inflammatory cell infiltrate is typically present in the superficial dermis.

In *molluscum contagiosum,* which is caused by a member of the poxvirus family, small waxy, dome-shaped epidermal nodules with central umbilication form. When the nodules are present on the eyelid margin, an associated follicular conjunctivitis may develop because of shedding of virus onto the conjunctival surface (Fig 13-5). Histologically, the lesions are distinctive in appearance (Fig 13-6).

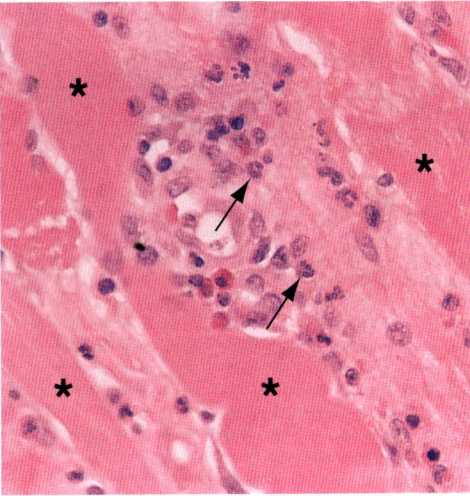

Figure 13-3 Biopsy from a case of preseptal cellulitis of the eyelid. Neutrophils *(arrows)* infiltrate between the skeletal muscle fibers *(asterisks)* of the orbicularis oculi muscle.

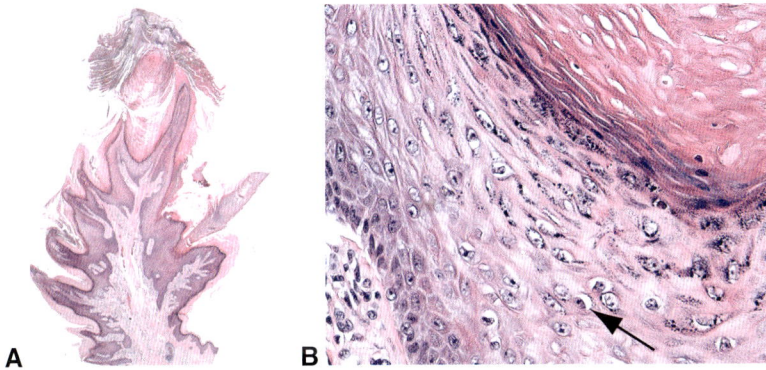

A   **B**

Figure 13-4 Verruca vulgaris. **A,** Verruca vulgaris is a form of human papillomavirus (HPV) infection of the eyelid epidermis. The resulting "wart" has a papillary growth pattern with fingerlike projections. **B,** Occasional koilocytes with nuclear contraction and cytoplasmic clearing are present *(arrow)*. *(Courtesy of Nasreen A. Syed, MD.)*

Parasitic infections

Infection of the eyelid with the mite *Demodex folliculorum* is increasingly recognized as a cause of chronic eyelid and conjunctival inflammation. The conditions caused by this parasite are discussed in more detail in BCSC Section 8, *External Disease and Cornea.*

Noninfectious Inflammatory Disorders

Chalazion

A chalazion is a chronic, often painless nodule of the eyelid that develops when the lipid secretions of the meibomian glands or, less often, the glands of Zeis are discharged into the surrounding tissues, inciting a lipogranulomatous reaction (Fig 13-7).

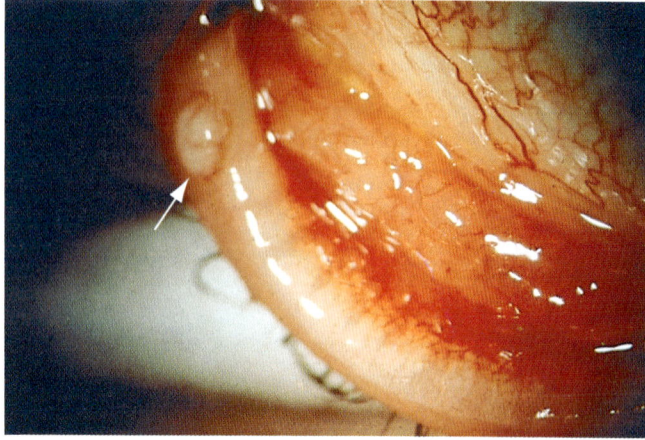

Figure 13-5 Molluscum contagiosum involving the eyelid margin *(arrow)*. Note the associated follicular conjunctivitis.

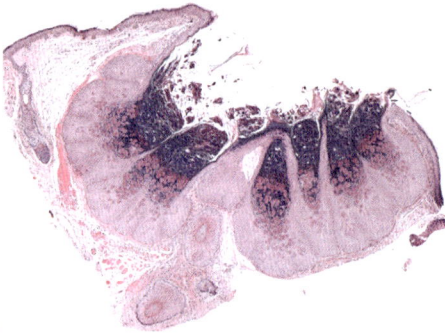

A

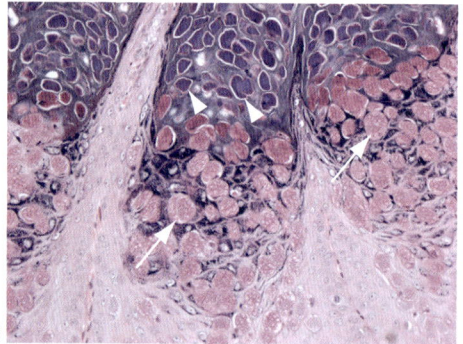

B

Figure 13-6 Molluscum contagiosum. **A,** Note the cup-shaped, thickened epidermis with a central crater. **B,** In the more central portion of the epidermis, cell nuclei are displaced peripherally by large eosinophilic viral inclusions known as *molluscum bodies (arrows)*. The molluscum bodies become more basophilic near the surface of the epithelium *(arrowheads)*. *(Courtesy of Nasreen A. Syed, MD.)*

Figure 13-7 Chalazion. Granulomatous inflammation consisting of epithelioid histiocytes and multinucleated giant cells *(arrows)* surrounds clear spaces (lipogranuloma). Because the lipid is dissolved by solvents during routine tissue processing, optically clear ("lipid dropout") spaces remain. Lymphocytes, plasma cells, and neutrophils are also often present.

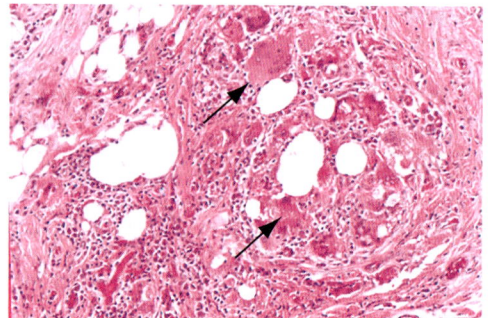

Degenerations and Deposits

Xanthelasma

A type of planar xanthoma, xanthelasma consists of single or multiple soft, yellow plaques that occur in the medial canthal region of the eyelids (Fig 13-8A). Associated hyperlipoproteinemic states, particularly hyperlipoproteinemia types II and III, are present in 30%–40% of patients with xanthelasma. Associated inflammatory signs are minimal. Histologically, eyelid xanthomas consist of aggregates of histiocytes with foamy, lipid-laden cytoplasm distributed diffusely and often around blood vessels within the dermis (Fig 13-8B). The histiocytes are postulated to phagocytose lipid that leaks from the blood vessels in the eyelid, although why the eyelid is often affected remains unclear.

Amyloidosis

The term *amyloid* refers to a heterogeneous group of extracellular proteins that structurally have a β-pleated sheet configuration and exhibit birefringence and dichroism under polarized light when stained with Congo red (see Chapter 5 and Fig 5-13). Amyloidosis is a group of diseases characterized by the deposition of specific amyloid proteins in various tissues and organs, often causing dysfunction of the affected tissues and organs. Common sources of amyloid proteins include

- immunoglobulin light chain fragments (AL amyloid), in plasma cell dyscrasias
- transthyretin, mutations in familial amyloid polyneuropathy types I and II
- gelsolin, mutations in familial amyloidosis, Finnish type (also known as *gelsolin amyloidosis* or *Meretoja syndrome*)

Amyloid deposits within the eyelid skin are highly indicative of a systemic disease process, either primary or secondary, whereas deposits elsewhere in the ocular adnexa are more likely to represent a localized disease process. Other systemic diseases with eyelid manifestations are listed in Table 13-1. See BCSC Section 8, *External Disease and Cornea,* which discusses the classification of amyloidosis.

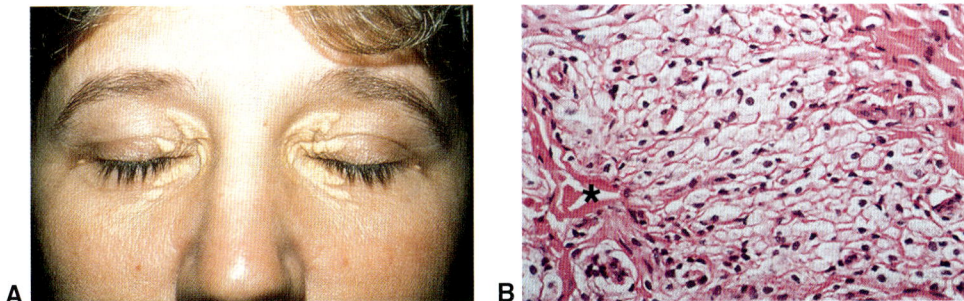

Figure 13-8   Xanthelasma. **A,** Patient with prominent xanthelasma. Note the yellow plaques on the medial upper and lower eyelids. **B,** Aggregates of foamy lipid-laden histiocytes are present in the dermis surrounding a venule *(asterisk)*. *(Part A from* External Disease and Cornea: A Multimedia Collection. *American Academy of Ophthalmology; 1994:slide 10.)*

Table 13-1 **Eyelid Manifestations of Systemic Diseases**

Systemic Condition	Eyelid Manifestations
Amyloidosis	Waxy papules/nodules, ptosis, purpura
Carney complex	Myxoma
Cryptophthalmos (Fraser) syndrome	Cryptophthalmos
Dermatomyositis	Edema, erythema
Erdheim-Chester disease	Xanthelasma, xanthogranuloma
Granulomatosis with polyangiitis (formerly Wegener granulomatosis)	Edema, ptosis, lower eyelid retraction
Hyperlipoproteinemia	Xanthelasma
Mandibulofacial dysostosis (Treacher Collins syndrome)	Lower eyelid coloboma
Neurofibromatosis 1	Cutaneous neurofibromas, plexiform neurofibroma of upper eyelid
Polyarteritis nodosa	Focal infarction
Relapsing polychondritis	Inflammatory papules
Sarcoidosis	Inflammatory papules
Scleroderma	Reduced mobility, taut skin
Systemic lupus erythematosus	Telangiectasias, edema
Thyroid eye disease	Swelling, retraction of the eyelids

Modified from Wiggs JL, Jakobiec FA. Eyelid manifestations of systemic disease. In: Albert DM, Jakobiec FA, eds. *Principles and Practice of Ophthalmology*. Saunders; 1994:1859.

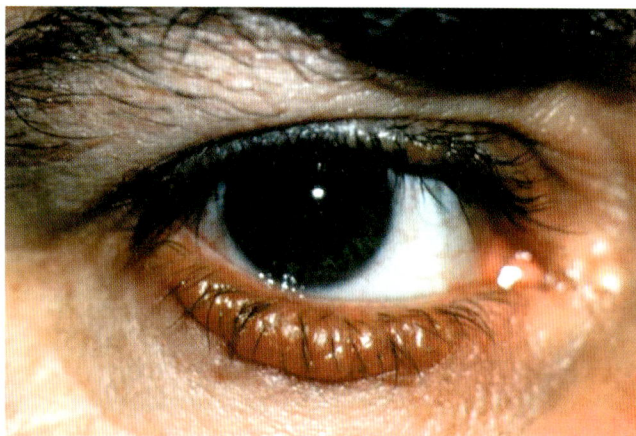

Figure 13-9 Cutaneous amyloidosis of the eyelid in multiple myeloma. Note the waxy elevation and the associated purpura of the lower lid, under the lesion. *(Courtesy of John B. Holds, MD.)*

Amyloid deposition in the skin is usually bilateral and symmetric and presents as multiple waxy yellow-white papules (Fig 13-9). The deposition of amyloid within blood vessel walls in the skin causes increased vascular fragility and often results in intradermal hemorrhages, accounting for the purpura seen clinically. On routine histologic sections, amyloid appears as an amorphous, eosinophilic extracellular deposit. Stains that are useful in demonstrating amyloid deposits include Congo red (see Chapter 10, Fig 10-12), crystal violet, and

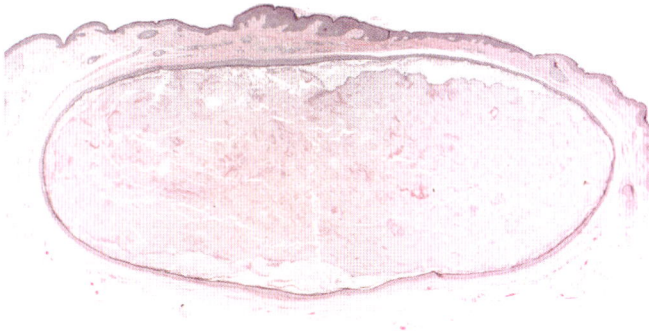

Figure 13-10 Epidermoid (epidermal inclusion) cyst in the dermis. The cyst lining resembles epidermis but does not contain skin appendages. The lumen contains keratin. *(Courtesy of Nasreen A. Syed, MD.)*

thioflavin T. Electron microscopy reveals that the deposits are composed of randomly oriented extracellular fibrils measuring 7–10 nm in diameter.

Cysts

See BCSC Section 7, *Oculofacial Plastic and Orbital Surgery,* for further information on the entities discussed in the following subsections.

Epidermoid Cysts

Epidermoid cysts, also called *epidermal inclusion cysts,* are common in the eyelids. They may arise spontaneously or as a result of the entrapment of epidermis beneath the skin surface following surgery or trauma. Epidermoid cysts are lined with keratinized stratified squamous epithelium and contain keratin (Fig 13-10).

Ductal Cysts

The eyelid contains the ducts of numerous structures, including the lacrimal gland and the apocrine and eccrine sweat glands. Cysts may develop in any of these ducts. A cyst arising from the duct of the lacrimal gland is called *dacryops.* Cysts arising from sweat ducts are referred to as either *apocrine* or *eccrine hidrocystomas* (Fig 13-11). Histologically, ductal cysts typically are lined with a double layer of cuboidal epithelium, as are the ducts from which they arise. The lumen of the cyst typically appears empty.

Neoplasia

Epidermal Neoplasms

Seborrheic keratosis

Seborrheic keratosis is a common benign epidermal proliferation typically occurring in middle age. Clinically, it is a well-circumscribed round to oval, dome-shaped verrucoid

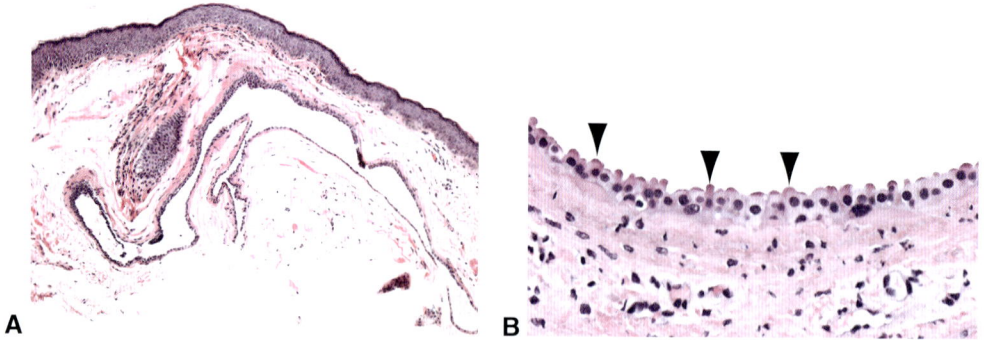

Figure 13-11   Apocrine hidrocystoma. **A,** Low-power photomicrograph shows a partially col-lapsed cyst that is lined by a double layer of epithelium (ie, an inner, low cuboidal layer and an outer, flattened myoepithelial layer). The lumen appears empty as the clear liquid contents are not visible on routine histologic examination. **B,** High magnification shows apocrine differentia-tion with cytoplasmic projections (snouts) on the inner surface *(arrowheads)* that are typical of decapitation secretion. *(Courtesy of Nasreen A. Syed, MD.)*

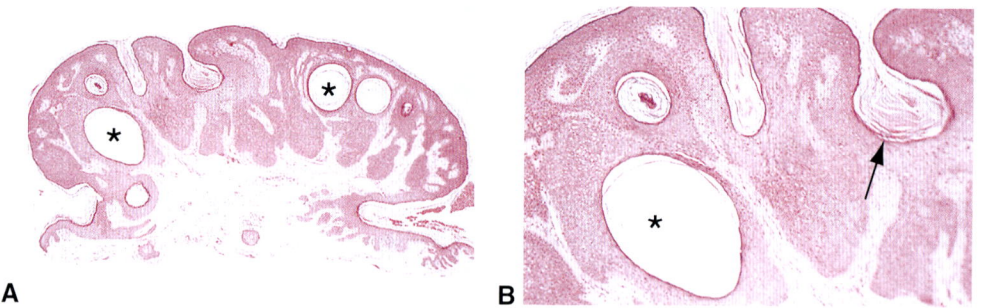

Figure 13-12   Seborrheic keratosis. **A,** The epidermis is acanthotic with a papillary configura-tion. Note the keratin-filled pseudohorn cysts *(asterisks).* **B,** When serial histologic sections are studied, pseudohorn cysts *(asterisk)* within the epidermis are found to represent crevices or infoldings of epidermis *(arrow)* rather than true cysts. *(Courtesy of Hans E. Grossniklaus, MD.)*

"stuck-on" papule, appearing tan pink to dark brown. Histologically, although several archi-tectural patterns are possible, all lesions demonstrate hyperkeratosis, acanthosis, and some degree of papillomatosis. The acanthosis is a result of the proliferation of either polygonal or basaloid squamous cells without dysplasia. In more pigmented lesions, the basal epidermal layer contains an increased amount of melanin. *Pseudohorn cysts,* concentrically laminated collections of surface keratin within an epidermal crypt, are a characteristic histologic find-ing in most types of seborrheic keratosis (Fig 13-12).

Irritated seborrheic keratosis, also termed inverted follicular keratosis, shows nonkera-tinized squamous epithelial whorling, or squamous "eddies," within the proliferating epider-mis (Fig 13-13). Sudden onset of multiple seborrheic keratoses is known as the *Leser-Trélat sign* and is associated with visceral malignancy, usually a gastrointestinal adenocarcinoma; these keratoses may in fact represent evolving acanthosis nigricans. Table 13-2 lists other systemic neoplastic syndromes with possible eyelid manifestations.

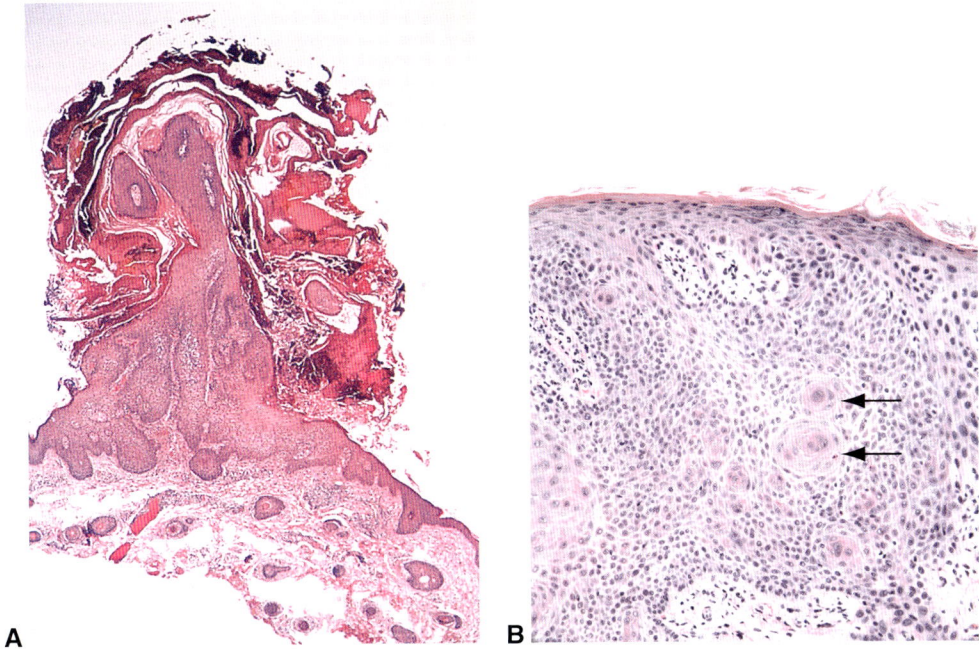

Figure 13-13 Irritated seborrheic keratosis (also known as *inverted follicular keratosis*). **A,** Low-magnification photomicrograph shows a papillary epidermal proliferation with hyperkeratosis on the surface. Clinically, this lesion appeared as a cutaneous horn. **B,** High-magnification photomicrograph of a different lesion. The epidermis often shows whorls of cells, known as squamous "eddies" *(arrows)*, and mild disorganization. *(Part B courtesy of Nasreen A. Syed, MD.)*

Table 13-2 Eyelid Neoplasms Associated With Systemic Neoplastic Syndromes

Syndrome	Eyelid Manifestations
Basal cell nevus syndrome (medulloblastoma, fibrosarcoma)	Multiple basal cell carcinomas
Cowden disease (breast carcinoma; fibrous hamartomas of breast, thyroid, gastrointestinal tract)	Multiple trichilemmomas
Muir-Torre syndrome (visceral carcinoma, usually colorectal)	Multiple sebaceous neoplasms (adenoma, carcinoma), keratoacanthoma

Modified from Wiggs JL, Jakobiec FA. Eyelid manifestations of systemic disease. In: Albert DM, Jakobiec FA, eds. *Principles and Practice of Ophthalmology.* Saunders; 1994:1859.

Actinic keratosis

Actinic keratoses are precancerous squamous lesions that typically occur starting in middle age. They appear clinically as erythematous, scaly macules or papules on sun-exposed skin, particularly the face and the dorsal surfaces of the hands. Actinic keratoses range from a few millimeters to 1 cm in diameter. Hyperkeratotic types of these lesions may form a cutaneous horn, and hyperpigmented types may clinically simulate lentigo maligna. Squamous cell carcinoma may develop from preexisting actinic keratosis, although most studies indicate that the risk is less than 15%. When squamous cell carcinoma arises in actinic keratosis, the risk of subsequent metastatic dissemination is very low (0.5%–3.0%).

Histologically, there are multiple variants, including a pigmented type. All types demonstrate changes in the epidermis with hyperkeratosis and parakeratosis. Cellular atypia (nuclear hyperchromatism and/or pleomorphism and an increased nuclear-to-cytoplasmic ratio) is present and ranges from mild (involving only the basal epithelial layers) to frank carcinoma in situ (full-thickness involvement of the epidermis). Loss of the granular cell layer, dyskeratosis (premature keratinization of individual cells), and mitotic figures above the basal epithelial layer are often found (Fig 13-14). The underlying dermis often shows solar elastosis (elastotic degeneration of collagen) (Fig 13-15), which manifests as fragmentation, clumping, and basophilic discoloration of the dermal collagen. A chronic inflammatory cell infiltrate is usually observed at the base of the lesion in the superficial dermis. Histologic

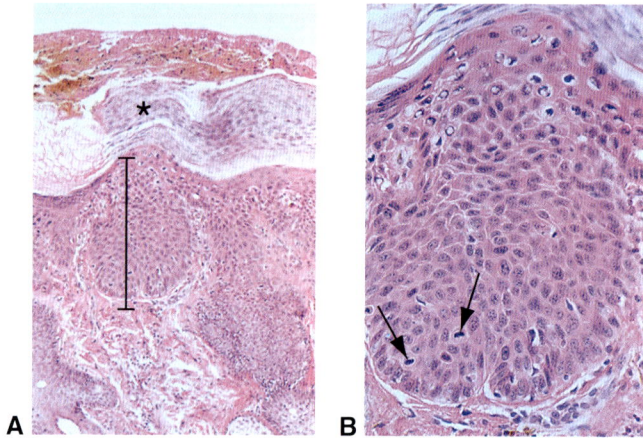

A   **B**

Figure 13-14   Actinic keratosis. **A,** Note the epidermal acanthosis *(bracket),* disorganization within the epidermis (dysplasia), parakeratosis *(asterisk),* and inflammation within the dermis. **B,** Higher magnification of part **A;** note the epidermal dysplasia and mitotic figures *(arrows).*

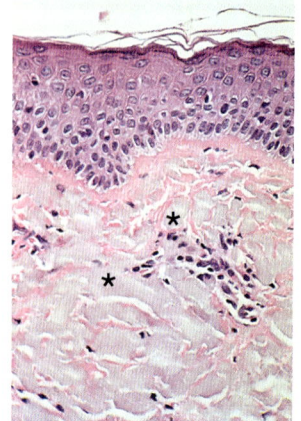

Figure 13-15   Solar elastosis of the dermis. The collagen of the dermis appears bluish *(asterisks)* instead of pink in this hematoxylin-eosin–stained section. This is a histologic indicator of ultraviolet light–induced tissue damage.

examination of the base of the lesion is necessary to determine whether invasion through the epidermal basement membrane, indicative of squamous cell carcinoma, is present.

Epidermal malignancies

Basal cell carcinoma Basal cell carcinoma (BCC), the most common malignant neoplasm of the eyelids, accounts for more than 90% of all malignant eyelid tumors. Although exposure to sunlight is the main risk factor, genetic factors can play a role in familial syndromes. The lower eyelid and medial canthus are the most common sites of involvement. Tumors in the medial canthal area are more likely to be deeply invasive and to involve the orbit.

Nodular BCC (the most common subtype) is a slow-growing, slightly elevated lesion, often with ulceration and pearly, raised, rolled edges (Fig 13-16A). The *morpheaform,* or sclerosing, variant of BCC is a flat or slightly elevated pale-yellow indurated plaque; this type is often infiltrative, and its extent is difficult to determine clinically. A small percentage of BCCs are pigmented or multicentric.

As the name implies, BCCs originate from the stratum basale, or stratum germinativum, of the epidermis and the outer root sheath of the hair follicle and occur only in hair-bearing tissue. Tumor cells are characterized by relatively bland oval nuclei and a high nuclear-to-cytoplasmic ratio. BCC forms cohesive islands with nuclear palisading of the peripheral cell layer, mimicking the hair matrix (Fig 13-16B). In the morpheaform type, thin cords and strands of tumor cells are set in a fibrotic stroma (Fig 13-17).

The treatment of choice is complete excision, and surgical margin evaluation is required. Typically, margin control is achieved with frozen sections or Mohs micrographic surgery. Morbidity in BCCs is almost always the result of local spread; metastasis is extremely unusual.

Squamous cell carcinoma Although *squamous cell carcinoma (SCC)* may occur in the eyelids, it is far less common than BCC of the eyelid. Like BCCs, most SCCs arise in solar-damaged

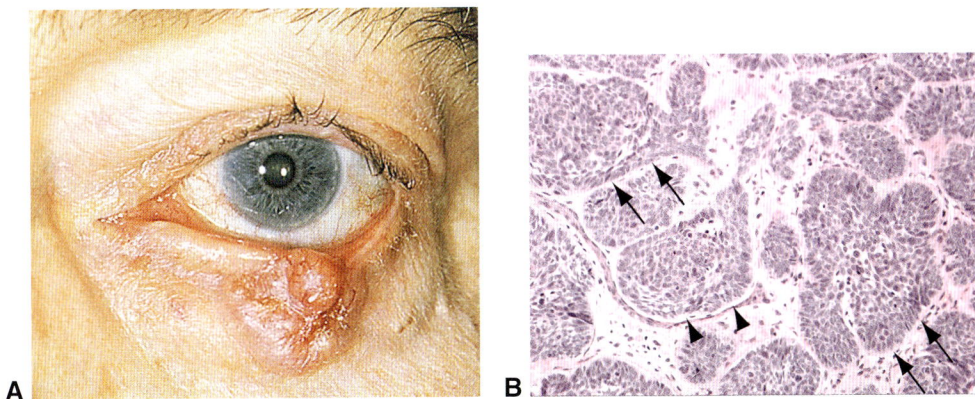

Figure 13-16 Basal cell carcinoma, nodular type. **A,** Clinical appearance with elevated, rolled edges and central ulceration. **B,** Histologic appearance. Note the characteristic palisading of the cells around the outer edges of the tumor islands *(arrows)* and the artifactitious separation (due to tissue processing) between the nests of tumor cells and the dermis (retraction artifact, *arrowheads*). *(Part B courtesy of Nasreen A. Syed, MD.)*

Figure 13-17 Basal cell carcinoma, morphea-form (sclerosing) type. Thin cords and strands of tumor cells infiltrating the dermis are surrounded by fibrotic (desmoplastic) dermal tissue.

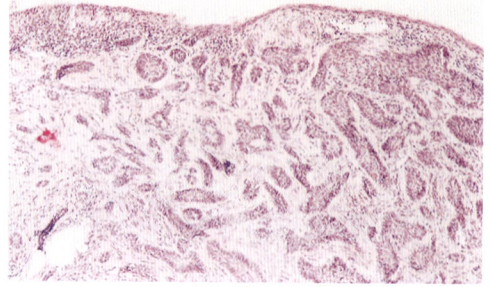

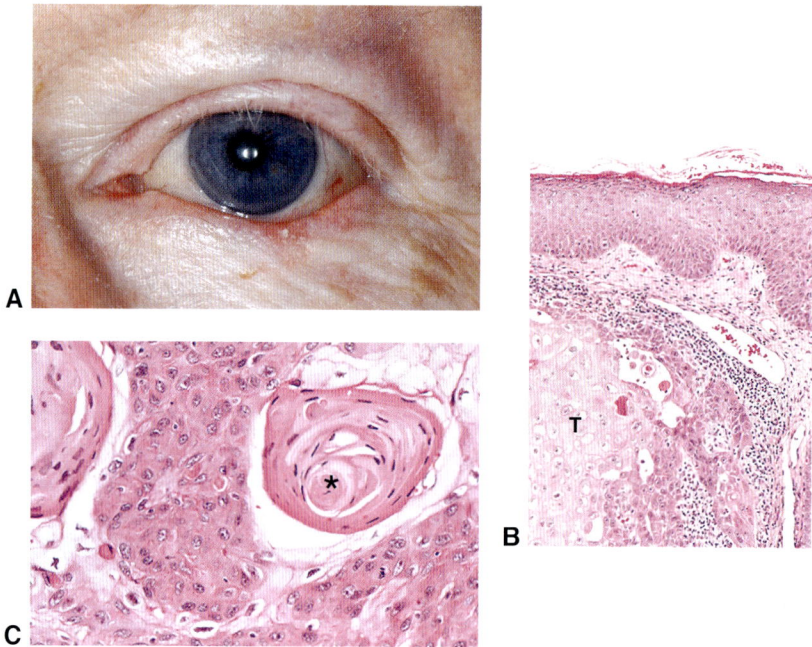

Figure 13-18 Squamous cell carcinoma. **A,** Clinical appearance. Note the focal loss of eyelashes (madarosis) and scaly appearance of the lower eyelid. **B,** Histologic appearance. Note the tumor cells (T) invading the dermis. **C,** A keratin pearl *(asterisk)*, a keratinized structure present within the epidermis rather than on the surface, is demonstrated in this well-differentiated squamous cell carcinoma. *(Part A courtesy of Keith D. Carter, MD.)*

skin, so the lower eyelid is more frequently involved than the upper eyelid. However, SCC is more likely to involve the upper eyelid than is BCC. The clinical appearance of SCC is diverse, ranging from ulcers to plaques to fungate or nodular growths. Accordingly, the clinical differential diagnosis is long; an accurate diagnosis requires pathologic examination of excised tissue.

Histologic examination shows atypical squamous cells that form nests and strands, extend beyond the epidermal basement membrane, infiltrate the dermis, and incite a fibrotic tissue reaction (Fig 13-18). Tumor cells may be well differentiated (forming keratin and easily recognizable as squamous), moderately differentiated, or poorly differentiated (requiring ancillary studies to confirm the nature of the neoplasm). When the diagnosis is in question, the pathologist should look for the presence of intercellular bridges. Perineural and lymphatic invasion may be present and is important to include in the pathology report when identified microscopically, as this finding may be associated with a less favorable prognosis. To treat this tumor adequately, frozen section (conventional or Mohs technique) or permanent section margin control is required. Regional lymph node metastasis may occur in patients with SCC of the eyelid.

> Chévez-Barrios P. Frozen section diagnosis and indications in ophthalmic pathology. *Arch Pathol Lab Med.* 2005;129(12):1626–1634.

KERATOACANTHOMA Keratoacanthoma is a rapidly growing epithelial proliferation with the potential for spontaneous involution. Strong evidence supports the idea that keratoacanthomas are a variant of a well-differentiated SCC. These dome-shaped nodules, which have keratin-filled central craters, may attain considerable size, up to 2.5 cm in diameter, within a matter of weeks to a few months (Fig 13-19). The natural history is typically spontaneous involution over several months, resulting in a slightly depressed scar. The incidence of keratoacanthoma is higher in immunosuppressed individuals because the health of the epidermis and epithelium of mucous membranes is supported by the immune system.

Histologically, keratoacanthomas show a cup-shaped invagination of well-differentiated squamous cells that proliferate in nests (squamous eddies) and acanthotic projections and incite a chronic inflammatory host response. The proliferating epithelial cells undermine the adjacent normal epidermis with a downward growth pattern. In the deeper portions of the proliferating nodule, mitotic activity, dykeratosis, and nuclear atypia may occur, similar to that seen in typical SCC. Many dermatopathologists and ophthalmic pathologists prefer to call this lesion *well-differentiated squamous cell carcinoma with*

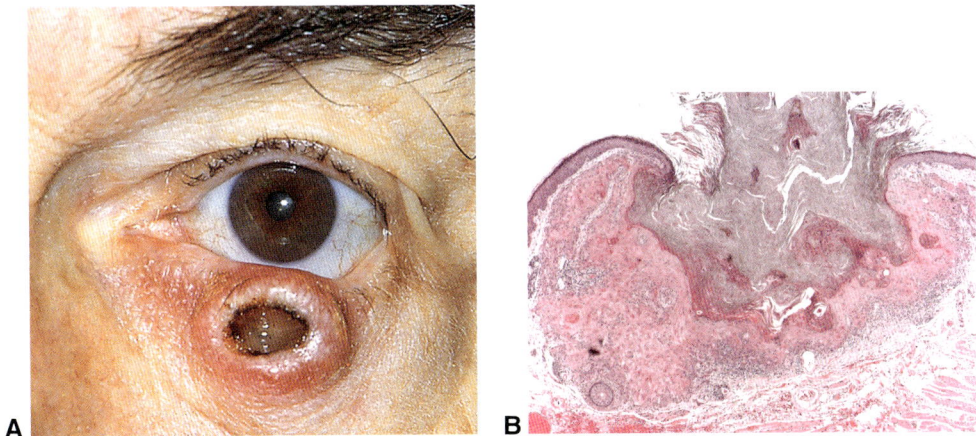

Figure 13-19 Keratoacanthoma. **A,** Clinical photograph. Note the elevated lesion with a central ulcerated crater and focal loss of eyelashes. In this case, the central crater was originally filled with keratin. **B,** Low-magnification histologic section illustrates the central keratin-filled crater and the downward (invasive) growth pattern. *(Part B courtesy of Nasreen A. Syed, MD.)*

keratoacanthoma-like differentiation because of the possibility of perineural invasion and metastasis.

If the lesion does not involute spontaneously, the lesion should be completely excised to permit optimal histologic examination of the lateral and deep margins of the tumor–host interface.

Dermal Neoplasms

Infantile (capillary) hemangiomas are common in the eyelids of children. They usually appear shortly after birth as a bright red lesion, grow over weeks to months, and involute by school age. Intervention is reserved for lesions that affect vision because of ptosis or astigmatism, leading to amblyopia.

The histologic appearance depends on the stage of evolution of the hemangioma. Early lesions may be very cellular, with solid nests of plump endothelial cells and correspondingly little vascular lumen formation. Established lesions typically show well-developed capillary channels lined with plump endothelial cells in a lobular configuration (Fig 13-20). Involuting lesions demonstrate increased fibrosis and hyalinization of capillary walls with luminal occlusion. β-Blockers are often used as first-line treatment of capillary hemangiomas, usually with significant reduction in size. Excision of these lesions should be performed with care because it can lead to significant blood loss from the large feeder vessels that are present within the hemangiomas.

Neoplasms and Proliferations of the Dermal Appendages

Dermal appendages of the eyelid include sebaceous glands, sweat glands, and hair follicles (see the section Topography, earlier in the chapter). They are also referred to as *adnexal appendages*, which, in this context, refers to skin appendages that are located within the dermis but communicate through the epidermis to the surface. Although meibomian glands technically are not dermal appendages, they are modified sebaceous glands embedded in the tarsus and may give rise to some of the neoplasms discussed in the following subsections, particularly sebaceous carcinoma.

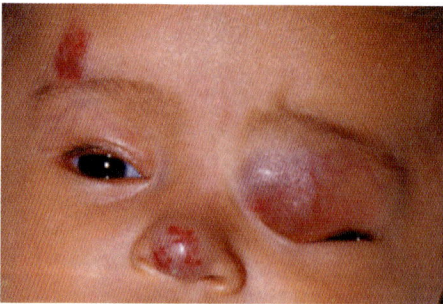

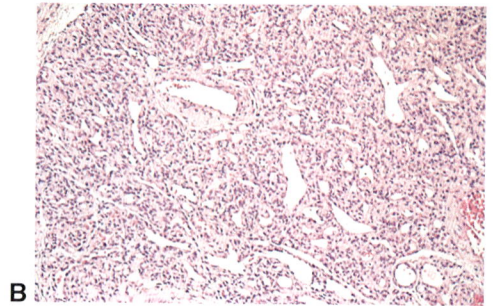

Figure 13-20 Infantile (capillary) hemangioma. **A,** Infant with multiple facial capillary hemangiomas, including a large lesion of the left upper eyelid. **B,** Histopathology. Note the small capillary-sized vessels and the numerous benign, proliferating, plump endothelial cells. *(Part A courtesy of Sander Dubovy, MD.)*

Syringoma

Syringoma, a common benign lesion derived from sweat glands, can occur in the eyelid, usually the lower eyelid, typically manifesting clinically as multiple tiny flesh-colored papules. Syringomas result from a malformation of the eccrine sweat gland ducts. Histologically, syringomas consist of multiple comma-shaped and/or round ductules lined with a double layer of epithelium and containing a central lumen, often with secretory material (Fig 13-21).

Sebaceous hyperplasia

Sebaceous hyperplasia is an uncommon benign lesion of the eyelid and face. Clinically, it appears as a small, yellow papule. Histologically, it is typically a single, enlarged sebaceous gland with an increased number of glandular lobules attached to a single central duct (Fig 13-22).

Sebaceous adenoma

Sebaceous adenoma is a benign lesion of the skin that can occur on the eyelid, though rarely. Sebaceous adenoma typically manifests as a circumscribed yellowish nodule. Histologically, it is composed of multiple sebaceous lobules that are irregularly shaped and incompletely differentiated (Fig 13-23). The possibility of Muir-Torre syndrome (a subtype

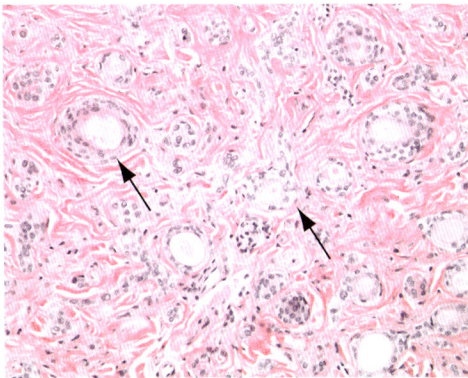

Figure 13-21 Syringoma. Note the round and comma-shaped epithelium-lined ductules *(arrows)*. *(Courtesy of Nasreen A. Syed, MD.)*

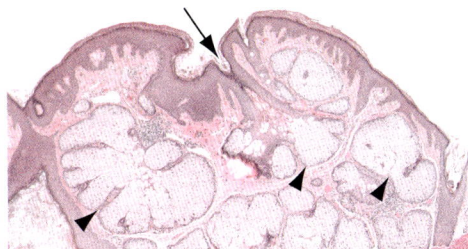

Figure 13-22 Sebaceous hyperplasia. Numerous sebaceous lobules *(arrowheads)* are seen surrounding a single hair follicle *(arrow)*. *(Courtesy of Nasreen A. Syed, MD.)*

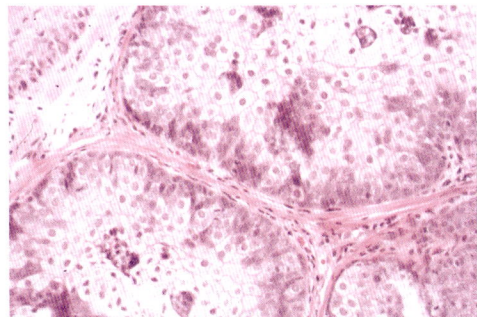

Figure 13-23 In sebaceous adenoma, sebaceous lobules demonstrate focal proliferations of immature basophilic (blue) sebocytes. This sebaceous proliferation is the one most commonly associated with Muir-Torre syndrome. *(Courtesy of Nasreen A. Syed, MD.)*

of Lynch syndrome, a hereditary cancer syndrome) should be considered when sebaceous adenoma is diagnosed, as it is the most common sebaceous neoplasm in this syndrome (see Table 13-2). Immunohistochemistry for DNA mismatch repair proteins may be useful in screening for cancer syndromes.

Sebaceous carcinoma

Sebaceous carcinoma is a malignancy with a propensity to occur on the eyelids. It most commonly involves the upper eyelid of individuals older than 65 years. It may originate in the meibomian glands of the tarsus, the glands of Zeis at the eyelid margin, or the sebaceous glands of the caruncle. Sebaceous carcinoma may be more common than SCC on the eyelid; however, the diagnosis is often missed or delayed because of this lesion's tendency to mimic other conditions, such as a chalazion or chronic unilateral blepharoconjunctivitis (Fig 13-24).

Histologically, well-differentiated sebaceous carcinomas are readily identified by the microvesicular foamy nature of the tumor cell cytoplasm, which resembles mature sebocytes. Moderately differentiated tumors may show some sebaceous features (Fig 13-25). Poorly differentiated tumors, however, may be difficult to distinguish from other, more common malignant epithelial tumors such as SCC or BCC. Special stains, such as oil red O or Sudan black B, may be used to diagnose sebaceous carcinomas because they reveal lipid within the cytoplasm of tumor cells. Tissue staining for lipids is performed on frozen tissue sections because the lipid constituents are often removed during paraffin processing. When sebaceous carcinoma is suspected clinically, the pathologist should be alerted so that tissue handling allows for any special stains needed. However, these stains are rarely used in clinical practice because of the technically difficult staining procedure. Although a variety of immunohistochemical stains have been investigated for their specificity in identifying sebaceous carcinoma, there is no single antibody or combination of antibodies that can consistently identify these tumors. An expert evaluation by an experienced pathologist may be required for an accurate diagnosis.

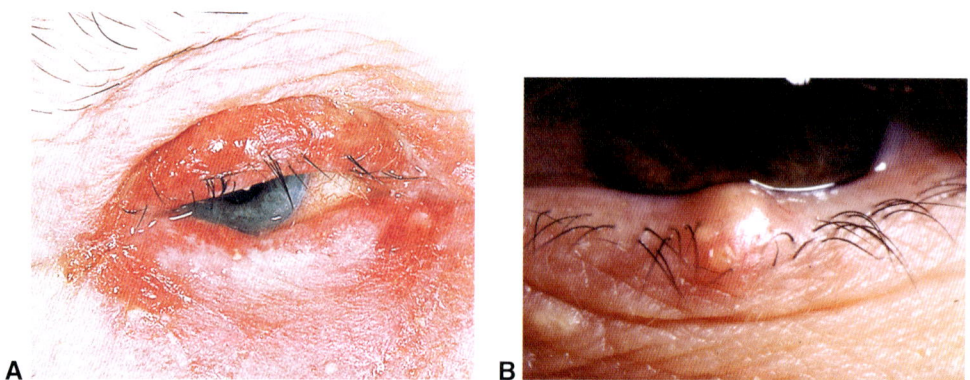

Figure 13-24 Sebaceous carcinoma, clinical appearance. **A,** This lesion mimics blepharoconjunctivitis with eyelid erythema, loss of eyelashes, ulceration, and irregular eyelid thickening. **B,** This lesion mimics a chalazion of the lower eyelid. Focal lash loss is present. *(Part B courtesy of Roberta E. Gausas, MD.)*

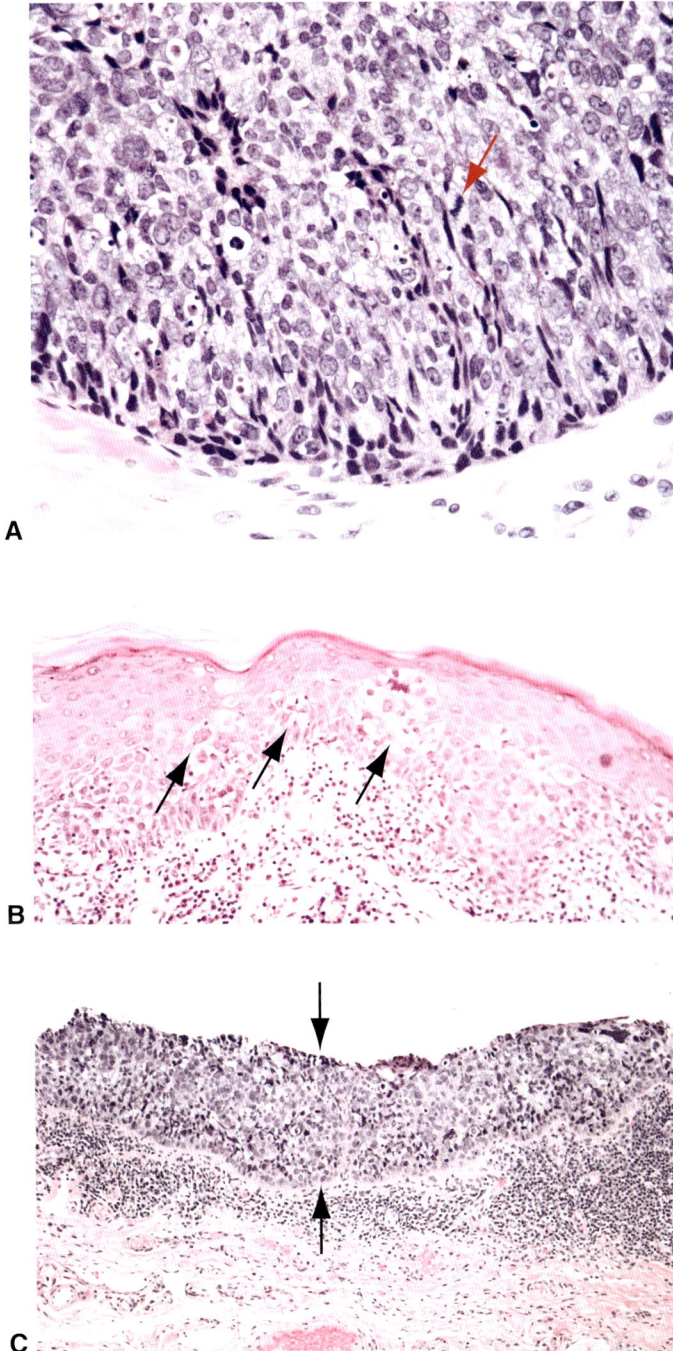

Figure 13-25 Sebaceous carcinoma, histologic appearance. **A,** Tumor cells often have dark, hyperchromatic, pleomorphic nuclei. The cytoplasm often has a foamy or vacuolated appearance. Note the mitotic figure *(arrow)*. **B,** Pagetoid invasion of epidermis by individual tumor cells and small clusters of tumor cells *(arrows)*. These areas are subtle and may be difficult to identify. **C,** Sebaceous carcinoma in situ, the complete replacement of normal conjunctival epithelium by tumor cells *(between arrows)*. *(Courtesy of Nasreen A. Syed, MD.)*

A primary characteristic of sebaceous carcinoma is *pagetoid spread,* the dissemination of both individual tumor cells and small clusters of tumor cells within the epidermis or conjunctival epithelium (see Fig 13-25B). The pagetoid areas do not have a direct connection to the main portion of the tumor. Another characteristic is the complete replacement of conjunctival epithelium by tumor cells, or *sebaceous carcinoma in situ* (see Fig 13-25C). This particular characteristic may make complete excision of sebaceous carcinoma challenging.

Treatment of sebaceous carcinoma typically involves wide local excision of the tumor. Widespread conjunctival epithelial involvement or deeply invasive tumors may require exenteration. Because it can be difficult to identify pagetoid spread or sebaceous carcinoma in situ on frozen sections, permanent sections are generally considered more reliable for evaluation of surgical resection margins than frozen sections of margins or Mohs technique. Before definitive excision, staging of tumor extent via routine processing of multiple small "map" biopsies, typically of the conjunctiva, may afford a more accurate assessment of the extent of spread of the carcinoma and, therefore, of the type of excision that is most appropriate for the patient. Adjunctive therapies for sebaceous carcinoma include the use of topical chemotherapy, cryotherapy, and radiotherapy.

Survival rates for patients with sebaceous carcinoma are worse than those for patients with SCC, but they have improved in recent years as a result of increased awareness, earlier detection, more accurate diagnosis, and more appropriate treatment. Typically, survival correlates with size and extent of the primary tumor. Spread of tumor may be local with direct invasion into the orbit and other adjacent structures. As metastases first involve regional lymph nodes, sentinel lymph node biopsy can be useful in tumor staging. Distant metastasis of tumor, usually to the liver and lung, may occur in rare cases.

Merkel Cell Carcinoma

Merkel cell carcinoma (MCC) is a rare neuroendocrine carcinoma of the skin, typically occurring in adults. It has an aggressive course with spread to regional lymph nodes and distant metastasis. The pathogenesis of MCC involves infection with the Merkel cell polyomavirus combined with other factors such as ultraviolet light exposure and immunosuppression. Clinically, the tumor often presents as a red or violaceous nodule with surface telangiectasia. Histologically, the tumor is composed of monotonous round, blue tumor cells with scant eosinophilic cytoplasm, vesicular nuclei with finely granular chromatin, and multiple nucleoli. There are numerous apoptotic nuclei and frequent mitoses (Fig 13-26). Immunohistochemical studies show that these tumor cells stain with cytokeratin 20 and neuroendocrine markers such as synaptophysin and chromogranin.

The management of MCC is primarily with wide local excision (at least 5-mm margins) and biopsy of regional lymph nodes. Resection requires evaluation of surgical margins with frozen section or Mohs technique. MCC has a high mortality rate compared with other eyelid tumors. The risk of regional and distant metastasis is approximately 30%, and local recurrences are common. Thus, the diagnosis of MCC requires prompt and complete surgical treatment and referral to the appropriate head and neck and oncology specialists.

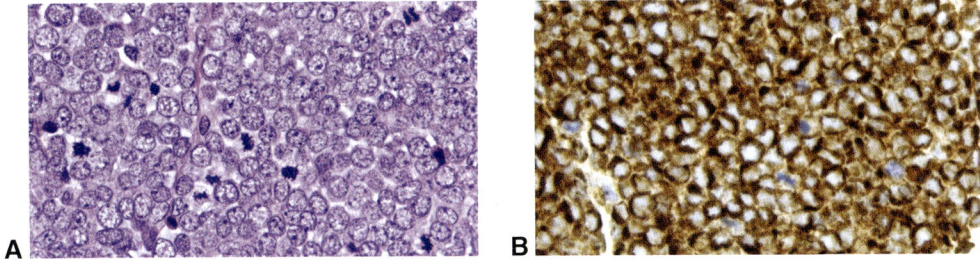

Figure 13-26 Merkel cell carcinoma (MCC). **A,** High-magnification photomicrograph shows that the tumor is composed of blue cells with round, granular-appearing nuclei and frequent mitoses. **B,** Immunohistochemistry with cytokeratin 20 shows the characteristic pattern of perinuclear dotlike staining. Molecular studies for Merkel cell polyomavirus (MCPyV) DNA are positive in approximately 80% of MCCs. *(Courtesy of Tatyana Milman, MD.)*

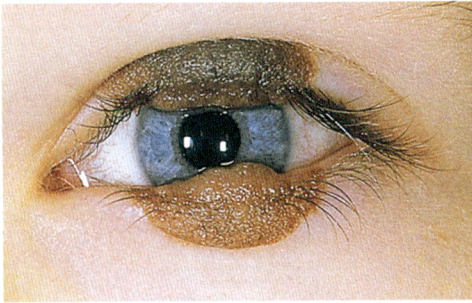

Figure 13-27 Congenital split, or kissing, nevus of the eyelid.

Melanocytic Neoplasms

Melanocytic nevus

Melanocytic nevi are benign proliferations of melanocytes that commonly occur on the eyelids. Melanocytic nevi may be visible at birth or shortly after birth (congenital nevi) or become apparent in adolescence or adulthood; congenital nevi tend to be larger than those appearing in later years. Nevi greater than 20 cm in diameter are called *giant congenital melanocytic nevi.* The risk for development of melanoma in congenital nevi is proportional to the size of the nevus; close follow-up and/or excision of congenital nevi is warranted. Congenital nevi of the eyelid may develop in utero before the separation of the upper and lower eyelids, resulting in matching nevi on these eyelids, termed a *kissing nevus* (Fig 13-27). Nevi in adults often appear as smooth dome-shaped, sometimes hyperpigmented, lesions on the eyelid margin. Other forms of nevi can occur on the eyelid, including blue nevi, Spitz nevi, and dysplastic nevi, though rarely.

Histologically, most nevi are composed of nevus cells, specialized melanocytes that have a round rather than dendritic shape and tend to cluster together in nests. The cytoplasm of the nevus cell contains a variable amount of melanin. Other characteristics of these cells include growth within and around adnexal structures, vessel walls, and the perineurium and extension into the deep reticular dermis or subcutaneous tissue. When a combination of round and spindle-shaped cells is seen in a lesion, the term *combined nevus* is used.

Nevi typically begin as macular (flat) lesions and evolve with age. In childhood, histologic examination reveals nests of nevus cells in the epidermis, along the dermal–epidermal junction, termed *junctional nevus* (Fig 13-28). Clinically, a junctional nevus is indistinguishable from an ephelis (freckle), but histologically, the latter demonstrates pigment in the basal layer of the epidermal epithelial cells. Typically in adolescence, the junctional nests of nevus cells continue to proliferate and migrate into the superficial dermis, and the nevus becomes increasingly elevated clinically. At this stage, the nevus may also increase in pigmentation. When both junctional and intradermal components are present, the histologic classification is *compound nevus* (Fig 13-29). Finally, sometime in adulthood, the junctional component disappears, leaving nevus cells only within the dermis, and, accordingly, the classification is *intradermal or dermal nevus* (Fig 13-30).

The cytologic appearance of nevus cells also evolves: the cells in the superficial portion of the nevus are round and have round to ovoid nuclei (type A nevus cells). Within

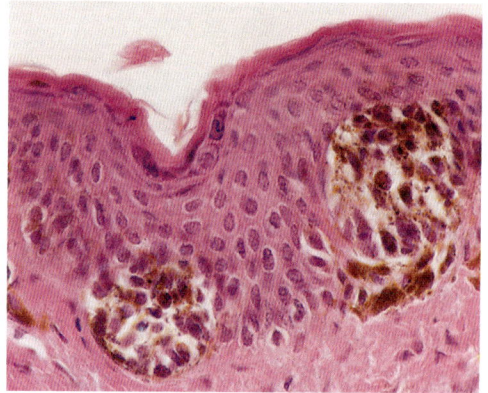

Figure 13-28 Junctional nevus. Nests of nevus cells (pigmented in this case) are apparent at the dermal–epidermal junction.

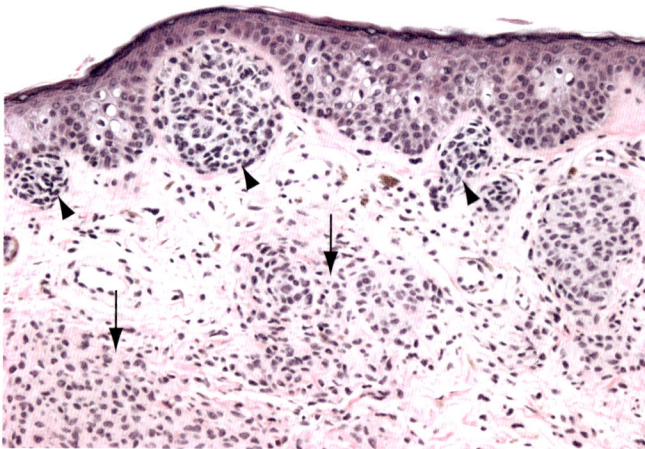

Figure 13-29 Compound nevus. Nests of nevus cells are present in the dermis *(arrows)* as well as at the dermal–epidermal junction *(arrowheads)*. *(Courtesy of Nasreen A. Syed, MD.)*

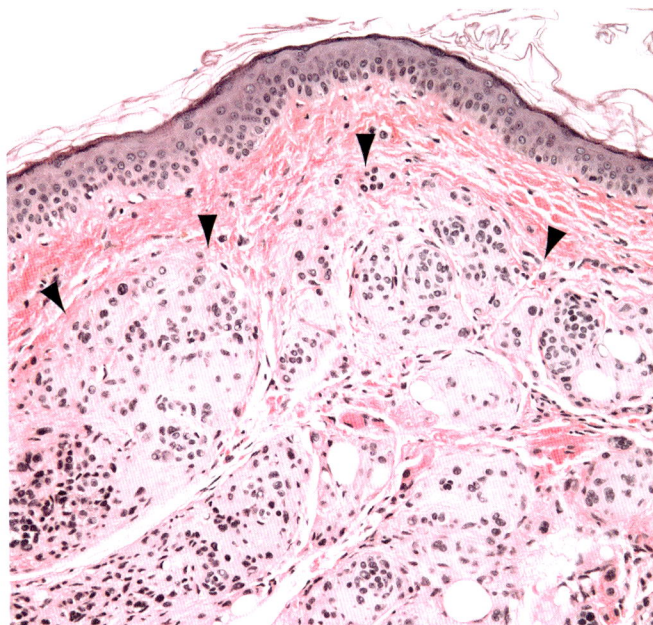

Figure 13-30 Intradermal nevus. The nests of nevus cells are confined to the dermis, and there is no junctional component. The superficial extent of the nevus cell nests is indicated with *arrowheads*. *(Courtesy of Nasreen A. Syed, MD.)*

the midportion, the cells are smaller, have less cytoplasm, and resemble lymphocytes (type B nevus cells). In the deepest portion, the nevus cells appear similar to Schwann cells of peripheral nerves with a spindle configuration (type C nevus cells). Recognition of this "maturation" is useful for classifying melanocytic neoplasms as benign. Multinucleated giant nevus cells and interspersed adipose tissue are common in older nevi.

Melanoma

Cutaneous melanoma occurs rarely on the eyelids. It may be associated with a preexisting nevus, develop de novo, or extend from a tumor elsewhere on the face. In a pigmented eyelid lesion, clinical features that suggest malignancy include asymmetry, border irregularity, color variegation, and diameter greater than 6 mm. Melanoma may be heralded by a vertical (perpendicular to the skin surface) growth phase. There are 3 main histologic subtypes of melanoma that occur on the eyelids (Fig 13-31):

- lentigo maligna
- superficial spreading
- nodular

Lentigo maligna melanoma, the most common type occurring on the eyelids, typically develops as an irregular pigmented macular lesion on the face in older adults and has a long preinvasive phase. Histologically, atypical melanocytes proliferate along the dermal–epidermal junction as single or small nests of cells in the epidermis, similar to primary

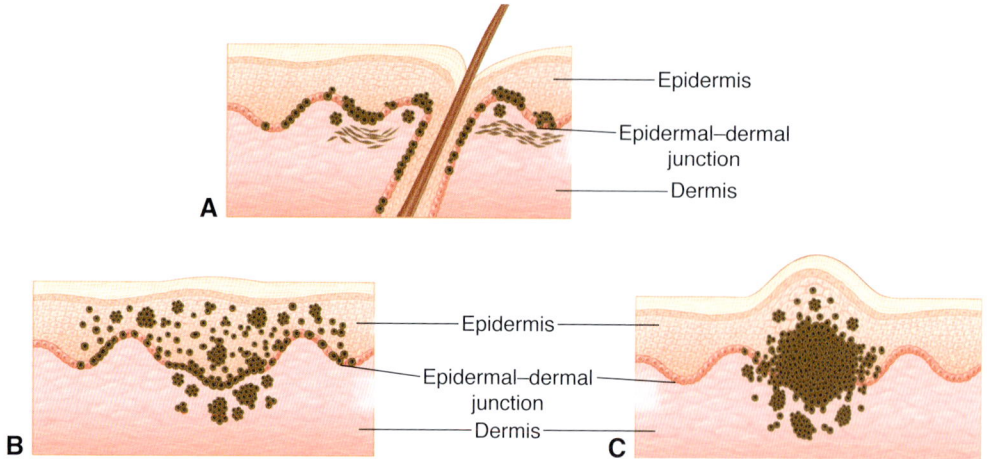

Figure 13-31 Schematic illustration of cutaneous melanoma types. **A,** Lentigo maligna melanoma. Atypical melanocytes (brown cells) proliferate predominantly in the basal layers of the epidermis in a linear or nested pattern, similar to primary acquired melanosis with atypia of the conjunctiva. Note the tendency of the melanocytes to involve the outer sheaths of the hair shafts. The invasive component is seen as brown cells (spindle and epithelioid) in the superficial dermis. **B,** In superficial spreading melanoma, tumor cell nests are present in all levels of the epidermis, often in a pagetoid fashion, with cells or clusters of cells scattered among epithelial cells. Lentigo maligna and superficial spreading melanomas spread horizontally (radial growth) through the skin, staying close to the dermal–epidermal junction. **C,** Nodular melanoma has a narrow intraepidermal component and more prominent vertical growth within the dermis; it is therefore more deeply invasive than the other types. *(Modified with permission from Spencer WH, ed.* Ophthalmic Pathology: An Atlas and Textbook. *Vol 4. Saunders; 1996:2270. Illustration by Christine Gralapp.)*

acquired melanosis with atypia of the conjunctiva. Superficial invasion of the dermis is also present. *Superficial spreading melanoma,* the most common type of cutaneous melanoma, demonstrates a radial (intraepidermal) growth pattern that extends beyond the invasive component. *Nodular melanoma* has a significant vertical growth phase that results in a raised or indurated mass.

The characteristic histologic features of melanoma include pagetoid intraepidermal spread of atypical melanocytic nests and single cells, nuclear abnormalities, lack of maturation in the deeper portions of the mass, and atypical mitotic figures. A bandlike lymphocytic host response along the base of the mass is more common in melanoma than in benign proliferations. Prognosis is correlated with tumor thickness (Breslow thickness) in stage I (localized) disease. Metastases, when they occur, typically involve regional lymph nodes first. Frozen sections are not typically used for making a diagnosis of melanocytic lesions, as these lesions are difficult to visualize with frozen techniques.

CHAPTER 14

Orbit and Lacrimal Drainage System

Highlights

- Nonspecific orbital inflammation is a heterogeneous group of noninfectious inflammatory processes that can affect any part of the orbit.
- Lymphoproliferative lesions are among the more common infiltrative processes in the orbit and can occur within the lacrimal gland or elsewhere in the orbit.
- Rhabdomyosarcoma is the most common orbital malignant tumor in children. When this neoplasm is suspected, urgent action is required in order to establish a diagnosis and prevent loss of orbital and ocular function.

Topography

Bony Orbit and Soft Tissues

Seven bones form the boundaries of the orbit (see Figs 1-1 through 1-3 in BCSC Section 7, *Oculofacial Plastic and Orbital Surgery*). They are the ethmoid, frontal, lacrimal, maxillary, palatine, sphenoid, and zygomatic bones.

The orbital cavity contains the globe, lacrimal gland, muscles, tendons, fat, fasciae, vessels, nerves, ciliary ganglion, and cartilaginous trochlea. Inflammatory and neoplastic processes that increase the volume of the orbital contents lead to *proptosis* (protrusion) of the globe and/or *displacement* (dystopia) from the horizontal or vertical position. The degree and direction of ocular displacement help localize the position of the mass.

The *lacrimal gland* is situated anteriorly in the superotemporal quadrant of the orbit. The gland is divided into orbital and palpebral lobes by the lateral portion of the aponeurosis of the levator palpebrae superioris muscle. The lacrimal gland is an eccrine gland, and the acini are round and composed of cuboidal epithelium. The nucleus is located toward the outer edge of the acinus. The ducts, which lie within the fibrovascular stroma, are lined by 2 layers: an inner, low cuboidal epithelium and an outer layer of low, flat myoepithelial cells. The histologic appearance of the lacrimal gland is very similar to that of the salivary glands. See BCSC Section 2, *Fundamentals and Principles of Ophthalmology,* and Section 7, *Oculofacial Plastic and Orbital Surgery,* for additional discussion.

Developmental Anomalies

Cysts

Orbital cysts may arise from a variety of ocular surface or orbital tissues and include cysts derived from the conjunctival or eyelid epithelium, teratomatous cysts, neural cysts, secondary cysts (mucoceles), inflammatory cysts (parasitic), and noncystic lesions with a cystic component. Orbital cysts can be developmental or acquired in origin. *Dermoid cyst* is a developmental lesion and the most common type of orbital cyst.

Dermoid cysts are believed to occur when surface ectodermal nests become entrapped in the bony sutures during embryogenesis. Most of these cysts manifest in childhood as a unilateral mass in the lateral brow. Histologically, a dermoid cyst is lined by keratinized stratified squamous epithelium and contains keratin, sebum, and hair. By definition, its walls contain dermal appendages, including sebaceous glands, hair follicles, and sweat glands (Fig 14-1). If the cyst wall does not have adnexal structures, the term *simple epithelial (epidermoid) cyst* is applied. Simple epithelial cysts may also be lined by respiratory, conjunctival, or apocrine epithelium.

Rupture of a dermoid cyst may cause a marked granulomatous reaction, largely due to the presence of sebum in the cyst lumen.

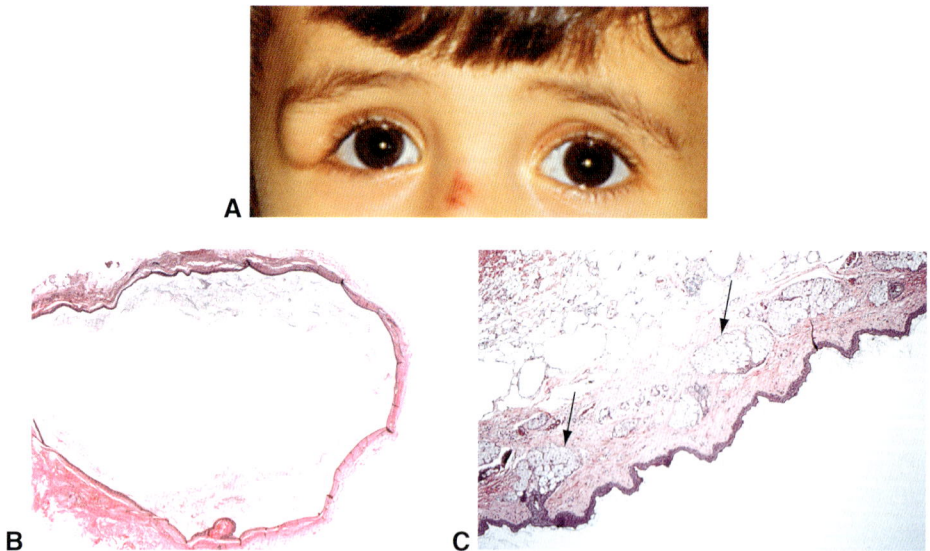

Figure 14-1 Orbital dermoid cyst. **A,** Clinical photograph of dermoid cyst of the right orbit. Note the typical superotemporal location. **B,** Low-magnification photomicrograph reveals a cyst lined by keratinized stratified squamous epithelium and containing keratin. The sebum dissolves out of the lumen during histologic processing. **C,** The cyst wall contains sebaceous glands *(arrows)* and adnexal structures. *(Part A courtesy of Sander Dubovy, MD; part B courtesy of Nasreen A. Syed, MD; part C courtesy of Hans E. Grossniklaus, MD.)*

Inflammation

Orbital inflammation can be idiopathic or secondary to a systemic inflammatory process (eg, granulomatosis with polyangiitis), retained foreign body, or infectious disease. It can be diffuse, involving multiple tissues (eg, sclerosing orbititis, diffuse anterior inflammation), or localized, involving specific orbital structures (eg, orbital myositis, optic perineuritis). Conditions masquerading as orbital inflammation include developmental orbital mass lesions and neoplastic disease, such as orbital lymphoma and rhabdomyosarcoma.

Noninfectious Inflammation

Nonspecific orbital inflammation

Nonspecific orbital inflammation (NSOI) refers to a space-occupying inflammatory disorder that simulates a neoplasm (it is sometimes known as *orbital pseudotumor* or *idiopathic orbital inflammatory syndrome*) but has no recognizable cause. This disorder accounts for approximately 5% of orbital lesions and can affect children and adults. Clinically, the onset is often abrupt, and patients usually report pain. The inflammatory response may be diffuse or compartmentalized. When localized to an extraocular muscle, the condition is called *orbital myositis* (Fig 14-2); when localized to the lacrimal gland, it is called *dacryoadenitis*.

In the early stages of NSOI, inflammation predominates, with a mixed inflammatory response (eosinophils, neutrophils, plasma cells, lymphocytes, and histiocytes [macrophages]) that is often perivascular and frequently infiltrates muscle and fat, causing fat necrosis. In later stages, fibrosis is the predominant feature, often with interspersed lymphoid follicles with germinal centers. The fibrosis may replace orbital fat and encase extraocular muscles and the optic nerve, restricting their function (Fig 14-3). Some cases that demonstrate

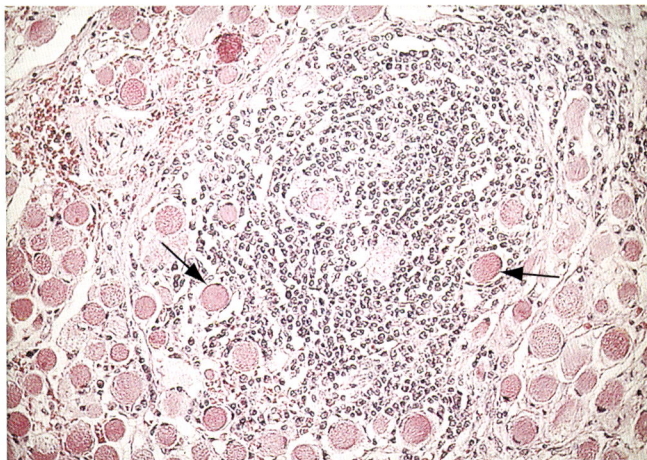

Figure 14-2 Nonspecific orbital inflammation (NSOI). NSOI can affect any orbital structure. In myositis, the skeletal muscle fibers *(arrows)* are surrounded by a dense infiltrate of chronic inflammatory cells. Unlike in thyroid eye disease, in myositis the muscle tendons are involved.

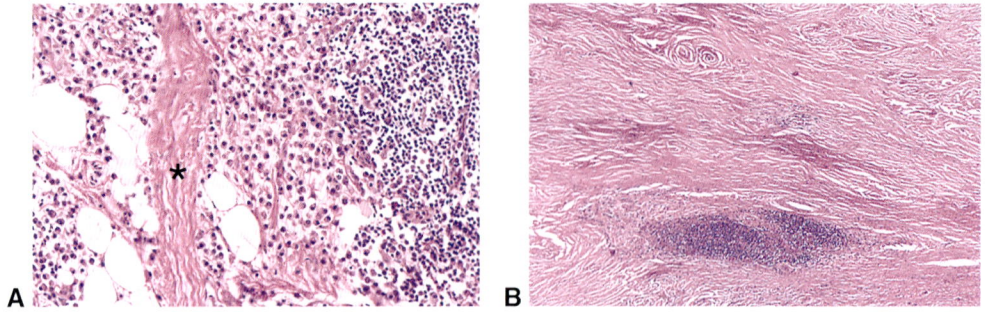

Figure 14-3 Nonspecific orbital inflammation. **A,** Note the mixture of inflammatory cells, mostly lymphocytes (small, blue) and plasma cells (larger, with pink cytoplasm), and the bundle of collagen *(asterisk)* running through the orbital fat. **B,** Diffuse fibrosis dominates the histologic picture of this fibrosing orbititis, representing a later stage of the condition in part **A.**

significant fibrosis and deposition of collagen as the dominant histologic feature early on seem to lack the inflammatory clinical signs usually associated with NSOI. Whether this "sclerosing" variant is a separate entity or a variant of NSOI remains controversial.

Often included in the differential diagnosis of NSOI is a lymphoproliferative process such as lymphoma. Immunophenotypic and molecular genetic analyses can differentiate NSOI from lymphoid tumors based on whether the infiltrate of lymphocytes is polyclonal (NSOI) or monoclonal (lymphoma). CD20 and CD25 receptors have been found in cases of NSOI and may provide the basis for treatment selection. Immunoglobulin (Ig) G4–positive lymphoplasmacytic infiltrates have recently become a marker for IgG4-related sclerosing disease (see "Immunoglobulin G4–related disease" later in the chapter). The nature of the pathologic findings dictates the recommended treatment. See BCSC Section 7, *Oculofacial Plastic and Orbital Surgery,* for further discussion.

Wallace ZS, Khosroshahi A, Jakobiec FA, et al. IgG4-related systemic disease as a cause of "idiopathic" orbital inflammation, including orbital myositis, and trigeminal nerve involvement. *Surv Ophthalmol.* 2012;57(1):26–33.

Thyroid eye disease

Thyroid eye disease (TED) (also known as *Graves disease, thyroid ophthalmopathy, thyroid-associated orbitopathy,* and *Basedow disease*) is related to thyroid dysfunction and is the most common cause of unilateral or bilateral proptosis (exophthalmos) in adults. The signs and symptoms of TED are related to inflammation of the orbital connective tissue, alterations in the extracellular matrix of the extraocular muscles, inflammation and fibrosis of the extraocular muscles, and adipogenesis. The muscles appear firm and white, and the tendons are usually not involved. Early in the disease, a cellular infiltrate of mononuclear inflammatory cells (eg, lymphocytes, plasma cells, mast cells) and fibroblasts permeates the interstitial tissues of the extraocular muscles, most commonly the inferior and medial rectus muscles (Fig 14-4). The fibroblasts synthesize hyaluronic acid (hyaluronan) and other glycosaminoglycans, resulting in enlargement of the muscles.

Because orbital fibrocytes (considered precursor cells of fibroblasts) are derived from the neural crest and are pluripotent, the enhanced cell signaling that occurs in TED

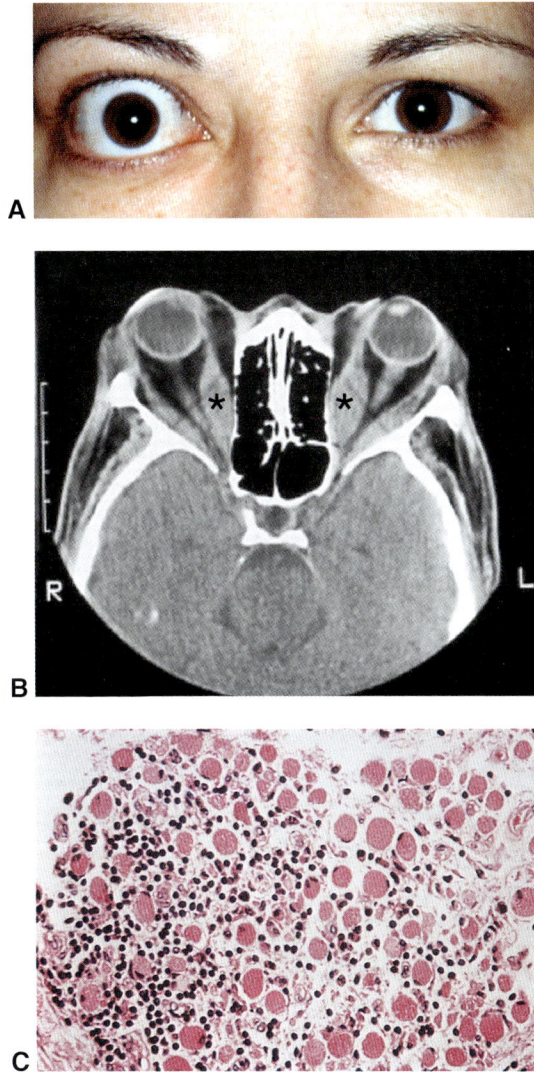

Figure 14-4 Thyroid eye disease (TED). **A,** Clinical photograph shows asymmetric proptosis and eyelid retraction, most prominent on the right. **B,** Computed tomography (CT) scan (axial view) shows fusiform enlargement of the extraocular muscles *(asterisks)* with sparing of the muscle tendons. **C,** The muscle bundles of the extraocular muscle are separated by fluid accompanied by an infiltrate of mononuclear inflammatory cells. *(Parts A and B courtesy of Sander Dubovy, MD.)*

promotes adipocyte differentiation and adipogenesis. These cellular changes lead to the characteristic features of TED.

As a result of the increased bulk within the orbit, the optic nerve may be compromised at the orbital apex, and optic nerve head swelling may result. The late stages of TED are associated with progressive fibrosis that results in restriction of ocular movement and severe eyelid retraction with resultant exposure keratitis.

See BCSC Section 7, *Oculofacial Plastic and Orbital Surgery*, for more detailed discussion of TED, including pathogenesis, clinical features, and treatment.

Shan SJ, Douglas RS. The pathophysiology of thyroid eye disease. *J Neuroophthalmol.* 2014; 34(2):177–185.

Immunoglobulin G4–related disease

Immunoglobulin G4–related disease (IgG4-RD) is an inflammatory condition that has characteristic features of tumefactive lesions in one or more organs; a lymphoplasmacytic infiltrate rich in IgG4-positive plasma cells; variable degrees of fibrosis, often in a storiform pattern (whorls of cells); obliterative phlebitis; and elevated serum IgG4 levels (Fig 14-5). Orbital and ocular adnexal involvement in IgG4-RD, also known as *IgG4-related ophthalmic disease,* was initially described as bilateral and symmetric, with persistent swelling of the lacrimal glands and infiltration of IgG4 plasma cells. However, IgG4-RD can manifest not only in the lacrimal glands, but also in the extraocular muscles, orbital nerves, sclerae, and eyelids. The proposed criteria for IgG4-related ophthalmic disease include

- imaging studies showing lacrimal gland enlargement or a mass lesion involving the lacrimal gland, trigeminal nerve, or various other ophthalmic tissues
- histologic examination showing lymphoplasmacytic infiltration with associated fibrosis, and with a ratio of IgG4-positive to IgG-positive plasma cells ≥40% or >50 IgG4-positive plasma cells per high-power field (40× objective)
- serum IgG4 level ≥135 mg/dL

The diagnostic criteria for IgG4-RD and its clinical implications continue to evolve.

Goto H, Takahira M, Azumi A; Japanese Study Group for IgG4-Related Ophthalmic Disease. Diagnostic criteria for IgG4-related ophthalmic disease. *Jpn J Ophthalmol.* 2015;59(1):1–7.

Infectious Inflammation

See BCSC Section 7, *Oculofacial Plastic and Orbital Surgery,* for additional discussion of orbital infectious diseases, and Section 8, *External Disease and Cornea,* for general discussion of microbial and parasitic infections.

Bacterial infections of the orbit

Bacterial infection of the orbit (orbital cellulitis) can occur through direct inoculation (trauma, surgery), spread from infection of adjacent structures (sinusitis), spread from a distant focus (bacteremia), or opportunistic infection (necrotizing fasciitis, mucormycosis). The most common cause of orbital cellulitis is paranasal sinus infection. Infection may be caused by a variety of organisms, including *Haemophilus influenzae, Streptococcus, Staphylococcus, Clostridium, Bacteroides, Klebsiella,* and *Proteus* species. The organism most commonly involved differs with age of the patient. Histologically, acute inflammation, necrosis, and abscess formation may be present. Tuberculosis, which rarely involves the orbit, produces a necrotizing granulomatous reaction.

Fungal and parasitic infections of the orbit

Fungal infections of the orbit generally produce severe, insidious orbital inflammation (Fig 14-6). Rhinocerebral or rhino-orbito-cerebral *mucormycosis (zygomycosis)* usually

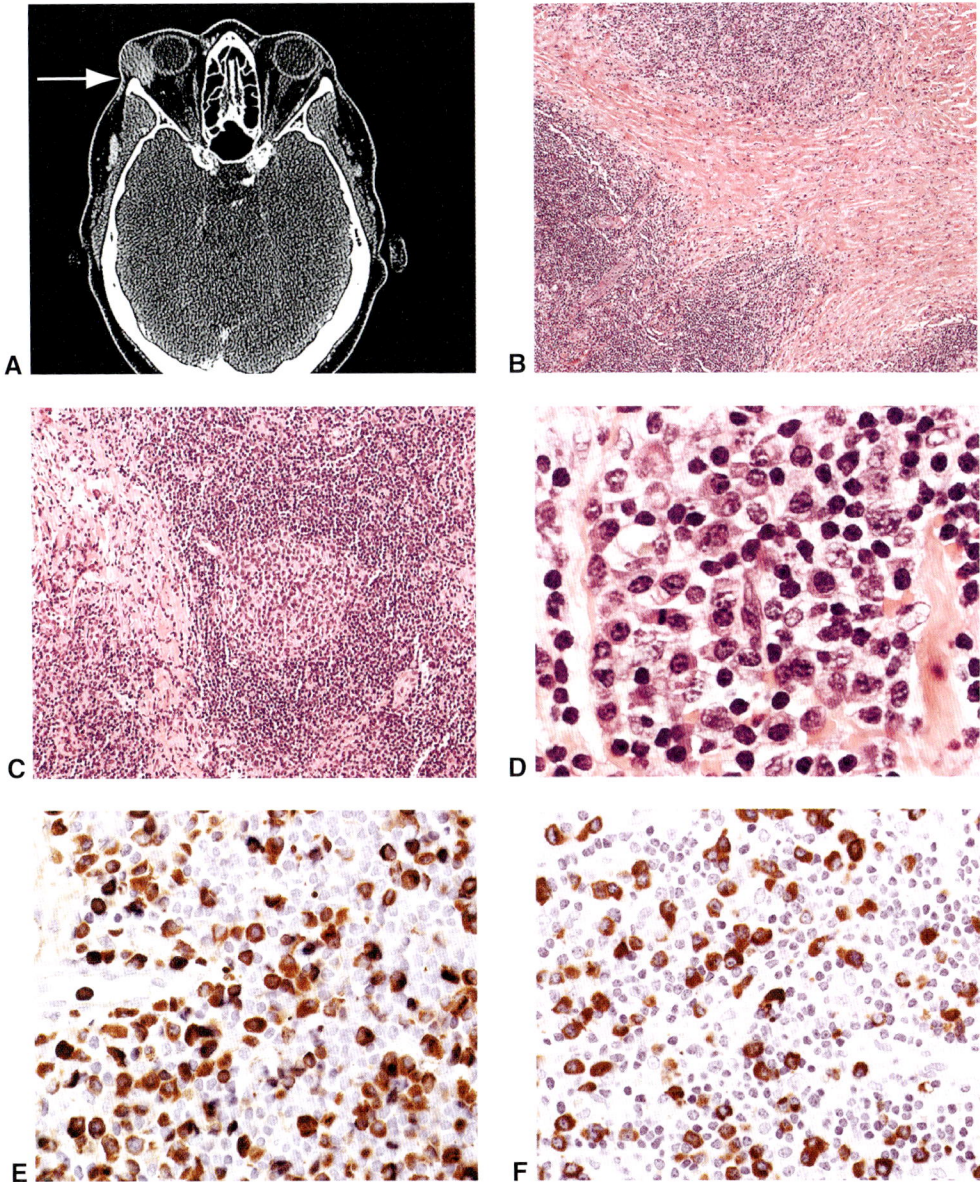

Figure 14-5 Immunoglobulin G4–related disease (IgG4-RD). **A,** CT image from a 67-year-old woman who presented with a 3-year history of an enlarging painless mass of the right lacrimal gland fossa, which was identified on CT as a homogeneously enhancing, circumscribed mass diffusely involving the right lacrimal gland *(arrow).* **B–D,** Photomicrographs show extensive collagenous fibrosis, lymphoid follicular hyperplasia, and markedly increased plasma cells. **E,** Immunohistochemistry reveals frequent IgG4 plasma cells, accounting for 40%–50% of total IgG-positive plasma cells. **F,** A different area of the lymphoid infiltrate stained for IgG4. A subsequent serum test showed an elevated serum IgG4 level. A diagnosis of IgG4-RD was made. *(Courtesy of Kirtee Raparia, MD.)*

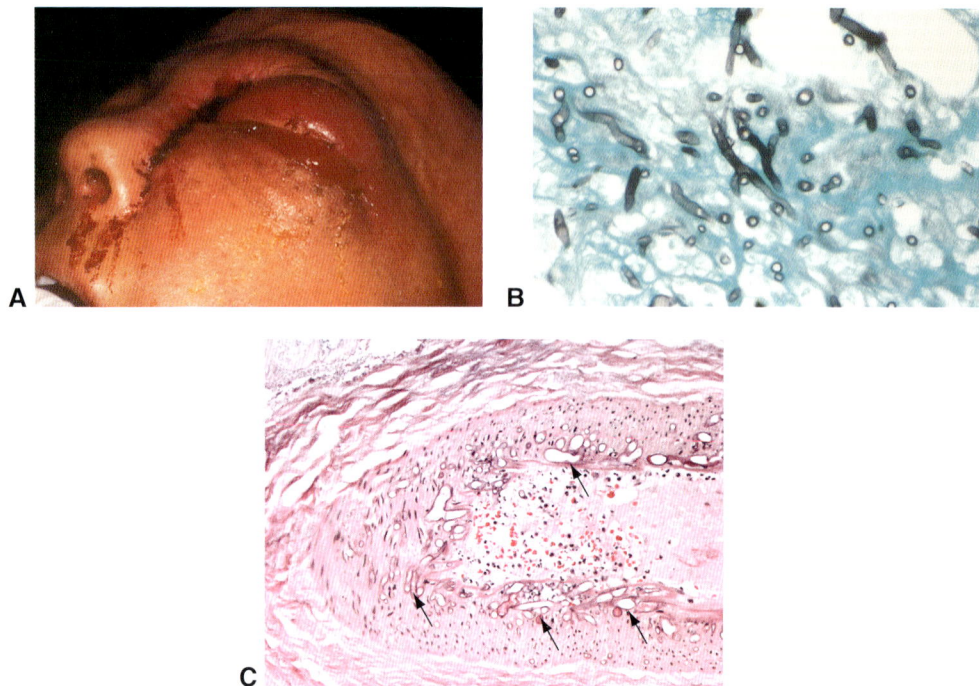

Figure 14-6 Fungal infections of the orbit generally produce severe, insidious orbital inflammation. **A,** Clinical appearance of *Aspergillus* orbititis, which is similar to the clinical presentation of mucormycosis. **B,** Microscopic section shows branching fungal hyphae *(Aspergillus)* on silver stain. **C,** Mucor hyphae are large and can often be seen on hematoxylin-eosin stain *(arrows).* The organisms are shown in the wall of the ophthalmic artery. *(Parts A and B courtesy of Hans E. Grossniklaus, MD; part C courtesy of Nasreen A. Syed, MD.)*

occurs in patients with poorly controlled diabetes mellitus (especially those with ketoacidosis), solid malignant neoplasms, or extensive burns; in patients undergoing treatment with corticosteroid agents; or in patients with severe neutropenia. Typically, mucormycosis represents spread from an adjacent sinus infection. The specific fungal genus involved is frequently *Mucor* or *Rhizopus.* Histologically, inflammation (acute and chronic) is present in a background of necrosis and is often granulomatous. Broad, nonseptate hyphae may be identified with hematoxylin-eosin (see Fig 14-6C), periodic acid–Schiff (PAS), and Gomori methenamine silver (GMS) stains. These fungi can invade blood vessel walls and cause a thrombotic vasculitis resulting in ischemic necrosis. The organisms have the potential for hematogenous spread to the central nervous system (CNS), resulting in stroke and death. Diagnosis is made by biopsy, often of necrotic-appearing tissues (eschar) in the nasopharynx.

Aspergillus infection of the orbit from the adjacent sinuses or hematogenous spread from other parts of the body may occur in immunocompromised or otherwise healthy individuals. With its slowly progressive and insidious symptoms, sino-orbital aspergillosis often goes unrecognized, resulting in a sclerosing granulomatous process. *Aspergillus* is often difficult to culture but may be observed in biopsied tissue as septate hyphae with 45° angle branching (see Fig 14-6A, B). Despite aggressive surgical therapy and adjunct therapy with antifungal agents, if extension into the brain occurs, orbital infections may be fatal.

Allergic fungal sinusitis is a form of noninvasive fungal disease resulting from an immunoglobulin E–mediated hypersensitivity reaction to the organisms in atopic individuals. Several species of fungi can cause the disease, which may extend into the orbit and intracranially in some cases.

Parasitic infections of the orbit are rare, especially in developed countries. They may be caused by *Echinococcus* species (orbital hydatid cyst), *Taenia solium* (cysticercosis), and *Loa loa* (ocular filariasis [loiasis]). These infectious diseases are seen mostly in patients who come from, or have traveled to, areas where the infections are endemic. Serologic studies for specific parasites may aid diagnosis.

Infections of the lacrimal drainage system

Infections can occur in various parts of the lacrimal drainage system and may be acute or chronic. The most commonly affected areas are the canaliculus, resulting in canaliculitis, and the lacrimal sac, resulting in dacryocystitis. Obstruction or the presence of foreign material (eg, dacryolith, punctal plug) may predispose to infection, but infection can develop in the absence of these factors. Bacteria, fungi, and viruses can all cause infection of the lacrimal drainage system, although the filamentous gram-positive bacterium *Actinomyces israelii* is the most common causative organism in canaliculitis. This organism may form a bacterial aggregate in the lacrimal drainage system, leading to dacryolith formation with a characteristic yellow color, known as a "sulfur granule." For more information on infections of the lacrimal drainage system, see BCSC Section 7, *Oculofacial Plastic and Orbital Surgery*.

Degenerations

Amyloid

Amyloid deposition in the orbit occurs in primary systemic amyloidosis and is usually benign. When amyloid deposition involves the extraocular muscles and nerves, it can cause ophthalmoplegia and ptosis. See Chapters 5, 6, 10, and 13 in this volume for more information on amyloid.

Neoplasia

Neoplasms of the orbit may be primary or secondary (extensions from adjacent structures or metastatic disease). Secondary tumors are slightly more common than primary tumors (see the section Secondary Tumors at the end of this chapter). The types of orbital tumors that occur in children differ from those that occur in adults. Developmental tumors are the primary orbital lesions most often encountered in children, whereas vascular and lymphoid tumors are the primary orbital lesions most often seen in adults.

In children, approximately 90% of orbital tumors are benign. Benign cystic lesions (dermoid or simple epithelial cysts) represent 50% of orbital lesions in childhood. Rhabdomyosarcoma is the most common primary orbital malignant tumor in childhood and represents 3% of all orbital masses. The orbit may be involved secondarily in cases of retino-blastoma, neuroblastoma, and leukemia/lymphoma.

See BCSC Section 7, *Oculofacial Plastic and Orbital Surgery,* for additional discussion.

Lacrimal Gland Neoplasia

Because the lacrimal gland is very similar to the salivary gland, epithelial lacrimal gland tumors are categorized according to the World Health Organization (WHO) epithelial salivary gland classification system. The most common types of epithelial lacrimal gland tumors are pleomorphic adenoma, adenocarcinoma arising from pleomorphic adenoma (carcinoma ex pleomorphic adenoma), and adenoid cystic carcinoma.

> von Holstein SL, Rasmussen PK, Heegaard S. Tumors of the lacrimal gland. *Semin Diagn Pathol.* 2016;33(3):156–163.

Pleomorphic adenoma

The most common epithelial tumor of the lacrimal gland is pleomorphic adenoma (also known as *benign mixed tumor*). Pleomorphic adenoma is slightly more common in men than in women and usually presents in the fourth or fifth decade of life. The tumor is pseu-doencapsulated and grows slowly by expansion. This progressive expansive growth may ex-cavate the bone of the lacrimal fossa. Tumor growth stimulates the periosteum to deposit a thin layer of new bone (ie, cortication). The adjacent orbital bone is not eroded. Typically, the patient experiences no pain.

Histologically, pleomorphic adenoma has a fibrous pseudocapsule and comprises a mixture of duct-derived epithelial and stromal elements, all arising from the lacrimal glan-dular epithelium. The epithelial component may form nests or tubules lined by 2 layers of cells, the outermost layer blending imperceptibly with the stroma (Fig 14-7). The stroma may appear myxoid and may contain heterologous elements, including cartilage and bone. Results of immunohistochemistry (IHC) reflect the epithelial and myoepithelial components, both derived from epithelium. The tumor cells are usually positive with IHC for keratin and epithelial membrane antigen in the ductal areas and positive with IHC for keratin, actin, myosin, fibronectin, and S-100 protein in the myoepithelial areas. Micro-scopic foci of carcinoma in situ may be identified in these lesions but are not a significant feature.

Malignant transformation may take place in a long-standing or incompletely excised pleomorphic adenoma in the form of adenocarcinoma (carcinoma ex pleomorphic ad-enoma), with relatively rapid growth after a period of relative quiescence. Malignancies, including adenocarcinoma (carcinoma ex pleomorphic adenoma) and adenoid cystic car-cinoma, may also develop in pleomorphic adenomas that recur in the orbit.

Adenoid cystic carcinoma

As mentioned previously, adenoid cystic carcinoma (ACC) can develop in a pleomorphic adenoma or, more commonly, arise de novo in the lacrimal gland. The tumor is slightly more common in women than in men, and the median age at presentation is about 40 years.

Unlike pleomorphic adenoma, ACC has no pseudocapsule; it tends to erode bone and invade orbital nerves, accounting for the pain that is frequently reported by patients

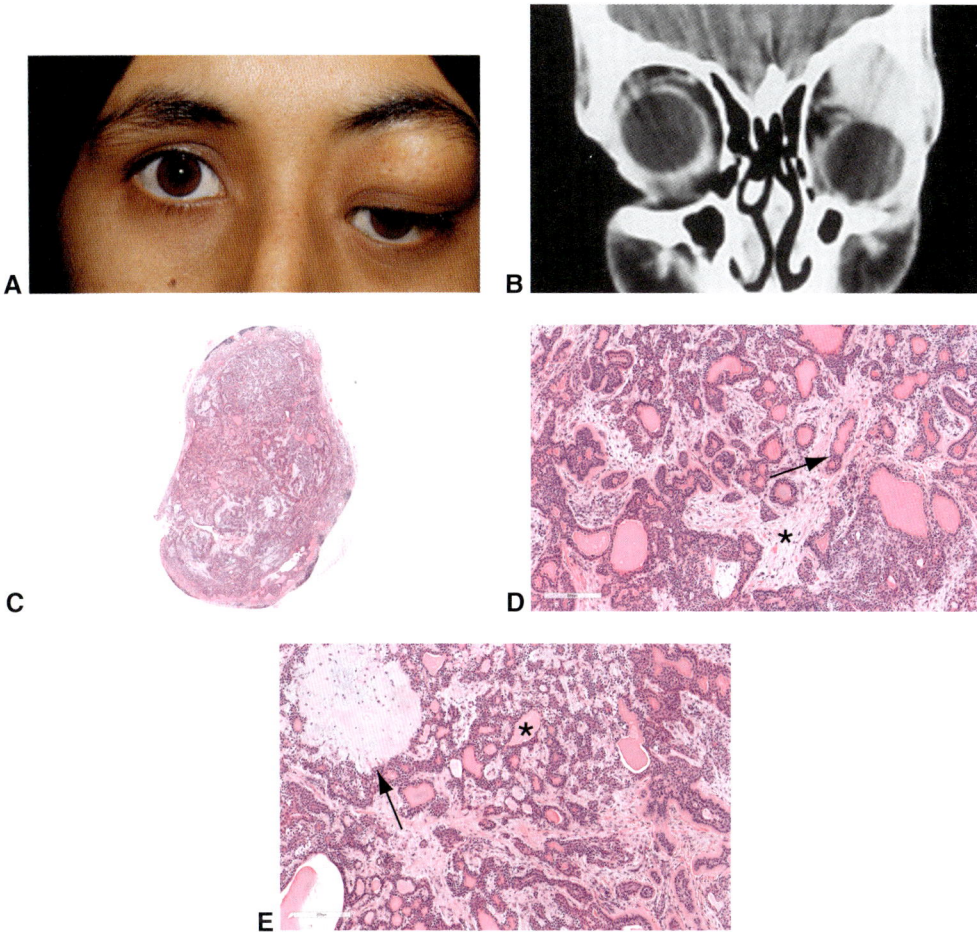

Figure 14-7 Pleomorphic adenoma (benign mixed tumor) of the lacrimal gland. **A,** Clinical photograph. A superotemporal orbital mass is present, causing proptosis and downward displacement of the left globe. **B,** CT scan (coronal view) demonstrates the left orbit tumor. **C,** Low-magnification photomicrograph shows the circumscribed nature of this pleomorphic adenoma. **D,** Note both the neoplastic epithelial elements *(arrow)* and the fibromyxoid stroma *(asterisk).* **E,** Frequent well-differentiated glandular structures with lumina *(asterisk)* are seen. The outer myoepithelial layer can become metaplastic and form other mesenchymal tissue (eg, bone, cartilage *[arrow]*). *(Parts A and B courtesy of Sander Dubovy, MD; parts C–E courtesy of Heather Potter, MD.)*

on presentation. The gross appearance is grayish white, firm, and nodular. Histologically, the tumor cells may grow in a variety of patterns: cribriform ("Swiss cheese"), which is the most common; basaloid (solid nests); comedo; sclerosing; and tubular (ductal) (Fig 14-8). Presence of the basaloid pattern has been associated with a worse prognosis (5-year survival rate of 20%) when compared with absence of a basaloid component (5-year survival rate of 70%). IHC staining for S-100 protein, keratin, and actin is typically positive within areas of myoepithelial differentiation. There is a correlation between expression of bcl-2 and BAX proteins and a more favorable prognosis. Expression of p53 is associated with a poor

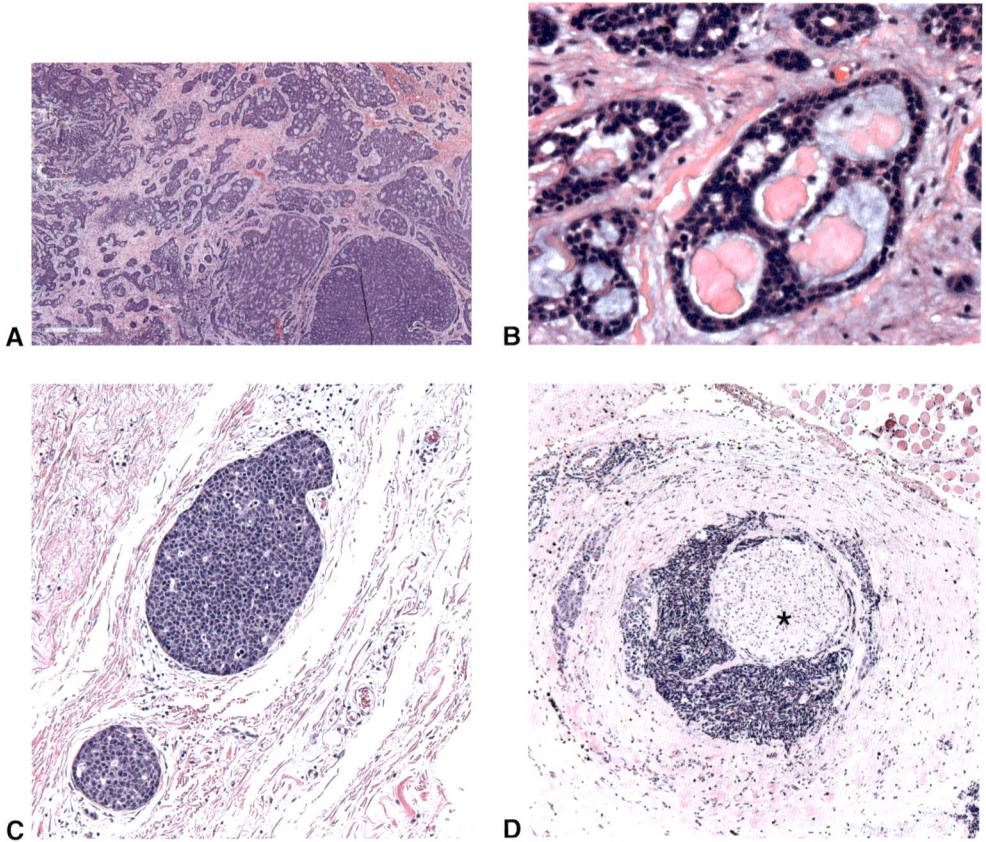

Figure 14-8 Adenoid cystic carcinoma of the lacrimal gland. **A,** Low-magnification photomicrograph shows numerous invasive tumor lobules. **B,** Note the characteristic cribriform ("Swiss cheese") pattern of growth. **C,** The solid lobules of tumor represent the basaloid pattern, which is associated with a less favorable prognosis. **D,** Perineural invasion of tumor. Blue tumor invades the perineurium and surrounds a peripheral nerve *(asterisk)*. *(Part A courtesy of Heather Potter, MD; parts B–D courtesy of Nasreen A. Syed, MD.)*

prognosis. Orbital exenteration is one of the currently accepted treatments for this tumor, but some advocate globe-sparing intra-arterial chemotherapy.

Ahmad SM, Esmaeli B, Williams M, et al. American Joint Committee on Cancer classification predicts outcome of patients with lacrimal gland adenoid cystic carcinoma. *Ophthalmology.* 2009;116(6):1210–1215.

von Holstein SL, Coupland SE, Briscoe D, Le Tourneau C, Heegaard S. Epithelial tumours of the lacrimal gland: a clinical, histopathological, surgical and oncological survey. *Acta Ophthalmol.* 2013;91(3):195–206.

Lymphoproliferative Lesions

Classification schemes for lymphoid neoplasms remain problematic, and classification of these lesions is a work in progress. Most classifications of lymphoid lesions have been based on lymph node architecture; such nodal classifications have therefore been difficult to apply to extranodal sites such as the ocular adnexa. Classification remains important with regard to selection of treatment protocols and prognostication. In general, diagnosis of lymphoma involves identifying a monoclonal population of lymphocytes. Because there are no lymph nodes in the orbit, it is problematic to classify these lesions according to the criteria used for lymph nodes.

Ocular adnexal lymphoproliferative lesions are traditionally divided into reactive lymphoid hyperplasia, atypical lymphoid hyperplasia, and ocular adnexal lymphoma (OAL). Many orbital lymphoid masses previously classified as reactive or atypical hyperplasia would now be considered neoplasia with newer, more specific diagnostic techniques such as IHC and flow cytometry, as well as with molecular testing. OAL is subtyped according to the *WHO Classification of Tumours of Haematopoietic and Lymphoid Tissues, 4th edition.*

Unlike patients with NSOI, those with orbital lymphoproliferative lesions present with gradual, painless progression of proptosis. Bilateral disease, which may occur, is suggestive of systemic disease. Staging of patients with orbital lymphoproliferative lesions should be done in collaboration with a medical oncologist. Studies may include positron emission tomography (PET) imaging and bone marrow biopsy.

When a biopsy of an orbital or conjunctival lymphoproliferative lesion is to be performed, the ophthalmologist should consult with the pathologist in advance to determine the optimal method for handling the tissue, including the type of fixative to use and the volume of tissue to obtain. It is very important that the tissue be handled gently; crush artifact can prevent the pathologist from rendering a diagnosis. Fresh (unfixed) tissue is required for touch preparations and flow cytometry. Exposure of the biopsy specimen to air for long periods should be avoided. Tissue samples may be wrapped in saline-moistened gauze or placed in tissue culture medium to slow autolysis. Gene rearrangement studies and IHC can be performed on fixed tissue. See Chapter 3, Table 3-1, for a checklist for requesting an ophthalmic pathology consultation.

Olsen TG, Heegaard S. Orbital lymphoma. *Surv Ophthalmol.* 2019;64(1):45–66.

Swerdlow SH, Campo E, Harris NL, et al. *WHO Classification of Tumours of Haematopoietic and Lymphoid Tissues.* 4th ed. International Agency for Research on Cancer; 2008.

Lymphoid hyperplasia

Reactive lymphoid hyperplasia (RLH) is characterized histologically by prominent lymphoid follicles with germinal centers (Fig 14-9), tingible body macrophages (containing apoptotic debris), and a polymorphous population of mature lymphocytes. Other inflammatory cells may be present in small numbers in the infiltrate. *Atypical lymphoid hyperplasia (ALH)* involves diffuse lymphoid proliferation, generally without reactive germinal centers. Histologically, it is characterized by an admixture of small, mature-appearing lymphocytes and larger lymphoid cells of unknown maturity. RLH and ALH are believed to represent one end of a continuum of lymphoproliferative lesions, with lymphoma at the other end.

Lymphoma

Lymphomas of the orbit may be a presenting manifestation of systemic lymphoma or may be a localized orbital neoplasm. Orbital lymphomas are generally non-Hodgkin low-grade

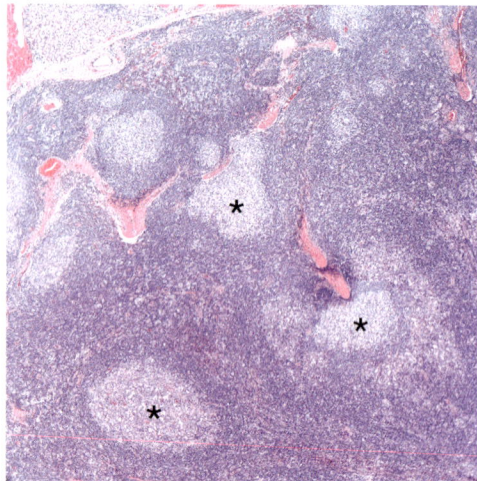

Figure 14-9 Reactive lymphoid hyperplasia of the orbit. The photomicrograph shows a dense infiltrate of lymphoid cells with a follicular pattern and well-formed germinal centers *(asterisks)*. A panel of immunohistochemical stains (not shown) demonstrated a polyclonal population of lymphocytes. *(Courtesy of Nasreen A. Syed, MD.)*

B-cell tumors with an excellent prognosis. Extranodal marginal zone B-cell lymphoma of mucosa-associated lymphoid tissue (MALT) is the most common type of lymphoma seen in the orbit. Other types of lymphoma, typically non-Hodgkin lymphomas such as follicular, large B-cell, and mantle cell, occur in the orbit but with a lower incidence. Each of these subtypes has a different prognosis for survival, and different treatment regimens tend to be used for each. Orbital lymphomas constitute one-half of the malignant tumors arising in the orbit and ocular adnexa.

Histologically, orbital lymphomas typically demonstrate a monomorphic sheet of lymphocytes and are composed of B-cells with immunopositivity for CD19 and CD20 (Fig 14-10). Immunophenotyping with different lymphocytic markers is used to further subclassify these tumors. T-cell lymphomas of the orbit are rare, more aggressive, and immunopositive for CD3, CD4, and CD8. The risk of secondary orbital involvement in systemic lymphoma is approximately 1%–2%; however, the risk of systemic lymphoma developing in a patient with orbital lymphoma is in the range of 30%–40%. The incidence of orbital lymphoma is increasing.

Soft-Tissue Tumors

In general, soft-tissue tumors are diagnosed both by recognition of the histologic patterns (ie, round cell, spindle cell, myxoid, epithelioid, pericytomatous, and pleomorphic) and by IHC. The characteristic pathologic features of soft-tissue tumors often overlap and are described on websites such as PathologyOutlines.com (www.pathologyoutlines.com/eye .html). Initially, a panel of IHC stains is used to narrow the differential diagnosis, and those results may direct further studies; however, it may be challenging to classify these tumors even with the assistance of an experienced soft-tissue pathologist.

Vascular Tumors

Orbital lymphatic malformations (previously termed *lymphangiomas*) typically present in childhood and are characterized by recurrent and fluctuating proptosis, often enlarging

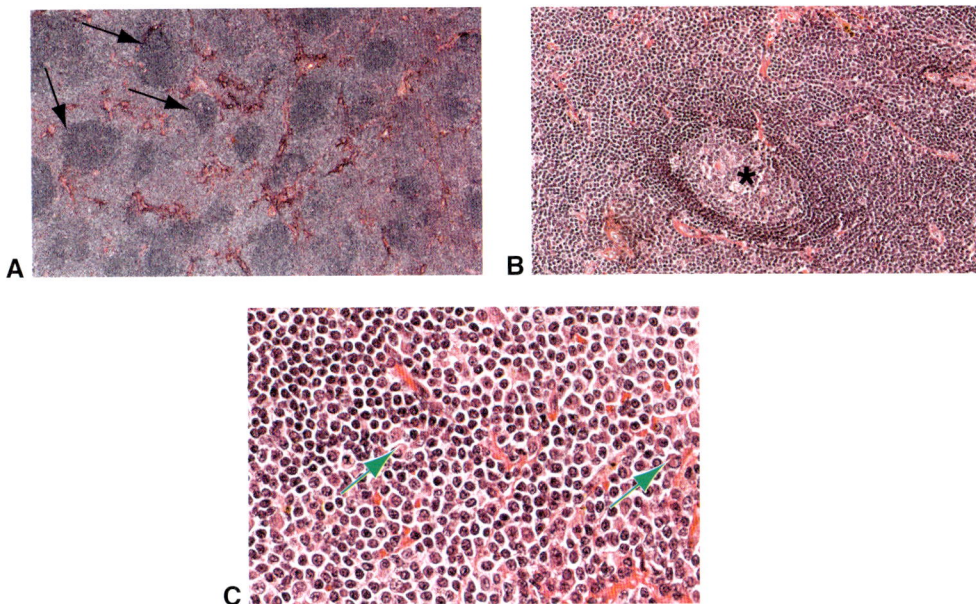

Figure 14-10 Low-grade B-cell lymphoma of the orbit. **A,** Low-magnification photomicrograph shows sheets of small, dense, uniform lymphocytes forming vague follicular arrangements *(arrows).* **B,** Higher magnification shows a lymphoid follicle with a germinal center *(asterisk).* **C,** Dutcher bodies, typical for marginal zone B-cell lymphoma of mucosa-associated lymphoid tissue (MALT), are seen within the nuclei *(arrows). (Courtesy of Heather Potter, MD.)*

in the setting of upper respiratory tract infection. They are unencapsulated, diffusely in-filtrating proliferations of vascular channels with lymphatic differentiation and scattered lymphoid aggregates with a fibrotic interstitium (Fig 14-11).

Orbital *hemangiomas* in adults are typically located intraconally and are encapsulated, consisting of large, irregular cavernous spaces *(cavernous hemangioma)* with relatively thin, fibromuscular walls (Fig 14-12). Vessels may show thrombosis and calcification. Cavern-ous hemangiomas are considered to be circumscribed, low-flow venous malformations. In contrast, hemangiomas in children are unencapsulated and more cellular, often with a cuta-neous component, and are composed of capillary-sized vessels *(infantile [capillary] heman-gioma).* See Chapter 13 for more information on infantile hemangioma.

Nassiri N, Rootman J, Rootman DB, Goldberg RA. Orbital lymphaticovenous malformations: current and future treatments. *Surv Ophthalmol.* 2015;60(5):383–405.

Tumors With Fibrous Differentiation

Solitary fibrous tumor

Solitary fibrous tumor (SFT) is the most common mesenchymal tumor of the orbit in adults. The superonasal orbit is a common site. The tumor most commonly presents in the fifth de-cade of life, but there is a wide age range. Most patients present with an orbital mass causing a combination of signs and symptoms, including proptosis, pain, diplopia, blurred vision, and epiphora.

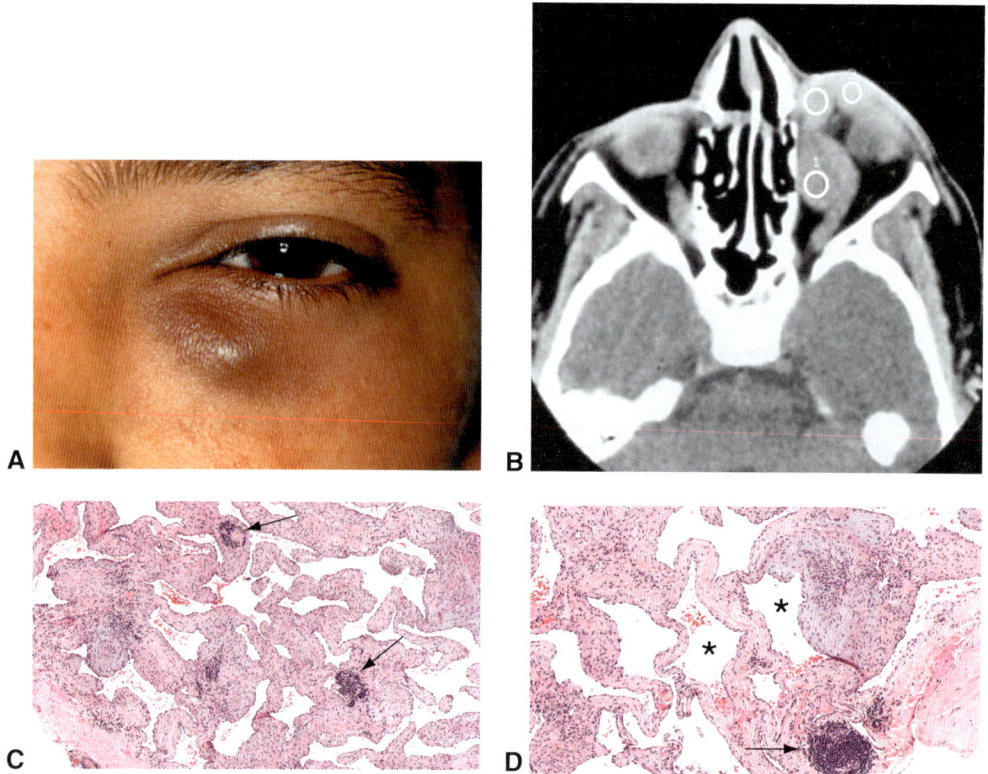

Figure 14-11 Orbital lymphatic malformation (lymphangioma). **A,** Clinical photograph shows an inferior orbital lesion extending anteriorly and nasally below the left lower eyelid of a young boy. **B,** CT scan (axial view) depicts a multilobulated mass *(white circles)* within the left orbit. **C,** Photomicrograph shows numerous vascular channels with lymphoid follicles *(arrows)* in between the vessels. **D,** Higher magnification demonstrates endothelium-lined vascular channels *(asterisks),* a lymphoid follicle *(arrow),* and scattered lymphocytes and plasma cells within the fibrous walls. *(Parts A and B courtesy of Sander Dubovy, MD; parts C and D courtesy of Heather Potter, MD.)*

Several studies have demonstrated that other soft-tissue tumors, such as hemangiopericytomas, fibrous histiocytomas, and giant cell angiofibromas of the orbit, share common histologic and immunophenotypic characteristics and may be more accurately classified as subtypes of orbital SFTs. Two commonalities among all these tumors are that (1) they are collagen rich and contain proliferating CD34-positive fibroblast-like cells; and (2) they often demonstrate strong nuclear STAT6 expression on IHC studies.

Classically, the presence of staghorn sinusoidal blood vessels (Fig 14-13) was used to distinguish hemangiopericytoma from other tumors; fibrous histiocytoma was differentiated by spindle-shaped, plump histiocyte-like cells with a focal storiform architecture (Fig 14-14); and giant cell angiofibroma was distinguished by the presence of multinucleated floret-type giant cells and ectatic vascular spaces. However, these findings overlap. For example, 87% of all fibrous tumors show staghorn vessels. Other shared histologic features may include mild hemorrhage, osteoclast-type cells, stromal myxoid change, mature

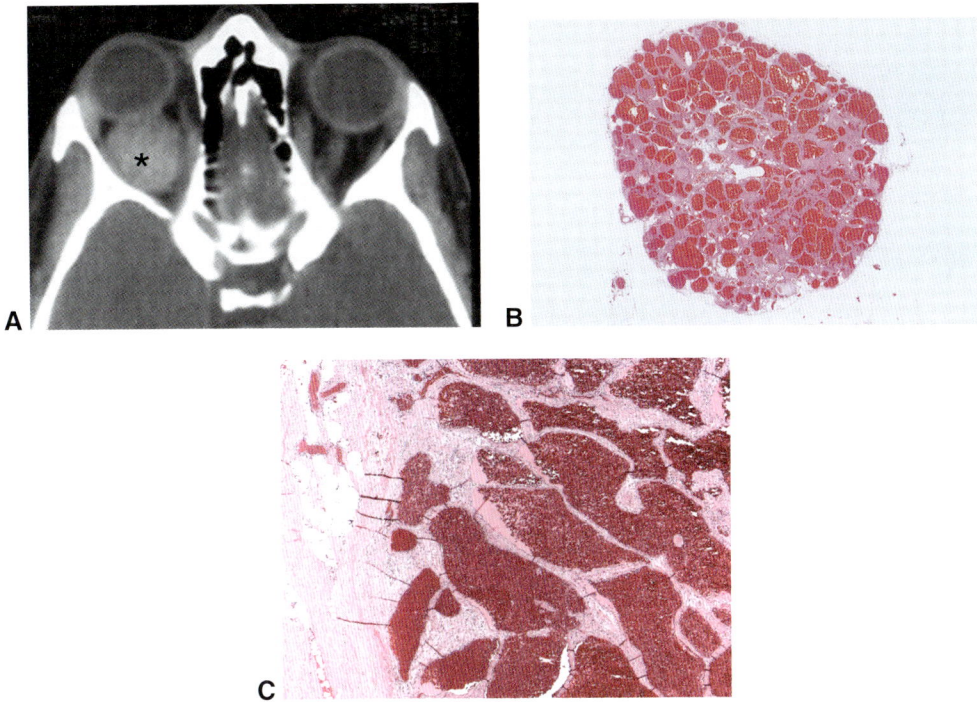

Figure 14-12 Orbital cavernous hemangioma. **A,** CT scan (axial view) shows a well-circumscribed retrobulbar intraconal mass *(asterisk)*. **B,** Low-magnification photomicrograph demonstrates large blood-filled spaces that are separated by relatively thin septa. **C,** Higher-magnification photomicrograph shows the large, irregular venous channels lined with flat endothelial cells and containing red blood cells. The collagenous capsule can be seen on the left side of the image. *(Part A courtesy of Sander Dubovy, MD; part B courtesy of Hans E. Grossniklaus, MD; part C courtesy of Nasreen A. Syed, MD.)*

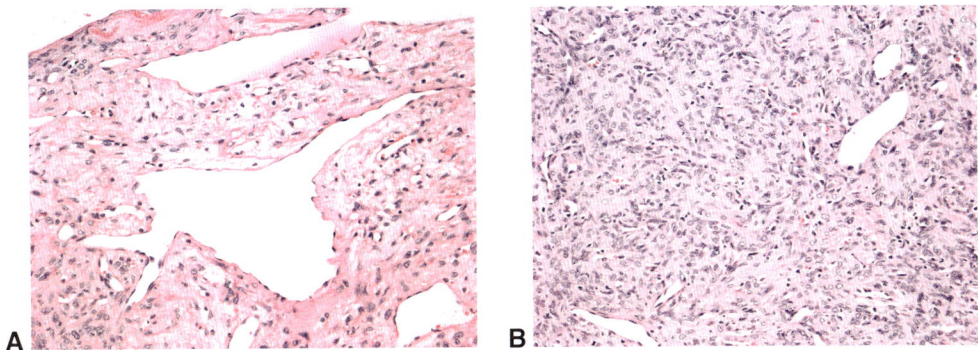

Figure 14-13 Solitary fibrous tumor (hemangiopericytoma-like). **A,** Photomicrograph demonstrates a cellular tumor with a characteristic slitlike and branching vascular (staghorn) pattern. **B,** Photomicrograph demonstrates closely packed cells with oval to spindle-shaped vesicular nuclei. *(Part A courtesy of Nasreen A. Syed, MD; part B courtesy of Ben J. Glasgow, MD.)*

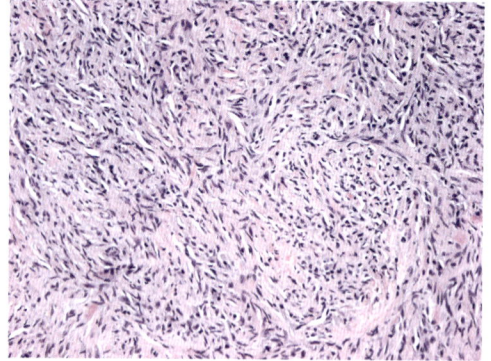

Figure 14-14 Fibrous histiocytoma. Photomicrograph illustrates the storiform (whorled and matlike) growth pattern. *(Courtesy of Nasreen A. Syed, MD.)*

adipocytes, and mineralization. The presence of overlapping features is the reason that the nomenclature of SFT is preferred to define all of these tumors.

Most SFTs are benign, although they do have a propensity for local recurrence. Marked cytologic atypia and increased mitotic activity, accentuated by strong IHC staining for Ki-67 and/or p53, support the designation of borderline or low-grade malignant behavior in these tumors.

Other primary tumors of fibrous connective tissue that may occur in rare cases in the orbit include nodular fasciitis, fibroma, and fibrosarcoma.

Demicco EG, Harms PW, Patel RM, et al. Extensive survey of STAT6 expression in a large series of mesenchymal tumors. *Am J Clin Pathol.* 2015;143(5):672–682.

Furusato E, Valenzuela IA, Fanburg-Smith JC, et al. Orbital solitary fibrous tumor: encompassing terminology for hemangiopericytoma, giant cell angiofibroma, and fibrous histiocytoma of the orbit: reappraisal of 41 cases. *Hum Pathol.* 2011;42(1):120–128.

Tumors With Muscle Differentiation

Rhabdomyosarcoma

Rhabdomyosarcoma is the most common primary malignant orbital tumor of childhood (average age at onset is 5–8 years). The typical presentation is a child with rapid-onset, progressive unilateral proptosis. Due to the extremely rapid growth of the tumor, these patients require immediate attention with urgent imaging and biopsy. There is often reddish discoloration of the eyelids that is *not* accompanied by local heat or systemic fever, as it is in cellulitis. Orbital rhabdomyosarcoma has a better prognosis (overall 5-year survival rate of about 90%) than does rhabdomyosarcoma occurring in other body sites.

Rhabdomyosarcoma arises from primitive mesenchymal cells that differentiate toward skeletal muscle. There are 3 recognized histologic types of orbital rhabdomyosarcoma (Fig 14-15):

- embryonal (most common)
- alveolar (worst prognosis)
- pleomorphic (best prognosis, least common)

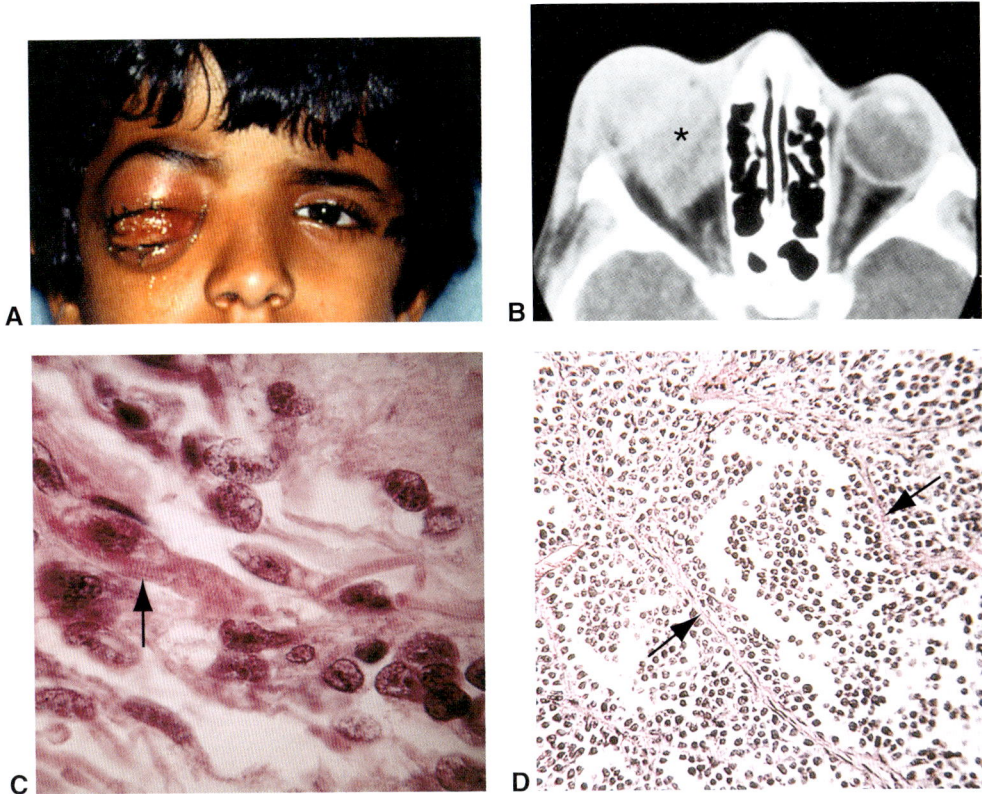

Figure 14-15 Rhabdomyosarcoma. **A,** Child with a large right orbital mass with apparent erythema of the eyelids. **B,** CT scan (axial view) shows a large, poorly circumscribed orbital tumor *(asterisk)* and proptosis. **C,** In this embryonal example, cross-striations *(arrow)* representing the Z bands of actin–myosin complexes within the cytoplasm of a tumor cell can be identified. **D,** Poorly cohesive rhabdomyoblasts separated by fibrous septa *(arrows)* into "alveoli" are low-magnification histologic features of the alveolar variant of rhabdomyosarcoma. This variant has a less favorable prognosis than the more common embryonal type. *(Parts A and B courtesy of Sander Dubovy, MD.)*

Embryonal rhabdomyosarcoma may develop in the conjunctival stroma and may present as grapelike submucosal clusters (ie, *botryoid variant*). Histologically, spindle cells are arranged in a loose syncytium with occasional elongated cells demonstrating cytoplasmic cross-striations (strap cells). These cross-striations are found in approximately 60% of embryonal rhabdomyosarcomas. Well-differentiated rhabdomyosarcomas feature numerous cells with well-defined cross-striations. Immunohistochemically, rhabdomyosarcoma typically is positive for desmin, muscle-specific actin, vimentin, and myogenin. Electron microscopy is helpful for demonstrating the typical sarcomeric banding pattern, especially in cases of embryonal rhabdomyosarcoma that are not as well-differentiated. Cytogenetic studies are important for identifying genetic translocations that have prognostic significance and may drive selection of treatment; this testing is routinely performed on these tumors. Presence of the fusion protein PAX3-FOXO1 is found in the alveolar subtype of the tumor and is associated with unfavorable outcomes.

See BCSC Section 6, *Pediatric Ophthalmology and Strabismus,* for additional discussion of rhabdomyosarcoma.

Hawkins DS, Gupta AA, Rudzinski ER. What is new in the biology and treatment of pediatric rhabdomyosarcoma? *Curr Opin Pediatr.* 2014;26(1):50–56.

Leiomyomas and leiomyosarcomas

Orbital tumors with smooth muscle differentiation are rare. *Leiomyomas* of the orbit are benign tumors that typically manifest with slowly progressive unilateral proptosis in patients in the fourth or fifth decade of life. Histologically, these spindle cell tumors show slender blunt-ended, cigar-shaped nuclei and trichrome-positive filamentous cytoplasm. IHC demonstrates smooth muscle differentiation. *Leiomyosarcomas* are malignant lesions that occur most commonly in patients in their seventh decade of life. Histologically, these tumors show more cellularity, necrosis, and nuclear pleomorphism than their benign counterparts. Mitotic figures appear in leiomyosarcomas but typically are absent in leiomyomas.

Peripheral Nerve Sheath and Central Nervous System Tumors

Neurofibroma

Neurofibroma, the most common peripheral nerve sheath tumor, is a slow-growing tumor that consists of a mixture of endoneurial fibroblasts, Schwann cells, and axons. Neurofibromas may be circumscribed but are not encapsulated. They are firm and rubbery. Microscopically, the spindle-shaped cells have slender, wavy nuclei. These nuclei are arranged in ribbons and cords in a matrix of myxoid tissue and collagen that contains axons. Cytogenetic studies indicate that the most frequent structural rearrangements involve chromosome arm 9p.

Isolated neurofibromas do not necessarily indicate a systemic syndrome, but they are more common in neurofibromatosis 1 (NF1). The plexiform type of neurofibroma is considered pathognomonic for NF1 (Fig 14-16). *Plexiform* refers to an intricate network, or *plexus,* classically described as a "bag of worms." Studies indicate that a limited number of pathways are potentially involved in tumorigenesis of the plexiform neurofibroma. The *CCN1* gene may be a useful diagnostic or prognostic marker and may serve as the foundation for new treatment strategies. The CCN1 and related gene products are cysteine-rich proteins that have been shown to play a role in intracellular signaling in the extracellular matrix.

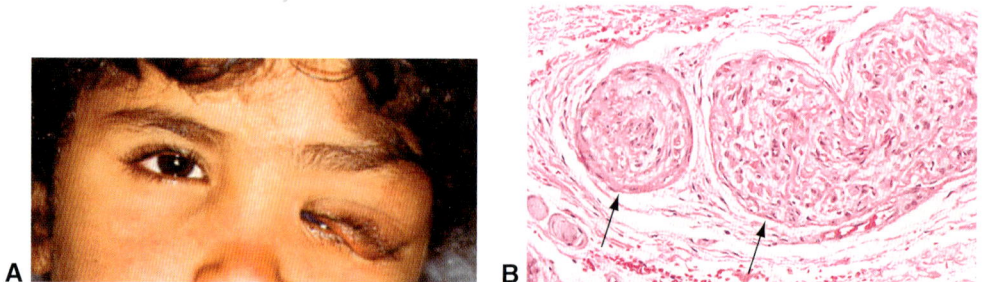

Figure 14-16 Plexiform neurofibroma. **A,** Clinical photograph depicting the typical S-shaped deformity of the upper eyelid. **B,** Note the thickened, tortuous nerves *(arrows)* with proliferation of endoneurial fibroblasts and Schwann cells. *(Part A courtesy of Sander Dubovy, MD.)*

Liu K, DeAngelo P, Mahmet K, Phytides P, Osborne L, Pletcher BA. Cytogenetics of neurofibromas: two case reports and literature review. *Cancer Genet Cytogenet.* 2010;196(1):
93–95.

Pasmant E, Ortonne N, Rittié L, et al. Differential expression of CCN1/CYR61, CCN3/NOV,
CCN4/WISP1, and CCN5/WISP2 in neurofibromatosis type 1 tumorigenesis. *J Neuropathol
Exp Neurol.* 2010;69(1):60–69.

Neurilemoma

A neurilemoma (also spelled *neurilemmoma;* also called *schwannoma*) arises from Schwann
cells of peripheral nerves. These are the most common nerve sheath tumors found in the
orbit of adults. Slow growing and encapsulated, this yellowish tumor may show cystic spaces
and areas of hemorrhagic necrosis. It may be solitary or associated with a genetic syndrome
such as neurofibromatosis or schwannomatosis. Histologically, neurilemomas can demonstrate one or more characteristic growth patterns. The Antoni A pattern consists of slender
spindle cells in which the nuclei are arranged in palisades that may form intervening Verocay
bodies (collections of fibrils resembling sensory corpuscles) (Fig 14-17). The Antoni B pattern is made up of stellate cells set in a mucoid stroma. Vessels are usually prominent and
thick walled, and no axons are present. IHC analysis of neurilemoma is relatively nonspecific, and typically the tumor is positive for S-100 protein and vimentin.

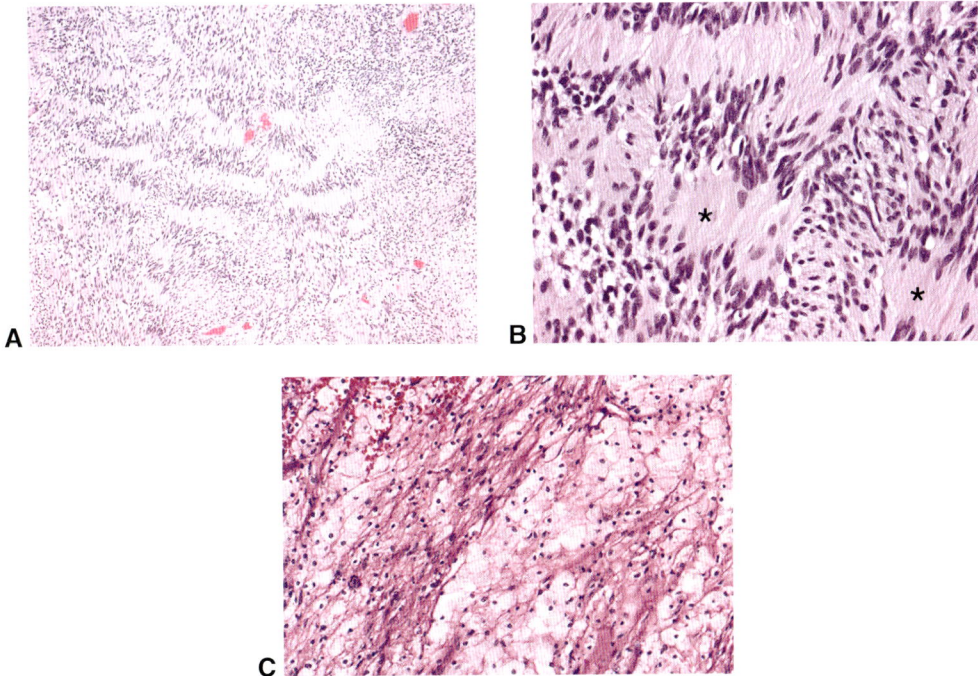

Figure 14-17 Neurilemoma (schwannoma). **A,** The Antoni A pattern. Spindle cell nuclei are
arranged in linear palisades. **B,** Palisading of nuclei may form a Verocay body *(asterisks).* **C,** The
Antoni B pattern consists of a loosely arranged, mucoid stroma and represents degeneration
within the tumor. *(Parts A and B courtesy of Nasreen A. Syed, MD.)*

Meningioma

Meningiomas are found in the CNS as they are derived from the meninges. Most meningiomas that affect the orbit are actually primary tumors of the intracranial cavity that invade through the orbital bones, typically the sphenoid bone, and behave as an infiltrative mass lesion in the orbit. A minority of meningiomas found in the orbit arise from the optic nerve sheath primarily. These tumors tend to stay within the sheath and result in compression of the optic nerve. For further discussion of meningioma and other CNS tumors occurring in the orbit, see Chapter 15.

Adipose Tumors

Lipomas are rare in the orbit. Their pathologic characteristics include encapsulation and a distinctive lobular appearance. Because lipomas are difficult to distinguish from normal or prolapsed fat histologically, their incidence may have been overestimated previously.

Like lipomas, *liposarcomas* are rare in the orbit. Liposarcomas are malignant tumors with adipose differentiation. They are categorized as several histologic variants. Histologic criteria for diagnosis depend on the type of liposarcoma, but the unifying diagnostic feature is the presence of lipoblasts. Cytogenetic and/or molecular studies for chromosome translocations and alterations in several genes, including *MDM2,* can be very useful for diagnosing and grading adipose tumors. Liposarcomas tend to recur before they metastasize.

Bony Lesions of the Orbit

Fibrous dysplasia of bone may involve one bone (monostotic) or more than one (polyostotic). When the orbit is affected, the condition is usually monostotic. However, the tumor may cross suture lines to involve multiple orbital bones. Patients often present during the first 3 decades of life. Narrowing of the optic canal and lacrimal drainage system can occur. Plain radiographic studies show a ground-glass appearance with lytic foci. Cysts that contain fluid also appear. As a result of arrest in the maturation of bone, trabeculae are composed not of lamellar bone but of woven bone with a fibrous stroma that is highly vascularized. Histologically, the bony trabeculae often have a C-shaped appearance (Fig 14-18).

Fibro-osseous dysplasia (juvenile ossifying fibroma), a variant of fibrous dysplasia, is characterized histologically by spicules of bone rimmed by osteoblasts (Fig 14-19). At low magnification, ossifying fibroma may be confused with a psammomatous meningioma.

Osseous and cartilaginous tumors of the orbit are rare; of these, *osteoma* is the most common. It is composed of mature bone and is slow growing and well circumscribed. Most commonly, an osteoma arises from the frontal sinus.

Other primary osseous and cartilaginous tumors that have been reported rarely in the orbit include both benign entities (eg, osteoblastoma) and malignant sarcomas (eg, Ewing sarcoma, osteogenic sarcoma).

Secondary Tumors

Secondary malignant orbital tumors are lesions that invade the orbit by direct extension from adjacent structures, such as the paranasal sinus, intracranial cavity, eye, eyelids, or ocular

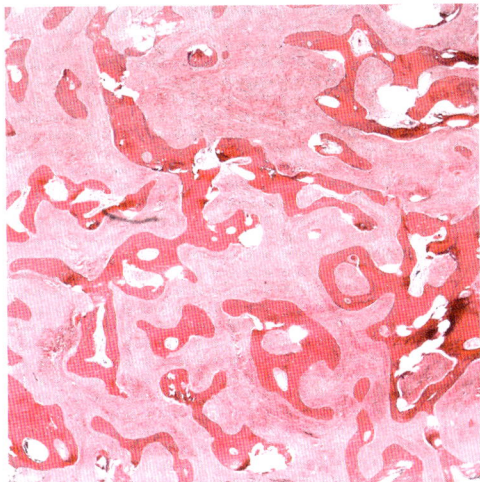

Figure 14-18 Fibrous dysplasia. The bony trabeculae are often C-shaped, composed of immature woven bone, and surrounded by a fibrous stroma. *(Courtesy of Nasreen A. Syed, MD.)*

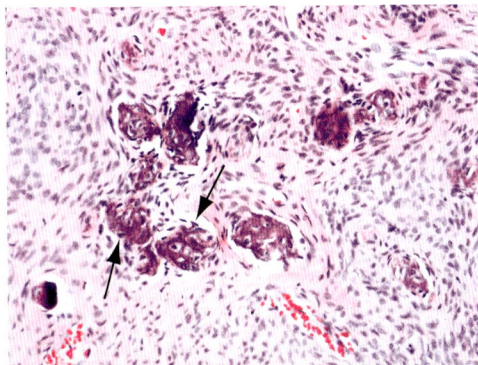

Figure 14-19 Fibro-osseous dysplasia (juvenile ossifying fibroma). Spicules of lamellar bone are set in a cellular fibrous stroma. Note the osteoblasts *(arrows)* lining the bony spicules. *(Courtesy of Tatyana Milman, MD.)*

surface. *Metastatic* tumors are malignant lesions that have spread from a distant primary site, usually by a hematogenous route. The most common primary tumor sites resulting in orbital metastasis are the breast in women and the prostate in men. In children, neuroblastoma is the most common primary tumor metastatic to the orbit.

Lacrimal Sac Neoplasia

Lacrimal sac neoplasms are rare and may mimic dacryocystitis clinically. In one study of patients undergoing dacryocystorhinostomy (DCR) for chronic nasolacrimal duct obstruction, neoplasm was the cause in only 5% of cases. As the lacrimal sac is lined with a transitional epithelium, similar to that in the bladder, squamous and transitional cell carcinomas may arise in the sac, though rarely. Most lacrimal sac tumors are benign papillomatous neoplasms that arise from the epithelial lining, but a wide variety have been reported.

Krishna Y, Coupland SE. Lacrimal sac tumors—a review. *Asia Pac J Ophthalmol (Phila).* 2017; 6(2):173–178.

CHAPTER 15

Optic Nerve

Highlights

- The optic nerve consists of retinal ganglion cell axons and glial cells.
- Because the optic nerve is contiguous with the brain, many of the conditions affecting the optic nerve are similar to those that affect the central nervous system.
- The optic nerve is vulnerable to disease processes extending from adjacent structures, including infections and neoplasms.
- Temporal artery biopsy is considered the gold standard for diagnosis of giant cell arteritis. Because skip lesions may be present in the artery, multiple stepped sections through the biopsy specimen are used to avoid missing affected areas.

Topography

The optic nerve is embryologically derived from the optic stalk and is continuous with the optic tract in the brain. Therefore, many diseases of the optic nerve reflect those of the central nervous system (CNS). The optic nerve measures 35–55 mm, extending from the eye to the optic chiasm, where the fibers decussate; from there, the fibers continue until they synapse in the lateral geniculate nucleus. The optic nerve is divided into 4 topographic areas (the length of each is given in parentheses):

- intraocular (0.7–1.0 mm)
- intraorbital (25–30 mm, with curvature and slack to accommodate eye movement)
- intracanalicular (4–10 mm)
- intracranial (average = 10 mm)

The clinically visible portion of the optic nerve inside the eye is known as the *optic disc*. The portion of the optic nerve inside the eye and anterior to the lamina cribrosa is known as the *optic nerve head (ONH)*. These terms are often used interchangeably.

The optic nerve consists of retinal ganglion cell axons and glial cells (Fig 15-1). Glial cells (*glia* = glue), including oligodendrocytes, astrocytes, and microglial cells, make up the supportive tissue of the CNS. Their functions are listed in Table 15-1.

The optic nerve becomes myelinated by oligodendrocytes just posterior to the lamina cribrosa of the sclera, making it larger in diameter than the optic nerve head. The optic nerve is also encased in a meningeal sheath consisting of the following: the external dense connective tissue sheath, or *dura* (which merges with the sclera anteriorly and the bony optic canal and the dura of the brain posteriorly); the cellular *arachnoid sheath* (which forms

285

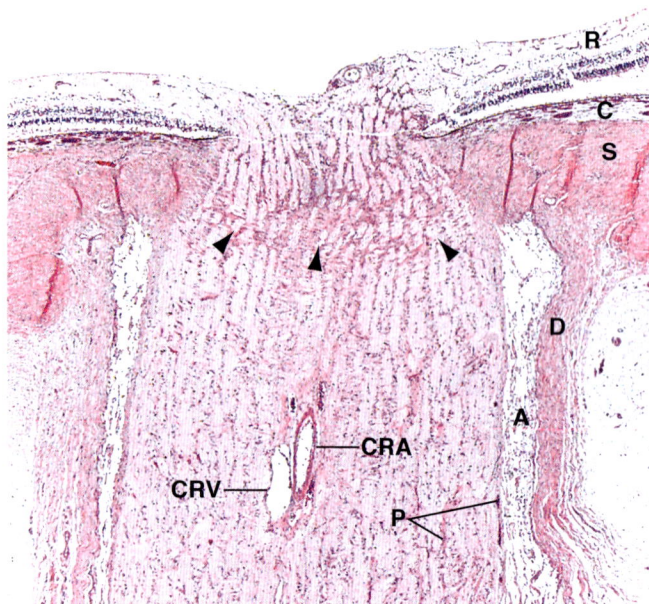

Figure 15-1 Longitudinal section of normal optic nerve. Axons of the retinal ganglion cells (R) travel in the nerve fiber layer toward the optic disc and make a 90° turn posteriorly to become the axonal fibers of the optic nerve. Optic nerve axons pass through the fenestrations in the lamina cribrosa *(arrowheads)*, a perforated area in the posterior sclera (S), and become myelinated, increasing the diameter of the retrolaminar nerve. Sclera surrounding the lamina cribrosa is continuous with the dura of the optic nerve (D). A=arachnoid; C=choroid; CRA=central retinal artery; CRV=central retinal vein; P=pial septa. *(Courtesy of Tatyana Milman, MD.)*

Table 15-1 Supporting Cells in the Central Nervous System

Cell Type	Function
Astrocytes	Provide support and nutrition for neurons like ganglion cells
Microglial cells	Perform phagocytic function similar to that of histiocytes
Oligodendrocytes	Produce and maintain myelin sheath of optic nerve

part of the internal sheath of the optic nerve and is the continuation of the arachnoidea mater around the brain); and the fibrovascular *pial sheath* (which also forms part of the internal sheath and is the continuation of the pia mater around the brain). The pial vessels and connective tissue extend into the optic nerve and divide the nerve fibers into fascicles. The subarachnoid space of the optic nerve sheath contains cerebrospinal fluid (Fig 15-2).

The vascular supply of the optic nerve stems predominantly from pial vessels, which are branches of the ophthalmic and superior hypophyseal arteries; the short posterior ciliary arteries mainly supply the optic nerve head. See BCSC Section 2, *Fundamentals and Principles of Ophthalmology,* and Section 5, *Neuro-Ophthalmology,* for additional discussion of the optic nerve and its vascular supply.

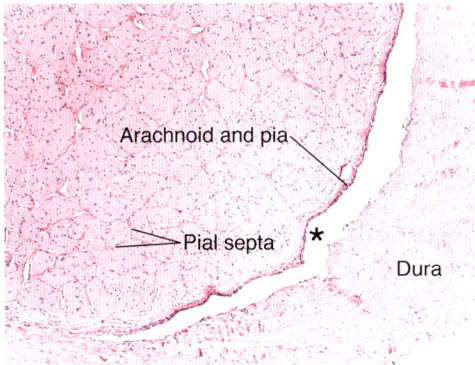

Figure 15-2 Cross section through a normal optic nerve. The axons of the optic nerve are segregated into fascicles by the delicate, fibrovascular pial septa. The nuclei of oligodendrocytes, astrocytes, and microglia are visible between the eosinophilic axons. The subdural space *(asterisk)* is relatively narrow in the normal optic nerve. *(Courtesy of Tatyana Milman, MD.)*

Developmental Anomalies

There are numerous developmental anomalies of the optic nerve, such as optic nerve hypoplasia, optic nerve colobomas, optic (nerve head) pits, morning glory disc anomaly, and Bergmeister papilla. Only those entities that have been well characterized histologically are discussed in this section. See BCSC Section 5, *Neuro-Ophthalmology,* and Section 6, *Pediatric Ophthalmology and Strabismus,* for additional discussion of developmental anomalies of the eye, including the optic nerve.

Colobomas

Colobomas of the optic nerve result from defective closure of the embryonic fissure. They are often inferonasal and may be associated with colobomatous defects of the retina and choroid, ciliary body, and iris (Fig 15-3A). Histologically, there is a large defect in the optic nerve, and atrophic, gliotic retina lines the defect. The sclera is commonly ectatic and bowed posteriorly (Fig 15-3B). The defect wall may contain adipose tissue and even smooth muscle.

Optic Pits

An optic pit is a developmental defect that is likely caused by incomplete embryonic fissure closure (Fig 15-3C). Clinically and histologically, there is a small depression in the optic disc that is associated with a defect in the lamina cribrosa. Histologically, herniation of dysplastic retina into the defect is typically found. Associated shallow serous macular detachments can be seen in 25%–75% of eyes with inferotemporal pits (Fig 15-3D). The source of the macular fluid remains unknown.

Inflammation

In general, *optic neuritis* is an all-encompassing term referring to inflammation of the optic nerve, which can be infectious or noninfectious. Neuritis may be isolated or one of a constellation of findings and may involve either the anterior or posterior segment of the eye.

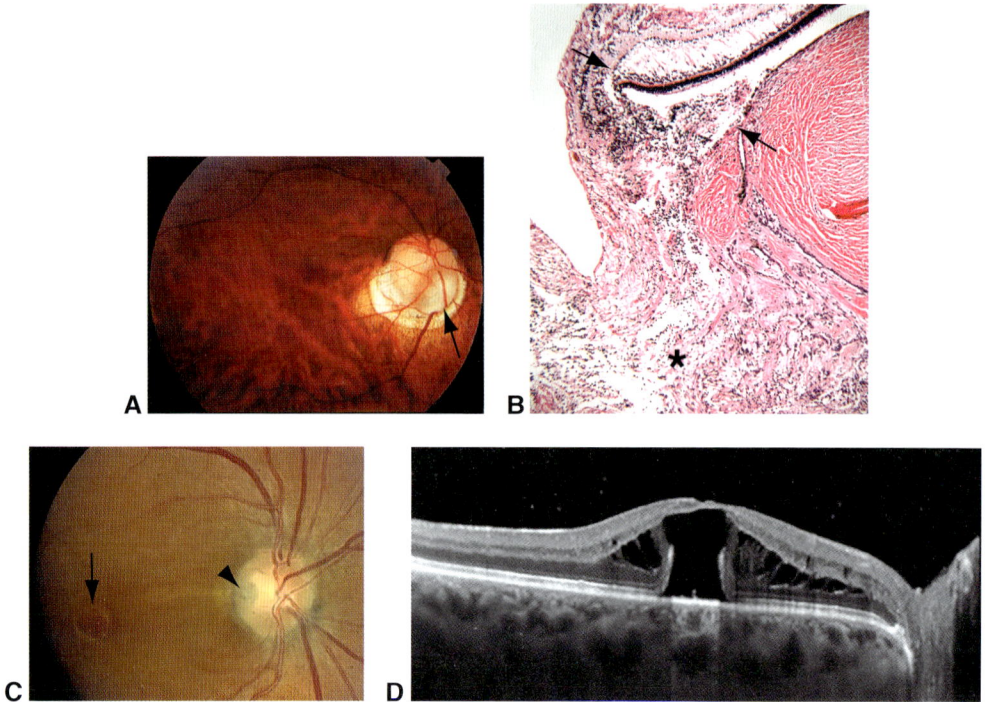

Figure 15-3 Optic nerve coloboma and pit. **A,** Fundus photograph of the right eye shows a colobomatous defect in the inferonasal optic nerve *(arrow).* **B,** Photomicrograph shows gliotic, disorganized retina *(asterisk)* that prolapses into the optic nerve head defect, which is lined by excavated sclera. Normal retina, retinal pigment epithelium, and choroid terminate at the edge of the colobomatous defect *(between arrows).* **C,** Fundus photograph (right eye, different patient) shows an optic pit *(arrowhead)* with associated macular edema *(arrow).* **D,** Optical coherence tomography image from the same patient shows an optic pit–associated maculopathy with intraretinal cystoid edema and subretinal fluid. *(Parts A and B courtesy of Tatyana Milman, MD; parts C and D courtesy of Benjamin J. Kim, MD.)*

Infectious Optic Neuritis

Bacterial, viral, or fungal infections of the optic nerve can occur because of spread of infection from adjacent anatomical structures or as part of a systemic infection, particularly in immunocompromised patients. *Bartonella henselae, Treponema pallidum,* and *Mycobacterium tuberculosis* are the organisms most often responsible for primary bacterial infections of the optic nerve. Examples of infectious diseases caused by viruses include herpes simplex (due to infection with human herpesvirus 1 or 2) and varicella (due to varicella-zoster virus infection). Acute disseminated encephalomyelitis (ADEM) is an immune-mediated demyelinating disease that often follows bacterial or viral infection. Histiocytes and microglia remove the damaged myelin, and astrocytic proliferation ultimately produces a glial scar, or *plaque.*

Fungal infections that can involve the optic nerve include mucormycosis, cryptococcosis, and coccidioidomycosis. Mucormycosis (also called *zygomycosis*) generally results

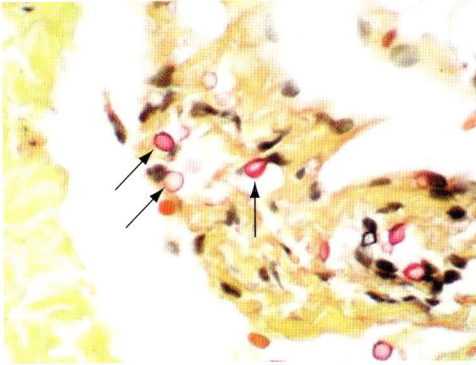

Figure 15-4 Cryptococcosis of the optic nerve in an immunocompromised patient. The dura is infiltrated by cryptococcal organisms *(arrows)*. This yeast has a mucopolysaccharide capsule that stains red with mucicarmine stain. No inflammatory infiltrate is observed. *(Courtesy of Tatyana Milman, MD.)*

from direct extension from nearby structures, usually a contiguous sinus infection. Cryptococcosis generally begins as a pulmonary infection, which can disseminate to the brain. Optic nerve involvement generally occurs via direct spread from the intracranial cavity and is commonly associated with multiple foci of necrosis with little inflammatory reaction (Fig 15-4). Coccidioidomycosis also begins as a primary pulmonary infection and can disseminate to other areas of the body, including the optic nerve and eye, producing necrotizing granulomas. Infectious optic neuritis is discussed further in BCSC Section 5, *Neuro-Ophthalmology.*

Noninfectious Optic Neuritis

Noninfectious inflammatory disorders of the optic nerve include classic optic neuritis in the setting of *multiple sclerosis, giant cell arteritis (GCA),* and *sarcoidosis.* Multiple sclerosis is a common inflammatory demyelinating disease of the CNS that causes optic neuritis. The histologic findings of optic neuritis from multiple sclerosis are similar to those of ADEM, with loss of myelin in the retrolaminar optic nerve and sectoral atrophy of the ganglion cells in more advanced cases (Fig 15-5). Further discussion on optic neuritis can be found in BCSC Section 5, *Neuro-Ophthalmology.*

Although GCA does not cause direct inflammation of the optic nerve, it is included here because it is a systemic inflammatory disorder that can cause optic nerve ischemia resulting in profound vision loss. GCA is characterized by inflammation that affects medium to large arteries. The gold standard for histologic diagnosis of GCA is a superficial temporal artery biopsy (Fig 15-6). It is critical to obtain a specimen of adequate length, approximately 2 cm, because areas of involvement can be patchy (ie, skip lesions). As such, a careful histologic examination requires stepped sections that sample the entire paraffin block; at minimum, 4 levels are evaluated.

Histologically, a chronic inflammatory infiltrate is seen in the vessel wall, often centered on the internal elastic lamina, resulting in its destruction. The inflammation is granulomatous with the presence of epithelioid histiocytes and sometimes multinucleated giant cells as well as lymphocytes. The intima is usually thickened and fibrotic, with broad disruption of the internal elastic lamina; the lumen may be thrombosed and subsequently recanalized.

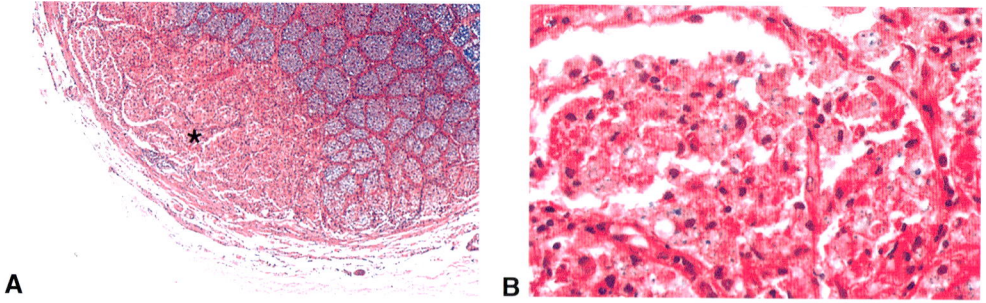

Figure 15-5 Demyelination of the optic nerve. **A,** Luxol fast blue stain for myelin. The blue-staining area indicates normal myelin. Note the sectoral absence of myelin in the lower left corner of the optic nerve *(asterisk),* corresponding to a focal area of demyelination. **B,** Higher magnification. The blue material (myelin) is engulfed by histiocytes (macrophages).

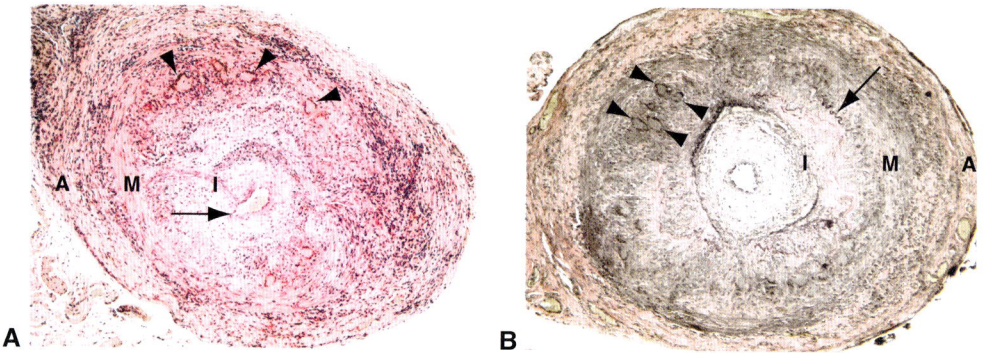

Figure 15-6 Temporal artery biopsy in giant cell arteritis. **A,** Vascular lumen *(arrow)* is markedly narrowed by intimal edema and inflammation. A prominent transmural inflammatory infiltrate with numerous multinucleated giant cells *(arrowheads)* is observed. **B,** Elastic stain highlights the diffuse loss of the internal elastic lamina. A short segment of the wavy internal elastic lamina remains *(arrow).* Giant cells *(arrowheads)* are noted at the level of the internal elastic lamina. A = adventitia; I = intima; M = media. *(Courtesy of Tatyana Milman, MD.)*

These same inflammatory features can affect the posterior ciliary arteries, resulting in their occlusion and liquefactive necrosis of the optic nerve. When the inflammation subsides, it can result in a scar in the vessel wall, primarily in the intima with focal loss of the muscularis layer (transmural scarring). This can be the primary finding in a biopsy specimen rather than active inflammation. Despite the name of the disease, the presence of giant cells is not required for diagnosis.

Corticosteroid therapy is the mainstay of treatment and should be initiated immediately when GCA is suspected. Temporal artery biopsy should be performed within 10–14 days because corticosteroid treatment can alter histologic findings, mainly diminishing the inflammation. Therefore, it is important to inform the pathologist of any corticosteroid treatment so that the findings can be interpreted appropriately. Bilateral temporal artery biopsies are rarely useful, increasing the yield at most by 2%–5%. Typically,

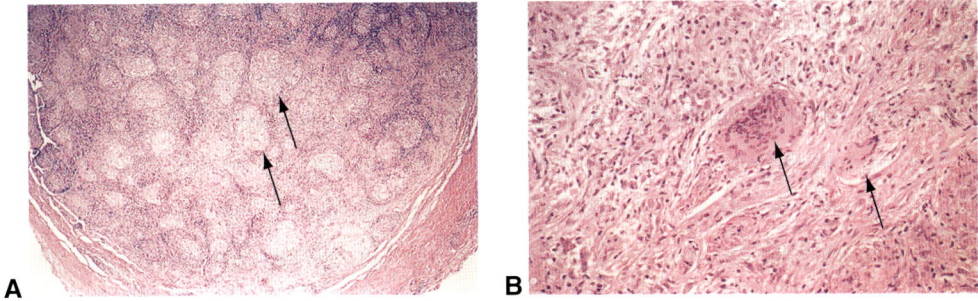

Figure 15-7 Sarcoidosis of the optic nerve. **A,** Low-magnification photomicrograph shows a cross section of the optic nerve with discrete noncaseating granulomas *(arrows)*. **B,** Higher magnification shows multinucleated giant cells *(arrows)* in the granulomas. *(Courtesy of Hans E. Grossniklaus, MD.)*

contralateral biopsies are employed when findings on the initial temporal artery biopsy are negative or atypical and there is high clinical suspicion for GCA. In the event of an unexpected biopsy result, a second opinion from a pathologist experienced in the interpretation of these biopsies may be helpful. Further discussion can be found in BCSC Section 5, *Neuro-Ophthalmology*.

Sarcoidosis, another systemic disorder that can involve the optic nerve, is often associated with retinal, vitreal, and uveal lesions (Fig 15-7; see also Chapter 12, Fig 12-10). Unlike the characteristic noncaseating granulomas in the eye, optic nerve lesions may show necrosis. Refer to BCSC Section 5, *Neuro-Ophthalmology,* and Section 9, *Uveitis and Ocular Inflammation*, for further discussion.

Degenerations

Optic Atrophy

Optic atrophy is the end-stage result of insults to the retinal ganglion cells and their axons. Although the etiology varies, the downstream sequence of events leading to optic atrophy is uniform: injury to the retinal ganglion cells and the axons of the anterior optic nerve (the portion of the nerve near the globe) results in axonal swelling, clinically apparent as ONH edema (Fig 15-8). Axonal swelling and loss of retinal ganglion cells are followed by retrograde degeneration of axons (ie, ascending atrophy, or Wallerian degeneration) toward the lateral geniculate body. Pathologic processes within the cranial cavity or orbit result in descending atrophy toward the retinal ganglion cell bodies (see BCSC Section 5, *Neuro-Ophthalmology,* for more on optic atrophy). Loss of myelin and oligodendrocytes accompanies axonal degeneration. The optic nerve also shrinks, despite the proliferation of astrocytes and fibroconnective tissue (gliosis) in the pial septa (Fig 15-9).

Glaucoma is a group of diseases characterized by optic neuropathy, resulting in optic atrophy. Histologically, there is early loss of retinal ganglion cell axons, blood vessels, and

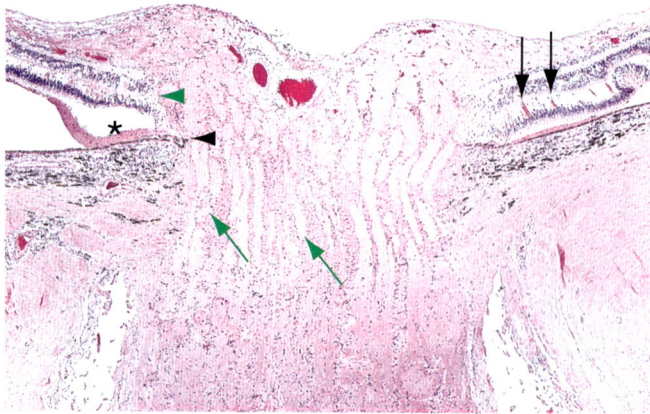

Figure 15-8 Optic nerve head edema. Swollen intralaminar axons demonstrate vacuolar alteration with pale staining *(green arrows)* and displace the retina laterally *(green arrowhead)* from its normal termination just above the end of Bruch membrane *(black arrowhead)*. Juxtapapillary serous intraretinal fluid *(black arrows)* and serous subretinal fluid *(asterisk)* are also present. *(Courtesy of Tatyana Milman, MD.)*

glial cells, particularly at the level of the lamina cribrosa. As the disease advances, the ONH becomes excavated, with posterior bowing of the lamina cribrosa (see Fig 15-9D). Evidence of optic nerve atrophy may precede detectable functional vision loss. See BCSC Section 10, *Glaucoma,* for further discussion.

Another example of optic atrophy is Schnabel cavernous optic atrophy, which is characterized microscopically by large cystoid spaces in the nerve posterior to the lamina cribrosa (Fig 15-10A). These spaces contain mucopolysaccharides, which stain with alcian blue (Fig 15-10B). Although the condition was initially observed in glaucomatous eyes after acute intraocular pressure elevation, it has been increasingly identified in elderly patients without glaucoma who have generalized arteriosclerotic disease. The source of mucopolysaccharides was originally thought to be vitreous, forced into the ischemic necrosis–induced cavernous spaces by elevated intraocular pressure; however, the mucopolysaccharides are more likely produced in situ, within the atrophic spaces of the optic nerve.

Optic Nerve Head Drusen

Drusen of the ONH are calcific bodies embedded within the parenchyma of the optic nerve. Evidence suggests that abnormal axonal metabolism leads to mitochondrial calcification and drusen formation. They are usually bilateral and associated with small, crowded ONHs with abnormal vasculature. When superficial, drusen appear on the optic disc as refractile, rounded pale-yellow or white deposits. Deeper ones may be mistaken for papilledema (pseudopapilledema). ONH drusen may cause visual field defects; in rare cases, they can cause an anterior ischemic optic neuropathy, resulting in significant vision loss. Most ONH drusen are located anterior to the lamina cribrosa and posterior to Bruch membrane (lamina choroidalis portion of the intraocular optic nerve).

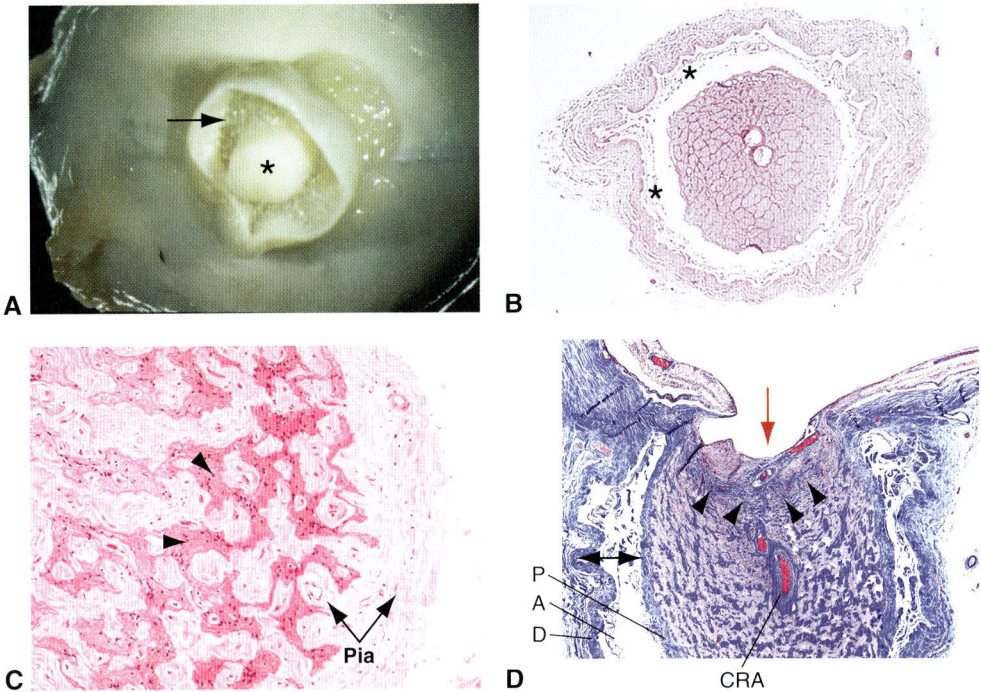

Figure 15-9 Optic nerve atrophy. **A,** Gross appearance of an optic nerve *(asterisk)* with widened subdural space *(arrow)* due to shrinkage of the nerve. **B,** Low-magnification photomicrograph also shows a widened subdural space *(asterisks)*. **C,** Cross section of an atrophic nerve shows loss of axons *(arrowheads)*, accompanied by glial proliferation and widening of fibrovascular pial septa *(arrows)*. **D,** Glaucomatous optic atrophy. Masson trichrome stains the collagen of the sclera, lamina cribrosa, and meninges dark blue and the axonal fascicles pink. The optic nerve demonstrates advanced cupping *(red arrow)*, accompanied by posterior bowing of the lamina cribrosa *(arrowheads)*. Axonal atrophy and thickening of pial septa are present. The subdural and subarachnoid spaces are widened owing to severe optic nerve atrophy *(double-ended arrow)*. A = arachnoid sheath; CRA = central retinal artery; D = dural sheath; P = pia. *(Part A courtesy of Debra J. Shetlar, MD; parts C and D courtesy of Tatyana Milman, MD.)*

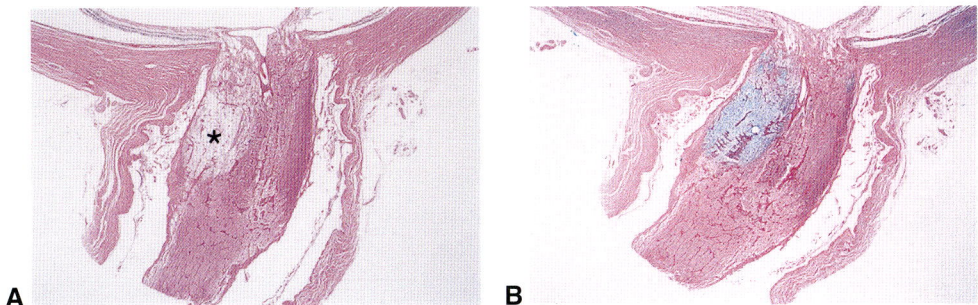

Figure 15-10 Schnabel cavernous optic atrophy. **A,** Photomicrograph shows atrophy resulting in cystoid spaces *(asterisk)* within the optic nerve. **B,** Photomicrograph shows cystoid spaces filled with alcian blue–positive material. *(Courtesy of Hans E. Grossniklaus, MD.)*

Figure 15-11 Histologically, optic nerve head (ONH) drusen appear as discrete basophilic calcified deposits *(arrows)* just anterior to the lamina cribrosa *(asterisk)*. The clear spaces in the ONH are histologic sectioning artifacts due to dropout of hard calcific material.

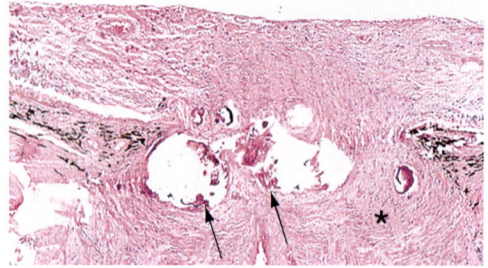

ONH drusen can be associated with the following:

- angioid streaks
- papillitis
- optic atrophy
- chronic glaucoma
- vascular occlusions

However, they are more commonly seen in otherwise normal eyes. Occasionally, they are dominantly inherited.

Histologically, ONH drusen appear as basophilic, irregular, calcified acellular deposits (Fig 15-11) that contain mucopolysaccharides, amino acids, DNA, RNA, and iron. For more information, see BCSC Section 5, *Neuro-Ophthalmology,* and Section 6, *Pediatric Ophthalmology and Strabismus.*

> Hamann S, Malmqvist L, Costello F. Optic disc drusen: understanding an old problem from a new perspective. *Acta Ophthalmol.* 2018;96(7):673–684.

Neoplasia

Tumors may affect the ONH (eg, melanocytoma, peripapillary choroidal melanoma, choroidal osteoma, and hemangioma) or the retrobulbar portion of the optic nerve (eg, glioma and meningioma). Invasion of the optic nerve can occur through direct extension of orbital or CNS tumors (eg, leptomeningeal carcinomatosis). Direct infiltration of the optic nerve may occur in hematologic malignancies (eg, leukemia). See BCSC Section 5, *Neuro-Ophthalmology,* and Section 7, *Oculofacial Plastic and Orbital Surgery*, for more information on these entities. The discussion in the following sections focuses on the histologic features of the more common optic nerve neoplasms.

Melanocytoma

Melanocytoma of the ONH is a benign, heavily pigmented (dark-brown to jet-black) melanocytic tumor located eccentrically on the ONH and adjacent choroid (Fig 15-12A; see also Chapter 17). It may be elevated and extend into the adjacent retina or extend posteriorly into the optic nerve. Melanocytomas may grow slowly, but malignant transformation

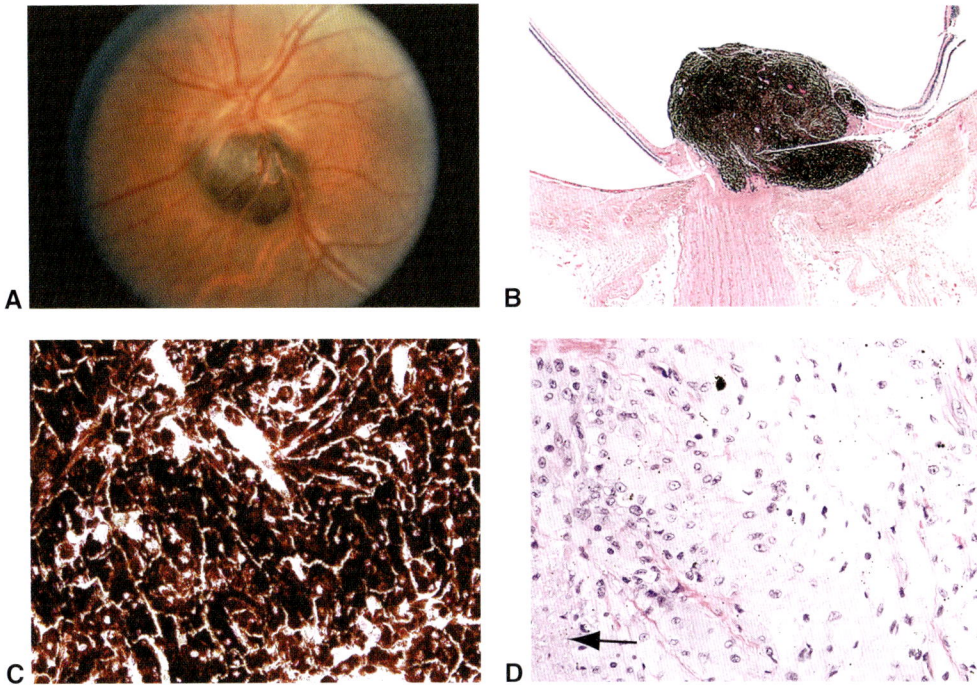

Figure 15-12 Melanocytoma of the optic nerve. **A,** Fundus photograph shows a dark mass on the inferior edge of the ONH. **B,** Low-magnification photomicrograph of melanocytoma shows a dome-shaped, jet-black mass involving the prelaminar optic nerve. The tumor also involves the juxtapapillary choroid and retina. **C,** Higher magnification shows darkly pigmented polyhedral melanocytes with dense intracytoplasmic pigment obscuring nuclear detail. **D,** Melanin bleach preparation shows the bland nuclear morphology and abundant cytoplasm of melanocytoma cells. Note the area of necrosis within the tumor *(arrow)*. *(Part A courtesy of Robert H. Rosa Jr, MD; parts B–D courtesy of Tatyana Milman, MD.)*

to melanoma is rare. Histologically, melanocytoma is a magnocellular nevus, composed of closely packed, heavily pigmented, plump polyhedral melanocytes. The dense pigment obscures nuclear detail (Fig 15-12B, C), so melanin bleach preparations (Fig 15-12D) are necessary to reveal the bland cytologic features, such as abundant cytoplasm, small nuclei with finely dispersed chromatin, and inconspicuous nucleoli. Necrosis and histiocytic infiltration are sometimes observed within melanocytoma and are not necessarily indicative of aggressive behavior. See also Chapters 12 and 17.

Glioma

A glioma (astrocytoma) may arise in any part of the visual pathway, including the ONH and optic nerve. Optic nerve gliomas are frequently associated with neurofibromatosis 1 (NF1). The tumors are low-grade juvenile pilocytic astrocytomas and commonly present in the first decade of life. Histologic examination of juvenile pilocytic astrocytoma shows proliferation of spindle-shaped astrocytes with delicate, hairlike (pilocytic) cytoplasmic processes that expand the optic nerve parenchyma (Fig 15-13). Enlarged, strongly eosinophilic filaments,

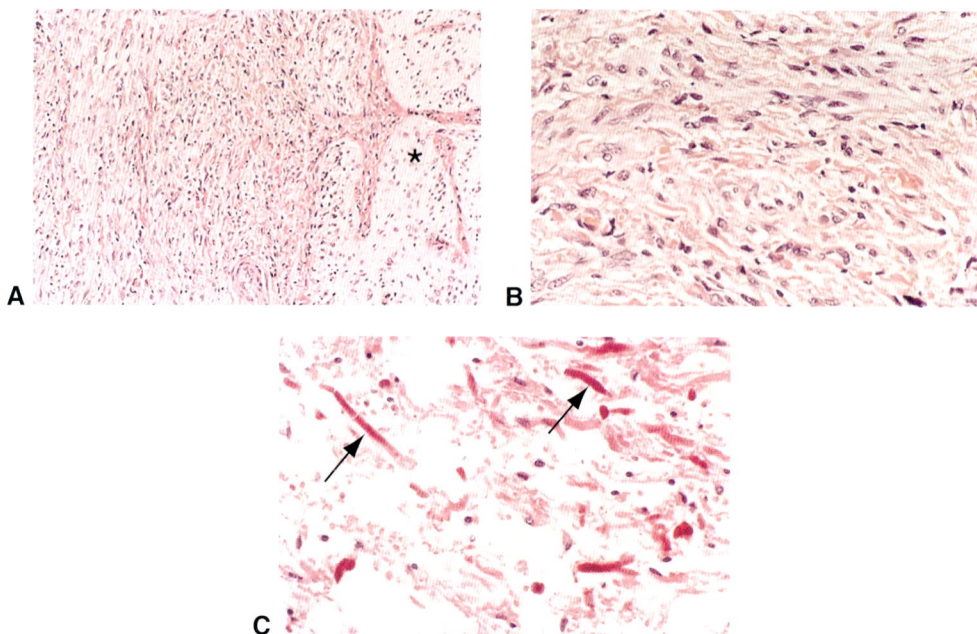

Figure 15-13 Astrocytoma of the optic nerve. **A,** The right side of this photomicrograph demonstrates a normal optic nerve *(asterisk);* the left side shows a pilocytic astrocytoma, which is more cellular in appearance. **B,** The neoplastic glial cells are elongated to resemble hairs (hence the term *pilocytic*). **C,** Degenerating eosinophilic filaments, known as *Rosenthal fibers (arrows),* may be observed in these tumors.

known as *Rosenthal fibers,* may be found in these tumors and represent degenerating cell processes (see Fig 15-13C). In addition, calcification and foci of microcystoid degeneration can be seen; the pial septa may be thickened. The meninges show reactive hyperplasia and astrocyte infiltration. Because the dura remains intact, the nerve exhibits fusiform or sausage-shaped enlargement within the sheath.

High-grade tumors (*grade IV astrocytomas,* also known as *glioblastoma multiforme*) rarely involve the optic nerve; when involvement of the optic nerve does occur, it usually is due to a primary brain tumor. Primary malignant glioma of the anterior visual pathway is rare and occurs mainly in adults. It is characterized histologically by nuclear pleomorphism, high mitotic activity, necrosis, and hemorrhage.

Meningioma

Primary optic nerve sheath meningiomas arise from the arachnoid layer of the optic nerve sheath (Fig 15-14). They are less common than secondary orbital meningiomas, which extend into the orbit from a primary intracranial site, usually through the sphenoid bone. Although optic nerve glioma is a more frequent hallmark of NF1, meningioma may also occasionally be associated with neurofibromatosis in younger patients. Primary optic nerve sheath meningiomas may invade the nerve and eye and, in rare cases, may extend through the dura to invade the orbit and extraocular muscles.

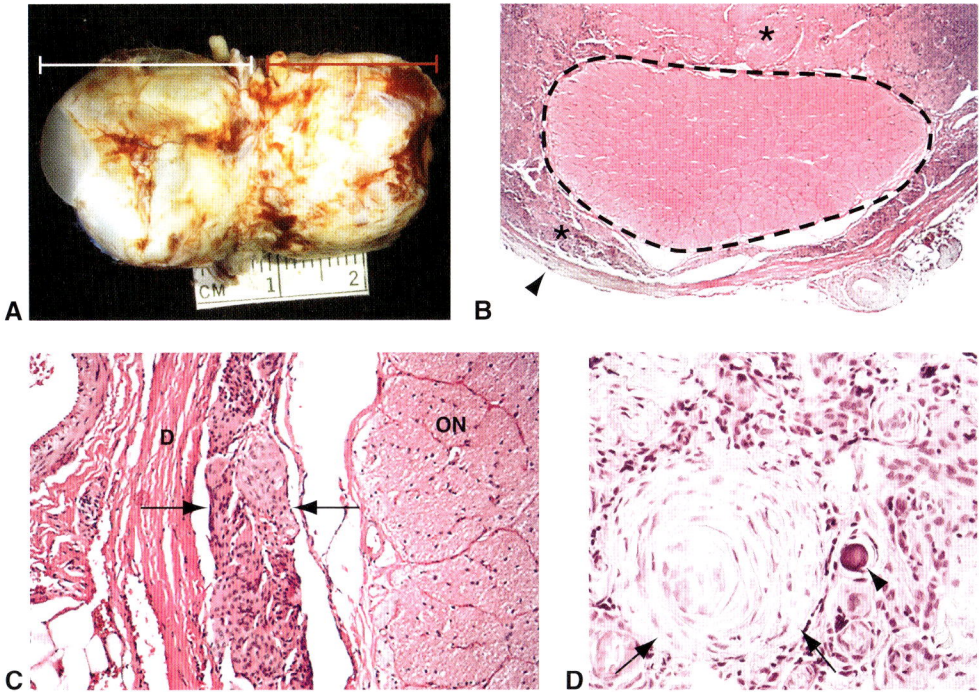

Figure 15-14 Optic nerve sheath meningioma. **A,** Gross photograph showing a globe *(white bracket)* with massive thickening *(red bracket)* of the optic nerve and sheath just posterior to the sclera, secondary to meningioma. **B,** This meningioma *(asterisks;* different from that shown in part A) has grown circumferentially around the optic nerve (outlined by *dashed line*), compressing and deforming it *(arrowhead* indicates the dura). **C,** Meningioma *(between arrows)* of the optic nerve sheath originates from the arachnoid layer of the meningeal sheath. D = dura; ON = optic nerve. **D,** High magnification of meningioma. Note the characteristic tumor whorl *(arrows)*. A calcified psammoma body is present adjacent to the whorl *(arrowhead)*. *(Parts A and D courtesy of Nasreen A. Syed, MD.)*

Histologically, the tumor (primary or secondary) is usually meningothelial, composed of plump cells with indistinct cytoplasmic margins (also called a *syncytial growth pattern*) arranged in whorls (see Fig 15-14D). *Psammoma bodies,* extracellular rounded calcifications surrounded by a cluster of meningioma cells, are variably present (see Fig 15-14D). Meningiomas are usually positive with the immunohistochemical stains epithelial membrane antigen (EMA) and somatostatin receptor 2a (SSTR-2). In addition, they also tend to express progesterone receptors.

PART II

Intraocular Tumors: Clinical Aspects

CHAPTER 16

Introduction to Part II

Intraocular tumors make up a broad spectrum of benign and malignant lesions that can lead to loss of vision and/or loss of life. Effective management of these lesions depends on accurate diagnosis. In most cases, experienced ophthalmologists diagnose intraocular neoplasms via clinical examination and ancillary diagnostic tests. When evaluating a patient with a tumor, the ophthalmologist should have sufficient knowledge to make an accurate diagnosis or at least to develop a differential diagnosis. In addition, there should be a low threshold for referral to a specialist when the diagnosis is not clear or treatment involves complex therapies and/or a multispecialty approach.

In the past 4 decades, significant advances have been made in understanding the biology of intraocular tumors and in managing these lesions. The Collaborative Ocular Melanoma Study (COMS) gathered important information concerning the most common primary intraocular malignant tumor in adults, choroidal melanoma. The study incorporated both randomized clinical trials for patients with medium and large choroidal melanomas and an observational study for patients with small choroidal melanomas. The COMS reported outcomes for enucleation versus brachytherapy for the treatment of medium-sized tumors and for enucleation alone versus enucleation preceded by external beam radiotherapy for large melanomas. In addition to the study's primary objectives, which were to evaluate the mortality outcomes after enucleation and globe-sparing radiotherapy for uveal melanoma, the COMS provided data regarding local tumor failure rates and visual acuity outcomes after iodine 125 brachytherapy. The results confirmed that eye-sparing plaque brachytherapy for well-selected patients does not adversely affect melanoma-related morbidity or mortality. The most common form of treatment for uveal melanoma is now eye-sparing radiation.

In recent years, there have been several other advances in the understanding and management of choroidal melanoma. Researchers have identified key cytogenetic aberrations that are associated with metastatic disease, including monosomy of chromosome 3, especially with gains in chromosome 8. Gene expression profile testing, another molecular technique, is highly predictive for late metastasis in uveal melanoma. Both forms of prognostic testing require tumor sampling obtained through fine-needle aspiration biopsy (FNAB) of the tumor or evaluation of paraffin-embedded tissue. Information gained from FNAB is useful for tumor prognostication and identification of patients at high risk for distant metastasis.

Retinoblastoma, the most common primary intraocular cancer in children, is most often caused by a mutation in the tumor suppressor gene *RB1*, which was isolated, cloned, and sequenced in the 1980s (the first tumor suppressor gene ever sequenced). As with choroidal melanoma, treatment of retinoblastoma has transitioned toward globe-conserving therapy with chemotherapy and local treatments, including laser therapy and cryotherapy. The trend away from external beam radiotherapy and toward chemotherapy has been fueled, in part, by growing recognition of the former's potential risk for increasing the incidence of second nonocular malignancies in children who harbor a germline mutation in the retinoblastoma gene. Advances in understanding the molecular genetics of retinoblastoma continue to enhance clinicians' ability not only to screen for this tumor in families with retinoblastoma, but also to provide appropriate counseling (see Chapter 19).

In the United States and Europe, most malignancies are staged using the classification system developed by the American Joint Committee on Cancer (AJCC). The AJCC system stages cancer in patients based on tumor size, lymph node status, and distant metastasis. Both clinical and pathologic data may be used to clinically stage a tumor. It is an important distinction that patients—not just a single organ, such as the eye—are staged. For certain tumors, such as retinoblastoma, other systems are used to stratify the level of disease within the eye and the risk of loss of the eye.

As with many other pathologic conditions of the eye, intraocular tumors may result in irreversible vision loss. Patient education and, if appropriate, referral for vision rehabilitation can be considered before loss of function and independence occur. The American Academy of Ophthalmology's Initiative in Vision Rehabilitation page on the ONE Network (www.aao.org/low-vision-and-vision-rehab) provides resources for low vision management, including patient handouts, and information about additional vision rehabilitation opportunities beyond those provided by the ophthalmologist.

CHAPTER 17

Melanocytic Tumors

▶ *This chapter includes related videos. Go to www.aao.org/bcscvideo_section04 or scan the QR codes in the text to access this content.*

Highlights

- Uveal melanomas may develop in the iris, ciliary body, or choroid. Ciliary body and choroidal melanomas carry a worse prognosis than iris melanomas because of their substantially higher risk for metastasis. The spread of uveal melanomas is typically hematogenous.
- Signs suggestive of iris melanoma include large size, prominent ectropion uveae, intratumoral vascularity, sectoral cataract, secondary glaucoma, seeding of the iris stroma and peripheral angle structures, extrascleral extension, and documented progressive growth.
- Because of the risk for malignant transformation, iris and choroidal nevi should be documented with photographs and observed for growth. Nevi of the ciliary body are infrequent in general and are often not identified clinically because of their location (ie, they are not typically visible on clinical examination).
- Posterior uveal melanomas arising from the ciliary body and choroid are associated with a high mortality rate. Referral to an ocular oncologist should be considered for patients with tumors displaying features suggestive of malignancy.
- Large ciliary body and choroidal melanomas may be associated with vision loss due to serous retinal detachment or vitreous hemorrhage; however, many uveal melanomas are asymptomatic.
- Features suggestive of choroidal melanoma include large size, presence of subretinal fluid, surface lipofuscin, vision symptoms, and documented growth.
- Uveal melanomas may be treated with enucleation, brachytherapy or proton beam therapy, or excision, depending on the size and location of the tumor.

Introduction

Intraocular melanocytic tumors develop from uveal melanocytes in the iris, ciliary body, and choroid. The 2 main groups of melanocytic tumors of the uveal tract (uvea) are benign nevi and melanomas. In contrast to melanocytic cancers of the skin and mucosal membranes, which usually initially spread through the lymphatics, melanocytic malignancies of the uvea that metastasize typically do so hematogenously. Pigmented intraocular tumors that originate from the pigmented epithelium of the iris, ciliary body, and retina constitute another group of melanin-containing tumors of neuroepithelial origin. These rare tumors are discussed separately at the end of this chapter. See also Chapter 12.

Iris Nevus

An iris nevus is a variably pigmented lesion of the iris stroma that causes minimal distortion of the iris architecture. It is a benign tumor, likely congenital in origin, that contains increased numbers of specialized melanocytes (nevus cells). Many of these lesions are small, produce no symptoms, and are recognized incidentally during routine ophthalmic examination. Their prevalence is uncertain, although iris nevi are thought to occur more frequently in patients with neurofibromatosis type I.

Iris nevi should be distinguished from iris freckles, which are flat lesions associated with an increased amount of melanin within cells and are not tumors (Fig 17-1A). Iris freckles may be associated with ultraviolet (UV) light exposure and are more prevalent in elderly individuals. Although iris freckles have no malignant potential, numerous iris freckles may be associated with increased risk for cutaneous melanoma, which is similarly associated with an elevated lifetime exposure to UV light. Individuals with more than 3 iris freckles may benefit from routine skin evaluation by a dermatologist.

Ophthalmoscopically, iris nevi present in 2 forms: (1) *circumscribed iris nevi,* which are flat to nodular, solitary or multiple, involving a discrete portion of the iris; and (2) *diffuse iris nevi,* which may involve an entire sector or, in rare instances, the entire iris. Iris nevi may cause ectropion uveae (Fig 17-1B) and, occasionally, a sectoral cataract.

Iris nevi are best evaluated by slit-lamp biomicroscopy coupled with gonioscopy. The clinician should pay specific attention to lesions involving the angle in order to rule out a ciliary body tumor, as the most important differential diagnosis is iris or ciliary body melanoma. High-frequency ultrasound biomicroscopy (UBM) is helpful in the evaluation of lesions that involve the angle as it can depict a ciliary body component. Examples of the clinical appearance of iris freckles and nevi are shown on page 306 in Figure 17-1.

Iris nevi do not usually require treatment beyond observation, including photographic documentation.

Iris Melanoma

Iris melanomas account for 3%–5% of all uveal melanomas (Fig 17-2; see p. 307). Small melanomas of the iris may be challenging to clinically differentiate from benign iris nevi.

Iris melanomas range in appearance from amelanotic (off-white) to dark-brown lesions, and three-quarters of them involve the inferior iris (see Fig 17-2A, C, D). In rare cases, their growth pattern is diffuse, resulting in unilateral acquired hyperchromic heterochromia (darker iris) and secondary glaucoma. One subtype grows in a pattern that resembles tapioca pudding (see Fig 17-2D, F).

Clinical evaluation of iris melanoma is identical to that for iris nevi. Signs suggesting malignancy include large size, prominent ectropion uveae and intratumoral vascularity (see Fig 17-2D), sectoral cataract, secondary glaucoma, seeding of the iris stroma (see Fig 17-2B) and peripheral angle structures, extrascleral extension, and documented progressive growth. The differential diagnosis of iris melanoma is listed in Table 17-1 and pictured in Figure 17-3.

Advances in high-frequency ultrasonography (echography) enable excellent characterization of iris tumor size and anatomical relationship to normal ocular structures (see Figs 17-1G, H and 17-2G, H). Anterior segment optical coherence tomography (OCT) may be helpful, but commercially available instrumentation often does not penetrate to the level of the posterior iris. Iris fluorescein angiography may document intrinsic vascularity; however, this finding is of limited value in narrowing the differential diagnosis. Biopsy may be considered when the diagnosis is not clear.

When there is documented growth or secondary glaucoma occurs, diagnostic/therapeutic excision of an iris melanoma is indicated. Alternatively, brachytherapy (radioactive plaque) or proton beam therapy may be used, particularly for larger lesions.

The prognosis for most patients with iris melanoma is excellent; the mortality rate is low (1%–4%), possibly because the tumor is usually small and likely because its biological behavior is distinct from that of ciliary body and choroidal melanomas. The main risk factor for metastatic death is invasion of the anterior chamber angle, which may present as poorly controlled glaucoma, mimicking pigmentary glaucoma.

Hau SC, Papastefanou V, Shah S, Sagoo MS, Restori M, Cohen V. Evaluation of iris and iridociliary body lesions with anterior segment optical coherence tomography versus ultrasound B-scan. *Br J Ophthalmol.* 2015;99(1):81–86.

Henderson E, Margo CE. Iris melanoma. *Arch Pathol Lab Med.* 2008;132(2):268–272.

Jakobiec FA, Silbert G. Are most iris 'melanomas' really nevi? A clinicopathologic study of 189 lesions. *Arch Ophthalmol.* 1981;99(12):2117–2132.

Khan S, Finger PT, Yu GP, et al. Clinical and pathologic characteristics of biopsy-proven iris melanoma: a multicenter international study. *Arch Ophthalmol.* 2012;130(1):57–64.

Laino AM, Berry EG, Jagirdar K, et al. Iris pigmented lesions as a marker of cutaneous melanoma risk: an Australian case-control study. *Br J Dermatol.* 2018;178(5):1119–1127.

Ciliary Body and Choroidal Nevi

Nevi of the ciliary body are rare, mostly small, and often first identified in histologic examination of globes enucleated for other reasons. Choroidal nevi may occur in up to 8% of the population (Fig 17-4; see p. 310). Similar to iris nevi, in most cases they cause no symptoms and are recognized incidentally on routine ophthalmic examination. Ophthalmoscopically, the typical choroidal nevus appears as a flat or minimally elevated, pigmented (gray to brown) choroidal lesion with soft margins (see Fig 17-4A–E). Some nevi are amelanotic (see Fig 17-4F).

Choroidal nevi are often associated with overlying retinal pigment epithelium (RPE) disturbance and drusen (see Fig 17-4A, D). These features are characteristic of a

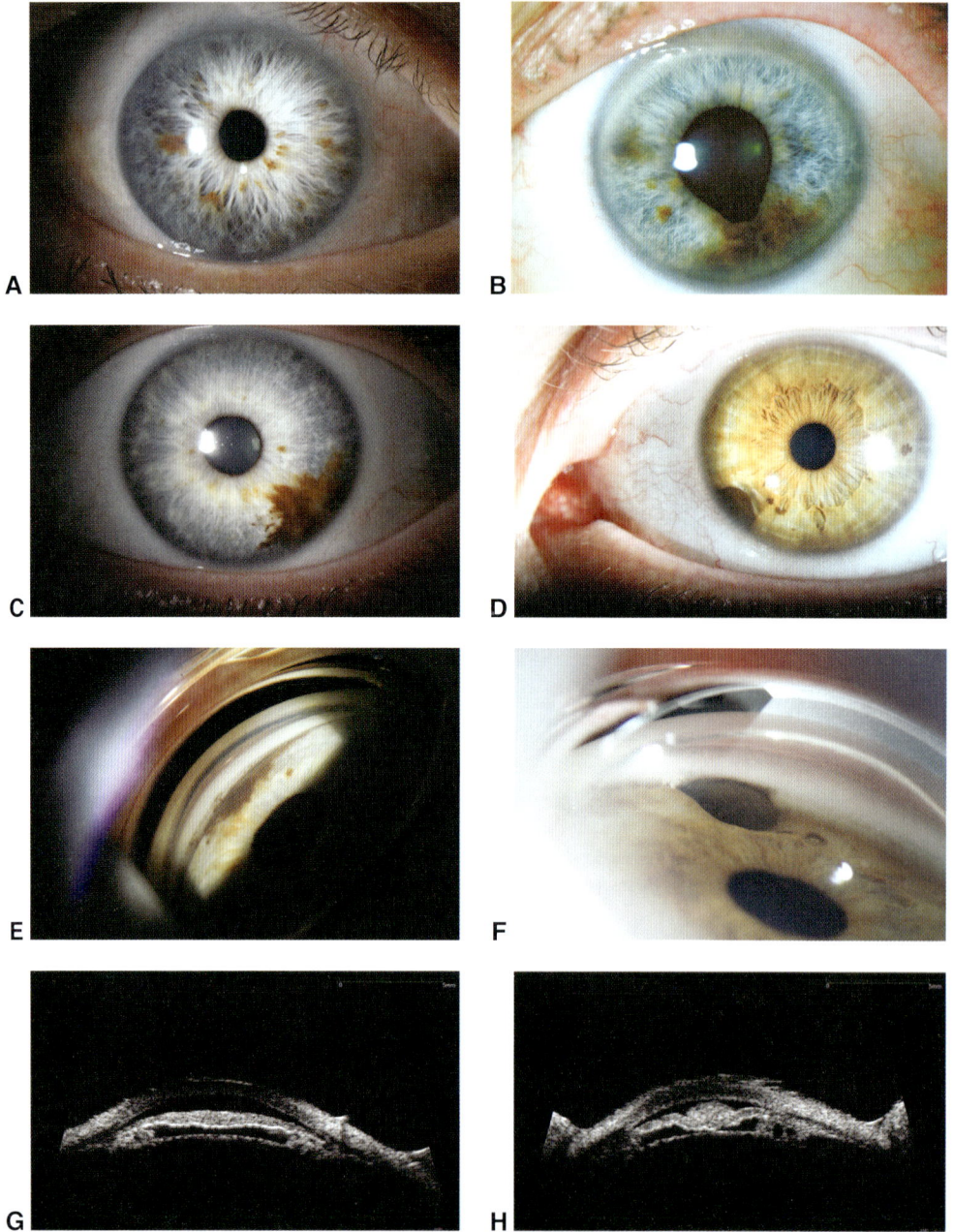

Figure 17-1 Benign iris melanocytic lesions, clinical appearance. **A,** Iris freckles are flat and often multiple. **B–D,** Iris nevi have a variable appearance and may be flat **(B, C)** or nodular **(D).** They may cause ectropion uveae **(B).** **C–H,** The slit-lamp **(C, D),** gonioscopic **(E, F),** and ultrasound biomicroscopic (UBM) **(G, H)** appearances of 2 long-standing iris nevi are shown. The lesion shown in parts **C, E,** and **G** is flat and diffuse and has remained stable for 15 years. The lesion shown in parts **D, F,** and **H** is nodular and has remained stable for 20 years. *(Parts A and C–H courtesy of Alison Skalet, MD, PhD; part B courtesy of Tero Kivelä, MD.)*

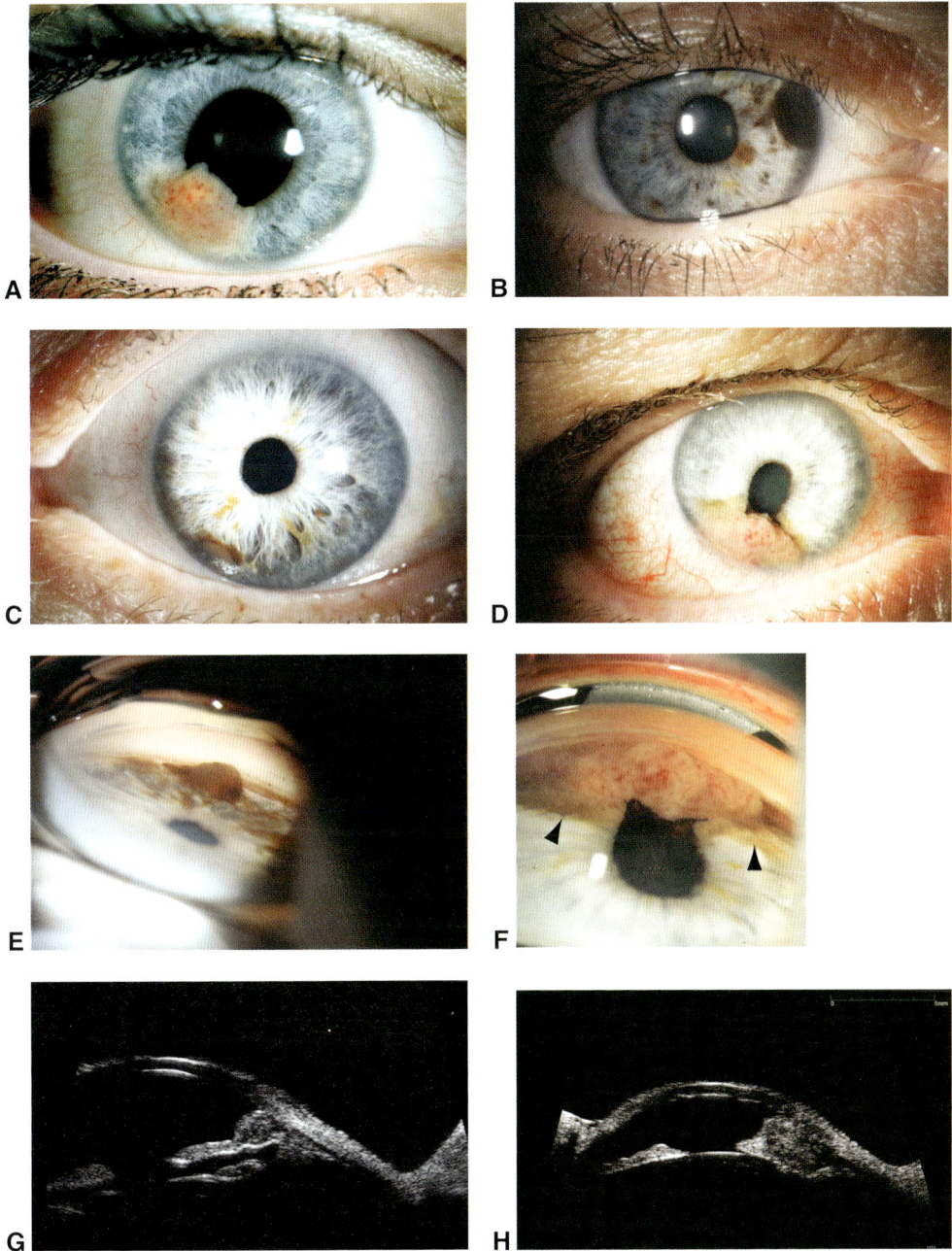

Figure 17-2 Iris melanoma, clinical appearance. **A,** The lesion can be amelanotic with visible intrinsic vascularity. **B,** Alternatively, it may be densely pigmented, obscuring any blood vessels (note the dispersed pigment on the iris stroma). **C–H,** The slit-lamp **(C, D),** gonioscopic **(E, F),** and UBM **(G, H)** appearances of 2 iris melanomas are shown. The melanoma shown in parts **C, E,** and **G** is a small nodular tumor involving the anterior chamber angle; fine-needle aspiration biopsy revealed a melanoma composed of mainly epithelioid cells. The tumor shown in parts **D, F,** and **H** is a large amelanotic melanoma with prominent vascularity. Note the flat pigmented portion of the tumor (*arrowheads* in part **F**) along the edges of the mass surrounding the amelanotic portion. *(Part A courtesy of Tero Kivelä, MD; parts B–H courtesy of Alison Skalet, MD, PhD.)*

Table 17-1 **Differential Diagnosis of Iris Melanoma**

Iris freckle (see Fig 17-1A)
Iris nevus (see Fig 17-1B–H)
Primary iris cyst (pigment epithelial or stromal) (see Fig 17-3A)
Iris melanocytoma
Lisch nodules (in neurofibromatosis, variably pigmented, multiple, small, flat, or nodular lesions) (see Fig 17-3B)
Congenital ocular or oculodermal melanocytosis (diffuse iris nevus) (see Figs 17-3D and 17-4G, H)
Iridocorneal endothelial (ICE) syndrome (Cogan-Reese iris nevus type)
Iris pigment epithelial proliferation (epithelial downgrowth after trauma or surgery)
Iris foreign body (secondarily pigmented)
Juvenile xanthogranuloma (amelanotic or tan colored)
Retained lens material simulating iris nodule (amelanotic)
Metastatic carcinoma to the iris (amelanotic) (see Fig 17-3C)

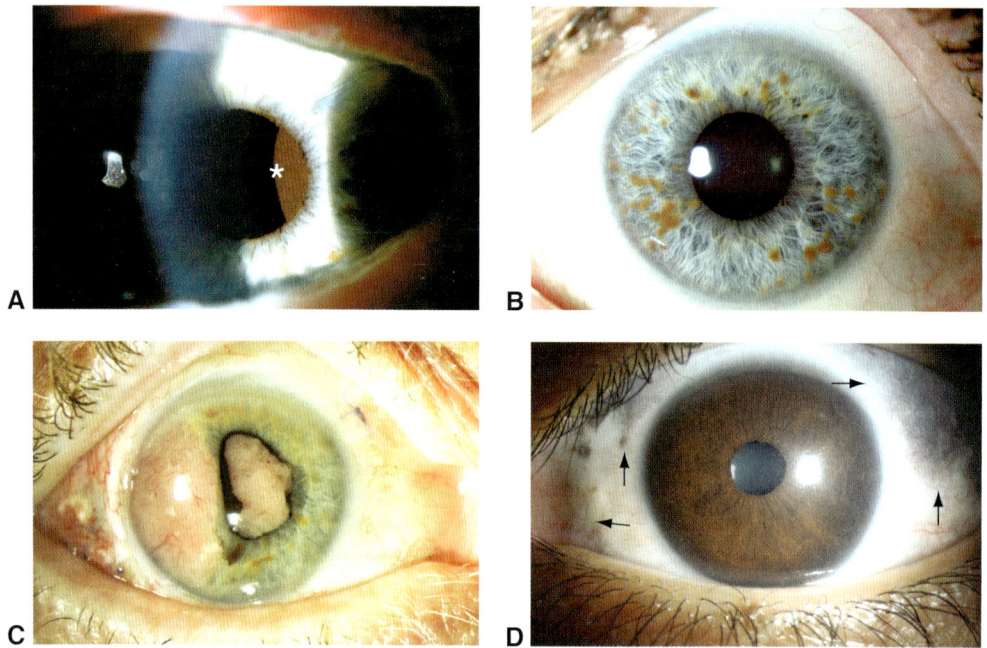

Figure 17-3 Differential diagnosis of iris melanoma. **A,** A pigment epithelial cyst *(asterisk)* can bow the iris forward focally. The cyst is visible after dilation. **B,** Multiple Lisch nodules in neurofibromatosis. Lisch nodules are melanocytic hamartomas that are typically tan to golden brown. **C,** Metastasis from a pulmonary carcinoma seen as an amelanotic mass on the temporal half of the iris and inside the pupil. The tumor distorts the pupil shape. **D,** Congenital ocular melanocytosis can cause a diffuse iris nevus but is associated with pigmented patches on the episclera and sclera *(arrows)*. Note the deeply pigmented, velvety stromal thickening in the iris. *(Parts A and B courtesy of Tero Kivelä, MD; parts C and D courtesy of Alison Skalet, MD, PhD.)*

long-standing, quiescent lesion. A minority develop atypical features such as localized serous retinal detachment over and around the nevus (see the section Melanoma of the Choroid and Ciliary Body), surface lipofuscin (see Fig 17-4E, F), or choroidal neovascular membranes. These atypical nevi may result in reduced vision, metamorphopsia, and visual field defects. Although these clinical features can be seen in the context of a benign lesion, they should also raise suspicion for malignant transformation, and careful follow-up for progression and lesion growth is indicated.

In the choroid, congenital ocular melanocytosis is similar in appearance to a diffuse nevus (see Fig 17-4G). This condition increases the lifetime risk for ciliary body and choroidal melanoma (1 in 400).

Findings on fluorescein angiography are not usually helpful for diagnosis; choroidal nevi may demonstrate either hypofluorescence or hyperfluorescence. Nevi are distinguished from choroidal melanomas and other pigmented fundus lesions by clinical evaluation and multimodal imaging, as described in the section Melanoma of the Choroid and Ciliary Body.

The management of choroidal nevi includes photographic documentation of all lesions; ultrasonographic measurement of lesions thicker than 1 mm; and lifelong, periodic reassessment for signs of growth or change consistent with transformation into choroidal melanoma (Fig 17-5). OCT can be helpful in excluding the presence of subclinical subretinal fluid.

Benign nevi may increase in diameter in the absence of malignant transformation. In a long-term study of choroidal nevi, nevi enlarged a median of 1 mm overall, but the median yearly rate of enlargement was less than 0.1 mm, and none of the enlarging nevi developed new orange pigment or subretinal fluid. Frequency of enlargement was reported to be 54% in patients younger than 40 years and 19% in patients older than 60 years. If rapid or more extensive enlargement is documented, especially in patients older than 40 years, malignant transformation should be suspected (Fig 17-6).

Mashayekhi A, Siu S, Shields CL, Shields JA. Slow enlargement of choroidal nevi: a long-term follow-up study. *Ophthalmology.* 2011;118(2):382–388.

Shields CL, Furuta M, Berman EL, et al. Choroidal nevus transformation into melanoma: analysis of 2514 consecutive cases. *Arch Ophthalmol.* 2009;127(8):981–987.

Melanocytoma of the Iris, Ciliary Body, and Choroid

Melanocytomas (magnocellular nevi) are rare tumors composed of characteristically large, polyhedral melanocytic cells that have small, bland nuclei and abundant cytoplasm filled with large melanin granules (see Chapter 15, Fig 15-12). Iris melanocytoma cells may seed to the anterior chamber angle, causing glaucoma. Melanocytomas of the ciliary body are usually not seen clinically because of their peripheral location. In some cases, extrascleral extension of a melanocytoma along an emissary canal appears as a darkly pigmented, fixed subconjunctival mass. Melanocytomas of the choroid appear as elevated, pigmented tumors, similar to a nevus or a melanoma. Malignant changes have been reported in some melanocytomas.

When a melanocytoma is suspected, photographic and ultrasonographic studies are appropriate. If growth is documented, biopsy should be considered to exclude melanoma.

Shields CL, Kaliki S, Hutchinson A, et al. Iris nevus growth into melanoma: analysis of 1611 consecutive eyes: the ABCDEF guide. *Ophthalmology.* 2013;120(4):766–772.

Shields JA, Shields CL, Eagle RC Jr. Melanocytoma (hyperpigmented magnocellular nevus) of the uveal tract: the 34th G. Victor Simpson lecture. *Retina.* 2007;27(6):730–739.

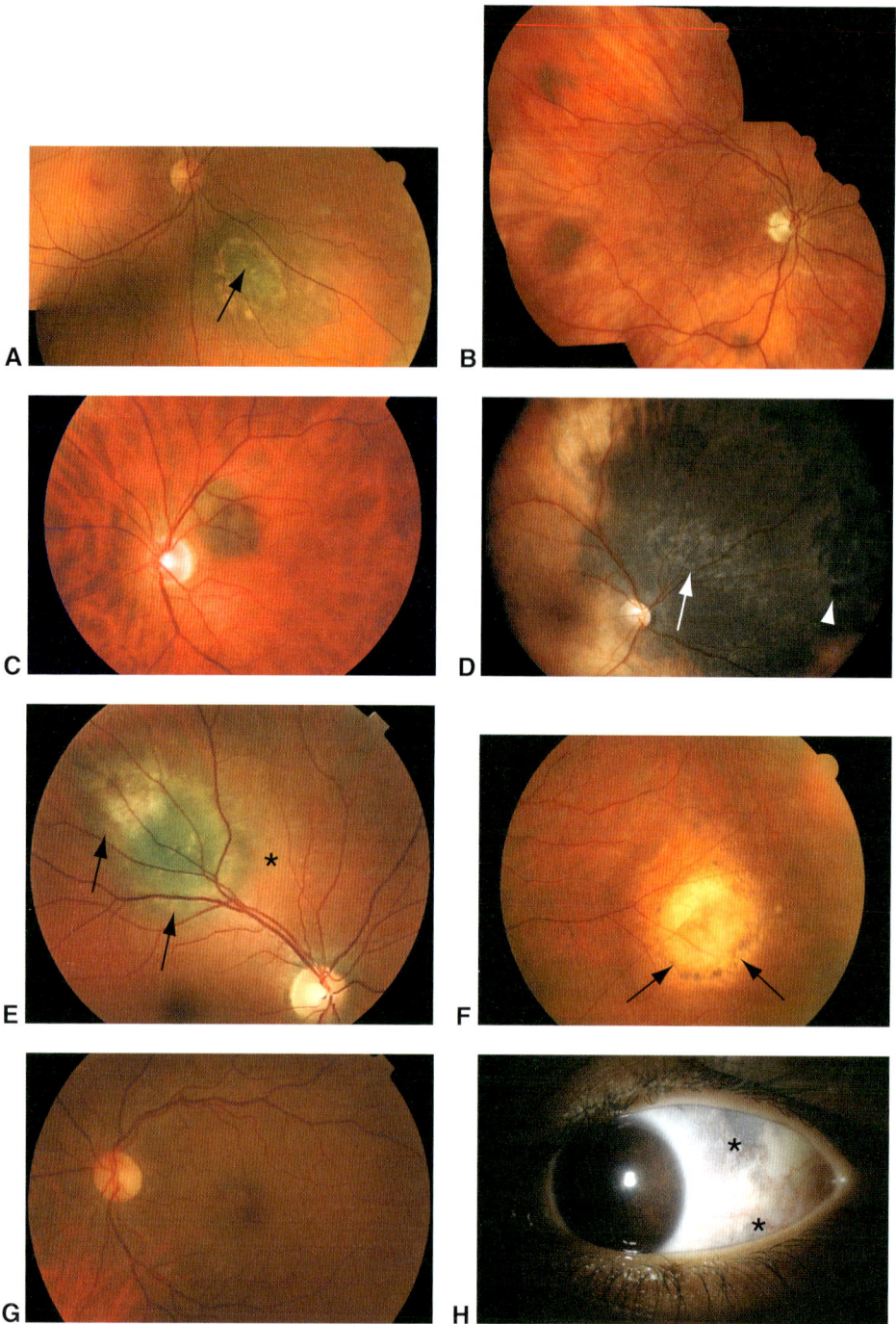

Figure 17-4 Choroidal nevi, clinical appearance. Choroidal nevi are generally thinner than 2 mm and variably brown. They may be solitary **(A)** or multiple **(B)**. Nevi may demonstrate drusen on their surface **(A,** *arrow*). **C,** Small nevi lack retinal pigment epithelial (RPE) changes. **D,** Large nevi usually exhibit RPE changes (note the drusen *[arrow]* and focal RPE hyperplasia *[arrowhead]*). **E–F,** Some nevi display surface lipofuscin, which appears as orange pigment on dark tumors **(E,** *arrows*), and pigmented melanolipofuscin on amelanotic tumors **(F,** *arrows*) and can be associated with subretinal fluid **(E,** *asterisk*). **G,** Congenital ocular melanocytosis has a diffuse nevus-like dark choroidal appearance. **H,** Appearance of patchy gray sclera *(asterisks)* and diffuse iris pigmentation associated with ocular melanocytosis. All of the lesions illustrated in this figure were followed for several years without evidence of growth. *(Parts A, B, F, and H courtesy of Alison Skalet, MD, PhD; parts C–E and G courtesy of Tero Kivelä, MD.)*

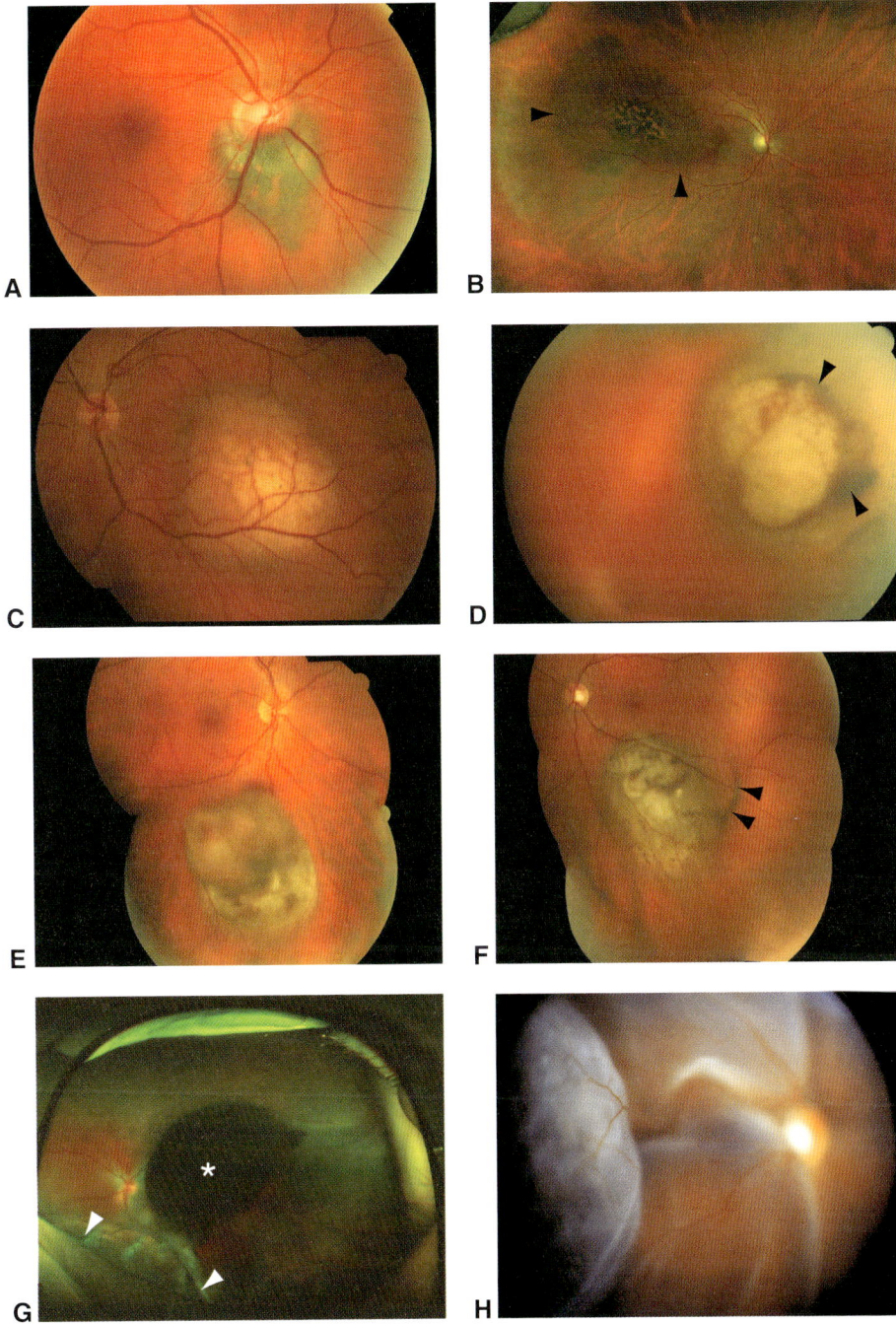

Figure 17-5 Choroidal melanoma, clinical appearance. **A, B,** Choroidal melanomas may be quite thin. Note the prominent surface lipofuscin in each case and the large area of flat involvement surrounding the elevated portion centrally in part **B** *(arrowheads);* however, they are more commonly elevated (>2 mm in height). Melanomas are usually pigmented **(A, B, E, F)** or, less commonly, amelanotic **(C, D).** Smaller melanomas typically have a dome shape, whereas larger tumors that have broken through Bruch membrane have a collar-button configuration **(D, E).** This is often accompanied by subretinal hemorrhage **(D,** *arrowheads).* **F,** Retinal invasion and vitreous seeding of a tumor may occur, with seeding seen as a dark streak *(arrowheads).* **G, H,** Very large tumors may be associated with large serous retinal detachments. In part **G,** the tumor apex is darkly pigmented *(asterisk),* and the retinal detachment is seen at the lower left *(arrowheads). (Parts A and H courtesy of Tero Kivelä, MD; parts B–G courtesy of Alison Skalet, MD, PhD.)*

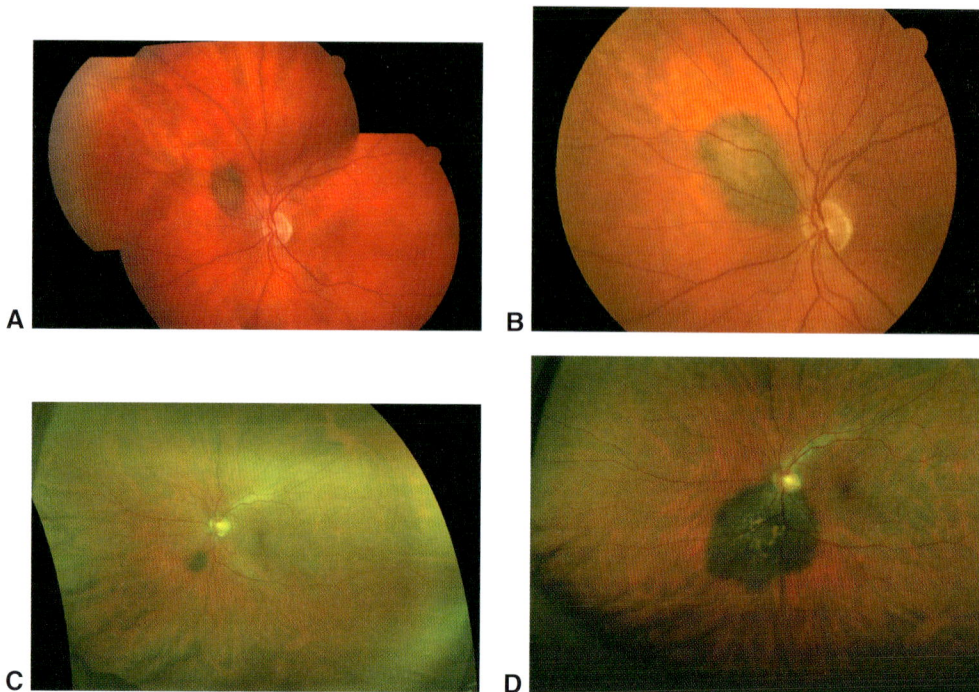

Figure 17-6 Malignant transformation of choroidal nevus to melanoma. **A,** Small choroidal nevus. **B,** After an observation period of 13 months, the nevus has expanded its borders and acquired surface lipofuscin. **C,** A different patient with a small peripapillary choroidal nevus. **D,** The nevus shown in part **C** demonstrated substantial growth and emergence of surface lipofuscin after an observation period of 6.5 years. *(Courtesy of Alison Skalet, MD, PhD.)*

Melanoma of the Choroid and Ciliary Body

Choroidal and ciliary body melanomas (posterior uveal melanomas) are the most common primary intraocular malignancies in adults. Approximately 6700–7100 new cases of uveal melanomas are reported annually worldwide, of which 65% affect non-Hispanic whites; 87,000–106,000 survivors are under follow-up care. The incidence varies by age, ethnicity, and latitude. The incidence based on ethnicity ranges from 0.4 cases per million people of Asian descent to 1.7 cases per million in Hispanics and 6.0 cases per million in non-Hispanic whites. Among whites, the incidence is higher in those living in regions at higher latitudes. From south to north, the incidence increases from 4.6 to 7.5 cases per million, respectively, in the United States and from 2.6 to 8.4 cases per million, respectively, in Europe.

Fewer than 1% of choroidal and ciliary body melanomas are diagnosed in children younger than 18 years. Approximately 80% of choroidal and ciliary body melanomas are found in adults between 45 and 80 years of age. In the United States and Europe, the mean age at diagnosis is 60–65 years, whereas in Asia it is 45–50 years.

Additional risk factors for posterior uveal melanoma include the following:

- light complexion (light skin, blue eyes, blond hair) and an inability to tan
- ocular melanocytic abnormalities including nevi (lifetime risk = 1 in 500) and congenital ocular and oculodermal melanocytosis (lifetime risk = 1 in 400)

- dysplastic nevus syndrome (three-fold risk)
- *BAP1* germline mutation or other genetic predisposition

The role of UV radiation as a risk factor for posterior melanoma remains unclear, although most studies conclude that UV light does not play a role. UV light may even be protective because it increases production of vitamin D, which is thought to lower the risk of cancers in tissues not exposed to direct sunlight.

Krantz BA, Dave N, Komatsubara KM, Marr BP, Carvajal RD. Uveal melanoma: epidemiology, etiology, and treatment of primary disease. *Clin Ophthalmol.* 2017;11:279–289.

Clinical Characteristics

The typical *choroidal melanoma* is a variably pigmented, elevated, dome-shaped mass (see Fig 17-5). Initial symptoms and signs may deceptively resemble those of vitreous detachment, although metamorphopsia, reduced vision, and a visual field defect from direct tumor growth or secondary retinal detachment may eventually develop depending on the location of the tumor. In many patients, however, choroidal melanomas are asymptomatic and are identified incidentally on routine dilated eye examination. Significant growth of a preexisting choroidal nevus or emergence of surface lipofuscin or subretinal fluid should prompt concern for malignant transformation into melanoma (see Fig 17-6).

The degree of pigmentation ranges from amelanotic to dark brown. At the RPE level, clumps of lipofuscin may be present over the surface of smaller tumors (see Figs 17-5A, B and 17-6B, D). Surface lipofuscin appears orange on pigmented tumors but is dark on amelanotic tumors. Localized subretinal fluid is common with melanomas, and larger tumors may be associated with more extensive serous detachment of the neurosensory retina (see Fig 17-5G, H). With time, 50% of tumors erupt through Bruch membrane and assume a mushroom or collar-button shape (see Fig 17-5D, E, G). This process may be associated with subretinal hemorrhage. Some tumors also erode through the retina, causing vitreous hemorrhage or vitreous seeding of a tumor (see Fig 17-5F). If extensive retinal detachment develops, anterior displacement of the lens–iris diaphragm and secondary angle-closure glaucoma occasionally occur. With larger tumors, neovascularization of the iris may occur.

Because they are located posterior to the iris, *ciliary body melanomas* often remain asymptomatic until they become rather large (Fig 17-7A). Symptoms and signs eventually include a dilated, often tortuous, episcleral vessel(s) (sentinel vessel) in the region of the tumor (Fig 17-7B); reduced vision from induced astigmatism or cataract when the tumor touches the lens; photopsia and visual field alterations from associated retinal detachment in more advanced cases; and, in rare cases, secondary glaucoma.

Ciliary body melanomas are not usually visible unless the pupil is widely dilated. Some erode through the iris root into the anterior chamber and become visible during gonioscopy (Fig 17-7C) or external examination (Fig 17-7D). Eventually, the tumor extends through the sclera along aqueous drainage channels, producing an epibulbar nodule (Fig 17-7E). Some ciliary body melanomas assume a diffuse growth pattern and extend up to 360° around the eye; in this case, they are known as *ring melanomas* (Fig 17-7F).

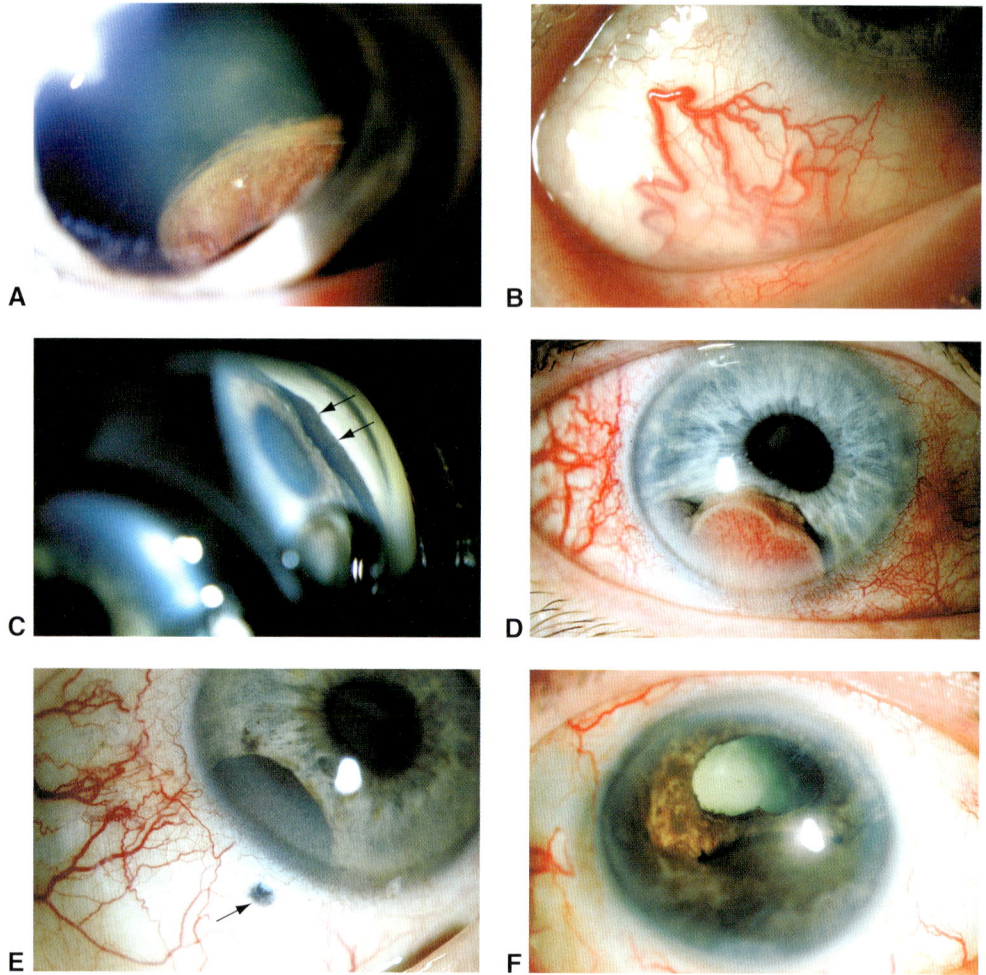

Figure 17-7 Ciliary body melanoma, clinical appearance. **A,** Ciliary tumors are often not evident unless the pupil is widely dilated. They may indent the lens. **B,** Sentinel episcleral vessels. **C,** Anterior extension of a ciliary body melanoma may be visible only with gonioscopy *(arrows).* **D,** The tumor may invade the anterior chamber. **E,** The tumor may extend through the sclera *(arrow)* via emissary channels. **F,** Ring melanoma grows circumferentially within the ciliary body and may extend into the anterior chamber. *(Courtesy of Tero Kivelä, MD.)*

Diagnostic Evaluation

Clinical evaluation of suspected posterior uveal melanomas includes obtaining a history (eg, personal and family histories of cancer), performing a full ophthalmic examination, and ordering multiple types of imaging studies (multimodal imaging) (Figs 17-8, 17-9; see pp. 316–317). When used appropriately, the tests described in this chapter enable accurate diagnosis of melanocytic tumors in most cases. Atypical lesions may need to be characterized via other testing modalities, including intraocular biopsy (see discussion later in this chapter and also in Chapter 3); alternatively, when appropriate, these lesions may be closely observed for characteristic changes in clinical behavior in order to establish a correct diagnosis.

The most important diagnostic technique for evaluating intraocular tumors is *indirect ophthalmoscopic examination*. It provides stereopsis and a wide field of view and facilitates visualization of the peripheral fundus, particularly when performed with scleral depression. Indirect ophthalmoscopy and wide-field fundus photography enable clinical assessment of tumor size and surface features. *Slit-lamp biomicroscopy* in combination with *gonioscopy* is the best method for clinically establishing the presence and extent of anterior involvement of the tumor (see Fig 17-7C), although high-frequency ultrasound biomicroscopy (UBM) also allows excellent visualization of anterior ocular structures (see Figs 17-1, 17-2). In addition, slit-lamp biomicroscopy enables a detailed assessment of surface features of posterior tumors, including the presence of lipofuscin, subretinal fluid, retinal tumor invasion, and vitreous involvement.

Multimodal imaging is the standard of care in the diagnosis and ongoing management of melanocytic tumors. *Fundus photography* is valuable for documenting the appearance of a choroidal tumor (see Figs 17-6A, B and 17-8A, B) and for identifying changes in its shape and basal dimensions over time (see Figs 17-6C, D and 17-8A, B). Wide-angle (60°–200°) fundus photographs (see Figs 17-6C, D and 17-9A, B) can reveal the full extent of many tumors and document their relationship to intraocular landmarks. Comparison with the optic disc can aid in approximating the size of tumors. The relative position of retinal blood vessels may be helpful markers of changes in the size of a lesion. Fundus photographs also allow clinicians to use intrinsic scales to measure the basal diameter of a choroidal melanoma.

Fundus autofluorescence (FAF) imaging helps highlight lipofuscin, which is brightly autofluorescent (see Fig 17-9C, D). In addition, recent leakage of subretinal fluid produces increased autofluorescence, whereas long-standing or past leakage may result in decreased autofluorescence from secondary RPE atrophy. *Enhanced depth imaging OCT* or *swept-source OCT* is helpful in developing the differential diagnosis because it can reveal degenerative RPE and photoreceptor changes in long-standing lesions, which are less likely to be small melanomas, as well as lipofuscin and subretinal fluid in suspicious melanocytic choroidal tumors.

Fluorescein angiography findings are not pathognomonic for choroidal melanoma but can be helpful in differentiating between tumors and hemorrhagic processes that may mimic tumors. *Indocyanine green angiography* is not more accurate than fluorescein angiography for diagnosis, but it does often show alterations in choroidal blood flow in the region of the tumor. However, neither technique is commonly used in diagnosing melanoma.

Standardized ultrasonography is the most important ancillary tool for evaluating ciliary body and choroidal melanomas (see Fig 17-9E–H). The growth and regression of an intraocular tumor can be documented with serial examinations. Standardized A-scan ultrasonography (see Fig 17-9G, H) usually reveals a solid tumor pattern with high-amplitude initial echoes and low-amplitude internal reflections (low internal reflectivity). Spontaneous vascular pulsations can be demonstrated in most cases. B-scan examination provides information about the size (thickness and basal diameter), general shape, and position of intraocular tumors (see Figs 17-8G, H and 17-9E, F). B-scan ultrasonography is also the best technique for detecting posterior extrascleral extension associated with intraocular malignancies. Occasionally, tumor shape and associated retinal detachment can be evaluated more easily with ultrasonography than with ophthalmoscopy. B-scan ultrasonography typically shows a dome-shaped (see Fig 17-9E) or collar button–shaped (see Fig 17-9F)

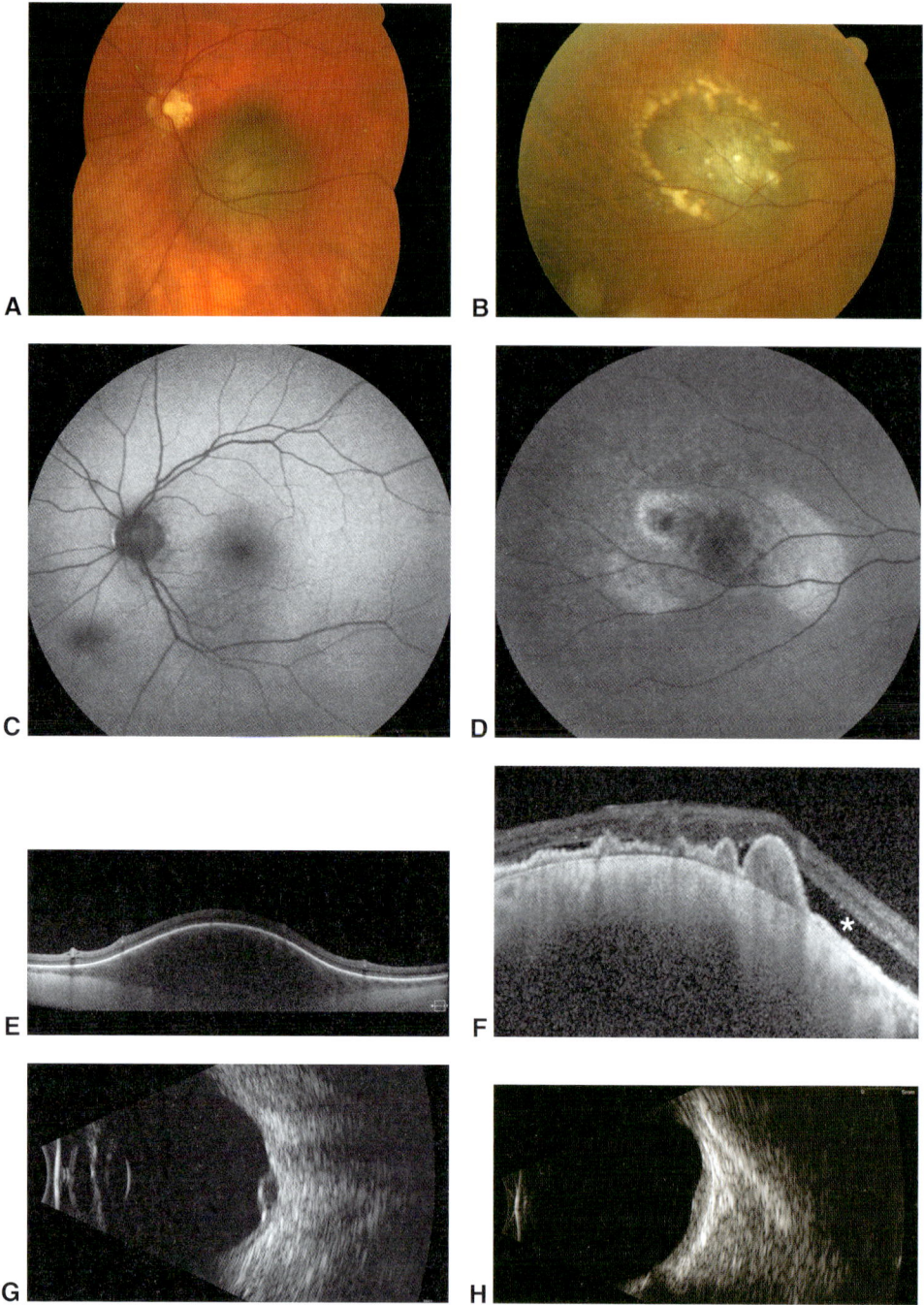

Figure 17-8 Multimodal imaging of choroidal nevi. **A, B,** Color fundus photographs document the tumor borders and surface appearance of 2 thin choroidal nevi. **C,** Fundus autofluorescence (FAF) reveals minimal RPE disturbance in the area of the choroidal lesion. **D,** FAF shows decreased autofluorescence centrally because of RPE loss as well as increased autofluorescence associated with more recent leakage, creating the appearance of a fluid gutter. **E,** Enhanced depth imaging optical coherence tomography (EDI-OCT) reveals no subretinal fluid associated with the lesion shown in parts **A** and **C. F,** EDI-OCT shows that the lesion shown in parts **B** and **D** has both numerous surface drusen and mild subretinal fluid *(asterisk).* **G, H,** B-scan ultrasonography reveals that both lesions are thin. *(Courtesy of Alison Skalet, MD, PhD.)*

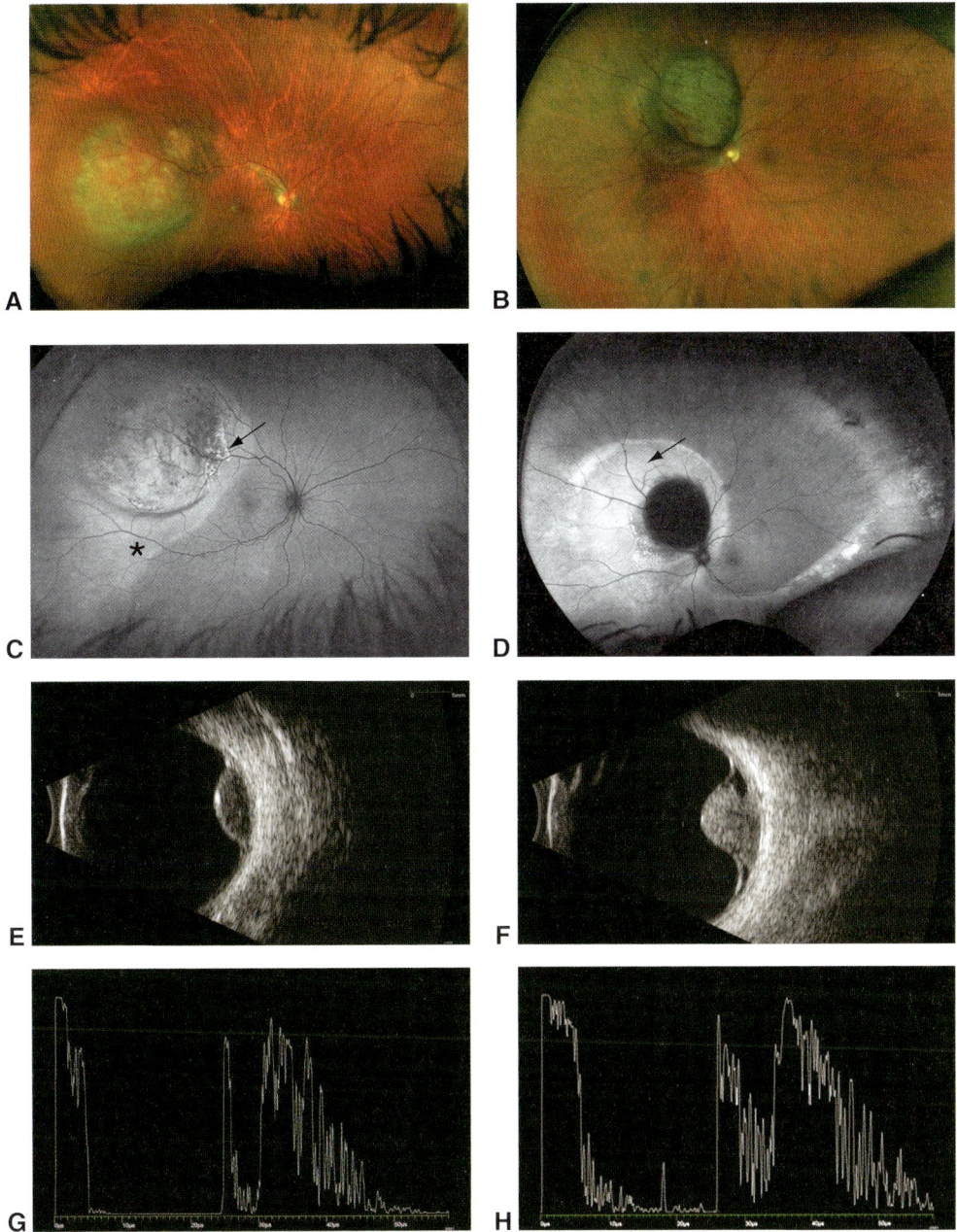

Figure 17-9 Multimodal imaging of choroidal melanomas. **A, B,** Wide-angle color fundus photographs document the tumor borders and surface appearance of 2 choroidal melanomas. **C,** FAF image of the lesion shown in part **A** reveals increased diffuse autofluorescence associated with subretinal fluid adjacent to the variably autofluorescent tumor *(asterisk).* Increased autofluorescence is associated with the lipofuscin *(arrow).* **D,** FAF image of the lesion shown in part **B.** The highly elevated tumor blocks underlying FAF. Diffusely increased autofluorescence is associated with subretinal fluid adjacent to the tumor *(arrow).* **E,** B-scan ultrasonography reveals the dome shape of the tumor shown in parts **A** and **C. F,** B-scan ultrasonography reveals the collar-button shape of the tumor shown in parts **B** and **D.** Images obtained from B-scan ultrasonography are helpful in measuring tumor size. **G, H,** Corresponding A-scan ultrasonographic image reveals a low, regular internal reflectivity associated with each melanoma. *(Courtesy of Alison Skalet, MD, PhD.)*

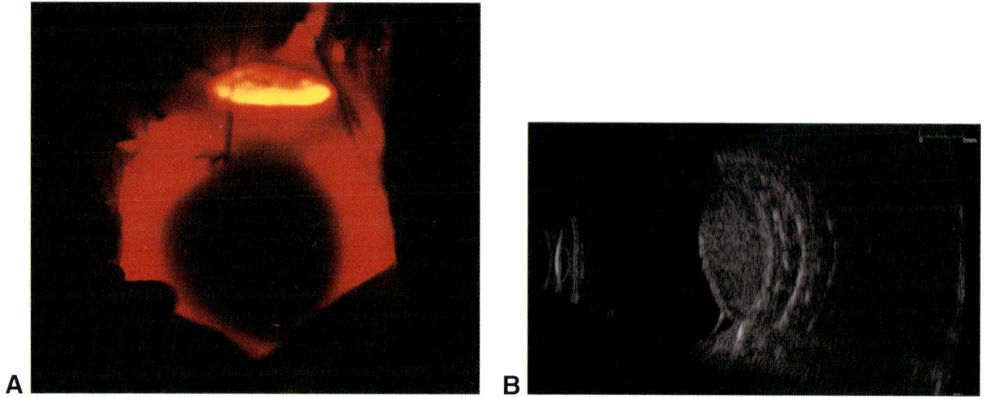

Figure 17-10 Intraoperative localization of melanoma for treatment purposes. **A,** Transillumination of the eye reveals a shadow at the site of a choroidal melanoma. This technique may be used to mark the tumor base to ensure accurate placement of a radioactive plaque. **B,** B-scan ultrasonography after placement of the radioactive plaque confirms optimal positioning. *(Part A courtesy of Tero Kivelä, MD; part B courtesy of Alison Skalet, MD, PhD.)*

choroidal mass that has a highly reflective anterior border, acoustic hollowness, and choroidal excavation. A serous retinal detachment is often associated with larger tumors.

The anterior location of ciliary body melanomas makes standard ultrasonography more difficult to perform (in contrast, high-frequency UBM, which does not share these limitations, enables excellent imaging of the anterior segment and ciliary body [see Fig 17-2G, H]). In addition, although ultrasonography is generally considered highly reliable in the differential diagnosis of posterior uveal melanomas, it may be difficult or impossible to differentiate a necrotic melanoma from a subretinal hemorrhage or a melanoma from an atypical metastatic tumor using this technology.

When high-frequency ultrasonography is not available, *transillumination* may be helpful in assessing the degree of pigmentation and in determining basal diameters of suspected ciliary body or anterior choroidal melanomas. The shadow of a tumor is visible with a bright, focused light source, preferably a high-intensity fiber-optic device, placed either on the surface of the topically anesthetized eye in a quadrant opposite the lesion or directly on the cornea, using a dark corneal cap. Fiber-optic transillumination is also routinely used to locate the uveal melanoma and delineate its borders during surgery for radioactive plaque insertion (Fig 17-10A). B-scan ultrasonography can be used after plaque placement to confirm appropriate positioning (Fig 17-10B).

Although *computed tomography (CT)* and *magnetic resonance imaging (MRI)* are not widely used to assess uncomplicated intraocular melanocytic tumors, they are useful in identifying tumors in eyes with opaque media and in possibly determining extrascleral extension as well as involvement of other organs. MRI may also help distinguish intraocular hemorrhage and atypical vascular lesions from melanocytic tumors.

Differential Diagnosis

This section describes the most common lesions considered in the differential diagnosis of posterior uveal melanoma.

Accurate diagnosis of a *choroidal nevus,* discussed earlier in this chapter, is associated with clinical experience and availability of ancillary testing modalities. For the evaluation and management of posterior pigmented lesions with characteristics predictive of growth, patients may be referred to ocular oncology centers. No single clinical factor is pathognomonic for benign versus malignant choroidal melanocytic lesions. Less than 10% of benign choroidal nevi have surface lipofuscin, and 15% or less are associated with subretinal fluid (see Fig 17-8B, D, F). In addition, 11%–58% of choroidal nevi have overlying drusen, a frequency that increases with the age of the patient. The presence of surface drusen reflects chronicity of a melanocytic choroidal tumor but can also be seen in melanomas that have transformed from a formerly quiescent nevus. More than 20% of choroidal melanocytic tumors thicker than 3 mm are melanomas, and far fewer than 1% of those thinner than 1 mm are melanomas. Tumors that are 1–3 mm in thickness are more difficult to classify with certainty on the basis of clinical evaluation alone; therefore, often close surveillance for growth is warranted. The risk of malignancy increases substantially for lesions with a basal diameter larger than 6 mm.

Risk factors for the growth of small choroidal melanocytic lesions have been well characterized; they include 5 clinical features that have given rise to the mnemonic "*to find small ocular melanomas*" (see Clinical Pearl).

CLINICAL PEARL

Clinical risk factors for growth of choroidal nevi: *"to find small ocular melanomas"*

- *T*hickness of the tumor greater than 2 mm
- *F*luid under the retina
- *S*ymptoms (eg, metamorphopsia, photopsia, visual field loss)
- *O*range pigmentation (lipofuscin) overlying the tumor
- *M*argin of the tumor touching the optic nerve head

The following factors are also concerning for melanoma:

- larger size at presentation
- absence of drusen or degenerative RPE changes
- homogeneous low internal reflectivity on ultrasonography
- hot spots on fluorescein angiography

To document growth of the tumor, the clinician may periodically photograph it and perform OCT and/or B-scan ultrasonography. Slow growth does not necessarily suggest or confirm malignancy. In a study of 284 benign choroidal nevi, 31% showed slow, progressive enlargement (median increase in diameter = 1 mm) over a long observation period (7 years or more). The frequency of enlargement may be higher in patients younger than 40 years (54%) than in those older than 60 years (19%). Enlarging nevi may not develop any new lipofuscin or subretinal fluid suggestive of malignant change. Thus, when rapid or progressive growth occurs or new risk factors appear, definitive treatment should be considered.

When risk factors for growth are identified, transscleral or transvitreal fine-needle aspiration biopsy (FNAB) for cytology and molecular testing is an alternative to observation. Cytologic evaluation of cells obtained by FNAB of a small melanocytic tumor requires an experienced cytopathologist, because cellularity of the FNAB specimen may be low and diagnosis based on samples that typically have limited cellularity is challenging. The role of prognostic molecular testing in this setting remains an area of debate.

Melanocytoma (magnocellular nevus) of the choroid or optic nerve head typically appears as a dark brown to black elevated lesion. Optic nerve melanocytoma is usually located eccentrically over the optic nerve head and may be elevated. It often has fibrillary or feathery margins as a result of extension into the nerve fiber layer (see Chapter 15, Fig 15-12). Because a melanocytoma rarely transforms into melanoma, it is important to differentiate the two. However, choroidal melanocytomas, particularly large ones, can be challenging to differentiate from choroidal melanomas without biopsy. As mentioned previously, for large or growing lesions, biopsy should be considered.

Congenital hypertrophy of the RPE (CHRPE) refers to sharply defined, flat, very darkly pigmented lesions that range from 1 mm to more than 10 mm in diameter. Patients are asymptomatic, and the lesion can be noted at any age. In younger patients, CHRPE often appears homogeneously black (Fig 17-11A); in older individuals, foci of depigmentation (lacunae) often develop (Fig 17-11B), and the lesion may slowly enlarge. The histologic findings are identical to those of *grouped pigmentation of the retina,* also known as *bear tracks* or *grouped CHRPE* (Fig 17-11C). In patients with *Gardner syndrome,* a subtype of *familial adenomatous polyposis,* the presence of multiple atypical CHRPE-like patches appears to be a marker for the development of colon carcinoma. These lesions are distinct from multifocal CHRPE in that they do not have sectoral distribution and have irregular depigmented margins (Fig 17-11D).

Patients with *age-related macular degeneration (AMD)* may present with macular or extramacular subretinal neovascularization, hemorrhage, and fibrosis, accompanied by varying degrees and patterns of pigmentation (Fig 17-12A). Hemorrhage, a finding commonly associated with neovascular (exudative) AMD, usually does not occur with melanomas unless the tumor has broken through Bruch membrane. Clinical evaluation of the fellow eye is helpful in documenting AMD. OCT shows predominantly subretinal and intraretinal abnormalities. Ultrasonography reveals high or heterogeneous reflectivity rather than low internal reflectivity, as well as a lack of intrinsic vascularity. When in doubt, the clinician may use fluorescein angiography to help reveal early hypofluorescence secondary to blockage from the hemorrhage, which is often followed by late hyperfluorescence in the distribution of the choroidal neovascular membrane (Fig 17-12B). Serial observation shows involutional alterations of the evolving disciform lesion.

Choroidal detachments can be hemorrhagic or serous. They are often associated with hypotony and may develop after ophthalmic surgery in the early postoperative period. Hemorrhagic detachments are often dome shaped, involve multiple quadrants, and may be associated with breakthrough vitreous bleeding. Ultrasonographic findings may closely resemble those of melanoma but may reveal absence of intrinsic vascularity and involution of the hemorrhage over time. Observational management is indicated in most cases. MRI with gadolinium contrast may be beneficial in diagnosing suspicious cases.

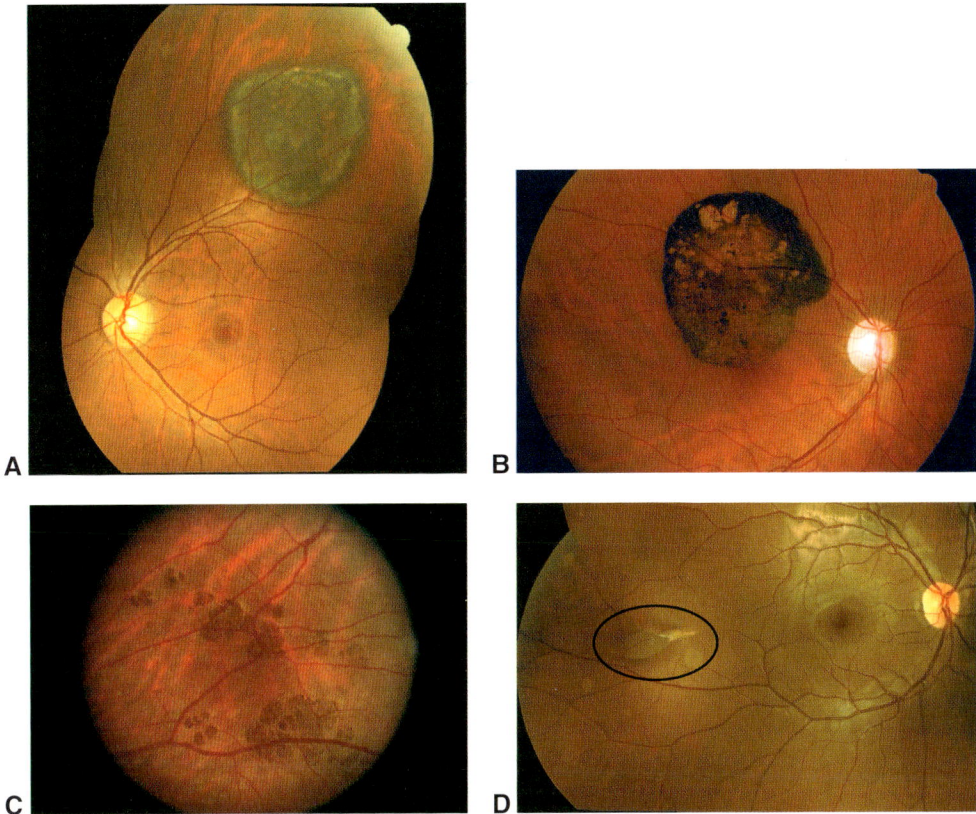

Figure 17-11 Congenital hypertrophy of the RPE (CHRPE), various clinical appearances. **A,** Large, homogeneously black CHRPE lesion. **B,** CHRPE with atrophic lacunae. **C,** Grouped pigmentation of the RPE represents a variant of CHRPE. **D,** Appearance of the RPE hamartoma associated with familial adenomatous polyposis. Note the depigmented margins and comma shape *(oval)*. *(Parts A and D courtesy of Alison Skalet, MD, PhD; parts B and C courtesy of Tero Kivelä, MD.)*

Peripheral exudative hemorrhagic chorioretinopathy (PEHCR) is a spontaneously developing, often asymptomatic, peripheral lesion in elderly individuals that resembles a choroidal detachment. It is often associated with suprachoroidal or subretinal bleeding and lipid exudation; associated retinal detachment is uncommon (Fig 17-12C). PEHCR is thought to be analogous to AMD, and the fellow eye often shows a similar or a nonexudative chorioretinal degeneration. PEHCR almost always involutes spontaneously.

Choroidal osteomas are benign, presumably acquired bony tumors that typically arise from the juxtapapillary choroid in young adults (more commonly in women) and are bilateral in 20%–25% of cases. The characteristic lesion appears yellow to orange and has well-defined margins (Fig 17-12D). Ultrasonography reveals a high-amplitude echo corresponding to the bony plate and loss of the normal orbital echoes behind the lesion (acoustic shadowing). CT can reveal calcification but is not needed for diagnosis. Choroidal osteomas typically enlarge slowly over many years and can decalcify with time. If they involve the macula, vision is generally impaired. Subretinal neovascularization is a common

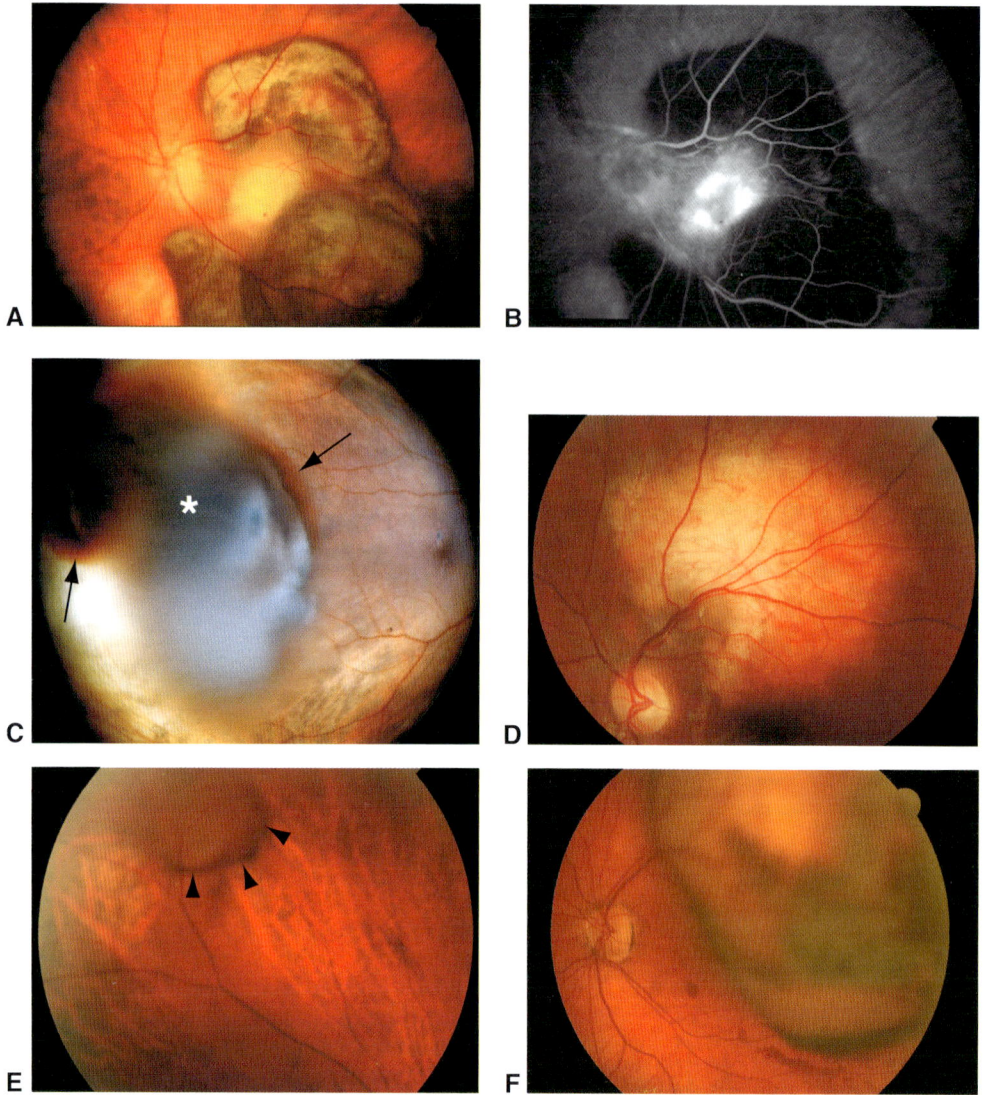

Figure 17-12 Conditions simulating posterior uveal melanoma. **A,** Subretinal hemorrhage secondary to neovascular (exudative) macular degeneration. **B,** Fluorescein angiography (same patient as in part **A**) reveals hyperfluorescence and late fluorescein leakage in the central macula associated with the choroidal neovascular membrane, and hypofluorescence associated with blockage of fluorescein transmission due to subretinal blood. **C,** Peripheral exudative hemorrhagic chorioretinopathy (PEHCR); note the red subretinal *(arrows)* and dark sub-RPE blood *(asterisk)*. **D,** Choroidal osteoma with yellow-orange color and well-defined pseudopod-like margins. **E,** Varix of the vortex vein *(arrowheads)*. This lesion is more likely to be developmental than degenerative. **F,** Metastasis to the choroid from lung cancer. Note the subretinal hemorrhage (patchy dark areas on the surface of the lesion). *(Parts A–E courtesy of Tero Kivelä, MD; part F courtesy of Alison Skalet, MD, PhD.)*

Table 17-2 Differential Diagnosis of Amelanotic Choroidal Mass

Amelanotic melanoma
Chorioretinal granuloma
Choroidal detachment
Choroidal hemangioma
Choroidal metastasis
Choroidal osteoma
Posterior scleritis
Sclerochoroidal calcification

Modified from Shields JA, Shields CL. *Intraocular Tumors: A Text and Atlas.* Saunders; 1992:137–153.

complication. The etiology of these lesions is unknown, but chronic low-grade choroidal inflammation has been suspected (see Chapter 12).

Choroidal hemangiomas (see Chapter 18) resemble the surrounding fundus in color and may appear to be lightly pigmented or orange. When a slit beam is passed over the lesion, it can appear to glow. These tumors are often better visualized on infrared imaging obtained with OCT than on fundus photographs. In infrared images, choroidal hemangiomas appear dark. Over time, a serous retinal detachment may develop. These lesions, which are often associated with overlying cystic retinal degeneration, are hyperechogenic on ultrasonography and show a characteristic vascular pattern on fluorescein and indocyanine green angiography.

Varix of the vortex vein (Fig 17-12E) is found predominantly in the nasal quadrants and can reach 4–5 mm in diameter. When filled with blood, it appears dark. The clinician can diagnose this condition by observing its coincidence with the vortex vein ampulla and by gently compressing the eye during indirect ophthalmoscopy, which causes the varix to deflate.

Intraocular metastases (Fig 17-12F; see also Chapter 20) are generally amelanotic and thus pale or yellowish, unless they originate from a cutaneous melanoma. Most show moderately high or heterogeneous reflectivity on ultrasonography. Table 17-2 lists additional conditions for consideration in cases with *amelanotic* choroidal masses.

Chien JL, Sioufi K, Surakiatchanukul T, Shields JA, Shields CL. Choroidal nevus: a review of prevalence, features, genetics, risks, and outcomes. *Curr Opin Ophthalmol.* 2017;28(3):228–237.

Mashayekhi A, Siu S, Shields CL, Shields JA. Slow enlargement of choroidal nevi: a long-term follow-up study. *Ophthalmology.* 2011;118(2):382–388.

Classification

Although classification of choroidal and ciliary body melanomas according to tumor volume would be logical, no simple and reliable method has been developed for doing this. Instead, several different systems are used to categorize these melanomas by size. The *Collaborative Ocular Melanoma Study (COMS)* classified posterior uveal melanomas as small, medium, or large on the basis of thickness and basal diameter. The recently revised, evidence-based, and validated tumor, node, metastasis (TNM) staging system developed by the American Joint Committee on Cancer (AJCC) is the classification most often used in clinical practice. The eighth edition, like the seventh, categorizes posterior uveal melanomas

Table 17-3 AJCC Tumor Size Categories for Ciliary Body and Choroidal Melanomas[a]

Tumor Thickness, mm	Largest Basal Dimension (Diameter) of Tumor, mm						
	≤3.0	3.1–6.0	6.1–9.0	9.1–12.0	12.1–15.0	15.1–18.0	>18.0
>15.0	4	4	4	4	4	4	4
12.1–15.0	3	3	3	3	3	4	4
9.1–12.0	3	3	3	3	3	3	4
6.1–9.0	2	2	2	2	3	3	4
3.1–6.0	1	1	1	2	2	3	4
≤3.0	1	1	1	1	2	2	4

[a] The numbers shown refer to categories of tumor size: 1 = small (T1); 2 = medium (T2); 3 = large (T3); very large (T4).

Adapted with the permission of the American College of Surgeons. Amin MB, Edge SB, Greene FL, et al (eds). *AJCC Cancer Staging Manual, 8th Edition.* Springer New York; 2017.

as small (T1), medium (T2), large (T3), or very large (T4) according to tumor thickness and basal diameter, extension to the ciliary body, and extrascleral growth (Table 17-3). These categories are used to assign melanomas to 7 stages (I, IIA, IIB, IIIA–C, and IV) that differ in prognosis (Table 17-4).

Metastatic Evaluation

The incidence of metastatic uveal melanoma is as high as 50% at 25 years after treatment for ciliary body or choroidal melanoma. The COMS reported an incidence of metastatic disease of 25% at 5 years after initial treatment and 34% at 10 years. However, metastatic disease at the time of initial presentation is rare and can be detected in fewer than 2% of patients. It is likely that a proportion of patients have undetectable micrometastases at the time of their primary treatment.

The liver is the primary organ involved in metastatic uveal melanoma; in 90% of patients, liver involvement is the first manifestation of metastatic disease. Other relatively frequent sites, generally after liver metastasis, include the lungs, bones, and skin. In cases that were autopsied, liver involvement was found in 100% of patients with metastases and lung involvement in 50%.

All patients benefit from metastatic evaluation before definitive treatment of intraocular melanoma (Table 17-5). The purpose of this evaluation is two-fold:

1. To determine whether the patient has any other medical conditions that contraindicate surgical treatment or need to be treated. For example, the COMS and smaller studies found a second primary cancer in approximately 10% of patients. If there is any question about whether the lesion in the eye is a metastatic tumor, the clinician should ensure a thorough medical evaluation to determine the site of primary malignancy.
2. To rule out the possibility of detectable metastatic melanoma from the eye, especially for AJCC T3 melanomas (metastasis found in 3%) and T4 melanomas

Table 17-4 AJCC Staging of Ciliary Body and Choroidal Melanoma

	Percentage of Patients	5-Year Survival	10-Year Survival
Stage I	21%–32%	96%–97%	88%–94%
Stage IIA	31%–34%	89%–98%	80%–84%
Stage IIB	22%–23%	79%–81%	67%–70%
Stage IIIA	9%–17%	66%–67%	45%–60%
Stage IIIB	3%–8%	45%–50%	27%–50%
Stage IIIC	1%	25%–26%	0%–10%
Stage IV (metastasis)	<2%	<5%	<1%

Modified from Kujala E, Damato B, Coupland SE, et al. Staging of ciliary body and choroidal melanomas based on anatomic extent. *J Clin Oncol.* 2013;31(22):2825–2831; and AJCC Ophthalmic Oncology Task Force. International Validation of the American Joint Committee on Cancer's 7th Edition Classification of Uveal Melanoma. *JAMA Ophthalmol.* 2015;133(4)376–383.

Table 17-5 Imaging Options for Staging and Surveillance of Metastases in Uveal Melanoma

Initial Staging
CT of the chest/abdomen/pelvis with IV contrast material
Non-contrast CT of the chest; MRI of the abdomen with gadolinium contrast
Chest x-ray and MRI of the abdomen with gadolinium contrast

Posttreatment Surveillance	
Liver Imaging	**Lung Imaging**
MRI of the abdomen with gadolinium contrast	Chest CT scan
CT scan with IV contrast material	2-View chest x-ray
Abdominal ultrasonography	

CT = computed tomography; IV = intravenous; MRI = magnetic resonance imaging.

Note: Options for imaging studies at initial staging and during surveillance after treatment of the primary uveal melanoma are shown. For lung and liver imaging, options are listed in the order of most to least sensitive. Decisions regarding the imaging technique used are multifactorial.

(metastasis found in 20%). When metastatic disease is clinically present during the pretreatment evaluation, treatment of the primary intraocular tumor will depend on patient and physician preference.

Initial staging evaluation for uveal melanoma should include a comprehensive physical examination and imaging of the lungs and liver. Chest/abdominal/pelvic CT with intravenous contrast material or, alternatively, MRI of the abdomen with gadolinium contrast or liver ultrasonography together with chest imaging with CT or an x-ray can evaluate the extent of the disease. Liver imaging is the most important component of the staging evaluation. Lung imaging is also usually performed at the time of diagnosis, although its yield is low. A positron-emission tomography (PET) scan typically is not performed for uveal melanoma staging or surveillance because these tumors may not be fluorodeoxyglucose avid; thus, this imaging modality has low sensitivity.

To detect metastatic disease in patients with uveal melanoma at an early phase, serial surveillance imaging is often performed over time. Strategies vary, with some centers imaging only the liver and others recommending imaging both the liver and the lungs. The same imaging modalities used in the initial staging may be used in surveillance imaging, with the recognition that exposure to ionizing radiation (ie, with CT scans) should be minimized. Liver function tests can be considered; however, they lack sensitivity and specificity and are not widely used in the modern era of uveal melanoma management. Possible novel blood markers for early detection of metastatic uveal melanoma are being explored.

In 2018, the first National Comprehensive Cancer Network (NCCN) clinical practice guidelines for uveal melanoma were published. NCCN guidelines recommend that surveillance imaging be considered for 10 years after treatment of the intraocular tumor and then as clinically indicated. Systemic imaging recommendations were stratified on the basis of expected risk of distant metastasis. For patients with a high risk for metastasis (eg, AJCC T4, gene expression profiling class 2), imaging is considered every 3–6 months for 5 years, and then every 6–12 months for 10 years. For patients at medium risk (eg, AJCC T2 and T3, class 1B), imaging is considered every 6–12 months for 10 years. No specific recommendations are made for low-risk patients (eg, AJCC T1, class 1A), and clinical practices vary considerably for this group. Some patients may choose to forgo asymptomatic surveillance imaging because of limited treatment options for advanced uveal melanoma and the anxiety caused by serial imaging.

If a lesion of concern is identified on surveillance imaging, a liver or other organ-site biopsy may confirm metastatic disease. Biopsy is appropriate before initiating treatment for metastatic disease.

The interval between the diagnosis of primary uveal melanoma and metastasis depends on many clinical, histologic, cytogenetic, and molecular genetic factors. It varies from a few months to more than 25 years. When metastatic disease is diagnosed early enough, the options for treatment include surgical resection; chemotherapy, including intra-arterial hepatic chemotherapy and chemoembolization; immunotherapy or biological therapy; and hepatic selective internal radiation therapy (SIRT, also known as *intrahepatic radioembolization*). However, it remains unclear how these therapies affect overall patient survival and quality of life.

AJCC Ophthalmic Oncology Task Force. International validation of the American Joint Committee on Cancer's 7th edition classification of uveal melanoma. *JAMA Ophthalmol.* 2015;133(4):376–383. [Erratum appears in *JAMA Ophthalmol.* 2015;133(9):1096.]

Francis JH, Patel SP, Gombos DS, Carvajal RD. Surveillance options for patients with uveal melanoma following definitive management. *Am Soc Clin Oncol Educ Book.* 2013:382–387.

Kujala E, Damato B, Coupland SE, et al. Staging of ciliary body and choroidal melanomas based on anatomic extent. *J Clin Oncol.* 2013;31(22):2825–2831.

Kujala E, Mäkitie T, Kivelä T. Very long-term prognosis of patients with malignant uveal melanoma. *Invest Ophthalmol Vis Sci.* 2003;44(11):4651–4659.

Mashayekhi A, Siu S, Shields CL, Shields JA. Slow enlargement of choroidal nevi: a long-term follow-up study. *Ophthalmology.* 2011;118(2):382–388.

NCCN Clinical Practice Guidelines in Oncology: Uveal Melanoma. Version1.2018. March 2018. National Comprehensive Cancer Network website. Accessed February 14, 2020. https://www.nccn.org/professionals/physician_gls/default.aspx

Treatment

For many years, management of posterior uveal melanomas was controversial for 2 reasons: (1) data on the natural history of untreated patients with posterior uveal melanoma were limited; and (2) there were insufficient data on patients who were matched for known and unknown risk factors and managed by different therapeutic techniques to compare their effectiveness. Currently, both surgical and radiotherapeutic techniques are used to treat posterior uveal melanoma. The choice of treatment depends on 4 factors:

1. size, location, and extent of the tumor
2. vision status of the affected eye and of the fellow eye
3. age and general health of the patient
4. patient and physician preference

Observation

Significant controversy persists regarding the diagnosis and management of small choroidal melanomas. Treatment should be considered for lesions with any of the 5 main risk factors for growth (thickness greater than 2 mm, subretinal fluid, symptoms, lipofuscin, or tumor margin touching the optic nerve head) and all lesions with documented growth. Short-term observation to verify growth of a suspected small uveal melanoma has traditionally been considered appropriate, especially when the tumor is located in the macular area. As mentioned earlier, FNAB can be an alternative but is technically challenging for small tumors and carries risks to vision. Observation of active and larger melanomas may be appropriate in very elderly patients and those with systemic illness who are poor candidates for any therapeutic intervention.

Enucleation

Historically, enucleation has been the gold standard in the treatment of malignant intraocular tumors. A past hypothesis that surgical manipulation of eyes containing a melanoma would lead to tumor dissemination and increased mortality is no longer accepted. Enucleation remains appropriate for some small to medium (T1 and T2) and many large (T3) and very large (T4) choroidal melanomas, especially when useful vision has been lost or when the patient declines other treatments. The COMS found no evidence that pre-enucleation external beam radiotherapy performed on patients with large choroidal melanomas improved 5-year survival. However, local orbital recurrence was more frequent after enucleation alone.

Hawkins BS; Collaborative Ocular Melanoma Study Group. The Collaborative Ocular Melanoma Study (COMS) randomized trial of pre-enucleation radiation of large choroidal melanoma, IV: ten-year mortality findings and prognostic factors. COMS report number 24. *Am J Ophthalmol.* 2004;138(6):936–951.

Brachytherapy with a radioactive plaque

The application of a radioactive plaque to the sclera overlying an intraocular tumor is the most common globe-sparing method to treat uveal melanoma. With this technique, which has been widely available since the 1950s, a very high dose of radiation can be delivered to the tumor (typically 80–100 gray [Gy] to the tumor apex and up to 1000 Gy to the tumor base), while a comparatively lower dose is delivered to the surrounding normal structures of the eye. Although various isotopes can be used (eg, cobalt 60, strontium 90, iridium 192, and palladium 103), the most common are iodine 125 (γ-rays) and ruthenium 106 (β-rays). In the United States, iodine 125 is the most frequently used isotope in the treatment of uveal melanomas of any size, whereas in Europe, ruthenium 106 is preferred for smaller melanomas. Advances in intraoperative localization, especially the use of ultrasonography (see Fig 17-10B), have increased local tumor control rates, which typically are greater than 90%. In most patients, the tumor decreases in size (Fig 17-13); in others, the result could be total flattening of the tumor or little change in size, although clinical and ultrasonographic changes may be evident. Though rare, local recurrence may occur; therefore, monitoring of treatment response with serial imaging, including photography and ultrasonography, is important. Regrowth may occur at the tumor margin or more diffusely.

American Brachytherapy Society–Ophthalmic Oncology Task Force. The American Brachytherapy Society consensus guidelines for plaque brachytherapy of uveal melanoma and retinoblastoma. *Brachytherapy.* 2014;13(1):1–14.

Bergman L, Nilsson B, Lundell G, Lundell M, Seregard S. Ruthenium brachytherapy for uveal melanoma, 1979–2003: survival and functional outcomes in the Swedish population. *Ophthalmology.* 2005;112(5):834–840.

Charged-particle radiation

High–linear energy transfer radiation with charged particles (protons or helium ions) is effective in managing ciliary body and choroidal melanomas, with local tumor control rates of up to 98% reported. The tumor response is similar to that observed after brachytherapy. In this technique, tantalum clips are surgically attached to the scleral surface before

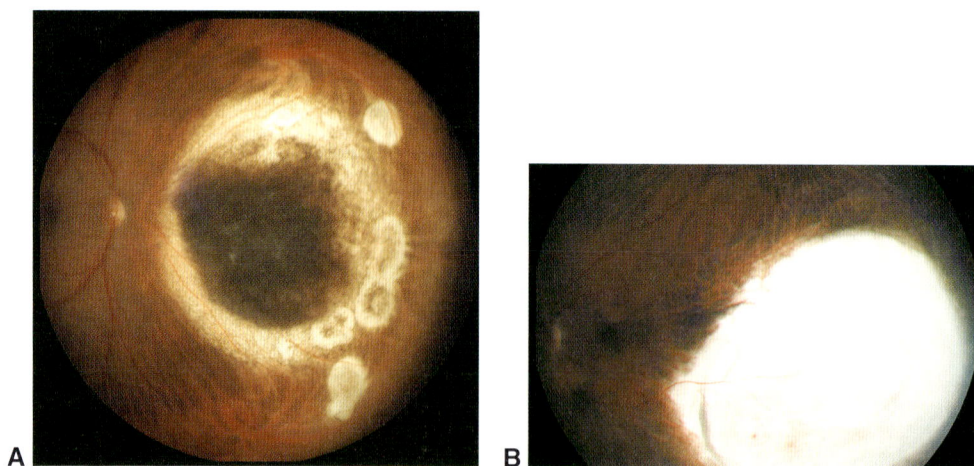

A   B

Figure 17-13 Choroidal melanoma, treated. **A,** Mildly elevated remnant of a melanoma surrounded by atrophic chorioretinal scarring nasal to the optic nerve head after plaque brachytherapy. **B,** After transscleral resection of a choroidal melanoma located temporal to the macula, the RPE and choroid are absent (and the outer retina is likely atrophic), but the inner retina is present, as evidenced by its blood vessels. *(Part A courtesy of Jacob Pe'er, MD; part B courtesy of Tero Kivelä, MD.)*

the first radiation fraction is delivered in order to allow localization of the tumor with MRI and CT guidance. The charged-particle beams deliver a more homogeneous dose of radiation energy to a tumor than a radioactive plaque would, and the lateral spread of radiation energy is less extensive. A specific charged-particle accelerator is required for this type of therapy and is not available in every treatment center.

Radiation-associated complications

Depending on tumor size and location, after treatment with either plaque brachytherapy or charged-particle radiation, more than 50% of patients experience radiation-related adverse effects that limit vision, especially optic neuropathy and maculopathy. These effects are often related to radiation-induced damage to the microvasculature. They may or may not respond to intravitreal anti–vascular endothelial growth factor (anti-VEGF) treatment; however, a trial of anti-VEGF is typically offered to patients. Future studies are needed to determine optimal patient selection and treatment interval for anti-VEGF therapy. After initial radiotherapy, large tumors may cause a chronic exudative retinal detachment or may become "toxic," often leading to neovascular glaucoma (NVG). Post-radiation NVG may also occur in the absence of exudative retinal detachment. Although NVG may be treatable with conservative therapies, eyes with NVG will sometimes be secondarily enucleated. Chronic dry eye may develop with either form of radiation. Charged-particle radiation may also be associated with cicatricial changes to the eyelid margins. When the tumor is anteriorly located, radiation cataract is common and can be managed with routine cataract extraction. These complications appear to be dose dependent and typically develop after a delay of 1 to several years.

Collaborative Ocular Melanoma Study Group. The COMS randomized trial of iodine 125 brachytherapy for choroidal melanoma, V: twelve-year mortality rates and prognostic factors: COMS report no. 28. *Arch Ophthalmol.* 2006;124(12):1684–1693.

External beam radiotherapy

Conventional external beam radiotherapy is ineffective for uveal melanoma. In recent years, some centers have used fractionated stereotactic radiotherapy and gamma knife radiosurgery as the primary treatment. Further study of these methods is warranted, but the published results and adverse effects are comparable to those of other irradiation methods.

Alternative treatments

Transpupillary thermotherapy and photodynamic therapy In the past, laser photocoagulation played a limited role in the treatment of melanocytic tumors. Today, transpupillary thermotherapy (TTT), in which a long-duration, large-spot-size, relatively low-energy infrared diode laser raises the temperature of the choroid, is used to manage selected small choroidal melanomas and, more frequently, to augment plaque brachytherapy or to control a local recurrence at the tumor margin. Studies suggest that TTT alone is associated with a higher rate of local tumor recurrence than is brachytherapy. Some of these recurrences are extraocular.

Surgical excision Surgical transscleral resection or endoresection during vitrectomy has been successfully performed in eyes with malignant and benign intraocular tumors (see Fig 17-13B). Concerns regarding surgical excision include the inability to evaluate tumor margins for residual disease, the high incidence of pathologically recognized scleral and retinal involvement in medium and large choroidal melanomas, and the possibility of spreading the tumor intraocularly and extraocularly. The surgical techniques are generally quite demanding, requiring an experienced surgeon with specialized training. Today, local excision of a uveal melanoma is coupled with adjuvant radiotherapy, such as brachytherapy or proton beam therapy, to reduce local recurrence rates to levels comparable to those after radiotherapy.

Chemotherapy Currently, chemotherapy is not effective in the treatment of primary uveal melanoma, nor is it routinely used in the treatment of metastatic disease.

Immunotherapy In immunotherapy, systemic cytokines, immunomodulatory agents, or vaccine therapy is used to try activating a tumor-directed T-cell immune response. This treatment is theoretically appropriate for uveal melanoma, because primary tumors arise in an immune-privileged organ and may express antigens to which the host is not sensitized. Currently, however, immunotherapy is not available for primary uveal melanoma. Immunotherapy for metastatic disease has been used with limited success.

Exenteration Traditionally advocated for patients with extrascleral extension of a posterior uveal melanoma, exenteration is rarely used today. Unless orbital invasion is very advanced, the current trend is toward more conservative treatment for these patients, with either enucleation plus a limited tenonectomy or modified plaque brachytherapy or proton beam therapy.

Prognosis and Prognostic Factors
There are 6 main clinical risk factors for melanoma-related mortality:

- larger tumor size (part of AJCC staging)
- ciliary body extension (part of AJCC staging)
- extraocular extension (part of AJCC staging)
- older age
- faster tumor growth
- tumor regrowth after globe-conserving therapy, especially radiotherapy

The histologic and molecular features associated with a higher rate of metastases include the following:

- epithelioid melanoma cells
- high mitotic or cell proliferation index
- specific extravascular matrix patterns (loops and networks of loops) and high microvascular density
- mean diameter of the 10 largest nucleoli
- large numbers of tumor-infiltrating lymphocytes and histiocytes (macrophages)

The prognostic factors most strongly associated with risk of metastasis are genetic:

- monosomy 3, especially with gains in chromosome 8
- gene expression profiling class 2 and, to a lesser extent, class 1B
- *BAP1* mutation within tumor tissue

See Table 17-4 (earlier in the chapter), which lists 10-year survival estimates according to the evidence-based staging system of the *AJCC Cancer Staging Manual, 8th Edition.* Stage IV implies that lymph node involvement or metastasis is present at the time of diagnosis of the primary tumor.

See Chapter 12 for a more detailed discussion of the histologic and molecular prognostic factors for uveal melanoma.

Damato B, Eleuteri A, Taktak AF, Coupland SE. Estimating prognosis for survival after treatment of choroidal melanoma. *Prog Retin Eye Res.* 2011;30(5):285–295.

Edge S, Byrd DR, Compton CC, Fritz AG, Greene FL, Trotti A, eds. Malignant melanoma of the uvea. In: *AJCC Cancer Staging Manual.* 7th ed. Springer; 2010:part X, pp 547–559.

Harbour JW. Molecular prognostic testing and individualized patient care in uveal melanoma. *Am J Ophthalmol.* 2009;148(6):823–829.

Shields CL, Furuta M, Thangappan A, et al. Metastasis of uveal melanoma millimeter-by-millimeter in 8033 consecutive eyes. *Arch Ophthalmol.* 2009;127(8):989–998.

Collaborative Ocular Melanoma Study

Data from the prospective, randomized, international COMS trial provide an additional framework for patient discussions concerning long-term survival and rates of globe conservation with enucleation and iodine 125 brachytherapy. See the sidebar on the following page for details.

Collaborative Ocular Melanoma Study (COMS). National Eye Institute. ClinicalTrials.gov. Last update posted June 2, 2006. Accessed January 3, 2020. https://clinicaltrials.gov/ct2 /show/NCT00000124

Epithelial Tumors of the Uveal Tract and Retina

Adenoma and Adenocarcinoma

Benign adenomas of the nonpigmented and pigmented ciliary epithelium may appear clinically indistinguishable from amelanotic and pigmented melanomas arising in the ciliary body. Benign adenomas of the RPE are rare. These lesions are oval, deeply pigmented tumors that arise abruptly from the RPE. Adenomas rarely enlarge and seldom undergo malignant change. Adenocarcinomas of the RPE are also very rare; only a few cases have been reported. They typically have feeder retinal vessels and may be associated with yellowish lipid exudates. Although these lesions display malignant features on histologic examination, their metastatic potential is minimal. Adenomas and adenocarcinomas show high internal reflectivity on ultrasonography.

Fuchs adenoma (also called *pseudoadenomatous hyperplasia*) is usually an incidental finding at autopsy and rarely becomes apparent clinically. It appears as an irregular, glistening, nonpigmented white or tan tumor arising from the inner surface of the pars plicata. It consists of benign proliferation of the nonpigmented ciliary epithelium with production of basement membrane material. See also Chapter 11.

COLLABORATIVE OCULAR MELANOMA STUDY (COMS)

Large Choroidal Melanoma Study Arm

- evaluated 1003 patients with choroidal melanomas greater than 16 mm in basal diameter and/or greater than 10 mm in apical height (greater than 8 mm if peripapillary)
- compared enucleation alone with enucleation preceded by external beam radiotherapy
- reported no significant difference in 5-year and 10-year all-cause mortality rates (approximately 40% and 60%, respectively)
- concluded that adjunctive radiotherapy did not improve overall survival but reduced the risk of orbital recurrence
- established the appropriateness of primary enucleation alone in managing large choroidal melanomas not amenable to globe-conserving therapy

Medium Choroidal Melanoma Study Arm

- evaluated 1317 patients with choroidal melanomas 6–16 mm in basal diameter and/or 2.5–10 mm in apical height (up to 8 mm if peripapillary)
- compared enucleation with iodine 125 brachytherapy
- reported no significant difference in 5-year and 10-year all-cause mortality rates (approximately 20% and 35%, respectively)
- reported no significant difference in 5-year and 10-year frequencies of histologically confirmed metastases (approximately 10% and 18%, respectively)
- reported the following ancillary findings: (1) only 2 of 660 enucleated eyes were misdiagnosed as having a choroidal melanoma; (2) at 5 years the local tumor recurrence rate was 10% and the secondary enucleation rate was 13%; and (3) at 3 years there was a decline in visual acuity to 20/200 in approximately 40% of patients, and the visual angle quadrupled (ie, there were 6 lines of vision loss) in approximately 50% of patients

Small Choroidal Melanoma Study

- observational study of 204 patients with tumors measuring 4–8 mm in basal diameter and/or 1.0–2.4 mm in apical height, but many of the tumors were nongrowing

Acquired Hyperplasia

Hyperplasia of the pigmented ciliary epithelium or the RPE usually develops in response to trauma, inflammation, or other ocular insults (Fig 17-14A). Because of their location, ciliary body lesions often do not become evident clinically. Occasionally, however, they may become large enough to simulate a ciliary body melanoma. Posteriorly located lesions may be more commonly recognized and can lead to diagnostic uncertainty. In the early management of these atypical lesions, observation to document their stability is often appropriate. In rare cases, adenomatous hyperplasia may mimic a choroidal melanoma.

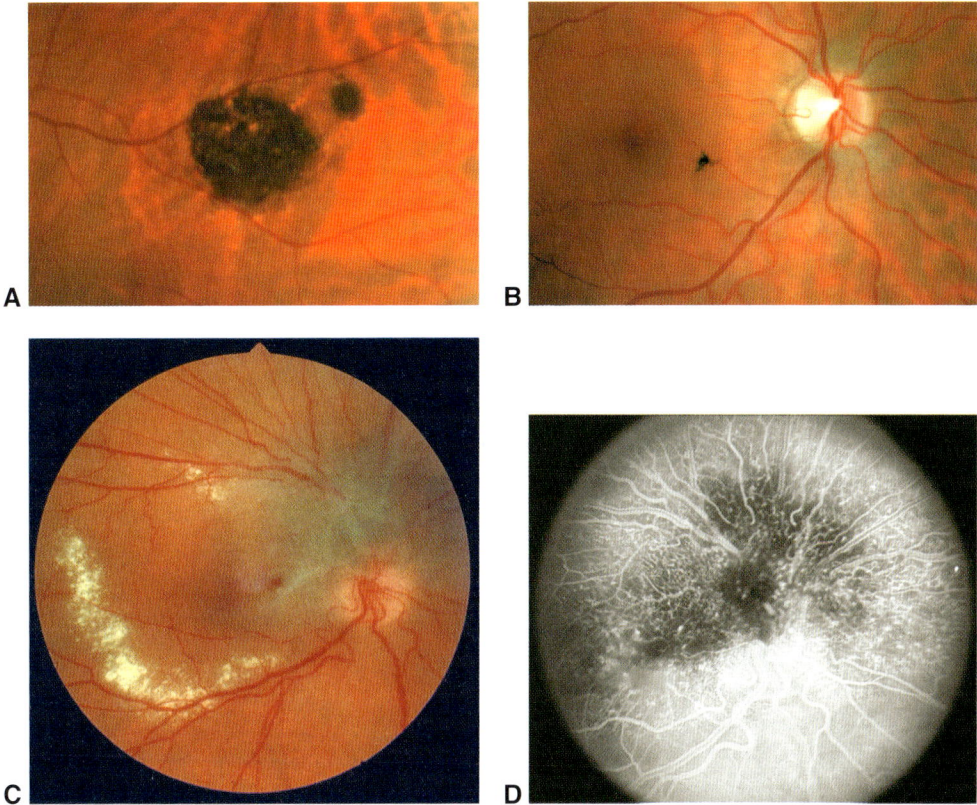

Figure 17-14 Lesions of the RPE. **A,** Reactive hyperplasia. **B,** Simple hamartoma. **C,** Clinical appearance of a peripapillary combined hamartoma of the retina and RPE. Note obscuration of the retinal vessels in the superior aspect of the lesion, moderate deep pigmentation, and secondary hard exudates. **D,** Fluorescein angiogram of the lesion shows the vascular component of the hamartoma, composed of small capillary-like telangiectatic vessels. Note the relative hypofluorescence superior to the optic nerve head, which is due to the RPE component of this lesion. *(Parts A and B courtesy of Tero Kivelä, MD; parts C and D courtesy of Robert H. Rosa Jr, MD.)*

Simple Hamartoma

Simple hamartoma of the RPE is a small (up to 1 mm), sharply demarcated, pigmented transretinal lesion that is located close to the center of the macula, arising from the RPE (Fig 17-14B). These lesions do not change over time.

Combined Hamartoma

Combined hamartoma of the RPE and retina is a rare disorder that occurs most frequently near the optic nerve head margin, although it may also be seen in the peripheral fundus. Typically, the hamartoma appears as a pigmented, slightly elevated lesion with vitreoretinal traction and tortuous retinal vessels (Fig 17-14C, D; see also Chapter 11, Fig 11-51). Glial cells within this lesion may contract, producing traction lines clinically visible in the retina. Exudative complications associated with the vascular component of the lesion may develop. These lesions have been mistaken for melanomas because of their pigmentation, slight elevation, and propensity to change in young individuals.

Kálmán Z, Tóth J. Two cases of congenital simple hamartoma of the retinal pigment epithelium. *Retin Cases Brief Rep.* 2009;3(3):283–285.

Shields CL, Thangappan A, Hartzell K, Valente P, Pirondini C, Shields JA. Combined hamartoma of the retina and retinal pigment epithelium in 77 consecutive patients: visual outcome based on macular versus extramacular tumor location. *Ophthalmology.* 2008;115(12):2246–2252.e3.

Fine-Needle Aspiration Biopsy

Intraocular fine-needle aspiration biopsy (FNAB) is not routinely used in the diagnosis of uveal tumors, as examination and use of noninvasive imaging techniques can accurately identify most tumors. In cases of diagnostic uncertainty or for genetic prognostic testing, FNAB can be employed. The procedure is performed under direct visualization through a dilated pupil, transvitreally (Video 17-1) or transsclerally (Video 17-2). Iris tumors may be accessible for FNAB through a transcameral approach. The cells obtained through FNAB can be evaluated for cytologic features to assist in diagnosis. More commonly, FNABs are performed for prognostic purposes in tumors clinically diagnosed as uveal melanomas. In this clinical scenario, cells obtained from FNAB are processed to extract the RNA or DNA for molecular testing and determine risk for metastasis. A variety of techniques may be used, including chromosomal analysis and gene expression profiling (see Chapter 3).

Intraocular FNAB may potentially allow tumor cells to exit the eye, although this concept is controversial. In general, a properly performed FNAB does not pose a major risk for seeding tumors. However, retinoblastoma is a notable exception. If a retinoblastoma is suspected, FNAB is avoided.

VIDEO 17-1 Transvitreal fine-needle aspiration biopsy.
Courtesy of Thomas Aaberg Jr, MD.
Go to www.aao.org/bcscvideo_section04 to access all videos in Section 4.

VIDEO 17-2 Transscleral fine-needle aspiration biopsy.
Courtesy of Thomas Aaberg Jr, MD.

Finn AP, Materin MA, Mruthyunjaya P. Choroidal tumor biopsy: a review of the current state and a glance into future techniques. *Retina.* 2018;38(Suppl 1):S79–S87.

McCannel TA, Chang MY, Burgess BL. Multi-year follow-up of fine-needle aspiration biopsy in choroidal melanoma. *Ophthalmology.* 2012;119(3):606–610.

CHAPTER 18

Vascular Tumors

Highlights

- Although vascular tumors do not have malignant potential, they can cause serious ocular morbidity that leads to permanent vision loss.
- Vascular tumors can be grouped by their primary location in the choroid or the retina and by whether they are prenatal or postnatal in origin.
- Prenatal (eg, congenital) retinal vascular tumors have tight junctions and do not have associated leakage or exudation.
- Vascular tumors can be associated with systemic disorders such as Sturge-Weber, Wyburn-Mason, and von Hippel–Lindau syndromes.

Introduction

Vascular tumors (also called *angiomatous tumors*) are benign lesions that can affect the retina and/or choroid. Some of these vascular lesions are not true neoplasms but rather are hamartomatous lesions or vascular malformations. Some are associated with systemic disorders. Although these vascular lesions do not have malignant potential, they can cause serious ocular morbidity, leading to permanent vision loss. Tumors in this category include choroidal hemangiomas (with circumscribed and diffuse variants) and retinal vascular tumors, such as retinal cavernous hemangioma, retinal arteriovenous malformations, retinal capillary hemangioblastoma, and retinal vasoproliferative tumor.

Choroidal Vascular Tumors

Choroidal Hemangiomas

Hemangiomas of the choroid occur in circumscribed and diffuse forms.

A *circumscribed choroidal hemangioma* typically occurs sporadically (without any systemic association) (Fig 18-1). This dome-shaped, often inconspicuous vascular hamartoma is generally located posterior to the equator, often in the macular area (see Fig 18-1A, B). Initially, it may be difficult to distinguish the tumor from the surrounding fundus because it blends with the adjacent normal choroid. Eventually, degenerative changes occur in the overlying retinal pigment epithelium (RPE), making the tumor more visible on clinical examination and fundus photography. These tumors also cause cystoid

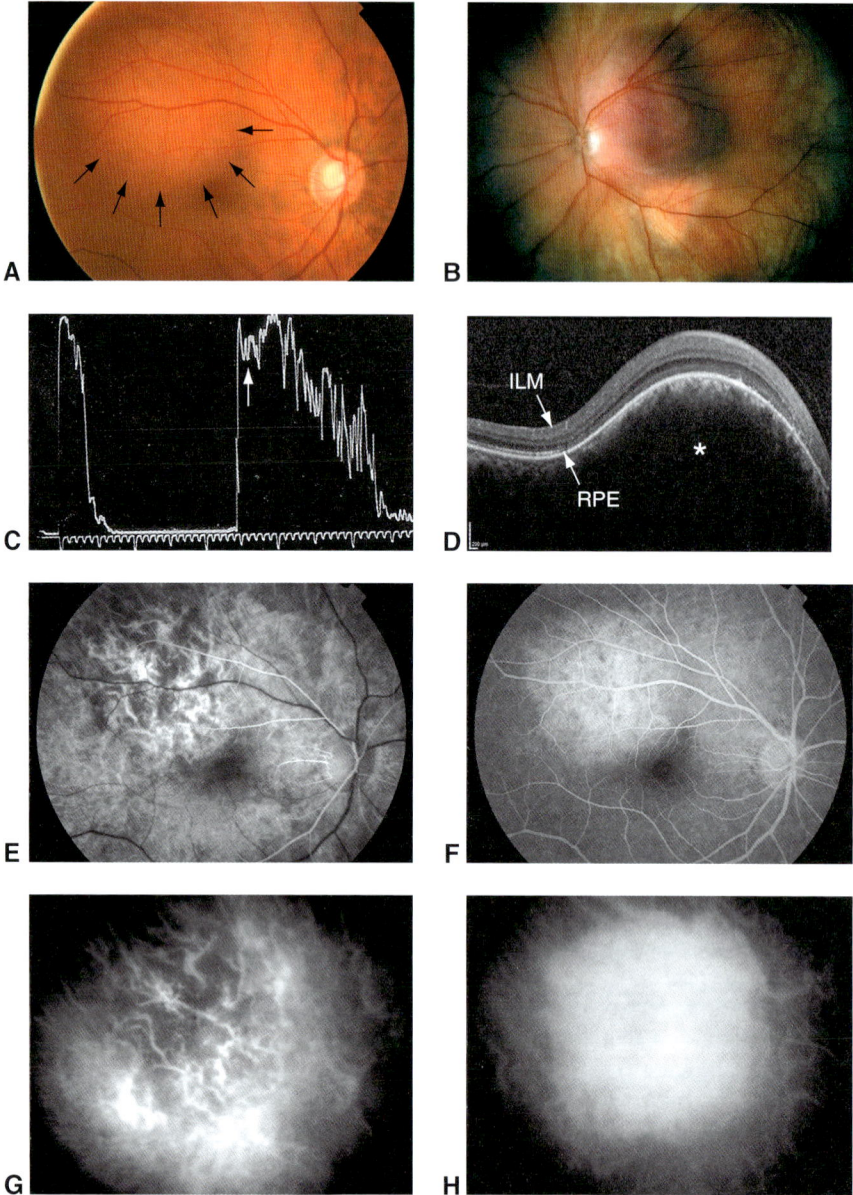

Figure 18-1 Circumscribed choroidal hemangioma. **A,** Dome-shaped tumor (inferior edge outlined by *arrows*) is similar in color to that of the surrounding fundus. **B,** Wide-angle fundus photograph in which the eye is illuminated transsclerally better highlights the reddish color of the hemangioma. **C,** A-scan ultrasonographic image shows characteristic high internal reflectivity *(arrow)*. **D,** Optical coherence tomography (OCT) shows a dome-shaped lesion with very low signal intensity *(asterisk)*. ILM = internal limiting membrane; RPE = retinal pigment epithelium. **E,** Early fluorescein angiogram (arterial phase) shows intratumoral choroidal vessels. **F,** In the late phase of the angiogram, the tumor is hyperfluorescent. **G, H,** Indocyanine green angiography demonstrates early hyperfluorescence, which is due to the choroidal location; the fluorescence increases in intensity during the angiogram. Compare parts **E–H** with part **A** (same lesion). *(Parts A, B, and E–H courtesy of Tero Kivelä, MD; part D courtesy of Robert H. Rosa Jr, MD.)*

degeneration in the overlying outer retinal layers. In some cases, the tumors cause a secondary exudative retinal detachment that often extends into the foveal region, resulting in blurred vision and metamorphopsia.

Circumscribed choroidal hemangioma may be difficult to diagnose because it can resemble other choroidal lesions, including

- amelanotic choroidal melanoma
- choroidal osteoma
- carcinoma metastatic to the choroid
- granuloma of the choroid

Diffuse choroidal hemangioma generally occurs in patients with Sturge-Weber syndrome (encephalofacial angiomatosis). In rare cases, it may occur in patients with congenital ocular melanocytosis (phakomatosis pigmentovascularis). Diffuse choroidal hemangioma produces diffuse homogenous reddish-orange coloration of the fundus, resulting in an ophthalmoscopic pattern referred to as *"tomato ketchup" fundus* (Fig 18-2). Secondary glaucoma and exudative retinal detachment develop in eyes with this lesion. For more information on Sturge-Weber syndrome, see BCSC Section 6, *Pediatric Ophthalmology and Strabismus.*

Ancillary diagnostic studies are helpful in evaluating both types of choroidal hemangiomas (circumscribed and diffuse). A-scan ultrasonography (echography) shows a high-amplitude initial echo and high-amplitude broad internal echoes (high internal reflectivity; see Fig 18-1C). B-scan ultrasonography reveals localized or diffuse choroidal thickening with prominent internal reflections but without choroidal excavation or acoustic shadowing. Optical coherence tomography (OCT) of circumscribed lesions typically shows minimal internal signal (see Fig 18-1D), a smooth surface, and tapered borders. Fluorescein angiography (FA) reveals hyperfluorescence of large choroidal vessels in the early choroidal filling phase; the fluorescence increases throughout the angiogram, with late staining of the tumor and late leakage or pooling in the cystoid spaces of the overlying retina (see Fig 18-1E, F). Indocyanine green (ICG) angiography, the preferred modality

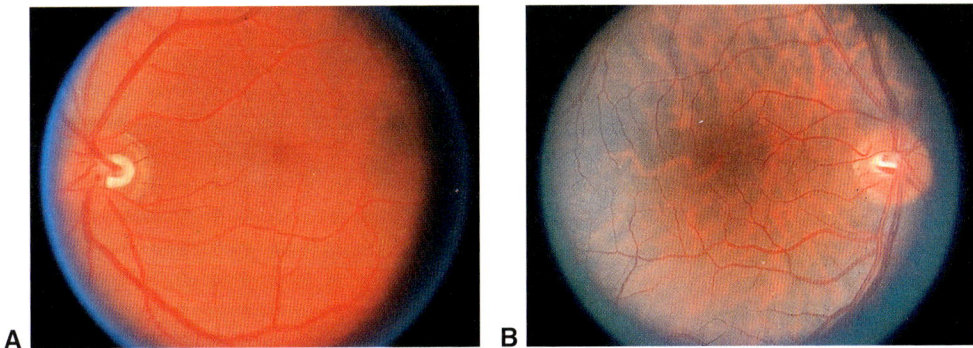

Figure 18-2 Diffuse choroidal hemangioma, clinical photographs. The saturated "tomato ketchup" red-orange color of the affected left fundus **(A)** contrasts markedly with the color of the unaffected right fundus **(B)** of the same patient.

for imaging choroidal vascular lesions, demonstrates early hyperfluorescence because of the intrinsic vascularity of these lesions. This hyperfluorescence peaks at around 3–4 minutes, and there is a classic "washout" of the dye in later frames, leaving a persistently hyperfluorescent rim (see Fig 18-1G, H). If this pattern is not seen, infiltrative lesions should be considered. Infrared imaging has recently been described as a method for identifying circumscribed choroidal hemangiomas, which appear dark in these images as compared with the surrounding tissue. Often, this method provides the clearest visualization of the lesion, allowing clinicians to determine the size and borders of circumscribed choroidal hemangiomas.

Asymptomatic choroidal hemangiomas require no treatment. The most common indication for treatment is exudative retinal detachment with subretinal fluid tracking toward the fovea and subsequent cystoid macular edema. Symptomatic circumscribed choroidal hemangiomas traditionally were managed with laser photocoagulation, which created chorioretinal adhesions. However, photocoagulation was often unsuccessful and created scars. Recurrent detachments were common.

The current treatment of choice for symptomatic circumscribed choroidal hemangioma is photodynamic therapy (PDT; see sidebar). Most choroidal hemangiomas respond to PDT, with resolution of the subretinal fluid and partial regression of the lesion, often with associated improvement in vision. However, cystoid macular edema may persist, particularly if chronic, and any degenerative changes in the overlying RPE may limit visual recovery; PDT may need to be repeated. See Chapter 9 in BCSC Section 12, *Retina and Vitreous*, for further discussion of choroidal hemangioma.

Therapeutic considerations   Photodynamic therapy (PDT) involves intravenous infusion of a photosensitive dye, verteporfin, which is activated with application of an infrared diode laser at 689-nm wavelength through the pupil, focused on the fundus. Once activated, the dye causes the release of free radicals, leading to vasoconstriction and thrombosis, which in turn induce regression of aberrant blood vessels. PDT was initially used to treat age-related macular degeneration (AMD) in the 1999 Treatment of Age-Related Macular Degeneration With Photodynamic Therapy (TAP) trial and the 2001 Verteporfin in Photodynamic Therapy (VIP) trial.

PDT for circumscribed choroidal hemangioma is given using the same standard laser parameters as those used in PDT for neovascular (exudative) AMD. The treatment involves slow intravenous administration of verteporfin, followed by direct application of the laser to the tumor. Standard-fluence ("full-fluence") PDT is used and refers to an energy of 50 J/cm^2 and light intensity of 600 mW/cm^2 over 83 seconds. Unlike procedures using an argon or diode laser, PDT is not painful.

After the procedure, patients should wear dark glasses and protective clothing and avoid direct sunlight because the verteporfin results in temporary photosensitivity of the skin and eyes.

Low-dose radiation (via brachytherapy or external radiotherapy methods such as charged-particle, stereotactic, or external beam) has been successfully used to treat choroidal hemangiomas, including those unresponsive to PDT. All these methods can be used to treat patients with circumscribed choroidal hemangioma; for diffuse choroidal hemangioma, because of the diffuse nature of the tumor, external beam radiotherapy techniques are used rather than plaque brachytherapy. Complications from radiation include dry eye, cataract, and radiation retinopathy. These complications, as well as the exudative retinal detachment, may limit visual recovery. In addition, fibrotic changes can occur over the lesion, affecting vision.

To date, there is little published evidence to support the use of vascular endothelial growth factor (VEGF) inhibitors to treat choroidal hemangioma.

Boixadera A, García-Arumí J, Martínez-Castillo V, et al. Prospective clinical trial evaluating the efficacy of photodynamic therapy for symptomatic circumscribed choroidal hemangioma. *Ophthalmology.* 2009;116(1):100–105.

Papastefanou VP, Plowman PN, Reich E, et al. Analysis of long-term outcomes of radiotherapy and verteporfin photodynamic therapy for circumscribed choroidal hemangioma. *Ophthalmol Retina.* 2018;2(8):842–857.

Retinal Vascular Tumors

Retinal vascular tumors include 4 distinct clinical entities:

- retinal cavernous hemangioma
- retinal arteriovenous malformations
- retinal capillary hemangioblastoma (RCH)
- retinal vasoproliferative tumor

These tumors can be further subdivided into vascular tumors of prenatal origin (retinal cavernous hemangioma, retinal arteriovenous malformations) and postnatal origin (RCH, retinal vasoproliferative tumor). Tumors of prenatal origin maintain vascular tight junctions and thus do not leak. This means that they do not present with subretinal fluid or exudation, in contrast to the postnatal tumors, which can be associated with exudative retinal detachments and visual impairment.

Prenatal Retinal Vascular Tumors: Non-Leaking Lesions

Retinal cavernous hemangioma

Cavernous hemangioma of the retina is an uncommon lesion that resembles a cluster of grapes (Fig 18-3). These lesions may also occur on the optic nerve head. In rare cases, retinal cavernous hemangioma may be associated with similar cavernous angiomatous lesions of the skin and central nervous system that are caused by a mutation in the gene *CCM1/KRIT1*. Patients with intracranial lesions may experience associated seizures. Given that these lesions are prenatal in origin, cavernous hemangiomas are not typically associated with exudation;

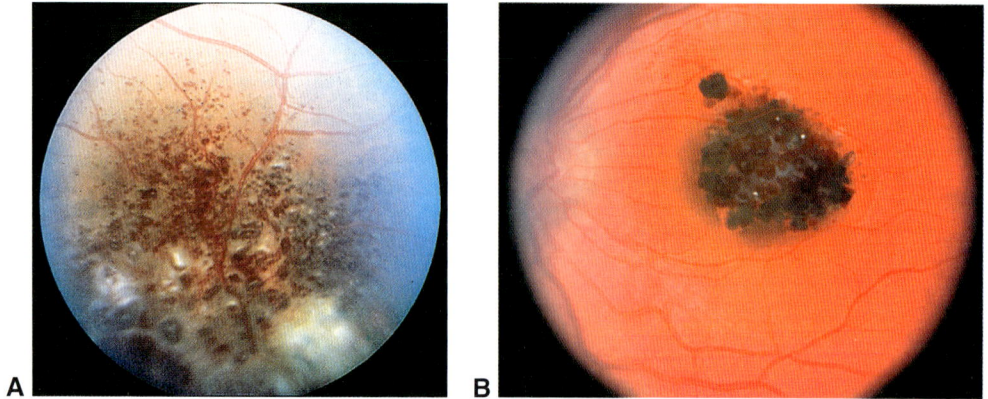

Figure 18-3 Retinal cavernous hemangioma, clinical photographs. **A,** Multiple tiny vascular saccules and associated white fibrotic tissue are seen in the retina. **B,** A smaller lesion consisting of a grapelike cluster of clumped vascular saccules is seen in the macula. *(Part B courtesy of Timothy G. Murray, MD.)*

thus, treatment is rarely required. However, small hemorrhages as well as gliotic and fibrotic areas may appear on the surface of the lesion. FA may reveal plasma–erythrocyte separation within the vascular spaces of the lesion; this separation is virtually diagnostic of cavernous hemangioma. In contrast to hemangioblastomas, retinal cavernous hemangiomas fill very slowly. The fluorescein remains in the vascular spaces for an extended period without leakage (see BCSC Section 12, *Retina and Vitreous*).

Choquet H, Pawlikowska L, Lawton MT, Kim H. Genetics of cerebral cavernous malformations: current status and future prospects. *J Neurosurg Sci.* 2015;59(3):211–220.

Gass JD. Cavernous hemangioma of the retina. A neuro-oculo-cutaneous syndrome. *Am J Ophthalmol.* 1971;71(4):799–814.

Retinal arteriovenous malformations

Congenital retinal arteriovenous malformation (also known as *racemose hemangioma*) is an anomalous artery-to-vein anastomosis that can occur in the iris, near the optic nerve head, or in the retinal periphery. Clinically, these malformations can range from a small, localized vascular communication to a prominent tangle of large, tortuous blood vessels throughout most of the fundus (Fig 18-4A, B). The term *racemose* refers to the clustered or bunched nature of the vessels. When associated with an arteriovenous malformation of the midbrain region, this condition is generally referred to as *Wyburn-Mason syndrome* (also known as *Bonnet-Dechaume-Blanc syndrome*; see BCSC Section 5, *Neuro-Ophthalmology*, and Section 6, *Pediatric Ophthalmology and Strabismus*). Arteriovenous malformations may also appear in the eyelid, orbit, and mandible.

An arteriovenous malformation of the retina is different from a congenital retinal macrovessel, which is a large aberrant retinal vessel that crosses the midline and, often, also the macular area (Fig 18-4C, D). Retinal macrovessels occasionally show arteriovenous communications.

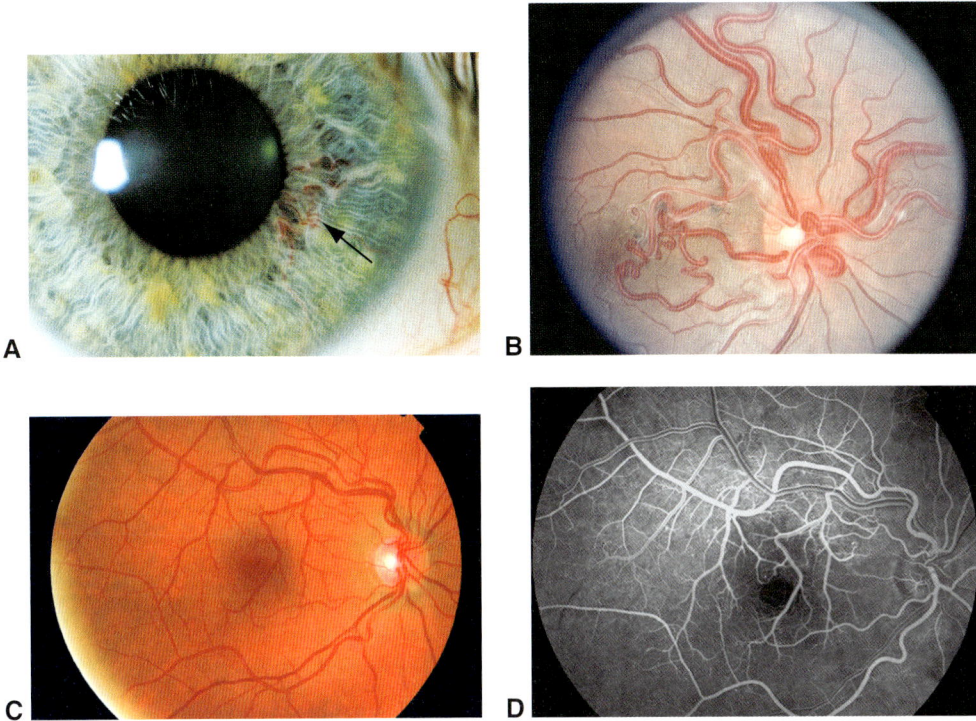

Figure 18-4 Intraocular arteriovenous malformations, clinical photographs. Arteriovenous malformation, or racemose hemangioma, in the iris (**A,** *arrow*) and the retina (**B**) in 2 patients. **C,** Although it can occasionally have an arteriovenous communication, a retinal macrovessel is distinct from racemose hemangioma. **D,** Fluorescein angiogram highlights the macrovessel, which crosses the macular area and the horizontal midline. Absence of leakage is characteristic of retinal arteriovenous malformations. *(Parts A, C, and D courtesy of Tero Kivelä, MD; part B courtesy of Robert H. Rosa Jr, MD.)*

Archer DB, Deutman A, Ernest JT, Krill AE. Arteriovenous communications of the retina. *Am J Ophthalmol.* 1973;75(2):224–241.

Heimann H, Damato B. Congenital vascular malformations of the retina and choroid. *Eye (Lond).* 2010;24(3):459–467.

Postnatal Retinal Vascular Tumors: Leaking Lesions

Retinal capillary hemangioblastoma

Retinal capillary hemangioblastoma (RCH) is a rare condition with a reported incidence of 1 in 40,000. It can be sporadic, occurring only in the retina, or it can be associated with a cerebellar and/or spinal hemangioblastoma, occurring as part of the *von Hippel–Lindau (VHL) syndrome* (Fig 18-5). A variety of names are used for RCH in the literature, including *angiomatosis retinae* and *retinal capillary hemangioma,* and sporadic lesions have also been called *von Hippel lesions,* a term meant to differentiate the nonsyndromic retinal lesions from those seen in the systemic disorder (VHL syndrome). This naming bias is

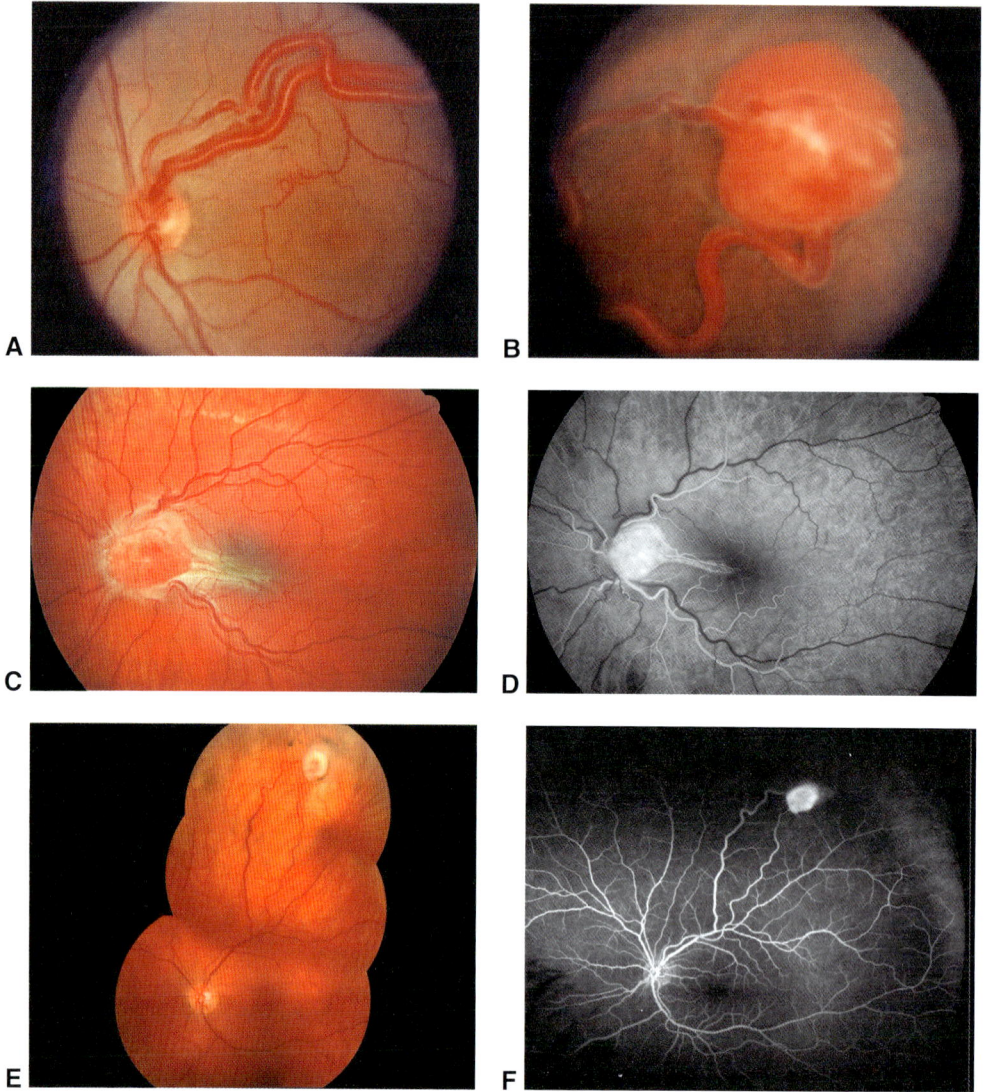

Figure 18-5 Retinal capillary hemangioblastoma (RCH), clinical photographs. Dilated, tortuous retinal feeder artery and draining vein emanate from the optic nerve head **(A),** leading to the red to orange peripheral retinal tumor **(B).** An optic nerve head hemangioblastoma causes traction in the macular area **(C).** In the early arterial phase of fluorescein angiography, the lesion is hyperfluorescent **(D). E,** Fundus photograph from a 48-year-old woman with von Hippel–Lindau syndrome, multiple cerebellar hemangioblastomas, and a typical-appearing RCH. **F,** Fluorescein angiogram from the same patient in part **D** demonstrates focal hyperfluorescence without leakage. *(Parts A and B courtesy of Robert H. Rosa Jr, MD; parts C and D courtesy of Tero Kivelä, MD; parts E and F courtesy of Mary Aronow, MD, Massachusetts Eye and Ear Infirmary.)*

historically derived: von Hippel, a German ophthalmologist, initially described the retinal lesions, and Lindau, a Swedish pathologist, recognized the overlap between the retinal and cerebellar lesions. In 1964, the term *von Hippel–Lindau* was adopted to recognize the contributions of both physicians and to unify the disease classification. The term *retinal capillary hemangioblastoma* most accurately reflects the pathogenesis of these lesions (see Chapter 11).

Although RCH may rarely be present at birth, the lesions typically are acquired and are usually diagnosed in the second to third decades of life. RCH may occur as a single lesion or as multiple ones. The lesions appear as red to orange tumors arising within the retina with large-caliber, tortuous afferent and efferent retinal blood vessels (see Fig 18-5A, B, E, F). As the lesions occur postnatally, leakage and exudation are common. Associated yellow-white retinal and subretinal lipid exudates, often involving the fovea, and exudative retinal detachments may occur. Atypical variations include tumors arising from the optic nerve head (see Fig 18-5C) and in the retinal periphery, where vitreous traction may elevate the tumor from the surface of the retina (see Fig 18-5B). FA demonstrates rapid arteriovenous transit (see Fig 18-5D, F), with immediate filling of the feeding arteriole, subsequent filling of the numerous fine blood vessels that constitute much of the tumor, and drainage by the dilated venule. Massive leakage of dye into the tumor and vitreous can occur.

RCHs are a common disease manifestation of VHL syndrome, wherein cerebellar and/or spinal hemangioblastomas may develop in patients but are less common. The VHL gene, which is located on chromosome 3, is mutated in the syndrome. Mutations in *VHL* cause overproduction of VEGF and other hypoxia-inducible factors, leading to the development of highly vascular tumors. A number of other tumors and cysts may develop in patients with this syndrome, the most serious of which are renal cell carcinoma and pheochromocytoma. For more information on VHL syndrome, see BCSC Section 6, *Pediatric Ophthalmology and Strabismus,* and Section 12, *Retina and Vitreous.* Chapter 11 in this volume discusses the histologic features of RCH.

When VHL syndrome is suspected, appropriate genetic consultation and ongoing screening are critical for early identification of the ocular and systemic manifestations of the disease. Patients with RCH can undergo genetic screening to determine whether they are at risk for developing systemic manifestations. More than 60% of patients with VHL syndrome have RCHs, which are often the first manifestation of the disease. Thus, by identifying the retinal lesions, the ophthalmologist is often the first medical specialist to diagnose VHL syndrome. Screening for systemic vascular anomalies (eg, cerebellar hemangioblastomas) and malignancies may reduce mortality, and aggressive screening for and early treatment of RCHs may reduce complications and improve long-term visual outcomes.

Treatment of RCH includes

- photocoagulation for small lesions, applied both to the lesion and the surrounding retina to create chorioretinal scarring and a blockade against expanding exudation
- cryotherapy for larger lesions located in the peripheral retina
- plaque brachytherapy or proton beam radiotherapy, or scleral buckling with cryotherapy for large lesions with more extensive retinal detachment

PDT has been used successfully to treat selected RCHs. The use of VEGF inhibitors in the treatment of RCH has been disappointing. Reports suggest that the principal efficacy of VEGF inhibitors is in reducing macular edema, but the impact on the size of the RCH has been variable. Although most optic nerve head lesions are rather resistant to treatment, some have responded to treatment with PDT, favored in this situation, or have been resected using vitrectomy-based techniques.

The visual prognosis remains guarded for patients with optic nerve head or large retinal lesions. The clinician should be aware that additional tumors may develop over time in patients with VHL syndrome, so careful serial examination of both eyes is required in order to identify and treat new tumors when they are small. Wide-field FA can be helpful in identifying small retinal hemangioblastomas in this setting.

Singh AD, Shields CL, Shields JA. von Hippel-Lindau disease. *Surv Ophthalmol.* 2001;46(2):117–142.

Retinal vasoproliferative tumors

Retinal vasoproliferative tumors (VPTs) are uncommon acquired retinal lesions that may be primary and idiopathic (74% of cases) or may develop because of preexisting ocular disease (26% of cases), including inflammatory, traumatic, and degenerative ocular conditions (eg, retinitis pigmentosa). These lesions were initially called *presumed acquired retinal hemangiomas* to differentiate them from RCH. Primary VPTs manifest in the third or fourth decade of life, and both sexes are equally affected. Most patients present with a single solitary lesion; however, in secondary cases, multiple tumors have been described.

Clinically, VPTs appear as an elevated pink and yellow vascular mass in the peripheral retina with associated subretinal exudation, which may be extensive. These lesions lack the prominent dilated feeder vessels typically seen in RCHs (Fig 18-6). Macular fibrosis, epiretinal membranes, cystoid macular edema, and subretinal fluid may lead to vision loss. Histologically, VPTs are composed of a mixture of glial cells and a network of fine capillaries with some larger dilated blood vessels.

Treatment of VPTs is notoriously difficult. Small peripheral VPTs that lack significant exudate or maculopathy may be managed with periodic observation. First-line treatment of symptomatic tumors generally involves triple freeze–thaw transconjunctival cryotherapy; repeated treatments are often required. Other treatment options include plaque brachytherapy, laser photocoagulation, and PDT. The use of anti-VEGF agents and intraocular steroids has been described. Chronic cases may require vitrectomy with membrane peel.

Shields CL, Shields JA, Barrett J, De Potter P. Vasoproliferative tumors of the ocular fundus. Classification and clinical manifestations in 103 patients. *Arch Ophthalmol.* 1995;113(5):615–623.

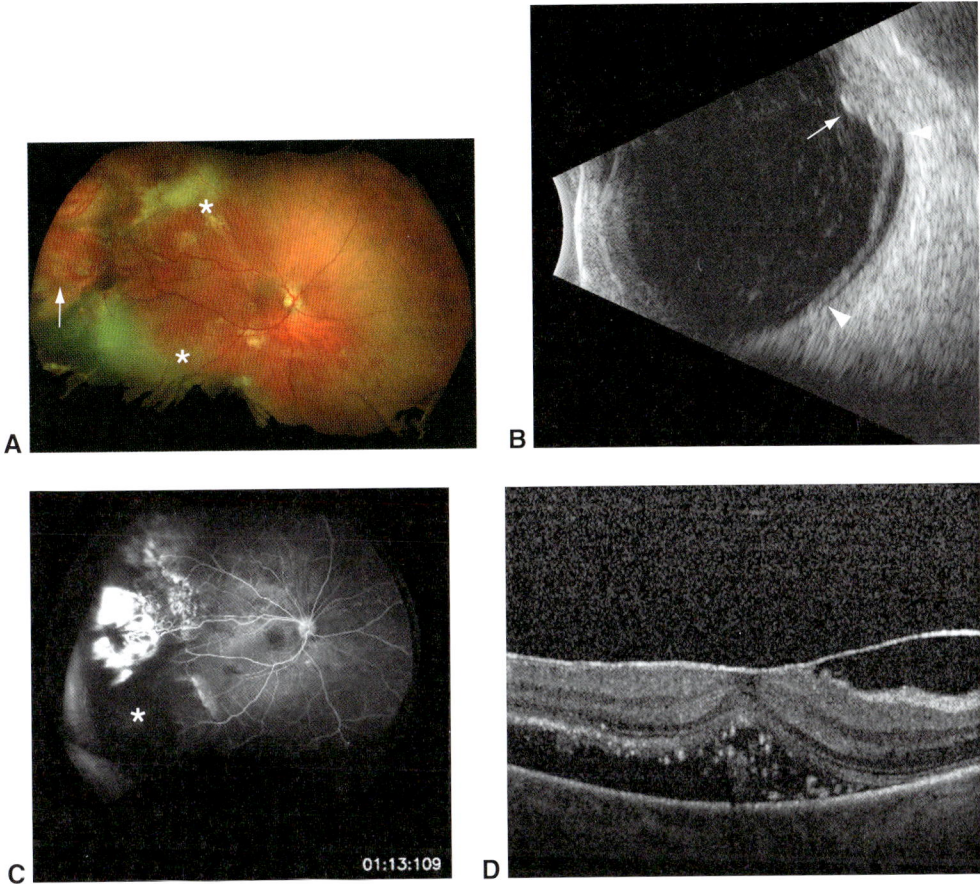

Figure 18-6 Vasoproliferative tumor (VPT). **A,** Color fundus photograph shows a VPT in the temporal periphery of the right eye *(arrow)*. The tumor appears as a pink and yellow elevated mass with tortuous internal vasculature and associated subretinal fibrosis and exudate *(asterisks)*. **B,** B-scan ultrasonographic image demonstrates a heterogeneous, amorphous elevated mass *(arrow)*. There is an associated retinal detachment *(between arrowheads)*, which is not uncommon. **C,** Fluorescein angiogram highlights the internal vascular component of the tumor that demonstrates significant hyperfluorescent staining; late leakage is common. Loss of retinal vasculature is seen in the area of previous cryotherapy treatment *(asterisk)*. **D,** OCT shows subretinal fluid tracking under the fovea, an epiretinal membrane, and significant foveal distortion. *(Courtesy of Jesse L. Berry, MD.)*

.

CHAPTER 19

Retinoblastoma

▶ *This chapter includes a related video. Go to www.aao.org/bcscvideo_section04 or scan the QR code in the text to access this content.*

Highlights

- Retinoblastoma is a rare tumor with an incidence of 250–300 cases annually in the United States. Despite its infrequent occurrence overall, retinoblastoma is the most common primary intraocular cancer in children.
- In the United States, children with retinoblastoma most often present with leukocoria and/or strabismus.
- Retinoblastoma typically is caused by a mutation in *RB1*, a tumor suppressor gene. The *RB1* mutation may be inherited from a parent who carries it or can result from a new germline (eg, heritable) or somatic mutation. The type of mutation—whether heritable or somatic—determines the patient's prognosis for secondary tumors and the type of counseling the family should receive.
- Unlike with most tumors, including other intraocular tumors, biopsy is contraindicated in retinoblastoma, and diagnosis and classification are based solely on clinical features.
- In advanced unilateral cases, enucleation traditionally is performed. However, recent therapeutic improvements have led to more children undergoing eye-sparing treatment with intravenous or intra-arterial chemotherapy.

Introduction

Retinoblastoma is the most common primary intraocular malignant tumor of childhood and is the second most common primary intraocular malignant tumor in all age groups (after uveal melanoma). The frequency of retinoblastoma in the United States and Europe ranges from 1 in 14,000 to 1 in 20,000 live births, with an estimated 250–300 new cases occurring each year. Both sexes and all races are affected equally, and the tumor occurs bilaterally in 30%–40% of patients. Approximately 90% of retinoblastoma cases are diagnosed in patients younger than 3 years. The mean age or age range at diagnosis is dependent on family history and disease laterality:

- patients with known family history of retinoblastoma: 4–8 months
- patients with bilateral disease: 12 months
- patients with unilateral disease: 24 months

The annual worldwide incidence of retinoblastoma is 8000–9000 cases, and the disease rate varies among countries by approximately 50-fold, mainly because of variances in birthrates. Disease registries indicate that the highest incidences of retinoblastoma occur in India, China, and countries in Africa.

Abramson DH, Beaverson K, Sangani P, et al. Screening for retinoblastoma: presenting signs as prognosticators of patient and ocular survival. *Pediatrics.* 2003;112(6 Pt. 1):1248–1255.

Orjuela M. Epidemiology. In: Rodriguez-Galindo C, Wilson MW, eds. *Retinoblastoma.* Springer; 2010:11–23. *Pediatric Oncology.*

Wong JR, Tucker MA, Kleinerman RA, Devesa SS. Retinoblastoma incidence patterns in the US Surveillance, Epidemiology, and End Results program. *JAMA Ophthalmol.* 2014;132(4):478–483.

Diagnostic Evaluation

The diagnosis of retinoblastoma is made clinically. Obtaining a biopsy specimen by fine-needle aspiration is contraindicated because of the risk of extraocular spread of tumor. In rare diagnostic dilemmas in which there is visual potential, an expert ocular oncologist may perform a biopsy procedure through the clear cornea followed by cryotherapy, although this is rarely done. If visual potential is poor and retinoblastoma is part of the differential diagnosis, the safest option for the child is enucleation.

Clinical Examination

The presenting signs and symptoms of retinoblastoma correspond to the extent and location of the tumor. In the United States, the most common presenting signs are leukocoria (white pupillary reflex), strabismus, and ocular inflammation (Fig 19-1, Table 19-1). Other presenting features, such as iris heterochromia, spontaneous hyphema, and orbital inflammation, are less common and are associated with more advanced tumors. A small retinoblastoma tumor may be identified on routine examination, but this is rare and generally limited to patients who receive screening evaluations because of a family history of

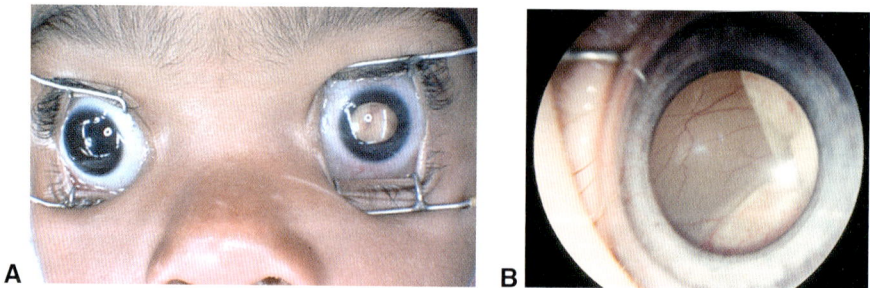

Figure 19-1 Retinoblastoma. **A,** Clinical photograph shows leukocoria and strabismus associated with an advanced intraocular tumor. **B,** Higher-magnification view through the pupil. Note the large retrolental tumor and secondary total exudative retinal detachment. *(Courtesy of Timothy G. Murray, MD.)*

the disease. Known vision problems at presentation are uncommon because most patients are very young children who cannot yet express the vision loss.

An examination under anesthesia (EUA) is necessary for all patients suspected of having retinoblastoma in order to completely assess the extent of ocular disease prior to treatment. The intraocular pressures and corneal diameters of the eyes should be determined, and the iris should be evaluated carefully for neovascularization with a portable slit lamp. In addition, the locations of retinal tumors, the occurrence of subretinal fluid or exudative detachment, and the presence of either vitreous or subretinal tumor seeds should be ascertained bilaterally and clearly documented. Fundus photography and ultrasonography (echography) should also be performed to document findings and allow serial comparisons.

Retinoblastoma begins as a round, translucent, gray to white tumor in the retina (Figs 19-2, 19-3, 19-4). As the tumor enlarges, necrotic foci with calcification emerge, giving the tumor its characteristic chalky white appearance. Larger tumors contain dilated, tortuous intratumoral vessels. Exophytic tumors grow beneath the retina and often involve serous

---

Table 19-1 Presenting Signs and Symptoms of Retinoblastoma

Leukocoria (most common)
Strabismus (approx. 20%)
Ocular and/or orbital inflammation (approx. 5%)
Pseudohypopyon
Hyphema
Iris heterochromia
Phthisis bulbi
Proptosis
Cataract
Glaucoma
Nystagmus
Tearing
Anisocoria

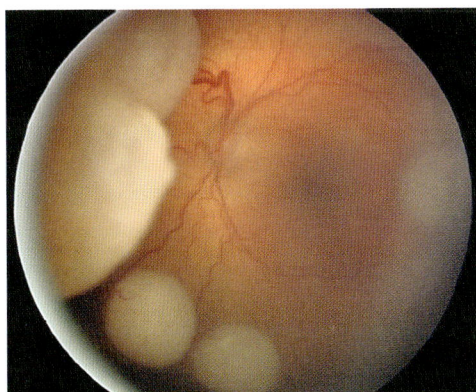

Figure 19-2 Retinoblastoma. Multiple tumor foci in an eye of a patient with a germline *RB1* mutation. *(Courtesy of Matthew W. Wilson, MD.)*

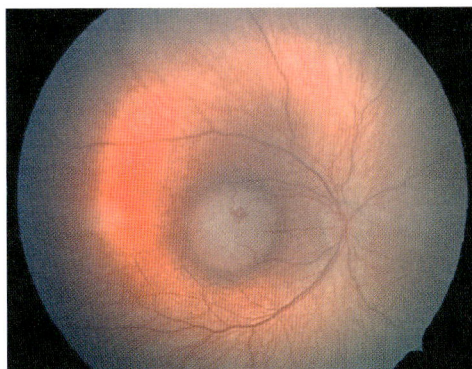

Figure 19-3 Retinoblastoma, clinical photograph. Discrete white macular tumor supplied by dilated retinal blood vessels. *(Courtesy of Timothy G. Murray, MD.)*

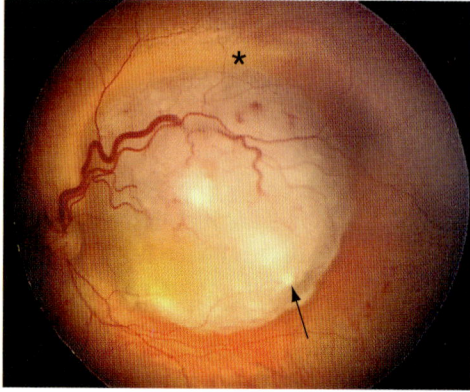

Figure 19-4 Endophytic retinoblastoma. Note the growth into the vitreous cavity, dilated retinal blood vessels, foci of calcification *(arrow)*, and cuff of subretinal fluid *(asterisk)*. *(Courtesy of Matthew W. Wilson, MD.)*

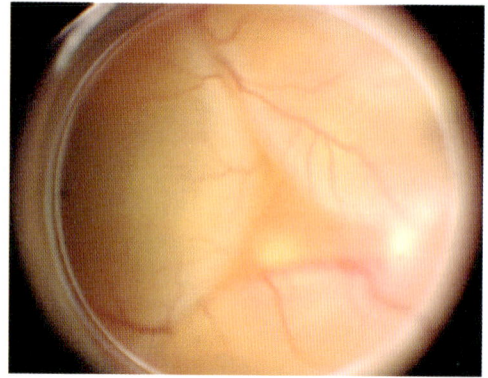

Figure 19-5 Exophytic retinoblastoma. Total exudative detachment due to tumor growth under the retina obscures tumor visualization. Note the normal-appearing retinal vessels, as opposed to those found in Coats disease. *(Courtesy of Matthew W. Wilson, MD.)*

retinal detachment. As these tumors grow, the retinal detachment may become extensive, obscuring clear visualization of the tumor (Fig 19-5). Endophytic tumors grow on the retinal surface and into the vitreous cavity; therefore, blood vessels may be more difficult to discern in these tumors. Exophytic tumors cause subretinal seeding, whereas endophytic retinoblastoma tumors are more likely to yield *vitreous seeds* (Fig 19-6; see also Fig 19-4); these cells shed from the tumor remain viable in the vitreous and may eventually become implanted in ocular tissue, resulting in new tumor foci within the eye. Vitreous seeds also may enter the anterior chamber; there, they may aggregate on the iris as nodules or settle inferiorly as a pseudohypopyon formed of tumor cells, rather than inflammatory cells (Fig 19-7). Secondary glaucoma and rubeosis iridis occur in approximately 50% of eyes with advanced disease. Most advanced tumors have mixed endophytic and exophytic growth.

Diffuse infiltrating retinoblastoma is a rare variant of retinoblastoma that is detected later in childhood (>5 years) and typically presents unilaterally. Diffuse infiltrating retinoblastoma presents a diagnostic challenge because dense vitreous cells impede visualization of the retina, and there is no isolated retinal mass. This variant often is mistaken for an intermediate or posterior uveitis of unknown etiology. A clue supporting a diagnosis of retinoblastoma is that the seeds are in clumps of various sizes, and some seeds may be spherical, which is atypical of vitritis.

Ancillary Imaging

In the initial staging EUA, patients with retinoblastoma may receive fundus photography, fluorescein angiography (FA), handheld optical coherence tomography (OCT), and B-scan ultrasonography. Results of color fundus photography enable documentation of the appearance and location of retinal tumors and the sites of vitreous and subretinal seeding; serial images over time are helpful for determining treatment efficacy and disease

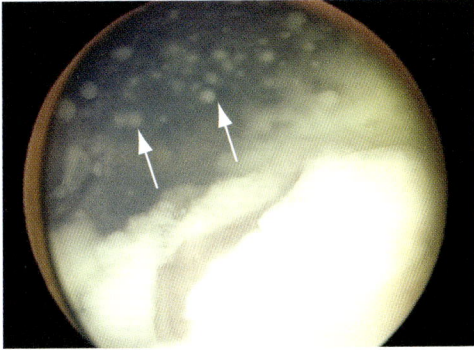

Figure 19-6 Retinoblastoma. Large endophytic tumor with extensive vitreous seeding *(arrows)*. *(Courtesy of Matthew W. Wilson, MD.)*

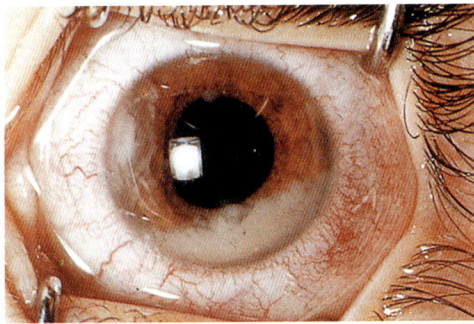

Figure 19-7 Retinoblastoma, clinical photograph. Pseudohypopyon resulting from migration of tumor cells into the anterior chamber. Note the clumped appearance of the cells, which is somewhat different from the appearance of inflammatory cells in a true hypopyon. Also note the tumor nodule on the iris surface at the 10 o'clock position, which is atypical for an inflammatory hypopyon.

recurrence. Common findings of retinoblastoma on FA include retinal vascular dilatation, capillary telangiectasia, intrinsic tumor vessel formation, and retinal venous leakage; subclinical iris neovascularization may also be seen.

In eyes with small tumors or a visible macula, OCT with a handheld device can be helpful in assessing macular anatomy and in identifying and monitoring retinal tumors. Small retinoblastoma tumors are smooth, round, cream-colored, homogeneous, and isodense on OCT. Small tumors may involve the inner nuclear layer (INL) and the outer nuclear layer (ONL), whereas very small tumors have been described as limited to the ONL, with draping of the overlying inner retinal layers beginning with the outer plexiform layer (Fig 19-8). So-called invisible tumors that are very early may be detected on OCT before ophthalmoscopic visualization is possible. OCT also can be used to evaluate the extent and morphology of vitreous seeds (Fig 19-9). Ultrasonographic findings of a dome-shaped retinal lesion with scattered intratumoral calcifications are critical for diagnosing retinoblastoma, particularly when ophthalmoscopic visualization of the tumor is limited (Fig 19-10). Results of EUA are used to classify each eye, as discussed in the Retinoblastoma Classification section. The group classification is useful in determining therapeutic options, visual prognosis, and potential for ocular salvage.

Retinoblastoma may invade the optic nerve head and spread through the lamina cribrosa into the central nervous system (CNS). Rarely, in bilateral cases, retinoblastoma can be associated with a separate CNS tumor called a *pinealoblastoma* (a condition

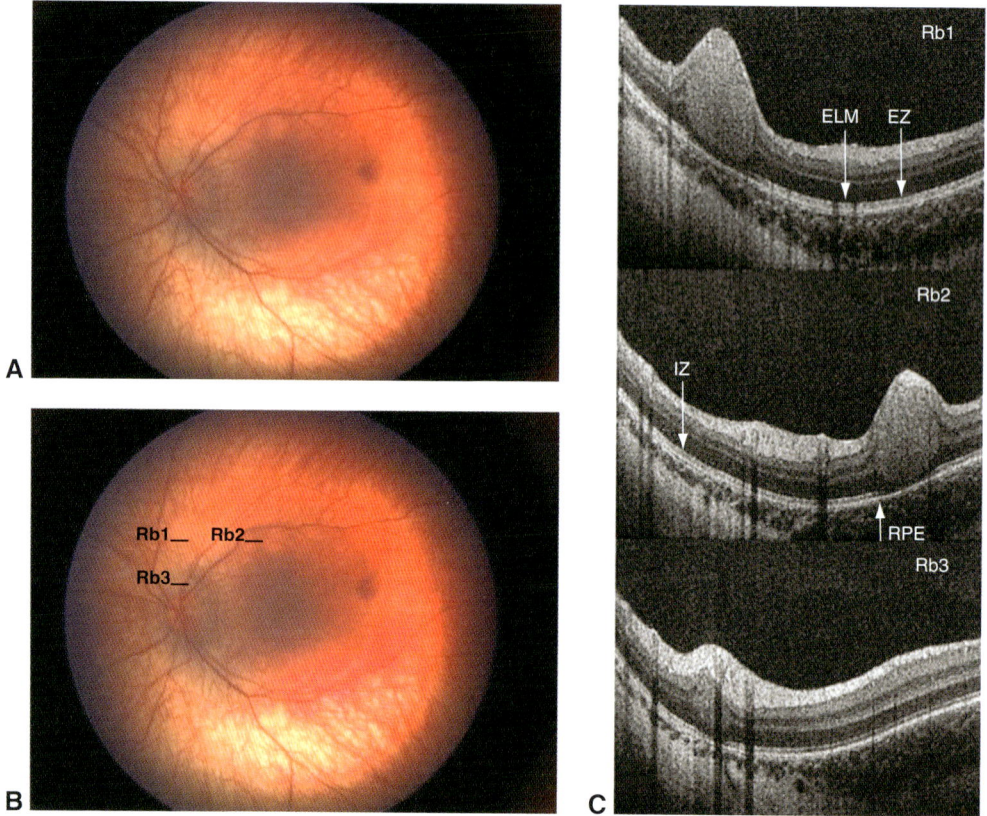

Figure 19-8 Optical coherence tomography (OCT) of retinoblastoma. **A,** Color fundus photograph of a left eye with 3 retinoblastoma tumors. **B,** Color fundus photograph of the same eye with the 3 retinoblastoma tumors labeled Rb1–3. The tumors are marked by lines through the body of the tumors correlating with the OCT slice. The smallest one, barely visible on ophthalmoscopy, lies just superior to the optic nerve. **C,** Spectral-domain OCT of the 3 tumors shows homogenous dome-shaped masses with overlying inner retinal draping. Tumor 3 is located in the outer retina involving the outer nuclear layer and possibly the outer plexiform layer. The inner nuclear layer and inner plexiform layer drape over the tumor. There is also an outer retinal abnormality in all tumors affecting the external limiting membrane (ELM), ellipsoid zone (EZ), and interdigitation zone (IZ). There is shadowing on OCT from the retinal vessels overlying the tumor, which are also seen clinically. RPE = retinal pigment epithelium. *(Reproduced with permission from Berry JL, Cobrinik DC, Kim JW. Detection and intraretinal localization of an 'invisible' retinoblastoma using optical coherence tomography. Ocul Oncol Pathol. 2016;2(3):149.)*

referred to as *trilateral retinoblastoma;* Fig 19-11). Hence, imaging studies of the optic nerve, orbits, and brain are essential for complete staging of a child with retinoblastoma. Magnetic resonance imaging (MRI) is the preferred diagnostic modality for this purpose. MRI enables better soft-tissue resolution than does computed tomography (CT) and does not expose the patient to potentially harmful radiation, which is especially important in children with a genetic cancer syndrome (see the Genetic Counseling section). Aside from MRI of the brain, systemic metastatic evaluation with bone marrow and lumbar puncture is not indicated in children without neurologic abnormalities or evidence of

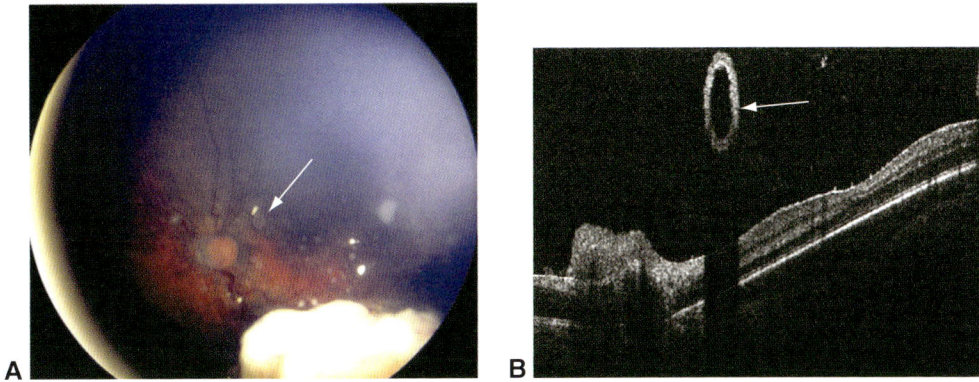

Figure 19-9 **A,** Clinical photograph shows a large, spherical vitreous seed *(arrow)* in retinoblastoma. **B,** OCT findings in a child with advanced retinoblastoma demonstrated an intact fovea, a dusting of small hyperreflective seeds on the retinal surface, and a hollow reflective cystic structure floating above the retina consistent with a spherical vitreous seed *(arrow).* *(Reproduced from Berry JL, Anulao K, Kim JW. Optical coherence imaging of large spherical seed in retinoblastoma. Ophthalmology. 2017;124(8):1208.)*

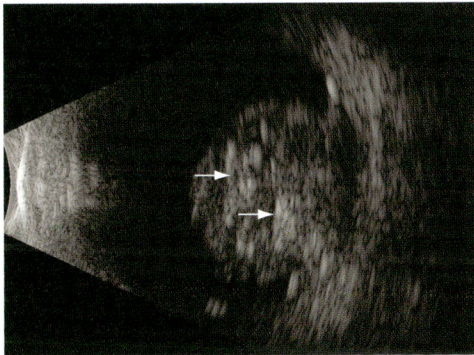

Figure 19-10 B-scan ultrasonographic findings demonstrate a dome-shaped retinal lesion with characteristic scattered calcifications within the tumor *(arrows).* *(Courtesy of Jesse L. Berry, MD, and Jonathan W. Kim, MD.)*

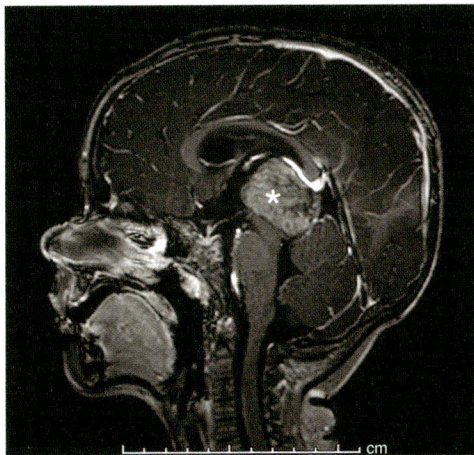

Figure 19-11 Contrast-enhanced sagittal T1-weighted magnetic resonance image of the brain demonstrates a large midline cerebral lesion *(asterisk)* involving the pineal region in a child with bilateral retinoblastoma; this is consistent with a pinealoblastoma (primitive neuroectodermal tumor [PNET]). The presence of the bilateral retinoblastomas and the pineal tumor is referred to as *trilateral retinoblastoma.* *(Courtesy of Jonathan W. Kim, MD.)*

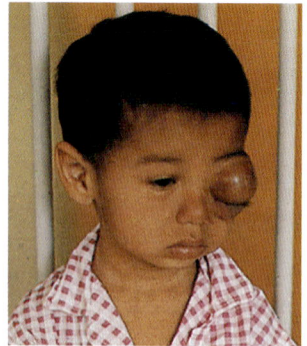

Figure 19-12 Advanced extraocular extension of retinoblastoma. Severe proptosis caused by retinoblastoma with orbital invasion.

extraocular extension. If extension of the retinoblastoma into the retrobulbar optic nerve is suspected, lumbar puncture and bone marrow biopsy may be performed as part of the workup, but they should not delay definitive enucleation or neoadjuvant chemotherapy.

In the United States, patients rarely present with metastases or intracranial extension at the time of diagnosis; in contrast, advanced presentations are common in resource-limited countries. The most frequently identified sites of metastatic involvement in children with retinoblastoma are the orbit, brain, distal bones, lymph nodes, skull bones, spinal cord, and abdominal viscera. Retinoblastoma cells may escape the eye by invading the optic nerve and extending into the cerebrospinal fluid. In addition, tumor cells may massively invade the choroid before traversing emissary canals, thereby spreading hematogenously or eroding through the sclera to enter the orbit. Extraocular extension may result in proptosis as the tumor grows in the orbit (Fig 19-12). In the anterior chamber, tumor cells may invade the trabecular meshwork, gaining access to the conjunctival lymphatics. Subsequently, palpable preauricular and cervical lymph nodes may develop.

Kim JW, Ngai LK, Sadda S, Murakami Y, Lee DK, Murphree AL. Retcam fluorescein angiography findings in eyes with advanced retinoblastoma. *Br J Ophthalmol.* 2014;98(12):1666–1671.

Differential Diagnosis

Leukocoria in children can result from many types of lesions, some of which masquerade as retinoblastoma (Table 19-2). The most common conditions that simulate retinoblastoma are persistent fetal vasculature, Coats disease, and ocular toxocariasis. Most of these conditions can be differentiated from retinoblastoma on the basis of a comprehensive history, clinical examination, and ancillary testing.

Persistent fetal vasculature

The most severe form of persistent fetal vasculature (formerly called *persistent hyperplastic primary vitreous*) is typically recognized within days or weeks of birth. The condition occurs unilaterally in two-thirds of cases and is associated with microphthalmia, a shallow or flat anterior chamber, a hypoplastic iris with prominent vessels, cataract with fibrovascular material adherent to the posterior capsule, and a retrolenticular fibrovascular

Table 19-2 Differential Diagnosis of Retinoblastoma

Persistent fetal vasculature
Coats disease
Toxocariasis (larval granuloma)
Astrocytic hamartoma (retinal astrocytoma)
Organizing vitreous hemorrhage
Medulloepithelioma
Cataract
Retinal dysplasia
Retinopathy of prematurity
Coloboma of choroid or optic nerve head
Macular toxoplasmosis (scar)
Posterior uveitis

mass that draws the ciliary body processes inward. On indirect ophthalmoscopy, a vascular stalk may be seen extending from the optic nerve head and attaching to the posterior lens capsule, or the remnants of a stalk at the capsule and optic nerve may be observed. Ultrasonographic findings that confirm that diagnosis include a microphthalmic eye (eg, short axial length) with persistent hyaloid remnants arising from the optic nerve head, usually in association with closed-funnel retinal detachment. This condition is not associated with retinal tumors, although small foci of calcification may be present. See also Chapter 10 in this volume and BCSC Section 6, *Pediatric Ophthalmology and Strabismus*.

Coats disease

Coats disease is clinically evident within the first decade of life and is more common in males. The Coats lesion is characterized by unilateral retinal telangiectasia associated with intraretinal yellow exudation without a distinct mass (Fig 19-13). The progressive leakage of fluid may result in extensive retinal detachment and neovascular glaucoma.

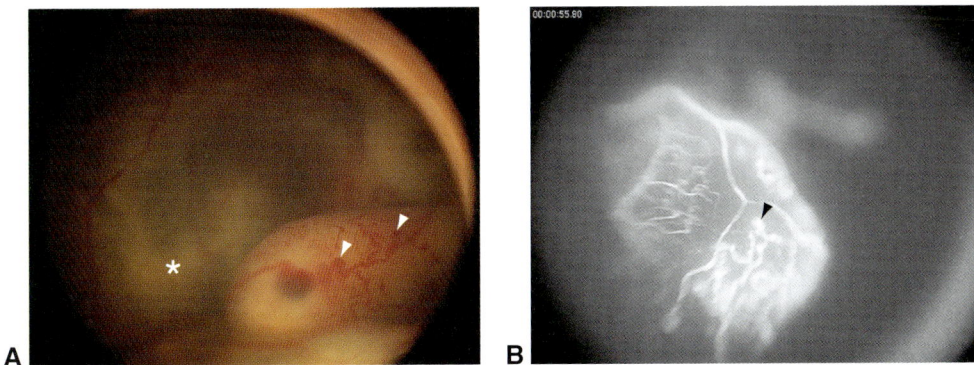

Figure 19-13 Coats disease. **A,** Clinical photograph demonstrating characteristic lightbulb aneurysms *(arrowheads)*. Note the associated exudative retinal detachment with subretinal exudate *(asterisk)*. **B,** Fluorescein angiogram showing classic telangiectatic vessels *(arrowhead)*. *(Courtesy of Matthew W. Wilson, MD.)*

On ultrasonography, retinal tumors are absent, and cholesterol accumulation is observed in the subretinal fluid. FA demonstrates the presence of telangiectatic vessels and areas of retinal ischemia. See BCSC Section 6, *Pediatric Ophthalmology and Strabismus,* and Section 12, *Retina and Vitreous,* for additional discussion.

Ocular toxocariasis

Ocular toxocariasis is a parasitic infection caused by *Toxocara canis* or *Toxocara cati* that typically occurs in older children with a history of soil ingestion or exposure to puppies or kittens. Toxocariasis presents with posterior and peripheral granulomas and associated uveitis. The granulomas often have a slightly elevated, circumscribed appearance. Exudative retinal detachment, organized vitreoretinal traction, and cataracts may be present. Ultrasonographic findings include vitritis, retinal detachment, granulomas, retinal traction, and an absence of calcium. See BCSC Section 6, *Pediatric Ophthalmology and Strabismus,* and Section 9, *Uveitis and Ocular Inflammation,* for further discussion.

Astrocytoma

Retinal astrocytoma, or astrocytic hamartoma, generally appears as a small, smooth, white, glistening tumor located in the nerve fiber layer of the retina (Fig 19-14). Retinal astrocytoma may present as 1 or multiple lesions occurring unilaterally or bilaterally. In some cases, the lesion grows and calcifies, yielding a "mulberry" appearance. Astrocytomas occasionally arise from the optic nerve head; such tumors often are referred to as *giant drusen.* Retinal astrocytomas commonly occur in patients with tuberous sclerosis and may be found in patients with neurofibromatosis; however, most cases are not associated with phakomatoses. Clinically, this lesion can masquerade as a small retinoblastoma, but handheld OCT imaging can be used to demonstrate that the tumor is confined to the nerve fiber layer. See BCSC Section 6, *Pediatric Ophthalmology and Strabismus,* for more information.

Medulloepithelioma

Medulloepithelioma usually appears as an off-white mass arising from the ciliary body (Fig 19-15A). However, in rare instances, this lesion also has been documented in the retina

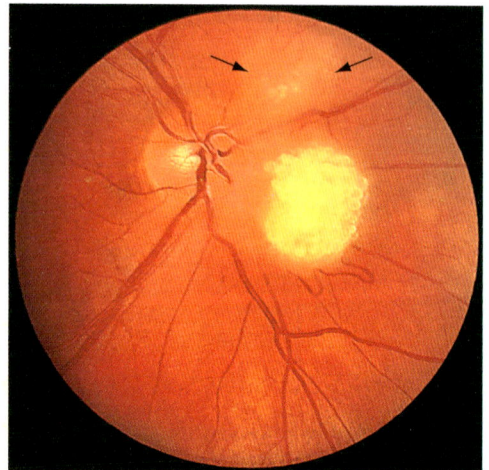

Figure 19-14 Retinal astrocytic hamartomas, clinical photograph. Note the more subtle opalescent lesion *(between arrows)* superonasal to the optic nerve head and the larger "mulberry" lesion that is inferonasal to the nerve head.

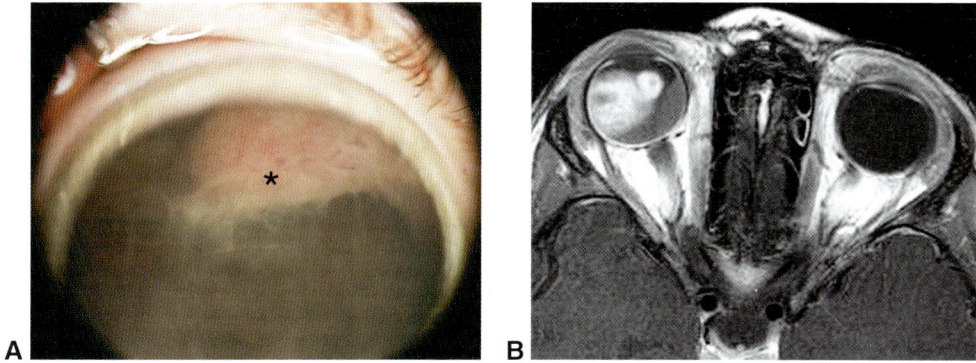

Figure 19-15 Medulloepithelioma. **A,** Pigmented lesion arising in the ciliary body, with an amelanotic apex *(asterisk).* The presence of melanin in these tumors is rare; most tumors are off-white to cream colored. **B,** T1-weighted magnetic resonance imaging with gadolinium; the image shows diffuse enhancement and multiple cystic spaces. *(Courtesy of Matthew W. Wilson, MD.)*

and optic nerve. Medulloepithelioma may be benign or malignant, although the benign form is far more common. In most cases, this type of tumor becomes clinically evident in children aged 4–12 years, but it may also occur in adults. Smaller lesions may present with unexplained neovascular glaucoma accompanied by iris heterochromia. The tumor may erode through the iris root or grow along the lens zonular fibers, extending into the anterior chamber. Diagnostic imaging may show large cysts on the surface of the tumor or within the lesion (Fig 19-15B). See Chapter 11 for a discussion of the histologic features of medulloepithelioma.

   Management of medulloepithelioma usually consists of enucleation or observation. Small lesions have been successfully treated with plaque brachytherapy, but in most eyes that have received this treatment, progressive degeneration eventually occurs, leading to enucleation. For most medulloepitheliomas, local surgical resection is avoided because of an association with late complications and metastases. Fortunately, metastasis is rare with appropriate management, even if the tumor appears frankly malignant on histologic examination.

Retinoblastoma Classification

The Reese-Ellsworth classification system for intraocular tumors is the traditional method for stratifying the intraocular extent of retinoblastoma. The system takes into account the number, size, and location of tumors and the presence or absence of vitreous seeding. Tumors are categorized from very favorable (group I) to very unfavorable (group V) by probability of eye preservation when treated with external beam radiotherapy (EBRT) alone. However, the Reese-Ellsworth classification does not stage extraocular disease, nor does it provide prognostic information about patient survival or vision. Moreover, in recent decades, EBRT has been supplanted by primary systemic and/or intra-arterial chemotherapy for treatment of retinoblastoma.

   In 2005, the first international classification system for intraocular retinoblastoma was introduced: the International Intraocular Retinoblastoma Classification (IIRC). The IIRC is now the most commonly used system worldwide. In this system, tumors are grouped in terms of size, proximity to critical anatomical structures, presence of subretinal fluid, and extent of vitreous and subretinal seeding. Eyes are assigned a letter from A to E, indicating those most to least salvageable with chemotherapy. Eyes with anterior chamber involvement, neovascular glaucoma, vitreous hemorrhage, or necrosis are classified as group E and are generally considered unsalvageable (Table 19-3).

The goal of the IIRC was to predict ocular salvage with systemic chemotherapy combined with local therapy and to provide a uniform classification scheme to be applied broadly across centers. Unfortunately, small inconsistencies in published grouping systems have undermined this. For instance, the classification system for Children's Oncology Group (COG) clinical trials includes a small deviation from the IIRC system in the allowed size of the fluid cuff for staging of group B eyes. The International Classification of Retinoblastoma (ICRB) described in 2006 differs from the IIRC in that tumor filling greater than 50% of the globe is a criterion for group E disease. Thus, some eyes classified as group D in the IIRC would be staged as group E in the ICRB scheme. This resulted in confusion in outcomes reporting, particularly in eyes with advanced disease.

The eighth edition of the American Joint Committee on Cancer TNM (tumor, node, metastasis) staging system was published in 2017 and introduced a comprehensive reclassification of intraocular disease in retinoblastoma. This clinical classification is based on a retrospective multicenter study of 1728 eyes diagnosed between 2001 and 2011, which addressed the proportion of eyes salvaged without EBRT. Notably, the system introduced a new specification, "H," indicating "hereditary trait" (see sidebar on p. 360). The classification schemes are summarized and compared in Table 19-3.

Mallipatna A, Gallie BL, Chévez-Barrios P, Lumbroso-Le Rouic L, Chantada GL, Doz F. Retinoblastoma. In: Amin MB, Edge SB, Greene FL, eds. *AJCC Cancer Staging Manual.* 8th ed. Springer; 2017:819–831.

Murphree AL. Intraocular retinoblastoma: the case for a new group classification. *Ophthalmol Clin North Am.* 2005;18(1):41–53.

Reese AB. *Tumors of the Eye.* 3rd ed. Harper & Row; 1976.

Shields CL, Shields JA. Basic understanding of current classification and management of retinoblastoma. *Curr Opin Ophthalmol.* 2006;17(3):228–234.

Treatment

Treatment of retinoblastoma has evolved dramatically in the last 100 years: from enucleation as the only option, to attempts at globe salvage with primary radiotherapy in the 1940s, to the modern chemotherapy era. Intravenous chemotherapy was introduced for this purpose in the 1990s, intra-arterial chemotherapy in the 2000s, and intravitreal chemotherapy in the 2010s.

The survival rate for retinoblastoma exceeds 95% when the disease is contained within the eye. In cases with extraocular spread, the survival rate is substantially lower. When determining the treatment strategy, the clinician's first goal must be preservation of life, then preservation of the eye, and finally preservation of vision. Modern management of intraocular retinoblastoma involves a combination of treatment modalities, including enucleation, local and systemic chemotherapy, laser therapy, cryotherapy, and plaque brachytherapy. EBRT is

Table 19-3 Comparison of Clinical Grouping Systems for Retinoblastoma

AJCC Clinical Staging 8th ed, 2017	IIRC Group Murphree, 2005	ICRB Group Shields, 2006
cT1 **Intra-retinal tumor(s)** with subretinal fluid ≤5 mm from base of any tumor		
cT1a Tumors ≤3 mm and further than 1.5 mm from disc and fovea	A, >3 mm to fovea or B, 1.5 to 3 mm	A, >3 mm to fovea or B, 1.5 to 3 mm
cT1b Tumors >3 mm or closer than 1.5 mm from disc or fovea	B	B, ≤3 mm or C, 3 to 5 mm
cT2 **Intraocular tumor(s)** with retinal detachment, vitreous seeding, or subretinal seeding		
cT2a Subretinal fluid >5 mm from the base of any tumor	C, >5 mm or D, >1 quadrant	C, or E, tumor >50% of eye volume
cT2b Vitreous seeding and/or subretinal seeding	C, "local" or D, "diffuse"	C, ≤3 mm or D, >3 mm or E, tumor >50% of eye volume
cT3 **Advanced intraocular tumor(s)**		
cT3a Phthisis or pre–phthisis bulbi	E	E
cT3b Tumor invasion of choroid, pars plana, ciliary body, lens, zonules, iris, or anterior chamber	E	E
cT3c Raised intraocular pressure with neovascularization and/or buphthalmos	E	E
cT3d Hyphema and/or massive vitreous hemorrhage	E	E
cT3e Aseptic orbital cellulitis	E	E
cT4 **Extraocular tumor(s)** involving orbit, including optic nerve		
cT4a Radiologic evidence of retrobulbar optic nerve involvement or thickening of optic nerve or involvement of orbital tissues		
cT4b Extraocular tumor clinically evident with proptosis and/or an orbital mass		

AJCC = American Joint Committee on Cancer; ICRB = International Classification of Retinoblastoma; IIRC = International Intraocular Retinoblastoma Classification.

Adapted from American College of Surgeons and Mallipatna A, Gallie BL, Chévez-Barrios P, Lumbroso-Le Rouic L, Chantada GL, Doz F. Retinoblastoma. In: Amin MB, Edge SB, Greene FL, eds. *AJCC Cancer Staging Manual.* 8th ed. Springer International Publishing; 2017:819–831. Also Murphree AL. Intraocular retinoblastoma: the case for a new group classification. *Ophthalmol Clin North Am.* 2005;18(1):42. Also Shields CL, Shields JA. Basic understanding of current classification and management of retinoblastoma. *Curr Opin Ophthalmol.* 2006;17(3):230, Table 1.

AJCC Clinical Staging: Additional Retinoblastoma Classifications

N1 Evidence of preauricular, submandibular, and cervical **lymph node involvement**

cM1 Clinical signs of **distant metastasis**

cM1a Tumor(s) involving any distant site (eg, bone marrow, liver) on clinical or radiologic tests

cM1b Tumor involving the CNS on radiologic imaging (not including trilateral retinoblastoma)

H **Hereditary trait**

HX Unknown or insufficient evidence of a constitutional *RB1* gene mutation

H0 Normal *RB1* alleles in blood tested with demonstrated high-sensitivity assays

H1 Bilateral retinoblastoma, retinoblastoma with an intracranial primitive neuroectodermal tumor (ie, trilateral retinoblastoma), patient with family history of retinoblastoma, or molecular definition of a constitutional *RB1* gene mutation

Adapted with permission from American College of Surgeons and Mallipatna A, Gallie BL, Chévez-Barrios P, Lumbroso-Le Rouic L, Chantada GL, Doz F. Retinoblastoma. In: Amin MB, Edge SB, Greene FL, eds. *AJCC Cancer Staging Manual. 8th ed.* Springer International Publishing; 2017:819–831.

now rarely performed. Metastatic disease is managed with intensive combinations of chemotherapy, radiation, and bone marrow transplantation. Recent findings of COG trials have demonstrated improved efficacy for curing patients who have regional extraocular retinoblastoma or metastatic retinoblastoma that does not involve the CNS. Treating children with retinoblastoma requires a team consisting of an ocular oncologist, a pediatric ophthalmologist, a pediatric oncologist, an interventional radiologist, and a radiation oncologist. For many of the therapeutic modalities, anesthesia is required in these young patients. Because new tumors may develop in an eye, particularly in patients with a germline mutation, serial EUAs are required for surveillance.

Enucleation

Enucleation remains a definitive treatment for retinoblastoma, enabling complete surgical resection of the disease in most cases. Enucleation often is curative in patients with unilateral disease and is considered an appropriate intervention in the following situations:

- Optic nerve involvement is suspected, and the surgeon can enucleate with a clear optic nerve margin (ie, complete tumor resection).
- Anterior segment involvement is present.
- Neovascular glaucoma is present.
- The eye has been otherwise anatomically or functionally destroyed by tumor.

- The affected eye has limited visual potential.
- The tumor persists or recurs despite attempts at globe salvage.

For eyes classified as group E in the IIRC system, enucleation is the typical treatment.

The goal of the tumor enucleation procedure is to minimize the potential for inadvertent globe penetration while obtaining the greatest possible length of resected optic nerve, typically at least 10 mm. Most surgeons place an implant postoperatively. Implants may be composed of nonporous silicone or an integrated porous material, such as hydroxyapatite or porous polyethylene.

Attempts at globe-conserving therapy should be undertaken only by ophthalmologists well versed in the management of this rare childhood tumor and in conjunction with similarly experienced pediatric oncologists. Failed attempts at eye salvage may place a child at risk of metastatic disease.

Chemotherapy

Chemotherapy is now the foundation of any globe-sparing regimen, either as a systemic intravenous treatment or as a selective intra-arterial modality.

Systemic intravenous chemotherapy typically includes 3–6 cycles of carboplatin, vincristine, and etoposide. This approach is highly successful in curing eyes classified as group A, B, or C when combined with local therapies, but it has only a 50% success rate in group D eyes. With chemotherapy, tumor regression occurs initially (chemoreduction), but adjunctive treatment with laser therapy, cryotherapy, and/or brachytherapy is necessary to completely treat the tumors; intravitreal injection of chemotherapy may also be needed to manage vitreous seeding (Fig 19-16). In addition, systemic chemotherapy often is given to patients with bilateral disease with at least IIRC group B or TNM group cT1b in the less affected eye. Although this treatment generally is well tolerated, even in very young children, complications can occur; these include cytopenia, ototoxicity, and potentially secondary acute myelogenous leukemia. Systemic chemotherapy without serial ophthalmoscopic examinations and without the use of adjunctive local therapies is not sufficient for treatment of intraocular retinoblastoma and may lead to extraocular spread and metastases.

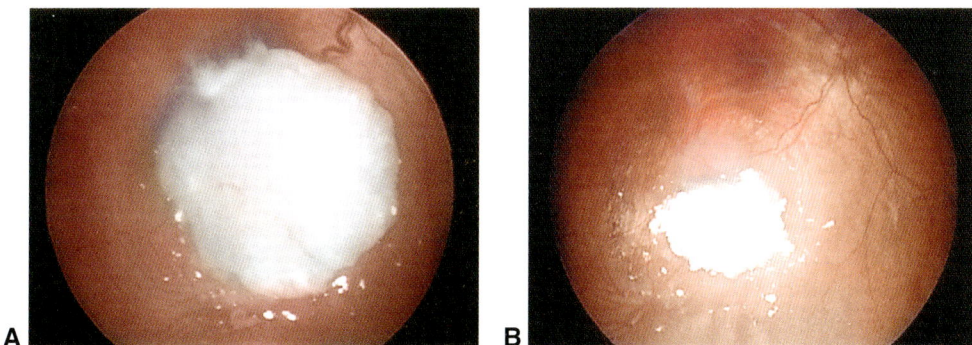

Figure 19-16 Retinoblastoma. **A,** Appearance before systemic chemotherapy. **B,** Reduced tumor volume after 2 cycles of systemic chemotherapy alone.

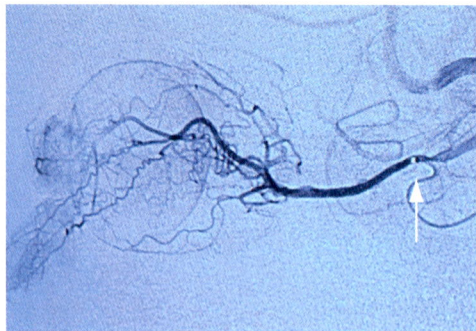

Figure 19-17 Angiogram of an eye with retinoblastoma under fluoroscopy during treatment with intra-arterial chemotherapy. *Arrow* demonstrates the location of the microcatheter injection into the ophthalmic vasculature. *(Courtesy of Dan S. Gombos, MD.)*

Due to the moderate success in treating more advanced eyes and systemic toxicities, *local intra-arterial chemotherapy* has gained popularity in the last 2 decades. Intra-arterial chemotherapy involves the selective infusion of chemotherapy into the ophthalmic artery via direct cannulation of the femoral artery (Fig 19-17). This modality usually involves administration of melphalan, topotecan, and/or carboplatin in 3 cycles. The effectiveness of intra-arterial chemotherapy is technique dependent and requires the expertise of an experienced interventional neuroradiologist. When this modality is used as primary therapy, cure rates of more than 90% have been reported for advanced-stage group D eyes. When it is used after previous treatment failure and tumor recurrence, the cure rate is approximately 50%. Intra-arterial chemotherapy typically is reserved for patients older than 3 months of age (>6 months in many centers) and/or at least 6 kg in weight. At some centers, intra-arterial therapy is reserved for children with unilateral disease; at others, tandem therapy is given to patients with bilateral disease.

Complications of intra-arterial chemotherapy include periorbital edema and erythema, nasal eyelash loss, a 3% per-infusion risk of ophthalmic vascular events (retinal nonperfusion, vitreous hemorrhage, subretinal hemorrhage, branch retinal vein occlusion, choroidal ischemia), and stroke. There is extensive debate about whether the risk for metastatic disease is increased in children with advanced retinoblastoma because of a lack of systemic chemotherapy. Most centers recommend adjuvant systemic chemotherapy after enucleation for children when pathologic evaluation of the globe reveals high-risk features for metastasis, such as massive choroidal invasion or tumor infiltration into the retrolaminar optic nerve. A recent COG study found that the highest risk for metastatic disease is the presence of concomitant peripapillary choroidal invasion of greater than 3 mm and postlaminar optic nerve invasion of 1.5 mm or greater, thus supporting adjuvant chemotherapy in this cohort. It should be noted that when eyes with advanced disease (which are more likely to have high-risk pathologic features) are salvaged, histologic information is not available to the medical team to prognosticate risk of systemic disease. For more information on the pathology of retinoblastoma, see Chapter 11.

Berry JL, Jubran R, Kim JW, et al. Long-term outcomes of group D eyes in bilateral retinoblastoma patients treated with chemoreduction and low-dose IMRT salvage. *Pediatr Blood Cancer.* 2013;60(4):688–693.

Chévez-Barrios P, Eagle RC Jr, Krailo M, et al. Study of unilateral retinoblastoma with and without histopathologic high-risk features and the role of adjuvant chemotherapy: a Children's Oncology Group study. *J Clin Oncol.* 2019;37(31):2883–2891.

Dalvin LA, et al. Ophthalmic vascular events after primary unilateral intra-arterial chemotherapy for retinoblastoma in early and recent eras. *Ophthalmology.* 2018;125(11):1803–1811.

Francis JH, Levin AM, Zabor EC, Gobin YP, Abramson DH. Ten-year experience with ophthalmic artery chemosurgery: ocular and recurrence-free survival. *PLoS One.* 2018;13(5):e0197081.

Local Consolidation Therapy

Laser Photocoagulation

Various types of laser treatments have been used to manage retinoblastoma. Lasers can be employed as a primary modality for group A/cT1a eyes with small tumors or as adjuvant treatment after systemic or intra-arterial chemotherapy. Most practitioners utilize an 810-nm infrared or 532-nm green laser for these purposes. The laser techniques vary, but for all treatments, the laser is applied to the tumor surface to elicit cytotoxic effects in tumor cells via photocoagulation or thermal injury. Multiple laser treatment sessions are necessary for tumor control, and complications of this modality include iris atrophy, cataracts, tumor seeding into the vitreous, retinal traction, and fibrosis.

Cryotherapy

Cryotherapy is an effective primary or adjunctive treatment for peripheral tumors with an apical thickness of up to 3 mm. The clinician directly visualizes the tumor with an indirect ophthalmoscope and applies cryotherapy transsclerally using a triple freeze–thaw technique. Typically, laser photoablation is chosen for smaller, posteriorly located tumors, and cryoablation is performed in larger, anteriorly located tumors. Close monitoring is necessary so that tumor regrowth or treatment complications can be managed promptly. Complications, including retinal tear and retinal detachment, are more likely to occur in large calcified tumors.

Plaque Radiotherapy

Radioactive plaque therapy (brachytherapy) may be used as a salvage therapy after globe-conserving treatments have failed to destroy all of the viable tumor; this therapy also can be applied as the primary treatment in eyes with small to medium tumors. The most commonly used isotopes for this procedure are iodine 125 and ruthenium 106. The plaque radiotherapy technique is generally applicable for tumors less than 16 mm in basal diameter and less than 8 mm in apical thickness. Ultrasound-assisted localization of the tumor intraoperatively enhances local tumor control. Compared with EBRT, plaque radiotherapy is associated with a greater likelihood of radiation optic neuropathy or retinopathy but a substantially lower risk of radiation-induced cancer.

Intravitreal Chemotherapy

Intravitreal chemotherapy was described as a treatment for retinoblastoma in the 1960s but was abandoned because of an association with extraocular tumor spread. The technique was re-introduced in 2012 with critical safety measures added to the procedure; this modality now is regarded as a highly effective adjuvant therapy for vitreous seeding. The safety measures include anterior ultrasonographic imaging to ensure that the injection is not made into a quadrant containing active tumor, reduction of intraocular pressure before the injection by means of anterior chamber paracentesis or ocular massage to prevent vitreous reflux, and cryotherapy during withdrawal of the injecting needle to kill any active tumor cells. The safety-enhanced technique is nearly 100% effective for vitreous seeding, and there have been no reports of extraocular tumor spread. Nevertheless, great care and attention to the safety precautions is imperative.

For most eyes, treatment is carried out in 3–6 injections based on the amount and type of seeding. Melphalan, the most frequently used agent for this purpose, is known to induce chorioretinal toxicity. Though not usually visually significant, this toxicity has been severe in some cases. Topotecan has also been used. Other adverse events associated with intravitreal injection include cataract, retinal detachment, and endophthalmitis. If any of these complications occur in a patient with retinoblastoma, enucleation may be required because intraocular surgery rarely is performed, given the risk of orbital seeding of active tumor. See Video 19-1 for a demonstration of intravitreal injection for retinoblastoma.

VIDEO 19-1 Intravitreal injection of melphalan for vitreous seeding in retinoblastoma.
Courtesy of Jesse L. Berry, MD.
Go to www.aao.org/bcscvideo_section04 to access all videos in Section 4.

Berry JL, Bechtold M, Shah S, et al. Not all seeds are created equal: seed classification is predictive of outcomes in retinoblastoma. *Ophthalmology.* 2017;124(12):1817–1825.
Francis JH, Abramson DH, Ji X, et al. Risk of extraocular extension in eyes with retinoblastoma receiving intravitreous chemotherapy. *JAMA Ophthalmol.* 2017;135(12):1426–1429.
Munier FL, Gaillard MC, Balmer A, et al. Intravitreal chemotherapy for vitreous disease in retinoblastoma revisited: from prohibition to conditional indications. *Br J Ophthalmol.* 2012;96(8):1078–1083.

External Beam Radiotherapy

Because retinoblastoma tumors are responsive to radiation, EBRT may be performed as a salvage technique; it is currently used only when chemotherapy has failed in the remaining eye. Two major concerns associated with EBRT have limited its use:

- Germline mutations in *RB1* are associated with a lifelong increased risk of subsequent independent primary malignancies (eg, osteosarcoma); this risk is exacerbated by exposure to EBRT, especially in children younger than 12 months.
- EBRT involves risk of radiation-related sequelae, such as orbital hypoplasia, midface hypoplasia, radiation-induced cataract, and radiation optic neuropathy and retinopathy.

Spontaneous Regression

In rare instances, very large retinoblastoma tumors can undergo complete and spontaneous necrosis. The mechanism by which spontaneous regression occurs is not well understood, but tumor growth exceeding the vascular supply likely plays a role. The incidence of spontaneous regression is unknown. Children with spontaneous regression can present with vitreous hemorrhage, a dislocated crystalline lens, or phthisis. For this reason, retinoblastoma should be part of the differential diagnosis for young children who present with unilateral phthisis without a history of trauma. The presence of calcification on imaging is highly suggestive of retinoblastoma, and prompt enucleation should be considered. Certain histologic features of the enucleated globe can suggest or confirm the diagnosis.

- The vitreous cavity is filled with islands of calcified cells embedded in a mass of fibroconnective tissue.
- Close inspection of the peripheral portions of the calcified islands reveals ghosted contours of fossilized tumor cells.
- Exuberant proliferation of retinal pigment and ciliary epithelia is present.

Genetic Counseling

Retinoblastoma is almost always caused by a mutation in both copies of the tumor suppressor gene *RB1*, located on the long arm of chromosome 13 at locus 14 (13q14); much less commonly, it is due to a deletion of part of this chromosomal arm. *RB1* was the first tumor suppressor gene to be identified. The wild-type protein product of *RB1*, pRB, serves as a cell-cycle regulator by inhibiting cell-cycle progression; thus, without a functional protein the cell cycle is unregulated. Both copies of *RB1* must be mutated (ie, "two hits") for retinoblastoma to occur, and additional mutations may be needed to promote tumorigenesis. Retinal cells are not terminally differentiated at birth; therefore, mutations in *RB1* can still occur in retinal cells over the first few years of life as the retina matures, resulting in tumor formation. Mutations in *RB1* and dysfunction of pRB can also be found in many different tumor types throughout the body because of their role in cell-cycle regulation.

Retinoblastoma may be inherited (10% of cases) or sporadic, owing to a new mutation (90%). Children with sporadic disease may have a solitary tumor related to a somatic event within a single retinal cell or may harbor a new spontaneous germline mutation, which can be inherited by their future children. Of the patients with sporadic disease, two-thirds have nonhereditary mutations in which both *RB1* mutations occur as a somatic event in a single retinal cell. The remaining one-third of patients have a new germline mutation present in all retinal cells or a mutation that occurred during embryogenesis in which the first *RB1* mutation is present in many but not all retinal cells (mosaicism). Thus, although these patients may have a family history of retinoblastoma (10% of them), it is more likely that the disease developed from a new sporadic mutation in a parental germ cell or in the developing embryo. These patients have a risk of passing a mutated copy of *RB1* to their offspring.

Patients with germline mutations in *RB1* often have bilateral or multifocal disease and an earlier presentation than do those with non-germline mutations. In addition, approximately 15% of patients with unilateral disease also have a germline mutation. Unless there are multiple tumors in the affected eye, clinical examination findings cannot distinguish patients with unilateral disease caused by germline versus non-germline mutations. Thus, it is crucial for children with retinoblastoma to undergo molecular testing for a germline *RB1* mutation.

Analysis of *RB1* mutations is done on DNA from peripheral leukocytes. Methods used for this analysis include next-generation sequencing, Sanger sequencing, karyotyping, fluorescence in situ hybridization (FISH), multiplex ligation-dependent probe amplification (MLPA), and RNA analysis. With these screening methods, there is a 96% chance of finding a tumor mutation in the peripheral blood, if one exists. This detection rate is higher when both blood and freshly harvested tumor are available for tumor-directed mutational analysis, as the results of each cell type can be compared in order to identify clinically relevant mutations.

In children younger than 6 months, 1%–3% of unilateral retinoblastomas are caused by amplification of the N-myc proto-oncogene *(MYCN)* and not by mutation in *RB1*. On clinical examination of a young child, it can be difficult to differentiate tumors driven by *MYCN* amplification from advanced unilateral disease owing to *RB1* mutation; enucleation is recommended if *MYCN* is the suspected etiology. When enucleation is performed, distinct histologic features of *MYCN*-associated tumors can be observed, including undifferentiated cells with prominent nucleoli and little calcification. These cellular features are similar to those seen in other *MYCN*-amplified tumors such as neuroblastoma. Tumors driven by *MYCN* amplification appear to be nonheritable. The exact mechanism of the amplification is still the subject of study.

Counseling with a genetic specialist is recommended for all families affected by retinoblastoma, and it is reasonable to examine parents and siblings of the patient for evidence of untreated retinoblastoma or retinocytoma, which would represent a hereditary predisposition to the disease. Genetic counseling for retinoblastoma can be complex. Owing to 90% penetrance of the disease-causing allele, a survivor of bilateral retinoblastoma has a 45% chance of having an affected child, whereas a survivor of unilateral disease (with a germline mutation) has a 7%–15% likelihood of having an affected child. Unaffected parents of a child with bilateral retinoblastoma have less than a 5% risk of having another child with retinoblastoma. If 2 or more siblings are affected, there is a 45% chance that another child will be affected, as this represents hereditary disease. Systematic screening for retinoblastoma by an ophthalmologist is recommended for children in families with retinoblastoma. In 2018, the first national guidelines for retinoblastoma screening in the United States were published (see the Skalet et al reference); these recommendations addressed practices and frequencies for screening for children at various risk levels. See also BCSC Section 6, *Pediatric Ophthalmology and Strabismus,* Table 25-8.

Abramson DH, Mendelsohn ME, Servodidio CA, Tretter T, Gombos DS. Familial retinoblastoma: where and when? *Acta Ophthalmol Scand.* 1998;76(3):334–338.

Murphree AL. Molecular genetics of retinoblastoma. *Ophthalmol Clin North Am.* 1995;8:155–166.

Rushlow DE, Mol BM, Kennett JY, et al. Characterisation of retinoblastomas without *RB1* mutations: genomic, gene expression, and clinical studies. *Lancet Oncol.* 2013;14(4):327–334.

Skalet AH, Gombos DS, Gallie BL, et al. Screening children at risk for retinoblastoma: consensus report from the American Association of Ophthalmic Oncologists and Pathologists. *Ophthalmology.* 2018;125(3):453–458.

Thériault BL, Dimaras H, Gallie BL, Corson TW. The genomic landscape of retinoblastoma: a review. *Clin Exp Ophthalmol.* 2014;42(1):33–52.

Associated Conditions

Retinocytoma

Retinocytoma is often clinically indistinguishable from retinoblastoma. In Chapter 11, the histologic features that distinguish retinocytoma from retinoblastoma are summarized (see Fig 11-48). The developmental biology of retinocytoma is controversial. Some authorities assert that retinocytoma is a completely differentiated form of retinoblastoma—analogous to ganglioneuroma, the differentiated form of neuroblastoma. Others contend that retinocytoma is a benign counterpart of retinoblastoma in which biallelic *RB1* mutations are present, but further genetic or genomic changes needed to promote tumorigenesis are absent. Though histologically benign, retinocytoma carries the same genetic implications as retinoblastoma. A child harboring a retinoblastoma in one eye and a retinocytoma in the other should be considered to have the same risk of transmitting an *RB1* mutation to future offspring as children with bilateral retinoblastoma.

Singh AD, Santos MM, Shields CL, Shields JA, Eagle RC Jr. Observations on 17 patients with retinocytoma. *Arch Ophthalmol.* 2000;118(2):199–205.

Primitive Neuroectodermal Tumor

Intracranial neoplasms known as *primitive neuroectodermal tumors (PNETs)* develop in some patients with bilateral retinoblastoma; PNETs represent the intracranial component of *trilateral retinoblastoma* (see Fig 19-11). The ectopic focus usually is located in the pineal gland or the parasellar region and traditionally is known as a *pinealoblastoma.* This tumor affects up to 5% of children with a germline *RB1* mutation. In rare cases, the PNET arises prior to ocular involvement. More commonly, this independent malignant tumor presents months or years after treatment of intraocular retinoblastoma.

Several observations support the concept that an intracranial PNET constitutes a primary tumor, as opposed to intracranial spread of retinoblastoma. In some patients with terminal retinoblastoma, CT findings have shown that intracranial tumor is anatomically separate from the ocular tumor(s). These intracranial tumors are not associated with metastatic disease elsewhere in the body and—unlike metastatic retinoblastoma—often have features of differentiation, such as *Flexner-Wintersteiner rosettes* (see Chapter 11, Fig 11-44A). Embryologic, immunologic, and phylogenic evidence of photoreceptor differentiation in the pineal gland further support the concept of trilateral retinoblastoma.

It is recommended that all patients with retinoblastoma undergo baseline neuroimaging studies to exclude intracranial involvement. Experts disagree on the role of serial imaging in screening for PNETs. Investigators have shown that the incidence of PNETs decreases over time. It is unclear whether this is due to the prophylactic effect of systemic chemotherapy or a decrease in the use of radiation therapy.

Friedman DN, Sklar CA, Oeffinger KC, et al. Long-term medical outcomes in survivors of extra-ocular retinoblastoma: the Memorial Sloan-Kettering Cancer Center (MSKCC) experience. *Pediatr Blood Cancer.* 2013;60(4):694–699.

Jubran RF, Erdreich-Epstein A, Butturini A, Murphree AL, Villablanca JG. Approaches to treatment for extraocular retinoblastoma: Children's Hospital Los Angeles experience. *J Pediatr Hematol Oncol.* 2004;26(1):31–34.

Moll AC, Imhof SM, Schouten-Van Meeteren AY, Kuik DJ, Hofman P, Boers M. Second primary tumors in hereditary retinoblastoma: a register-based study, 1945–1997: is there an age effect on radiation-related risk? *Ophthalmology.* 2001;108(6):1109–1114.

Prognosis

Children with intraocular retinoblastoma who have access to modern medical care have a very good prognosis for survival (>95% in industrialized countries). The main risk factor associated with death is extraocular extension of the tumor, either directly through the sclera or, more commonly, by invasion of the optic nerve, especially to the surgically resected margin (see Chapter 11, Fig 11-46). Massive choroidal invasion ($\geq$3 mm of invasion), extrascleral extension, or postlaminar optic nerve disease increase the risk that metastatic disease could develop. The highest risk of developing metastatic disease is in the setting of active tumor at the cut end of the optic nerve; this clinical situation requires adjuvant chemotherapy and radiation therapy. There is evidence that bilateral tumors may increase the risk of death because of the association with primary intracranial PNET.

Historically, children with extraocular retinoblastoma had a very poor prognosis for survival. However, in a recent COG report, the authors demonstrated that intensive multimodal therapies—including high-dose chemotherapy, radiation, and bone marrow transplantation—have enabled improved efficacy for curing patients with regional extraocular retinoblastoma (87% event-free survival [EFS] at 36 months) and metastatic retinoblastoma not involving the CNS (79% EFS at 36 months), while rates for patients with CNS disease continue to be dismal (8% EFS at 36 months).

Children who survive bilateral retinoblastoma have an increased incidence of a second-primary nonocular malignancy later in life. The mean latency for tumor development of a second tumor is approximately 9 years from management of the primary retinoblastoma. A patient with a germline *RB1* mutation has an approximately 0.5%–1% incidence of second-primary tumor development per year of life; thus, the risk exceeds 25% at 50 years of age. This risk is elevated further in patients who were treated with EBRT. The most common type of second-primary cancer in these patients is osteosarcoma (also called *osteogenic sarcoma*). Other relatively common second malignancies include soft-tissue sarcomas, cutaneous melanoma, PNETs, other brain tumors, and primitive unclassifiable tumors (Table 19-4).

Table 19-4 Second-Primary Malignant Neoplasms in Retinoblastoma Survivors

Tumors Arising in the Field of Ocular Radiation		Tumors Arising Outside the Field of Ocular Radiation	
Pathologic Type	Percentage	Pathologic Type	Percentage
Osteosarcoma	40	Osteosarcoma	36
Fibrosarcoma	10	Cutaneous melanoma	12
Other soft-tissue sarcoma	8	Primitive neuroectodermal tumor	9
Anaplastic and unclassifiable	8	Ewing sarcoma	6
Squamous cell carcinoma	5	Papillary thyroid carcinoma	6
Rhabdomyosarcoma	5	Assorted other	30
Assorted other	24		

Information from Moll AC, Imhof SM, Schouten-Van Meeteren AY, Kuik DJ, Hofman P, Boers M. Second primary tumors in hereditary retinoblastoma: a register-based study,1945–1997: is there an age effect on radiation-related risk? *Ophthalmology.* 2001;108(6):1109–1114. Also Abramson DH, Frank CM. Second nonocular tumors in survivors of bilateral retinoblastoma: a possible age effect on radiation-related risk. *Ophthalmology.* 1998;105(4):573–579. Also Abramson DH, Ellsworth RM, Kitchin FD, Tung G. Second nonocular tumors in retinoblastoma survivors. Are they radiation-induced? *Ophthalmology.* 1984;91(11): 1351–1355.

Up to 20% of patients with bilateral retinoblastoma treated with chemotherapy will present with a second nonocular tumor within 20 years, and in up to 40% of those who were irradiated, a second or third nonocular tumor will develop. The 5-year survival rate in patients with sarcomas after retinoblastoma treatment is less than 50%. It is recommended that patients with germline *RB1* mutations adhere to lifelong risk-modification practices, such as not smoking, avoiding unnecessary radiation exposure, and applying sunscreen. An international consensus panel convened by the American Association of Cancer Research recently gave recommendations for second-primary tumor surveillance in hereditary retinoblastoma; these include an annual physical examination, with an assessment of the skin to identify second-primary skin cancers, as well as education regarding the signs and symptoms of bone and soft-tissue sarcomas. Although it may be feasible to conduct annual whole-body MRI procedures on patients with *RB1* germline mutations beginning at age 8–10 years (when general anesthesia would no longer be required), there is no consensus on the use of whole-body imaging as a surveillance tool. Effective screening strategies for second-primary nonocular cancers in this population is an area of active research.

Dunkel IJ, Krailo MD, Chantada GL, et al. Intensive multi-modality therapy for extra-ocular retinoblastoma (RB): a Children's Oncology Group (COG) trial (ARET0321). *J Clin Oncol.* 2017;35(15 Suppl):10506–10506.

Kamihara J, Bourdeaut F, Foulkes WD, et al. Retinoblastoma and neuroblastoma predisposition and surveillance. *Clin Cancer Res.* 2017;23(13):e98–e106.

CHAPTER 20

Ocular Involvement in Systemic Malignancies

Highlights

- The most common tumor occurring in the adult eye is a secondary metastatic tumor. This generally presents as a choroidal mass, disseminated from a carcinoma elsewhere in the body.
- The most common intraocular site for metastatic tumors is the posterior choroid, owing to its rich blood supply.
- Lymphoma can affect a single ocular tissue or multiple tissues, from the ocular adnexa to various parts of the eye, and there may be systemic involvement.
- Ocular involvement in leukemia is frequent and most commonly manifests clinically as retinal hemorrhages and cotton-wool spots.

Secondary Tumors of the Eye

Metastatic Carcinoma

Since the first report in 1872 of a metastatic tumor in the eye of a patient with carcinoma, ocular metastases have been described as the most common intraocular tumor in adults. However, they may not be the lesions that are most commonly seen by ophthalmologists, as much of the data regarding the incidence of these tumors are derived not from clinical studies but from evaluation of the eyes at the time of autopsy. As long-term survival rates for patients with primary systemic malignancies continue to improve and the incidence of intraocular and orbital metastatic disease increases, so will the need for prompt recognition and appropriate diagnostic and therapeutic management by the ophthalmologist.

Metastases to the eye are being diagnosed with increasing frequency for various reasons, including

- increased incidence of certain tumor types that metastasize to the eye (eg, breast, lung)
- prolonged survival of patients with certain cancer types (eg, breast cancer)
- increased awareness among medical oncologists and ophthalmologists of the pattern of metastatic disease

Ferry AP, Font RL. Carcinoma metastatic to the eye and orbit: I. A clinicopathologic study of 227 cases. *Arch Ophthalmol.* 1974;92(4):276–286.

Mechanism of metastasis to the eye

The most common mechanism of intraocular metastasis is the hematogenous dissemination of tumor cells. The anatomy of the arterial blood supply to the eye dictates the location of tumor cell deposits within the eye. The posterior choroid, with its rich vascular supply, is the most common site of intraocular metastases; it is affected 10–20 times as frequently as the iris or ciliary body. The retina and optic nerve head, which are supplied by the single central retinal artery, are rarely the sole site of involvement. Bilateral ocular involvement has been reported in approximately 25% of cases of metastatic disease, and multifocal involvement is frequently seen within an eye. Many patients with ocular metastases also have concurrent central nervous system (CNS) (Fig 20-1) and other metastases. Ocular metastatic lesions are sometimes found before a primary tumor is detected; this is most often seen with lung adenocarcinoma.

Primary tumor sites

The medical literature contains many reports of ocular metastases representing a wide variety of primary tumor types. Most metastatic solid tumors to the eye are carcinomas from various organs. In a survey of 520 eyes with uveal metastases, the most common primary tumors to metastasize to the eye were breast (47%), lung (21%), and gastrointestinal tract (4%). In females, the breast is the most common primary tumor site; in males, the lung. In contrast, cutaneous melanoma is rarely described as metastasizing to the eye. Table 20-1 shows the most common primary tumors that metastasize to the choroid.

Clinical features and diagnosis

The clinical features of intraocular metastases depend on the location within the eye and are discussed in the following sections. Metastatic tumors can be mistaken for other

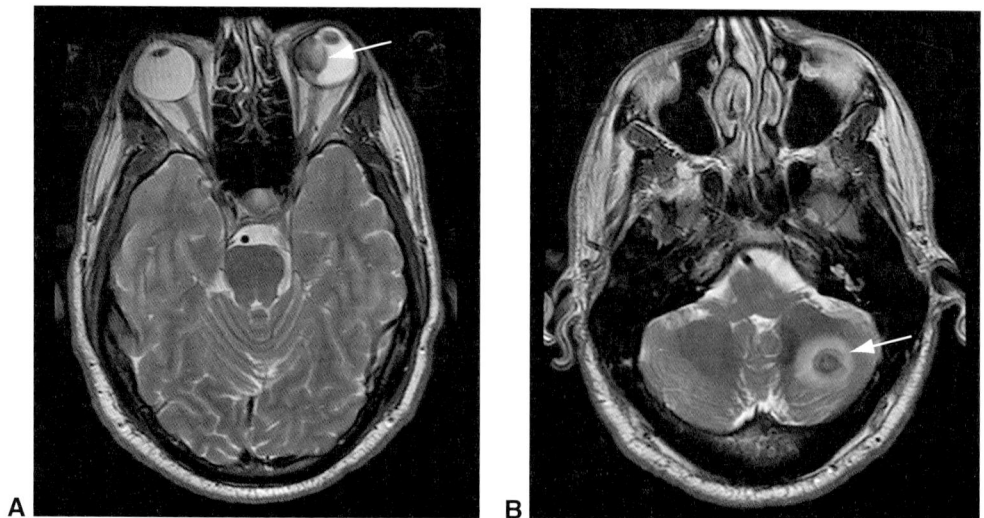

Figure 20-1 Axial T2-weighted magnetic resonance images of central nervous system (CNS) metastases. **A,** Metastatic intraocular tumor in the left eye *(arrow)*. **B,** Concurrent left cerebellar mass with surrounding edema *(arrow)*. *(Courtesy of Dan S. Gombos, MD.)*

Table 20-1 Primary Solid Tumors That Metastasize to the Uveal Tract (in Decreasing Order of Frequency)

Males (*n* = 137)	Females (*n* = 287)
Lung (40%)	Breast (70%)
Unknown (30%)	Lung (10%)
Gastrointestinal tract (10%)	Unknown (10%)
Kidney (5%)	Other (<5%)
Prostate (5%)	Gastrointestinal tract (<5%)
Skin (<5%)	Skin (1%)
Other (<5%)	Kidney (<1%)
Breast (1%)	

Modified from Shields CL, Shields JA, Gross NE, et al. Survey of 520 eyes with uveal metastases. *Ophthalmology.* 1997;104:1265–1276.

ocular lesions, including primary tumors. The steps involved in making an accurate diagnosis include taking a thorough medical history, performing a careful ocular examination, and using ancillary ophthalmic tests. The selection of ancillary ophthalmic testing is determined by the location of the tumor(s). Review of patient medical records, including previous pathology reports, may be necessary to determine the origin of metastatic tumors. In a minority of cases, biopsy of the lesion may be needed to make the diagnosis of metastatic tumor rather than primary intraocular tumor. When the ocular diagnosis is unclear, the clinician should consider referral to an ocular oncologist as this specialist has extensive experience in the diagnosis and management of ocular metastatic tumors.

Anterior segment: iris and ciliary body Metastases to the iris and ciliary body usually appear as gray-white to tan-pink gelatinous nodules (Figs 20-2, 20-3, 20-4). Metastases to the anterior uvea may include the following clinical features:

- iridocyclitis (sometimes before the tumor becomes clinically evident)
- secondary glaucoma
- iris neovascularization (rubeosis iridis)
- hyphema
- irregular pupil
- pseudohypopyon

Anterior segment tumors are best evaluated with slit-lamp biomicroscopy coupled with gonioscopy. High-frequency ultrasonography (eg, ultrasound biomicroscopy) may quantify tumor size and anatomical relationships.

Posterior segment: choroid, retina, and optic nerve With tumors in the posterior pole, patients commonly report painless loss of vision. Indirect ophthalmoscopy may reveal an exudative retinal detachment associated with a placoid or "lumpy bumpy" amelanotic tumor mass (Figs 20-5, 20-6, 20-7). These lesions are usually minimally elevated and ill defined, often amelanotic, gray, yellow, or off-white, with secondary alterations at the level of the retinal pigment epithelium (RPE) presenting as clumps of brown pigment ("leopard spots"; Fig 20-8).

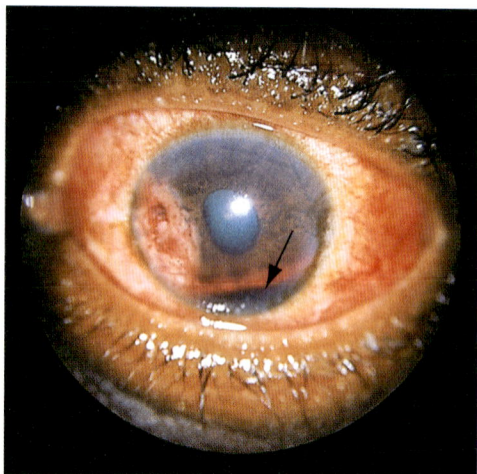

Figure 20-2 Metastatic tumor in the iris with associated hyphema *(arrow).*

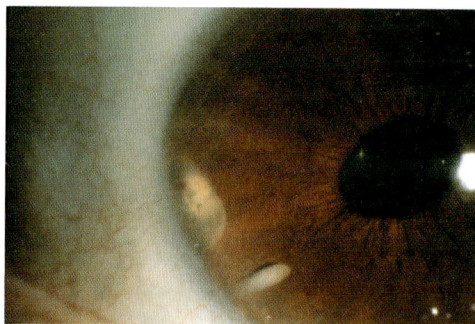

Figure 20-3 Metastasis from breast carcinoma to the iris. Note the 2 gray-white lesions on the iris surface. *(Courtesy of Timothy G. Murray, MD.)*

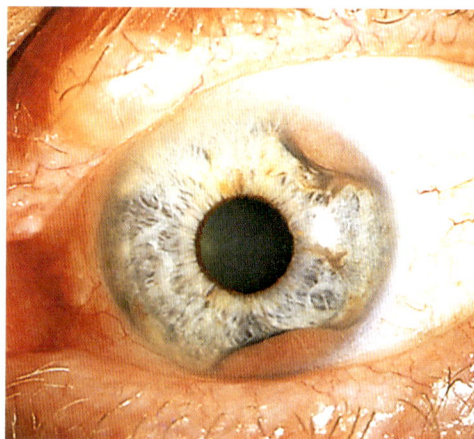

Figure 20-4 Metastatic cutaneous melanoma to the iris. Note the 2 lesions located peripherally and lacking pigmentation.

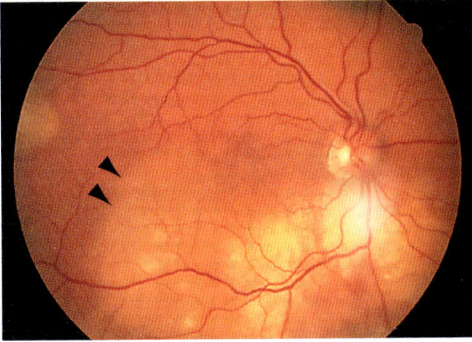

Figure 20-5 Multiple metastatic lesions in the choroid. Note the pale-yellow color, "lumpy bumpy" configuration, and shallow subretinal fluid *(arrowheads)*.

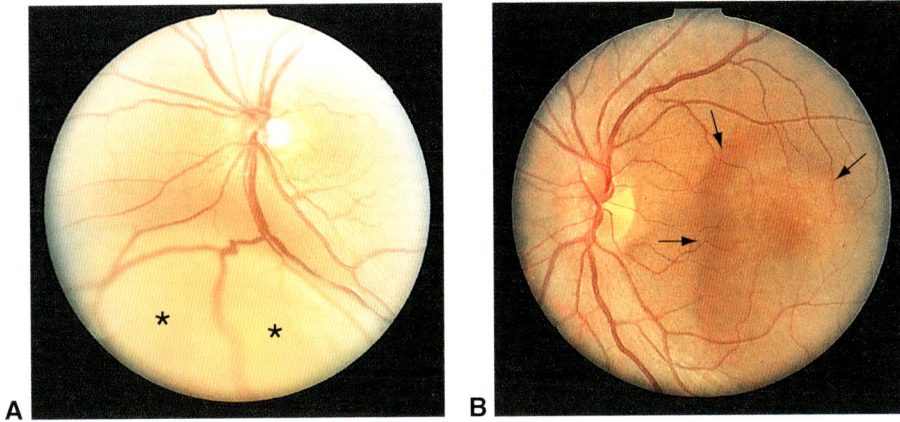

A

B

Figure 20-6 Choroidal metastases. **A,** Metastatic lesion to the choroid inferiorly, associated with bullous retinal detachment *(asterisks)*. **B,** Subtle metastatic lesion to the choroid *(arrows)* in the macula, associated with serous effusion.

The mushroom configuration seen in primary choroidal melanoma from invasion through Bruch membrane is rarely present in uveal metastases. The retina overlying the metastasis may appear opaque and often can detach because of the accumulation of subretinal fluid. Rapid tumor growth with necrosis and uveitis are occasionally seen. Dilated epibulbar vessels may be seen in the quadrant overlying the metastasis. For a differential diagnosis of choroidal metastasis, see Table 20-2.

Although *fluorescein angiography* may be helpful in defining the margins of a metastatic tumor, it is typically less useful in differentiating a primary intraocular neoplasm from a metastasis. The double circulation pattern from an intrinsic intratumoral blood supply and prominent early choroidal filling often seen in choroidal melanomas are rarely found in metastatic tumors because of their rapid growth (ie, versus slow growth in choroidal melanomas, which allows for the development of an intratumoral vascular supply).

Ultrasonography (echography) is diagnostically valuable in patients with choroidal lesions. In the setting of a metastatic tumor, B-scan ultrasonography shows an echogenic choroidal mass with an ill-defined, sometimes lobulated or lumpy bumpy outline (see

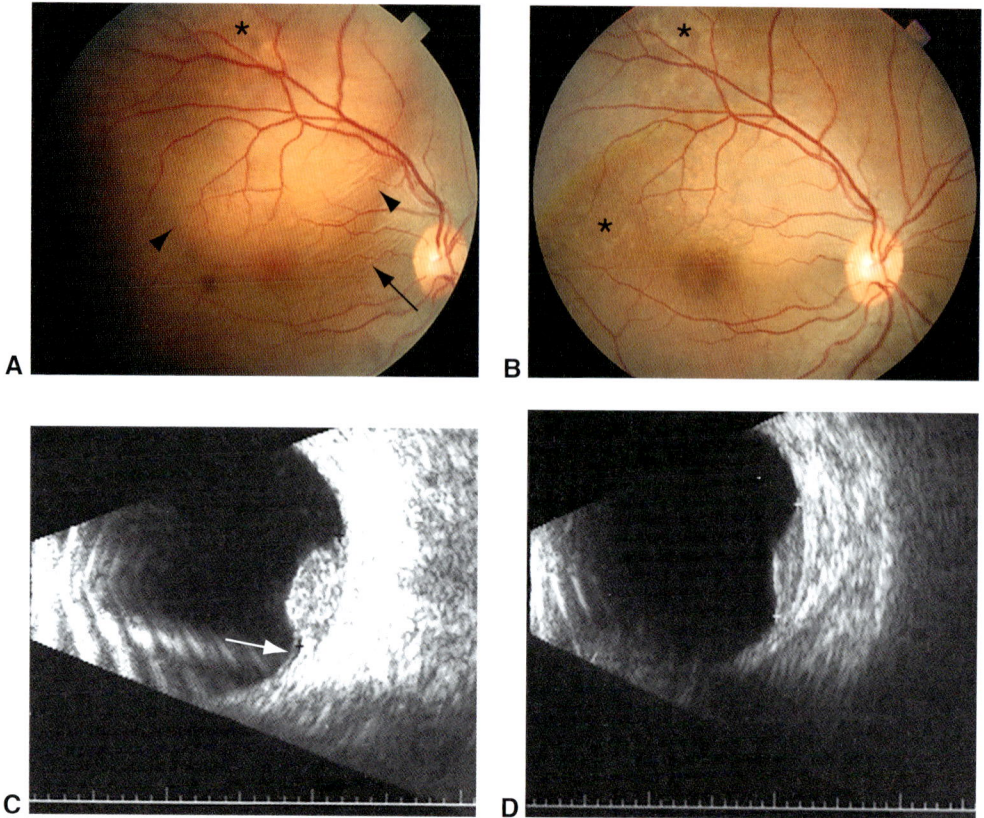

Figure 20-7 Metastatic breast carcinoma to the choroid before and after external beam radiotherapy. **A,** Clinical photograph of metastatic breast carcinoma to the choroid. Note the yellowish choroidal lesion *(between arrowheads)* with focal retinal striae *(arrow)* and pigmentary change *(asterisk).* **B,** After radiation, note the yellowish focal drusenoid lesions *(asterisks)* and resolution of the retinal striae in the macular region. **C,** B-scan ultrasonography shows the choroidal mass demonstrated in part **A** with shallow exudative retinal detachment *(arrow).* **D,** B-scan ultrasonography shows reduction in the size of the choroidal mass after radiation therapy and resolution of the exudative retinal detachment corresponding to part **B.** Classically, metastatic lesions show high internal reflectivity on A-scan ultrasonography. *(Courtesy of Dan S. Gombos, MD.)*

Fig 20-7C). Overlying secondary exudative retinal detachment is commonly detected. A-scan ultrasonography demonstrates irregular and generally high reflectivity.

Enhanced depth imaging optical coherence tomography (EDI-OCT) may demonstrate a lumpy bumpy contour, choriocapillaris compression, and photoreceptor loss in the overlying retina.

Metastases to the optic nerve may produce edema of the optic nerve head, decreased vision, and visual field defects. Because metastases may involve the parenchyma or the optic nerve sheath, magnetic resonance imaging (MRI) and ultrasonography may be valuable in detecting the presence of additional lesions and identifying their location.

Metastases to the retina, which are quite rare, appear as white noncohesive lesions, often distributed in a perivascular location suggestive of cotton-wool spots (Fig 20-9). Because of

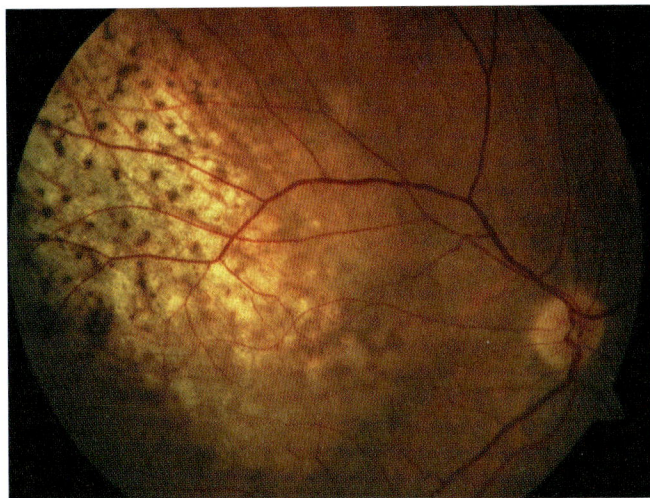

Figure 20-8 Clinical fundus photograph of metastatic breast carcinoma to the choroid. Note the amelanotic infiltrative choroidal mass with secondary overlying retinal pigment epithelial changes accounting for the characteristic leopard spots. *(Courtesy of Matthew W. Wilson, MD.)*

Table 20-2 Differential Diagnosis of Choroidal Metastasis

Amelanotic nevus	Vogt-Koyanagi-Harada syndrome
Amelanotic melanoma	Central serous retinopathy
Choroidal hemangioma	Infectious/inflammatory lesions, granuloma
Choroidal osteoma	Organized subretinal hemorrhage
Choroidal detachment	Extensive neovascular membranes
Posterior scleritis	Rhegmatogenous retinal detachment

secondary vitreous seeding of tumor cells, these metastases sometimes resemble retinitis rather than a tumor. Vitreous aspirates for cytologic studies may confirm the diagnosis (see Fig 20-9C).

Other diagnostic factors

One of the most important diagnostic factors in the evaluation of suspected ocular metastatic tumors is a history of systemic malignancy (see the section "Primary tumor sites"). At the time the ocular metastasis is diagnosed, most patients have a known systemic malignancy, although the interval between the diagnosis of the primary tumor and that of the ocular metastasis can be many years. For example, in a study of 264 patients with uveal metastases from breast cancer, greater than 90% of patients had a history of treatment before the development of ocular involvement. The ocular metastasis was the initial manifestation of the breast cancer in only 3% of patients, but the eye was the first site of metastatic disease in 16% of patients in this study, many of whom had been in remission for years.

For some patients, however, often there is no history of systemic malignancy. Various studies have shown that in patients in whom an ocular metastatic lesion(s) was diagnosed, the ocular lesion was the first manifestation of cancer in about 30% of cases; that is, 30% of

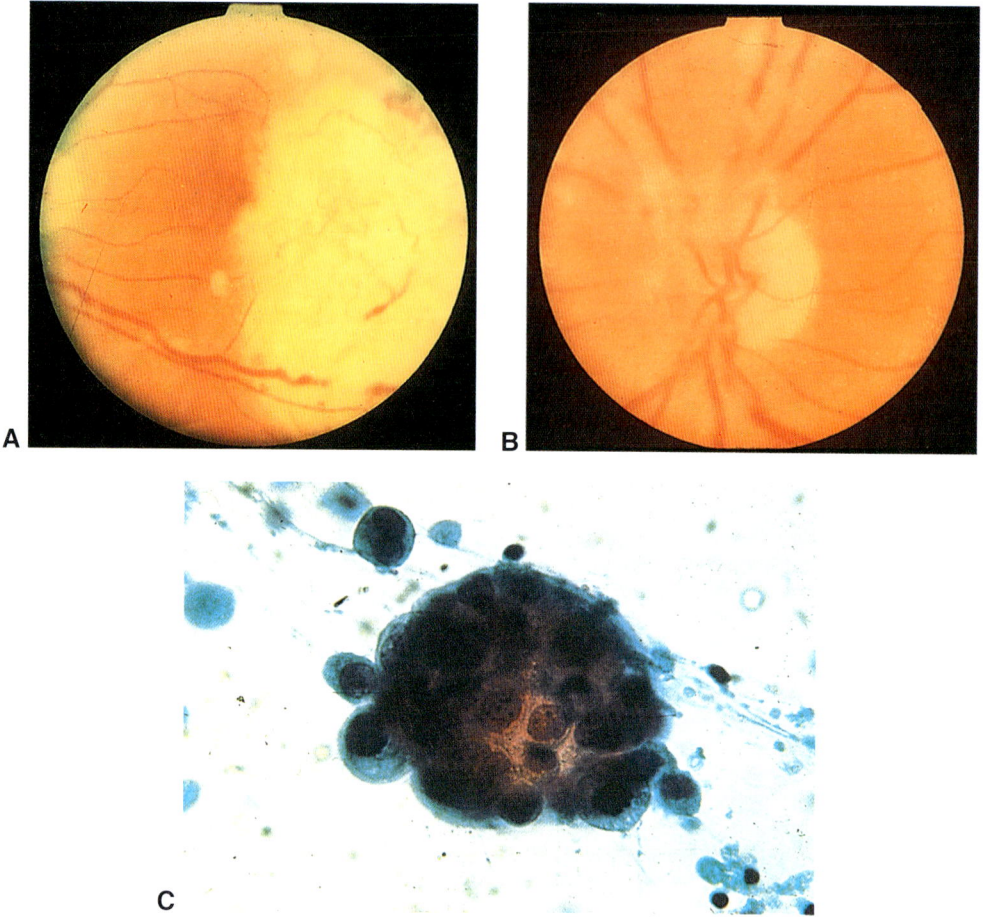

Figure 20-9 Metastatic lung carcinoma to the retina. **A,** Metastatic lung carcinoma involving the macula. Vision was reduced to finger counting. **B,** Same eye, showing the characteristic perivascular distribution of metastases. **C,** Vitreous aspirate from the same eye, showing clumping of tumor cells that is characteristic of carcinoma.

patients with an ocular metastatic lesion have an unknown primary tumor at the time of the ocular diagnosis. This is especially true of patients with ocular metastasis from lung cancer. A study of 194 patients with uveal metastases from lung carcinoma demonstrated that diagnosis of the uveal metastasis preceded the diagnosis of primary lung cancer in nearly half of the patients (44%). Thus, any patient with an amelanotic fundus mass suspected of being a metastatic focus should be referred for a thorough systemic evaluation, including imaging of the breast, chest, abdomen, and pelvis. Suspicious lesions identified on systemic evaluation often require biopsy before further management can be determined.

Fine-needle aspiration biopsy (FNAB) of the choroidal lesion may be helpful in rare cases when the diagnosis cannot be established by noninvasive procedures. Although metastatic tumors may recapitulate the histology of the primary tumor, they are often less differentiated. For this reason, special histochemical and immunohistochemical stains facilitate the diagnosis of metastatic tumors. It may not always be possible to narrow the differential to just one primary tumor type, but FNAB with appropriate special studies may reduce the list to a few likely primary sites. FNAB may be helpful even when the primary cancer is known. For example, breast cancer may demonstrate a change in receptor status during metastatic spread that warrants biopsy of new metastatic disease and often changes the therapeutic options for the patient. Communication between the patient's ophthalmologist and medical oncologist is paramount throughout the diagnostic workup.

Demirci H, Shields CL, Chao AN, Shields JA. Uveal metastasis from breast cancer in 264 patients. *Am J Ophthalmol.* 2003;136(2):264–271.

Shah SU, Mashayekhi A, Shields CL, et al. Uveal metastasis from lung cancer: clinical features, treatment, and outcome in 194 patients. *Ophthalmology.* 2014;121(1):352–357.

Shields CL, Shields JA, Gross NE, Schwartz GP, Lally SE. Survey of 520 eyes with uveal metastases. *Ophthalmology.* 1997;104(8):1265–1276.

Prognosis

The diagnosis of an ocular metastasis is typically associated with a poor prognosis for survival because widespread dissemination of the primary tumor has usually occurred. In one report, survival time after the diagnosis of metastasis to the uvea ranged from 1 to 67 months, depending on the primary cancer type. Overall, the average survival of patients with ocular metastases is less than 1 year. Although the overall survival rate for women with breast cancer has improved, patients with breast carcinoma metastatic to the uvea have historically survived an average of 9–13 months after the metastasis was detected. The 5-year survival rate in patients with metastatic ocular disease in the setting of breast cancer is approximately 25% across studies. Shorter survival time is typically seen in patients with ocular metastases from lung carcinoma, with about half of patients deceased at 1 year.

Treatment

The goal in ophthalmologic management of ocular metastases is preservation or restoration of vision whenever possible and palliation of pain. Radical surgical procedures and treatments with risks that exceed the desired benefits should be carefully considered in the context of the patient's overall health status. All treatment should be coordinated with the patient's primary oncologists and should reflect the goals of the care plan.

Indications for treatment include decreased vision, pain, diplopia, and severe ocular proptosis. The patient's age and health status and the condition of the fellow eye are also critical in the decision-making process. When ocular metastases are concurrent with widespread metastatic disease, systemic chemotherapy alone or in combination with local therapy is reasonable. In patients manifesting metastases in the eye alone, confirmed after careful workup and systemic imaging, local therapeutic modalities may be sufficient, allowing conservation of visual function with minimal systemic morbidity.

In patients with susceptible tumors, chemotherapy or hormonal therapy may induce a prompt response in the ocular lesion as well. In such patients, no additional ocular treatment may be indicated. However, when vision is endangered by choroidal metastases in spite of systemic therapy, additional forms of local therapy, such as external beam radiotherapy, brachytherapy, photodynamic therapy, or transpupillary thermotherapy, may be indicated.

Radiotherapy is frequently associated with rapid improvement of the patient's symptoms, along with resolution of exudative retinal detachment and often direct reduction in tumor size. Possible adverse effects of the radiation include cataract, radiation retinopathy, and radiation optic neuropathy; ocular surface irritation and dry eye are expected and should be aggressively treated, as they can cause significant discomfort. Sometimes, enucleation is performed because of severe, unrelenting pain.

Cohen VML. Ocular metastases. *Eye (Lond).* 2013;27(2):137–141.

Jardel P, Sauerwein W, Olivier T, et al. Management of choroidal metastases. *Cancer Treat Rev.* 2014;40(10):1119–1128.

Direct Intraocular Extension

In contrast to intraocular metastases, direct extension of extraocular tumors into the eye is rare because the sclera is usually an effective barrier to such invasion. Intraocular extension occurs most commonly with conjunctival squamous cell carcinoma and less frequently with conjunctival melanoma and basal cell carcinoma of the eyelid. Only a small minority of carcinomas of the conjunctiva penetrate the globe, and these are often aggressive variants of squamous cell carcinoma: mucoepidermoid, adenoid, and spindle cell carcinoma. These neoplasms usually recur several times after local excision before they invade the eye. For more information on conjunctival tumors, see BCSC Section 8, *External Disease and Cornea.*

Lymphoid Tumors

Ocular lymphomas are most often of a non-Hodgkin B-cell type; in rare cases, they are T cell in origin. They may arise in different parts of the eye, expressing various clinical manifestations, and their nomenclature is as varied as the areas of anatomical involvement. Ocular lymphomas are classified as *primary intraocular lymphomas (PIOLs; also known as primary vitreoretinal lymphomas [PVRLs]), primary uveal lymphomas, primary ocular adnexal lymphomas,* and *secondary lymphomas* from systemic disease. PIOL (PVRL) is the most aggressive type of lymphoma involving the eye and is often associated with primary central nervous system lymphoma (PCNSL); in fact, it is considered a variant of PCNSL with overlapping cytologic and clinical features.

Primary Intraocular Lymphoma

Clinical evaluation

Primary intraocular lymphoma (PIOL), more accurately termed *primary vitreoretinal lymphoma (PVRL)* to differentiate it from primary uveal lymphoma, is considered the most aggressive of the ocular lymphomas. It is a non-Hodgkin diffuse large B-cell lymphoma (DLBCL). Ocular signs and symptoms may occur before, concurrently with, or subsequent to CNS disease. When the eye is involved first, the disease may be mistaken for a nonspecific posterior uveitis. PIOL is considered a masquerade syndrome because it simulates many

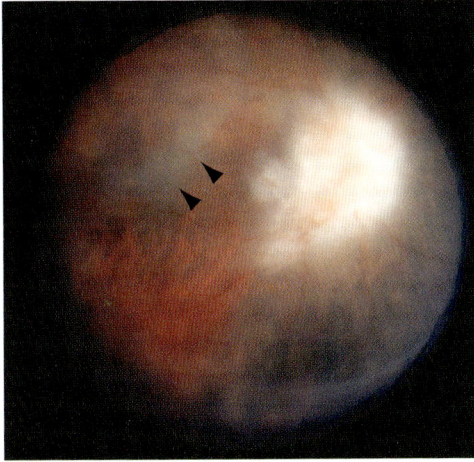

Figure 20-10 Fundus photograph from a patient with primary intraocular (vitreoretinal) lymphoma (PIOL). Note the vitreous haze, optic nerve head involvement, and subretinal infiltrate *(arrowheads)*. *(Courtesy of Jacob Pe'er, MD.)*

diagnoses, most commonly posterior uveitis. In patients older than 50 years with onset of bilateral posterior uveitis, PIOL should be considered in the differential diagnosis. Although 30% of patients present with unilateral involvement, delayed involvement of the second eye occurs in approximately 85% of patients. Approximately 25% of patients with PCNSL will have PIOL at some point, and at least 60% of patients who present with PIOL will develop CNS disease.

Patients with PIOL often report decreased vision and floaters. They present with diffuse vitreous cells and haze, which may be associated with deep subretinal and/or sub-RPE yellow-white infiltrates (Fig 20-10). Often, fine details of the retina are obscured by the density of the vitritis. Retinal vasculitis and/or vascular occlusion may be noted. The RPE may reveal characteristic clumping overlying the sub-RPE infiltrates (see Chapter 10, Fig 10-14). Anterior chamber reaction may be absent or minimal. See the discussion of cytologic findings of PIOL in Chapter 10.

Imaging

In patients with PIOL, fluorescein angiographic findings can be variable; however, most often hypofluorescent spots are persistent from early to late frames of the angiogram. This is thought to be secondary to tumor cell aggregates between Bruch membrane and the RPE, which do not absorb fluorescein owing to an intact overlying cell membrane. Hypofluorescent window defects can also be present because of damaged RPE. Indocyanine green (ICG) angiography is rarely indicated for PIOL but may show hypocyanescent spots. Ultrasonographic examination may reveal discrete nodular or placoid infiltration of the subretinal space, associated retinal detachment, and vitreous syneresis with increased reflectivity. Although ocular coherence tomography (OCT) findings are not diagnostic, amorphous nodular lesions at the level of the RPE may be seen. If the diagnosis is suspected, consultation with a neurologist and/or an oncologist should be considered, coupled with CNS imaging studies and lumbar puncture. Diagnostic vitrectomy is often performed to confirm PIOL even when the CNS imaging and/or cerebrospinal fluid analysis reveals lymphoma.

Pathologic studies

Diagnostic confirmation of ocular involvement requires sampling of the vitreous and, when appropriate, the subretinal space. Coordinated presurgical planning with the ophthalmic pathologist regarding sample handling is critical to clarify all the steps needed for obtaining the vitreous specimen and transporting it to the laboratory. The pathology laboratory to which the vitreous sample is submitted must be skilled in the processing of small-volume cytologic specimens and experienced in the cytologic evaluation of vitreous samples. If the laboratory lacks the skills to process these samples, the opportunity to diagnose PIOL may be missed and a second biopsy, after cells have re-accumulated in the vitreous, may be required. Even in cases where the biopsy and laboratory evaluation are executed as planned, the diagnosis may be elusive. After consultation with the pathologist, diagnostic pars plana vitrectomy can be performed to obtain the vitreous specimen. When a subretinal nodule is accessible in a region of the retina that is unlikely to compromise visual function, subretinal aspiration of the lesion can be done. Expedited transport of the vitreous to the pathology laboratory is important to ensure cell viability.

The methodology for evaluation of the vitreous and subretinal specimens varies depending on the laboratory. Cytopathology (see Chapter 10, Fig 10-16), including immunohistochemical studies for subclassification of the cells, flow cytometry, and polymerase chain reaction or fluorescence in situ hybridization analysis for gene rearrangements and mutations, and the ratio of interleukin-10 to interleukin-6 are all possible methods of pathologic analysis for lymphoma; see Chapter 3 for a discussion of some of these methods. Specimens with atypical, large lymphocytic cells (Fig 20-11) and characteristic cell surface markers establish the diagnosis of large B-cell lymphoma.

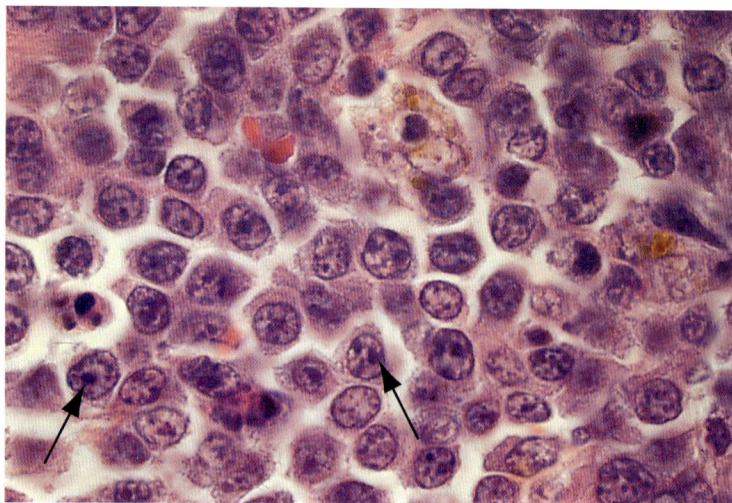

Figure 20-11   Large cell lymphoma, histology. Note the nuclear atypia with irregular nuclear contours and prominent nucleoli *(arrows)* of these neoplastic lymphoid cells, which were obtained by fine-needle aspiration biopsy.

Treatment

In general, high-dose intravenous methotrexate is given for PCNSL and may also be effective for PIOL. When there is only ocular involvement, intravitreal injections of methotrexate or rituximab or external beam radiotherapy is usually employed. Because the blood–ocular barriers may limit penetration of chemotherapeutic agents into the eye, these modalities may be used in addition to high-dose intravenous methotrexate when there is minimal response of the ocular disease after systemic therapy for the CNS disease. There is no consensus as to whether irradiation of the affected eye using fractionated external beam radiation is more efficacious for the treatment of intraocular lymphoma than intravitreal injection of methotrexate or rituximab. However, although radiotherapy may induce ocular remission, the tumor can recur, and further irradiation places the patient at risk for vision loss due to radiation retinopathy. Radiotherapy to the eye is also associated with substantial ocular surface discomfort. Intravitreal injection of methotrexate or rituximab tends to produce very good local tumor response and low ocular recurrence rates; however, retinal toxicity may occur. CNS or systemic lymphoma is treated in parallel with the intraocular disease by a medical oncologist.

Prognosis

Although the prognosis for patients with PIOL is poor, particularly with CNS involvement, advances in early diagnosis have produced a cohort of long-term survivors. Serial follow-up with the ophthalmologist and an experienced medical oncologist is critical in the management of this disease. Patients with PCNSL without ocular involvement should be observed longitudinally by an experienced ophthalmologist for possible ocular involvement, even after remission of the CNS disease.

Coupland SE, Bechrakis NE, Anastassiou G, et al. Evaluation of vitrectomy specimens and chorioretinal biopsies in the diagnosis of primary intraocular lymphoma in patients with Masquerade syndrome. *Graefes Arch Clin Exp Ophthalmol.* 2003;241(10):860–870.

Kim MM, Dabaja BS, Medeiros J, et al. Survival outcomes of primary intraocular lymphoma: a single-institution experience. *Am J Clin Oncol.* 2016;39(2):109–113.

Sagoo MS, Mehta H, Swampillai AJ, et al. Primary intraocular lymphoma. *Surv Ophthalmol.* 2014;59(5):503–516.

Primary Uveal Lymphoma

Many cases of uveal lymphoid infiltration, formerly known as *reactive lymphoid hyperplasia,* are now recognized as low-grade B-cell marginal zone mucosa-associated lymphoid tissue (MALT) lymphomas of the uveal tract. Primary uveal lymphoma, though also a form of intraocular lymphoma, is distinct from PIOL, discussed earlier in the chapter. These lesions, which typically present in patients in the sixth decade of life, can occur in any part of the uveal tract (Fig 20-12). There is an overlap between uveal lymphoma and similar lymphoid proliferations in the conjunctiva and orbit, termed *ocular adnexal lymphoma.* For information on the pathology of ocular adnexal lymphoma, see Chapter 5 for conjunctival lymphoma and Chapter 14 for orbital lymphoma.

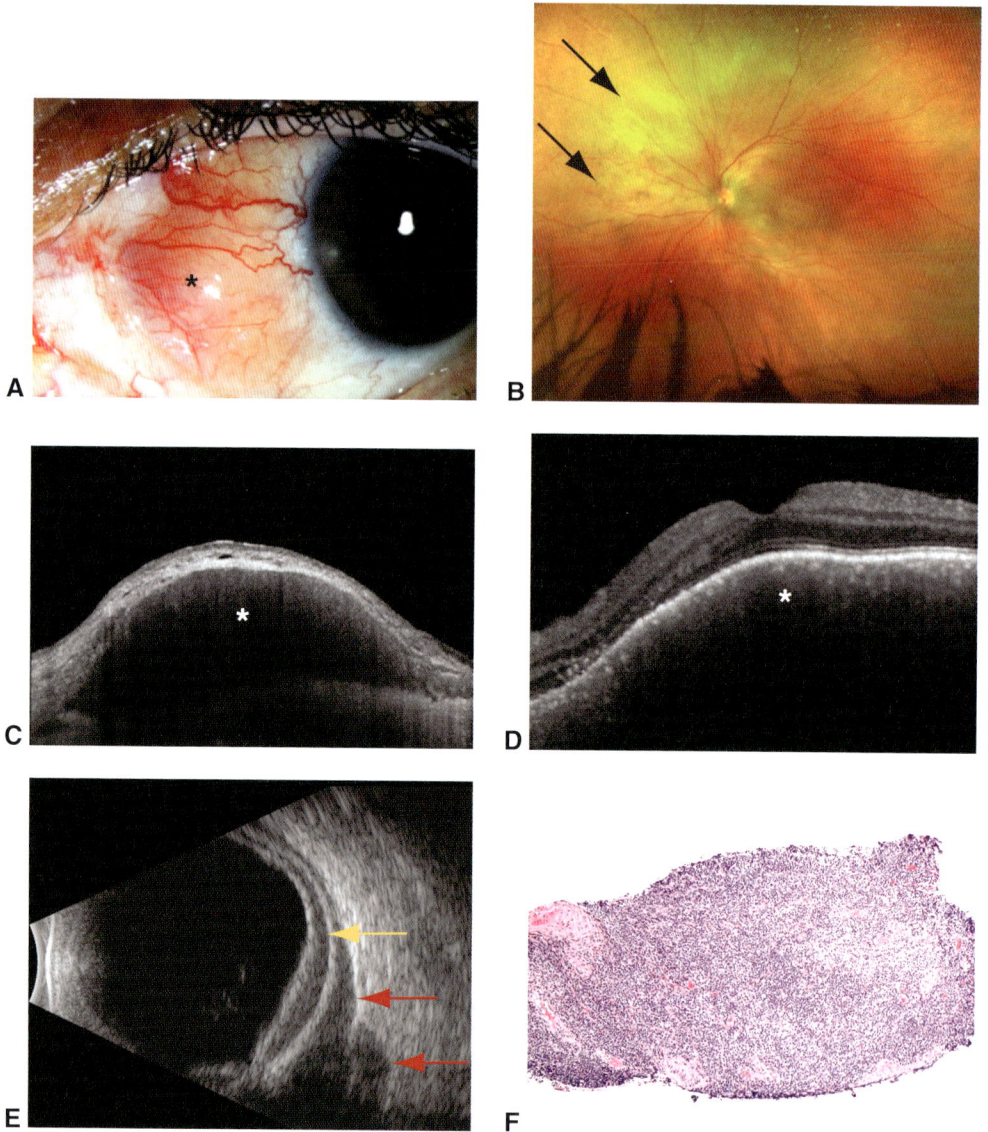

Figure 20-12 Uveal lymphoma, with concomitant ocular adnexal involvement. **A,** Slit-lamp photograph of a raised pink-orange "salmon patch" conjunctival lesion *(asterisk)* showing B-cell lymphoma. **B,** Multifocal creamy-yellow amelanotic choroidal lesions are seen ophthalmoscopically *(arrows)*. **C,** Anterior segment optical coherence tomography (OCT) of the conjunctival lesion demonstrates a homogenous subepithelial mass *(asterisk)*. **D,** OCT through the macula shows a diffusely thickened and irregular choroid *(asterisk)*. **E,** B-scan ultrasonography shows a diffusely thickened choroid *(yellow arrow)* and crescentic, extrascleral lucencies *(red arrows)* that are pathognomonic for uveal lymphoma and represent extraocular collections of lymphoid cells. **F,** Histologic examination of the conjunctival biopsy specimen demonstrates a monomorphic sheet of small lymphocytes consistent with extranodal marginal zone B-cell lymphoma, as determined with additional special pathologic studies. *(Courtesy of Jesse L. Berry, MD.)*

Clinical evaluation

Patients with uveal lymphoma typically notice painless, progressive vision loss. Ophthalmoscopically, the presence of multifocal creamy-yellow amelanotic choroidal lesions tends to be most helpful in establishing the diagnosis (see Fig 20-12B); similar lesions may be seen in PIOL, although those lesions are located between the RPE and Bruch membrane and *not* in the choroid. Associated subretinal fluid is seen in some eyes, and diffuse uveal thickening is common. Secondary glaucoma may be present. Frequently, the delay between the onset of symptoms and diagnostic intervention is significant.

This rare disorder is characterized pathologically by localized or diffuse infiltration of the uveal tract by relatively mature lymphoid cells. Clinically, this condition can simulate posterior uveal melanoma, metastatic uveal carcinoma, sympathetic ophthalmia, Vogt-Koyanagi-Harada syndrome, and posterior scleritis. Proptosis of the affected eye may occur in a small proportion of patients who develop simultaneous episcleral orbital infiltration. Of note, the component on the external surface of the sclera can be a polyclonal "reactive" lymphoid infiltrate.

Aronow ME, Portell CA, Sweetenham JW, Singh AD. Uveal lymphoma: clinical features, diagnostic studies, treatment selection, and outcomes. *Ophthalmology.* 2014;121(1): 334–341.

Imaging

Fluorescein angiography depicts variable findings in patients with uveal lymphoma involving the choroid; ICG angiography provides superior characterization. Classically, multiple scattered hypocyanescent lesions are present, which correspond to the area of choroidal infiltration by the lymphoma. OCT, specifically EDI-OCT, reveals placoid or irregular lesions and thickening of the inner choroid, often associated with subretinal fluid (see Fig 20-12D). B-scan ultrasonography, the modality of choice for evaluation of choroidal lymphoma, typically reveals diffuse, homogenous choroidal thickening with associated secondary retinal detachment. A pathognomonic feature of uveal lymphoma is crescent-shaped areas of acoustically hollow extrascleral extension (see Fig 20-12E).

Pathologic studies

Biopsy confirmation should be targeted to the most accessible tissue. When extraocular involvement is present, biopsy of the involved conjunctiva or orbit may be considered. For isolated uveal involvement, FNAB or pars plana vitrectomy with biopsy may be indicated. Dense lymphoid infiltrates are seen on histologic evaluation. Coordination with the ophthalmic pathologist is crucial, as it increases the likelihood of diagnosis with appropriate specimen handling and cell marker studies.

Treatment

Historically, eyes with uveal lymphoid infiltration were generally managed by enucleation. Current management emphasizes globe-conserving therapy aimed at vision preservation. Early intervention with low-dose ocular and orbital fractionated external beam radiotherapy may definitively manage the disease.

Prognosis

The prognosis for survival is excellent for patients with uveal lymphomas, as these are typically low-grade lymphomas, unlike PIOL. Preservation of visual function appears related to primary tumor location and secondary sequelae, including exudative retinal detachment or dysfunction from chronic tissue infiltration. Early intervention appears to improve the chances of visual preservation.

Secondary Involvement of Systemic Lymphoma

Ocular lymphoma may represent spread from systemic disease.

Clinical evaluation

Ocular involvement in systemic lymphoma has a variable presentation. Features may include uveitis; infiltration of any portion of the uveal tract; or a discrete mass of the conjunctiva, eyelid, or orbit. Diagnostic biopsy is directed to the most accessible region of the eye where a large amount of tissue can be obtained. Ideally, the pathologist will be able to compare the results of the ocular biopsy with those of biopsies from other sites.

Treatment

Treatment is dictated by the type of lymphoma and extent of disease; when the site of tumor involvement is new, restaging may be necessary. Treatment may include systemic chemotherapy, orbital radiation, or bone marrow transplantation. Such cases are managed in collaboration with a medical oncologist.

Ocular Manifestations of Leukemia

Ocular manifestations of leukemia are common, occurring in as many as 80% of eyes from patients with the disease examined at autopsy. Clinical studies have documented ophthalmic findings in as many as 40% of patients at diagnosis of the leukemia. Patients may be asymptomatic, or they may report blurred or decreased vision.

Clinically, the retina is the most commonly affected intraocular structure. Leukemic retinopathy is characterized by intraretinal and subhyaloid hemorrhages, hard exudates, cotton-wool spots, and white-centered retinal hemorrhages, also known as pseudo–Roth spots (Fig 20-13). (Classically, white-centered hemorrhages associated with endocarditis are termed *Roth spots;* they may be called *pseudo–Roth spots* when associated with other diseases.) In leukemia, these findings are usually the result of associated anemia, hyperviscosity, and/or thrombocytopenia. True leukemic infiltrates are less common and appear as yellow-white deposits in the retina and the subretinal space. Perivascular leukemic infiltrates produce gray-white streaks in the retina. Vitreous involvement by leukemia is rare and most often results from direct extension via retinal hemorrhage. If necessary, a diagnostic vitrectomy can be performed to establish a diagnosis.

Although the retina is the most commonly affected ocular structure clinically, histologic studies have shown that the uveal tract is more commonly affected by leukemia than is the retina. The uveal tract may serve as a "sanctuary site" for leukemic cells, making the eye more likely to be a site of recurrent disease. Choroidal infiltrates may be difficult to detect

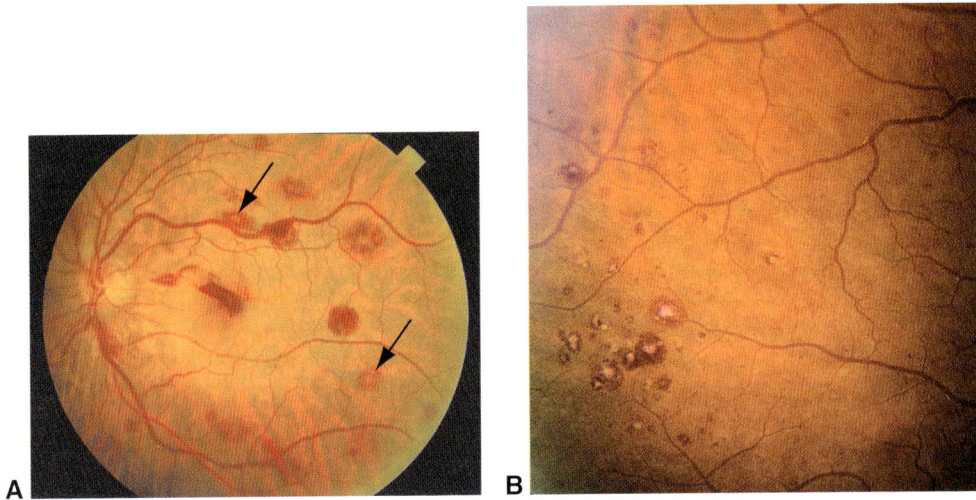

Figure 20-13 Retinal involvement in leukemia. **A,** Clinical photograph of leukemic retinopathy demonstrates scattered intraretinal hemorrhages, some of which have white centers *(arrows)*. **B,** White-centered hemorrhages, also known as *pseudo–Roth spots*. *(Part A courtesy of Robert H. Rosa Jr, MD; part B courtesy of Jacob Pe'er, MD.)*

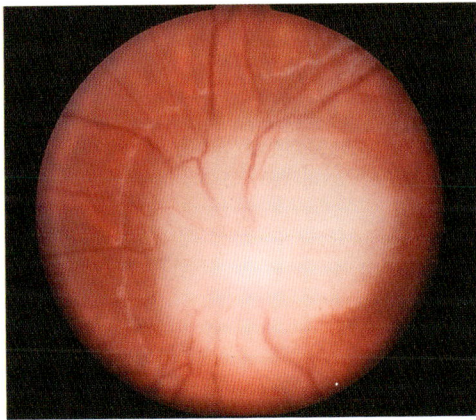

Figure 20-14 Leukemic infiltration of the optic nerve, an ophthalmic emergency. *(Courtesy of Robert H. Rosa Jr, MD.)*

with indirect ophthalmoscopy; they may be better detected on ultrasonography as diffuse thickening of the choroid. Serous retinal detachments may overlie these infiltrates. Leukemic involvement of the iris manifests as a diffuse thickening with loss of the iris crypts, and small nodules may be seen at the margin of the pupil in some cases. Leukemic cells may invade the anterior chamber, forming a pseudohypopyon. Infiltration of the angle by these cells can give rise to secondary glaucoma.

With leukemic infiltration of the optic nerve (Fig 20-14), the patient may present with severe vision loss and optic nerve edema. One or both eyes may be affected. This is an ophthalmic emergency that requires immediate treatment to preserve as much vision as possible. Systemic imaging, CNS assessment including lumbar puncture with cytology, and bone marrow evaluation are necessary to confirm the diagnosis. Urgent external beam radiation to the optic nerves is typically used along with combined systemic and intrathecal chemotherapy.

Leukemic infiltrates may also involve the orbital soft tissue, with resultant proptosis. These rare tumors are referred to as *granulocytic sarcomas* or *chloromas* because they are solid masses of granulocytic precursors, including myeloblasts and myelocytes from myelogenous leukemias. The tumors appear to have a greenish hue on direct visualization. The term *granulocytic sarcoma* is a misnomer as this tumor is not a true sarcoma. These tumors have a predilection for the lateral and medial walls of the orbit.

Involvement of the eye may be seen at initial diagnosis or relapse of leukemia; treatment typically consists of systemic chemotherapy. Depending on the response, low-dose radiation to the eye may be included; however, this should be done with caution as it may limit future use of radiation therapy. The exception is optic nerve infiltration with acute vision loss, for which radiotherapy is mandatory for treatment. The prognosis for vision depends on the particular subtype of leukemia and the extent of ocular involvement.

Rosenthal AR. Ocular manifestations of leukemia: a review. *Ophthalmology.* 1983;90(8): 899–905.

Additional Materials and Resources

Related Academy Materials

The American Academy of Ophthalmology is dedicated to providing a wealth of high-quality clinical education resources for ophthalmologists.

Print Publications and Electronic Products

For a complete listing of Academy products related to topics covered in this BCSC Section, visit our online store at:

https://store.aao.org/clinical-education/topic/comprehensive-ophthalmology.html

Or call Customer Service at 866.561.8558 (toll free, US only) or +1 415.561.8540, Monday through Friday, between 8:00 a.m. and 5:00 p.m. (PST).

Online Resources

Visit the Ophthalmic News and Education (ONE®) Network at aao.org/onenetwork to find relevant videos, online courses, journal articles, practice guidelines, self-assessment quizzes, images, and more. The ONE Network is a free Academy-member benefit.

Access free, trusted articles and content with the Academy's collaborative online encyclopedia, EyeWiki, at aao.org/eyewiki.

Basic Texts and Additional Resources

American Academy of Ophthalmology. *Pathology Atlas.* Available at:
store.aao.org/clinical-education/topic/ocular-pathology-oncology.html
Cummings TJ. *Ophthalmic Pathology: A Concise Guide.* Springer-Verlag; 2013.
Dutton JJ. *Atlas of Clinical and Surgical Orbital Anatomy.* 2nd ed. Elsevier/Saunders; 2011.
Eagle RC Jr. *Eye Pathology: An Atlas and Text.* 3rd ed. Lippincott Williams & Wilkins; 2017.
Font RL, Croxatto JO, Rao NA. *Tumors of the Eye and Ocular Adnexa.* American Registry of Pathology; 2006.
Grossniklaus HE, Bergstrom C, Baker Hubbard G, Wells JR, Singh AD, eds. *Pocket Guide to Ocular Oncology and Pathology.* Springer-Verlag; 2012.
Grossniklaus HE, Eberhart CG, Kivelä TT, eds. *WHO Classification of Tumours of the Eye.* 4th ed. International Agency for Research on Cancer (IARC); 2018.
Heegaard S, Grossniklaus HE, eds. *Eye Pathology: An Illustrated Guide.* Springer-Verlag; 2015.
Karcioglu ZA, ed. *Orbital Tumors: Diagnosis and Treatment.* 2nd ed. Springer-Verlag; 2015.
McLean IW, Burnier MN, Zimmerman LE, Jakobiec FA. *Tumors of the Eye and Ocular Adnexa.* Armed Forces Institute of Pathology; 1995.

Naumann GOH, Holbach L, Kruse FE, eds. *Applied Pathology for Ophthalmic Microsurgeons.* Springer-Verlag; 2008.

Roberts F, Thum CK. *Lee's Ophthalmic Histopathology.* 3rd ed. Springer-Verlag; 2014.

Shields JA, Shields CL. *Eyelid, Conjunctival, and Orbital Tumors: An Atlas and Textbook.* 3rd ed. Wolters Kluwer; 2015.

Shields JA, Shields CL. *Intraocular Tumors: An Atlas and Textbook.* 3rd ed. Lippincott Williams & Wilkins; 2015.

Singh AD, Dolan B, Biscotti CV, eds. *FNA Cytology of Ophthalmic Tumors.* Karger Publishers; 2012.

Spencer WH, ed. *Ophthalmic Pathology: An Atlas and Textbook.* 4th ed. Elsevier/Saunders; 1996.

Yanoff M, Sassani JW. *Ocular Pathology.* 7th ed. Elsevier/Saunders; 2015.

Requesting Continuing Medical Education Credit

The American Academy of Ophthalmology is accredited by the Accreditation Council for Continuing Medical Education (ACCME) to provide continuing medical education for physicians.

The American Academy of Ophthalmology designates this enduring material for a maximum of 10 *AMA PRA Category 1 Credits™*. Physicians should claim only the credit commensurate with the extent of their participation in the activity.

To claim *AMA PRA Category 1 Credits™* upon completion of this activity, learners must demonstrate appropriate knowledge and participation in the activity by taking the posttest for Section 4 and achieving a score of 80% or higher.

This Section of the BCSC has been approved as a Maintenance of Certification (MOC) Part II self-assessment CME activity and is also approved by the American Board of Pathology as an MOC CME activity.

To take the posttest and request CME credit online:

1. Go to www.aao.org/cme-central and log in.
2. Click on "Claim CME Credit and View My CME Transcript" and then "Report AAO Credits."
3. Select the appropriate media type and then the Academy activity. You will be directed to the posttest.
4. Once you have passed the test with a score of 80% or higher, you will be directed to your transcript. *If you are not an Academy member, you will be able to print out a certificate of participation once you have passed the test.*

CME expiration date: June 1, 2023. *AMA PRA Category 1 Credits™* may be claimed only once between June 1, 2020, and the expiration date.

For assistance, contact the Academy's Customer Service department at 866.561.8558 (US only) or +1 415.561.8540 between 8:00 a.m. and 5:00 p.m. (PST), Monday through Friday, or send an e-mail to customer_service@aao.org.

Study Questions

Please note that these questions are not part of your CME reporting process. They are provided here for your own educational use and identification of any professional practice gaps. The required CME posttest is available online (see "Requesting Continuing Medical Education Credit"). Following the questions are answers with discussions. Although a concerted effort has been made to avoid ambiguity and redundancy in these questions, the authors recognize that differences of opinion may occur regarding the "best" answer. The discussions are provided to demonstrate the rationale used to derive the answer. They may also be helpful in confirming that your approach to the problem was correct or, if necessary, in fixing the principle in your memory. The Section 4 faculty thanks the Resident Self-Assessment Committee for drafting these self-assessment questions and the discussions that follow.

1. What histologic description best describes a hamartoma?
   a. normal mature tissue at an abnormal location
   b. abnormal mature tissue at a normal location
   c. stereotypic, monotonous new growth of a specific tissue phenotype
   d. abnormal tissue derived from all 3 embryonic germ cell layers

2. What is the mechanism of bone formation in phthisis bulbi?
   a. cataract formation
   b. dystrophic calcification of Bowman layer
   c. metaplasia of the retinal pigment epithelium
   d. serous retinal detachment

3. What is the most commonly used tissue fixative?
   a. absolute ethanol
   b. formalin
   c. Bouin solution
   d. glutaraldehyde

4. During gross examination, which extraocular muscle is a helpful landmark in determining the laterality of a globe?
   a. superior oblique muscle
   b. inferior rectus muscle
   c. inferior oblique muscle
   d. superior rectus muscle

5. Which immunohistochemical stain is helpful in identifying lesions that arise from cells with a neuroectodermal origin?

    a. HMB-45

    b. CD20

    c. actin

    d. S-100

6. Which layer of the cornea is not replaced when it is destroyed?

    a. Bowman

    b. stroma

    c. Descemet membrane

    d. epithelium

7. What type of cells in the retina proliferate in response to trauma?

    a. epithelial cells

    b. fibroblasts

    c. glial cells

    d. photoreceptors

8. Which is the most characteristic description of the histologic findings in a pterygium?

    a. basophilic degeneration

    b. squamous metaplasia

    c. eosinophilic deposits

    d. nuclear atypia

9. A corneal scraping from a patient with keratitis demonstrates cysts and trophozoites. What is the etiology of the keratitis?

    a. *Pseudomonas*

    b. herpes simplex virus

    c. *Acanthamoeba*

    d. *Fusarium*

10. On slit-lamp examination, aggregates of translucent, golden-brown globular deposits are noted in the interpalpebral superficial cornea in both eyes. A histologic stain for what material may be helpful in visualizing the deposits?

    a. calcium

    b. elastin

    c. glycosaminoglycan

    d. hyaline

11. On gonioscopy, which anatomical landmark marks the termination of Descemet membrane?

    a. scleral spur

    b. Schwalbe line

    c. trabecular meshwork

    d. iris root

12. In hemolytic glaucoma, which characteristic material accumulates in the trabecular meshwork?

    a. rigid hemolyzed erythrocytes

    b. pigmented epithelioid melanocytes

    c. hemosiderin-laden histiocytes

    d. eosinophilic protein-laden histiocytes

13. Polymorphisms in what gene are associated with pseudoexfoliation syndrome?

    a. *LOXL1*

    b. *FOXC1*

    c. *PAX6*

    d. *PITX2*

14. Which histologic feature best explains the opaque appearance of the sclera?

    a. loose fibrovascular tissue

    b. presence of melanocytes

    c. sparse vascularization

    d. variable collagen orientation

15. Where in the lens are new cortical fibers produced?

    a. nucleus

    b. anterior capsule

    c. equator

    d. posterior capsule

16. Which pathologic findings characterize the inflammation in phacoantigenic uveitis (also known as *lens-induced granulomatous endophthalmitis* and previously called *phacoanaphylactic endophthalmitis*)?

    a. nongranulomatous inflammation

    b. zonal granulomatous inflammation

    c. nodular granulomatous inflammation

    d. diffuse granulomatous inflammation

17. Which degenerative lens change is caused by migration of lens epithelium along the posterior capsule, followed by enlargement or swelling of those epithelial cells?

    a. posterior subcapsular cataract

    b. duplication cataract

    c. nuclear sclerosis

    d. cortical cataract

18. What is the most prominent cell type that is found in the vitritis associated with bacterial endophthalmitis?

    a. neutrophils

    b. epithelioid histiocytes

    c. T and B lymphocytes

    d. eosinophils

19. What is the composition of asteroid bodies in the vitreous?

    a. keratin

    b. hyaline

    c. amyloid

    d. calcium

20. Which primary cellular element is observed histologically in the periretinal membranes found in proliferative vitreoretinopathy?

    a. RPE cells

    b. amacrine cells

    c. bipolar cells

    d. choroidal melanocytes

21. Which fundus finding is associated with Gardner syndrome?

    a. combined hamartoma of the retina and RPE

    b. congenital hypertrophy of the RPE

    c. hyperplasia of the RPE

    d. osseous metaplasia of the RPE

22. An area of peripheral retina demonstrates pathologic changes of inner retinal atrophy, retinal vascular sclerosis, and condensation and adherence of vitreous at the margins with an overlying pocket of liquefied vitreous. What is the diagnosis?

    a. paving-stone degeneration

    b. cystoid degeneration

    c. lattice degeneration

    d. retinoschisis

23. Which layer of the iris is responsible for determining the color of the iris?
    a. anterior border layer
    b. stromal layer
    c. anterior iris pigment epithelium
    d. posterior iris pigment epithelium

24. What is the predominant cell type found in Dalen-Fuchs nodules?
    a. histiocytes
    b. lymphocytes
    c. retinal pigment epithelial cells
    d. neutrophils

25. What is the most common primary intraocular malignancy found in adults?
    a. retinoblastoma
    b. intraocular lymphoma
    c. iris melanoma
    d. choroidal melanoma

26. Which gene is associated with mutations that occur within uveal melanoma tissue and correlate with increased risk of metastasis?
    a. *BAP1*
    b. *GNAQ*
    c. *EIF1AX*
    d. *SF3B1*

27. A 13-year-old boy presents with redness of the right eye; constant epiphora; and umbilicated, nodular, waxy lesions on the eyelid margin. Which kind of conjunctivitis does this patient most likely have?
    a. bacterial
    b. follicular
    c. pseudomembranous
    d. giant papillary

28. Which is the most likely periocular location for basal cell carcinoma to develop?
    a. upper eyelid margin
    b. lower eyelid margin
    c. lateral canthus
    d. medial canthus

29. Keratoacanthoma is a variant of which other eyelid malignancy?
    a. basal cell carcinoma
    b. squamous cell carcinoma
    c. melanoma
    d. sebaceous carcinoma

30. Which is the most common epithelial tumor of the lacrimal gland?
    a. mucoepidermoid carcinoma
    b. squamous cell carcinoma
    c. pleomorphic adenoma
    d. adenoid cystic carcinoma

31. Which abnormality of embryologic development is responsible for the formation of optic nerve colobomas?
    a. failure of neural crest differentiation
    b. incomplete regression of the primary vitreous
    c. failed induction of the surface ectoderm lens placode
    d. incomplete closure of the embryonic fissure

32. What is the approximate mortality rate for patients with iris melanoma?
    a. 4%
    b. 15%
    c. 30%
    d. 55%

33. What is the most likely location for metastasis from uveal melanoma?
    a. bone
    b. brain
    c. liver
    d. lung

34. A patient presents with blurry vision and is noted to have a change in refraction. Slit-lamp examination reveals a large and engorged episcleral vessel, and gonioscopy shows a pigmented lesion in 1 clock-hour of the iridocorneal angle. What is the most likely cause of the refractive change?
    a. corneal astigmatism
    b. lenticular astigmatism
    c. axial hyperopia
    d. axial myopia

35. What is the most common secondary tumor in retinoblastoma survivors with a germline *RB1* mutation?

    a. fibrosarcoma

    b. melanoma

    c. pinealoblastoma

    d. osteosarcoma

36. Clinically, which intraocular structure is most commonly affected in patients with leukemia?

    a. cornea

    b. iris

    c. retina

    d. optic nerve

Answers

1. **b.** Hamartomas are developmental anomalies that can be described as hypertrophy (abnormal size) and hyperplasia (abnormal amount) of mature tissue in a normal location. A choristoma consists of normal, mature tissue at an abnormal location and can contain 1 or 2 embryonic germ layers. A teratoma is a tumor that consists of a proliferation of tissue derived from all 3 embryonic germ cell layers. A neoplasm is a stereotypic, often monotonous new growth of a specific tissue phenotype.

2. **c.** *Phthisis bulbi* is defined as atrophy, shrinkage, and disorganization of the eye and intraocular contents. In the end stage of this process, osseous metaplasia of the retinal pigment epithelium (RPE) with bone formation may be a prominent feature. The sclera becomes markedly thickened, particularly posteriorly. Extensive dystrophic calcification of Bowman layer, lens, retina, and drusen usually occurs.

3. **b.** The most commonly used fixative is 10% neutral-buffered formalin. Formalin is a 40% solution of formaldehyde that stabilizes proteins, lipids, and carbohydrates and prevents enzymatic destruction of the tissue (autolysis). Bouin solution is a fixative that is sometimes used for small biopsy specimens such as conjunctival tissue. Glutaraldehyde is a fixative used for electron microscopy. Absolute ethanol is a fixative used for crystals such as corneal urate crystals.

4. **c.** When the laterality of the globe is being determined, the inferior oblique muscle is a very helpful landmark. This muscle inserts onto the sclera temporally over the macula, with its fibers running inferiorly. Because of the posterior location of the inferior oblique insertion, the inferior oblique muscle is not typically cut flush with the sclera at the time of enucleation. The rectus muscles usually are cut flush with the sclera during enucleation to attach them to the prosthetic orbital implant, so the rectus muscles are not typically seen on the surface of an enucleated globe. The superior oblique is present only as a tendon at its insertion on the globe. This tendon, which is more anterior than the inferior oblique muscle, varies in the amount excised and is thus less likely to be consistently identified on an enucleated globe.

5. **d.** Immunohistochemical (IHC) stains are widely used in ophthalmic pathology. They take advantage of the specific antigens expressed by specific types of cells. An antibody to a specific antigen is linked to a chromogen (a compound that produces a particular color as a result of a chemical reaction) or color. When the stain is applied, the antibody binds to the cells that produce that specific antigen and the cell is stained by the chromogen.

   Different antibodies can be used to identify different cell types and the lesions that arise from them. For example, epithelial cells produce cytokeratins. Therefore, a cytokeratin IHC stain can be used to identify adenomas or carcinomas that are derived from epithelial cells. S-100 is an antigen produced by cells that arise from neuroectoderm. The nervous system, including the retina and optic nerve, arises from neuroectoderm. Neural tumors such as schwannomas and neurofibromas stain with S-100. Melanocytes also arise from neuroectoderm, so melanocytic lesions are positive with S-100 as well.

   HMB-45 and Melan-A are more specific stains for melanocytes and melanocytic lesions. These stains are positive in nevi, primary acquired melanosis, and melanoma. But unlike S-100, they will not stain tumors of neural origin. CD antigens are used to subtype white blood cells. T lymphocytes stain with CD3; B lymphocytes with CD20. This is helpful in diagnosing reactive lymphoid hyperplasia and lymphoma. Actin, desmin, and myoglobin are used for lesions with smooth or skeletal muscle features, including leiomyoma and rhabdomyosarcoma.

6. **a.** Bowman layer is not replaced once it is incised or destroyed. The endothelial and epithelial layers are critical to corneal wound healing. The epithelium should cover the defect within days of injury to prevent permanent corneal weakness. Stromal keratocytes (fibroblast-like cells) migrate across the wound, laying down collagen and fibronectin. The endothelial cells adjacent to the wound slide across the posterior cornea and lay down a new thin layer of Descemet membrane.

7. **c.** The retina is made of terminally differentiated cells that typically do not regenerate when injured. Because the retina is part of the central nervous system (CNS), glial cells (eg, Müller cells, astrocytes), rather than fibroblasts, proliferate in response to retinal trauma.

8. **a.** The most characteristic histologic finding in a pterygium is basophilic degeneration of collagen (also called *elastotic degeneration*) within the substantia propria, due to actinic damage. The degenerated collagen stains positively with histochemical stains for elastin, such as Verhoeff–van Gieson. Squamous metaplasia (eg, surface keratinization and loss of goblet cells) may be seen in a subset of pterygia, but it is not a universal finding. Nuclear atypia is a finding in ocular surface squamous neoplasia, which may occur in association with a pterygium, but the atypia is a neoplastic, not degenerative, change. Eosinophilic deposits are characteristic histologic findings of amyloid deposits, not pterygia.

9. **c.** *Acanthamoeba* protozoa have a cyst morphology, and these cysts are difficult to eradicate from the corneal stroma. Less commonly, trophozoite forms may also be identified. Epithelial cells infected with herpes simplex virus may display intranuclear inclusions; these are rarely seen histologically because corneal grafting is not generally performed during the acute phase of infection. *Fusarium* is a genus of filamentous fungi. *Fusarium* keratitis manifests histologically as hyphae, best seen on Gomori or Grocott methenamine silver (GMS) stain. *Pseudomonas* is a gram-negative bacterium and is rod shaped (bacillus).

10. **b.** The clinical findings are characteristic of actinic keratopathy, also known as *spheroidal degeneration,* Labrador keratopathy, and *climatic droplet keratopathy.* This keratopathy is characterized by aggregates of translucent, golden-brown spheroidal deposits in the interpalpebral superficial cornea. The condition is generally bilateral and is more common in males. Smaller spheroidal deposits may mimic calcific band keratopathy; this phenomenon has been described as "actinic" band keratopathy. Histologic examination reveals irregular basophilic globules deep to the epithelium in the region of Bowman layer and the anterior stroma. Analogous to the actinic degeneration of collagen in pingueculae and pterygia, the deposits stain black with special stains for elastin, such as Verhoeff–van Gieson. Calcium stains such as von Kossa and alizarin red are helpful in visualizing the deposits seen in calcific band keratopathy. Glycosaminoglycan deposits stain with alcian blue or colloidal iron and are seen in macular corneal dystrophy. Hyaline stains with Masson trichrome and is seen in granular corneal dystrophy.

11. **b.** The termination of Descemet membrane is manifested gonioscopically as the Schwalbe line. The scleral spur, a triangular extension of the sclera, appears gonioscopically as a white band. Anterior to the scleral spur in an internal indentation of the sclera are the trabecular meshwork and Schlemm canal. The iris root inserts into the anterior ciliary body posterior to the scleral spur.

12. **c.** Hemolytic glaucoma is characterized by the accumulation of hemosiderin-laden histiocytes in the trabecular meshwork. Rigid hemolyzed erythrocytes are seen after intraocular hemorrhage in ghost cell glaucoma. Pigmented epithelioid melanocytes can invade the trabecular meshwork in the setting of uveal melanomas. In phacolytic glaucoma, eosinophilic protein-laden histiocytes are seen within the trabecular meshwork.

13. **a.** Polymorphisms in the lysyl oxidase–like 1 gene *(LOXL1)* are associated with pseudoexfoliation syndrome. Lysyl oxidase is a pivotal enzyme in extracellular matrix formation; it catalyzes covalent crosslinking of collagen and elastin. *FOXC1* and *PITX2* mutations are associated with Axenfeld-Rieger syndrome. *PAX6* mutations are associated with developmental abnormalities, such as aniridia and Peters anomaly.

14. **d.** In comparison to the collagen lamellae of the corneal stroma, scleral collagen fibers are thicker and more variable in thickness and orientation, resulting in the opaque appearance of the sclera. Loose fibrovascular tissue is present in episcleral and lamina fusca layers but does not contribute to the opacity of the sclera. Melanocytes are found in the lamina fusca. The scleral stroma has sparse vascularization.

15. **c.** In the equatorial, or *bow,* region of the lens, the epithelial cells move centrally, elongate, produce crystalline proteins, lose organelles, and transform into lens fibers. As the lens epithelial cells differentiate, new fibers are continuously laid down over existing fibers, compacting them in a lamellar arrangement. Thus, the outermost fibers, derived from postnatally differentiated lens epithelial cells, are the most recently formed and make up the cortex of the lens, while older layers are located toward the center. The center of the lens contains the oldest fibers, the *embryonic and fetal lens nucleus.* Lens fibers are densely compacted in the nucleus. The anterior capsule is lined by a monolayer of lens epithelial cells. Epithelial cells are not typically observed posterior to the lens equator; thus, lens cortical fibers cannot be produced along the posterior capsule.

16. **b.** Phacoantigenic uveitis (lens-induced granulomatous endophthalmitis) is usually associated with penetrating ocular injuries with rupture of the lens capsule. The exposed lens material provokes granulomatous inflammation. Histologically, there is a central nidus of degenerating lens material, surrounded by concentric layers of inflammatory cells *(zonal granuloma).* Neutrophils are present in the innermost zone of inflammation. The intermediate zone consists primarily of epithelioid histiocytes and multinucleated giant cells. Lymphocytes and plasma cells are present in the outer zone. The inflammatory cells may be surrounded by fibrovascular connective tissue, depending on the duration of the inflammatory response.

17. **a.** Posterior subcapsular cataract is a result of epithelial disarray at the lens equator, followed by posterior migration of the lens epithelial cells along the posterior capsule. As the cells migrate, they can enlarge significantly. These swollen cells are called *Wedl,* or *bladder,* cells. If they involve the center of the lens in the visual axis, they can cause significant decrease in vision. A duplication cataract occurs after injury to the lens epithelium. The lens epithelium undergoes metaplasia and forms anterior subcapsular fibrous plaques. After the resolution of the inciting stimulus, the lens epithelium may produce another capsule that completely surrounds the fibrous plaque. The earliest sign of focal cortical degeneration is hydropic swelling of the lens fibers with decreased intensity of eosinophilic staining. Eosinophilic globules (morgagnian globules) accumulate in the slitlike spaces between the lens fibers. Ultimately, the entire cortex can become liquefied. Nuclear cataracts take on a subtle homogeneous eosinophilic appearance and are difficult to assess histologically.

18. **a.** Because the vitreous is acellular and avascular, it is not often a primary site of inflammation. However, it commonly becomes secondarily involved in inflammation of adjacent tissues. Vitritis is the presence of white blood cells, either benign or malignant, in the vitreous. Vitreous inflammation due to infectious agents is referred to as *infectious endophthalmitis.* In bacterial endophthalmitis, the vitritis consists predominantly of an infiltrate of neutrophils (polymorphonuclear leukocytes), which are acute inflammatory cells. Epithelioid histiocytes represent granulomatous inflammation. T and B lymphocytes are chronic inflammatory cells. The vitreous infiltrate in noninfectious uveitis is typically composed of chronic inflammatory cells, including lymphocytes. Eosinophils are commonly found in allergic reactions but may be present in some chronic inflammatory processes, such as sympathetic ophthalmia.

19. **d.** Asteroid hyalosis is a condition with a dramatic clinical appearance but little clinical significance. Histologically, asteroid bodies are rounded structures, typically attached to vitreous fibrils. The bodies are basophilic with hematoxylin-eosin stain. They are usually positive with stains for calcium such as alizarin red and von Kossa. Occasionally, they will be surrounded by a foreign body giant cell reaction, but the condition is not generally associated with vitreous inflammation. Studies have shown that asteroid bodies are composed of complex lipids and also have a component with structural and elemental similarity to hydroxyapatite, a calcium phosphate complex. There is an association between asteroid hyalosis and both diabetes mellitus and systemic hypertension.

20. **a.** Proliferative vitreoretinopathy (PVR) membranes form as a result of the proliferation of retinal pigment epithelium (RPE) cells and other cellular elements, including glial cells (Müller cells, fibrous astrocytes), histiocytes, fibroblasts, and myofibroblasts. Amacrine and bipolar cells, which are found in the inner nuclear layer of the retina, are not a major constituent of PVR membranes. Unless there is rupture of Bruch membrane, choroidal melanocytes do not have access to the subretinal space or vitreous cavity and therefore are not typically observed in PVR membranes.

21. **c.** Hyperplastic RPE lesions that mimic congenital hypertrophy of the RPE (CHRPE) can be present in Gardner syndrome and in carriers of the *APC* gene mutation. The presence of 4 or more of these lesions in each eye of a patient with a family history of Gardner syndrome or the *APC* mutation identifies that patient as a carrier. A mutation in *APC* confers an increased lifetime risk of developing colon polyps, benign tumors, and cancer. In combined hamartoma of the retina and RPE, the RPE is hyperplastic and frequently migrates into the retina in a perivascular distribution. Vitreous condensation and fibroglial proliferation may be present on the surface of the tumor. Osseous metaplasia of the RPE with bone formation can be a prominent feature in phthisis bulbi.

22. **c.** Histologically, lattice degeneration of the peripheral retina demonstrates pathologic findings of a localized area of inner retinal atrophy with loss of the internal limiting membrane, adherent vitreous at the edges of the lesion with an overlying pocket of liquefied vitreous, and sclerosis of the remaining retinal vessels. Lattice degeneration may present as prominent sclerotic vessels in a wicker or lattice pattern. The clinical presentation has many variations. The vitreous directly over lattice degeneration is liquefied, but formed vitreous remains adherent at the margins of the degenerated area. The internal limiting membrane is discontinuous, and the inner retinal layers are atrophic.

23. **a.** Iris color is determined by the number and size of melanin granules in the melanocytes of the anterior border layer.

24. **a.** A characteristic finding in sympathetic ophthalmia is the presence of Dalen-Fuchs nodules, which are accumulations of epithelioid histiocytes and lymphocytes between the RPE and Bruch membrane, usually beneath the peripheral retina. The histiocytes may demonstrate pigment phagocytosis. Other characteristic pathologic findings in sympathetic ophthalmia include a diffuse granulomatous panuveitis, histiocytes and giant cells in the choroid with pigment phagocytosis, preservation of the choriocapillaris, exudative retinal detachments, and retinal perivasculitis. Sympathetic ophthalmia is described after perforating ocular trauma and ocular surgery, including vitrectomy, glaucoma procedures, and cataract extraction, and noninvasive procedures such as cyclophotocoagulation. Ninety percent of cases occur within 1 year of injury, but the range of reported cases is 2 weeks to 50 years.

25. **d.** Choroidal melanoma is the most common primary intraocular malignancy in adults. The most common secondary intraocular malignancy in adults is metastatic breast cancer in females and lung cancer in males. Retinoblastoma is the most common primary intraocular malignancy in children but is extraordinarily rare in adults. Intraocular lymphoma can occur in adults but is not as common as choroidal melanoma. Iris melanomas are far less common.

26. **a.** Frequent mutations have been described in the following 5 genes in uveal melanoma: *BAP1, EIF1AX, GNA11, GNAQ,* and *SF3B1*. Mutations in *BAP1, SF3B1,* and *EIF1AX* are almost mutually exclusive with each other, which suggests alternative downstream molecular events during tumor progression. *BAP1* (*BRCA1*-associated protein-1) mutations are associated with poor prognostic factors and high metastatic risk. In contrast, *EIF1AX* and *SF3B1* mutations are associated with favorable prognostic factors. *GNAQ* and *GNA11* have been shown to occur early in tumor formation and are not associated with prognosis.

27. **b.** Molluscum contagiosum, which is caused by a member of the poxvirus family, is characterized by dome-shaped, waxy epidermal nodules with a central umbilication. If present on the eyelid margin, these nodules may cause a secondary follicular conjunctivitis. Histologically, the epithelial nuclei are displaced peripherally by large eosinophilic (pink) viral inclusions known as *molluscum bodies*. As the infected cells migrate to the surface, the viral inclusions become more basophilic (blue/dark purple). Bacterial conjunctivitis is associated with a papillary reaction and purulent discharge. In pseudomembranous conjunctivitis, the fibrin network is easily peeled off, leaving the conjunctiva intact; pseudomembranes form on the conjunctiva. Giant papillary conjunctivitis (GPC) occurs in primary and secondary forms, all of which are at least partially caused by chronic ocular allergy. Primary forms of GPC include vernal and atopic keratoconjunctivitis. Secondary GPC is caused by contact lenses, ocular prostheses, or exposed sutures.

28. **b.** Basal cell carcinoma (BCC) is the most common malignant tumor of the eyelid, accounting for more than 90% of all eyelid tumors. BCC occurs most commonly on the lower eyelid (50%–60%), followed in frequency by the medial canthus (25%–30%), upper eyelid, and lateral canthus. There are many different clinical manifestations of BCC of the eyelid, including nodular, ulcerative, pigmented, and morpheaform. The morpheaform type, which is less common, behaves more aggressively and the margins are difficult to determine on clinical examination. Complete excision including pathologic evaluation of excision margins is the treatment of choice for BCCs of the eyelid.

29. **b.** Keratoacanthoma occurs most commonly on facial skin as a single, large, elevated growth with a central crater. There is usually a history of rapid growth over 4 to 8 weeks,

and often a history of spontaneous regression over several months. There is strong evidence that keratoacanthomas are a variant of a well-differentiated squamous cell carcinoma. In fact, many dermatopathologists and ophthalmic pathologists prefer to call this lesion *well-differentiated squamous cell carcinoma with keratoacanthoma-like differentiation* because of the possibility of perineural invasion and metastasis.

30. **c.** Pleomorphic adenoma (also called *benign mixed tumor*) is the most common epithelial lacrimal gland tumor; it constitutes approximately 50% of this category. This tumor grows slowly and may mold the bone of the lacrimal fossa. Tumor growth stimulates the periosteum to deposit a thin layer of new bone (ie, cortication). The adjacent orbital bone is not eroded. The slow growth causes gradual proptosis without pain. Although this is usually a benign tumor, recurrences are difficult to manage and can occur with incomplete excision or by seeding of the orbit from incisional biopsies. Surgical therapy is thus directed at complete removal with an adequate margin within the tumor pseudocapsule. Histologically, pleomorphic adenoma is a combination of epithelial and stromal elements that are derived from normal lacrimal epithelium. The epithelial component may form nests or tubules lined by 2 layers of cells, the outermost layer blending imperceptibly with the stroma. The stroma may be myxoid and demonstrate occasional heterologous findings of cartilage or bone.

31. **d.** Optic nerve coloboma results from defective closure of the posterior embryonic or choroidal fissure. It is often inferonasal and may be associated with colobomatous defects of the retina and choroid, ciliary body, and iris. Failure of neural crest differentiation profoundly affects development of the ocular structures and results in cryptophthalmos (absence of the eyelids, conjunctiva, cornea, and lens). The primary vitreous consists of fibrillar material, mesenchymal cells, and vascular components. The tunica vasculosa lentis surrounds the developing lens, the vasa hyaloidea propria is a network of vessels posterior to the lens, and the hyaloid artery connects the vasa hyaloidea propria to the optic nerve. Failure of these vessels to regress results in persistent fetal vasculature and often microphthalmia. Early in embryogenesis, the optic vesicle influences the specific region of head ectoderm to form the lens placode. The lens placode later invaginates to become the lens vesicle. Failure of induction of the lens placode results in primary congenital aphakia.

32. **a.** Iris melanomas account for 3%–5% of all uveal melanomas and are associated with a distinctly lower mortality rate (1%–4%) than melanomas of the ciliary body and choroid.

33. **c.** The liver is the primary organ involved in metastatic uveal melanoma, and liver involvement is commonly the first manifestation of metastatic disease. Other relatively frequent sites, generally after liver metastasis, are the lungs, bones, and skin. All patients require metastatic evaluation prior to definitive treatment of intraocular melanoma.

34. **b.** Because they are located posterior to the iris, ciliary body melanomas often remain asymptomatic until they become rather large. Patients may note reduced vision from induced astigmatism or cataract when the tumor touches the lens (ie, lenticular astigmatism). Additional signs and symptoms include dilated, often tortuous, episcleral vessel(s) (sentinel vessel); photopsia and visual field alterations from associated retinal detachment (in more advanced cases); and, in rare cases, secondary glaucoma. Corneal astigmatism is unlikely to result from a ciliary body melanoma but may be caused by ocular surface neoplasia. Orbital tumors that flatten the posterior surface of the globe may induce axial hyperopia. Axial myopia is unlikely to develop in an adult with neoplasm.

35. **d.** In patients previously treated for retinoblastoma, osteosarcomas represent 40% of tumors that arise within the field of radiation and 36% of those arising outside the field of radiation.

36. **c.** Clinically, the retina is the most commonly affected intraocular structure in leukemia. Ocular manifestations of leukemia are common, occurring in as many as 80% of eyes from patients with the disease examined at autopsy. Leukemic retinopathy is characterized by intraretinal and subhyaloid hemorrhages, hard exudates, cotton-wool spots, and white-centered retinal hemorrhages (pseudo–Roth spots). These findings in leukemia are usually the result of associated anemia, hyperviscosity, and/or thrombocytopenia. Although the retina is the most commonly affected ocular structure clinically, histologic studies have shown that the uvea is more commonly affected by leukemia than is the retina. A patient with leukemic infiltration of the optic nerve may present with severe vision loss and optic nerve edema. One or both eyes may be affected. This is an ophthalmic emergency and requires immediate treatment to preserve as much vision as possible.

Index

(*f* = figure; *t* = table)

A-scan ultrasonography. *See* Standardized ultrasonography
AA amyloid, 67
Abrasion, of cornea, 45, 188
Abscess, 240, 266
Abusive head trauma, 189–191, 190*f*
Acanthamoeba keratitis, 27*t*, 95, 96*f*
Acantholysis, 238
Acanthosis, 238, 240, 246, 248*f*
Acanthosis nigricans, 246
ACC (adenoid cystic carcinoma), 17*f*, 270–272, 272*f*
Accessory lacrimal glands, 88, 238
Acellular capillaries, 181–182, 182*f*, 187
Acquired hyperplasia, 332, 333*f*
Actin, 32, 32*t*
Actinic keratitis, 99, 247–249, 248*f*
Actinic keratopathy, 100–101, 101*f*
Actinic keratosis, 247–249, 248*f*
Actinomyces israelii, 269
Acute disseminated encephalomyelitis (ADEM), 288, 289
Acute retinal necrosis (ARN), 171, 172*f*
Adenoid cystic carcinoma (ACC), 17*f*, 270–272, 272*f*
Adenomas and adenocarcinomas
    of ciliary body, 210, 210*f*, 211, 331
    of eyelid, 253–254, 253*f*
    gastrointestinal, 170, 246
    of lacrimal gland, 88, 88*f*, 270, 271*f*
    of retinal pigment epithelium, 170–171, 211, 331
    sebaceous, 253–254, 253*f*
Adenoviruses, 59
Adipose tissue, 57, 58*f*, 259, 282
Adipose tumors, 282
Adult-onset foveomacular vitelliform dystrophy (AFMVD), 197–198, 201*f*
Age-related macular degeneration (AMD)
    about, 191
    clinical characteristics, 191–195, 191–196*f*
    differential diagnosis, 177, 320, 321, 322*f*
    drusen and, 191–193, 191–193*f*, 192*t*
    photodynamic therapy for, 338
Aging. *See* Degenerations
AIDS/HIV infection, 70, 171
AJCC. *See* American Joint Committee on Cancer staging system
Albinism, 167–168, 168*f*
Alcian blue stain, 27*t*
ALH. *See* Atypical lymphoid hyperplasia
Alizarin red stain, 27*t*
Alkapton, 104
Allergic reactions
    fungal sinusitis, 269
    inflammation and, 8
    noninfectious conjunctivitis and, 60
Alport syndrome, 140
Alveolar rhabdomyosarcoma, 278, 279, 279*f*
Amblyopia, 140, 168, 252
AMD. *See* Age-related macular degeneration

Amelanotic choroidal masses, 323, 323*t*, 337, 384*f*, 385
Amelanotic nevus, 75
American Academy of Ophthalmology's Initiative in Vision Rehabilitation, 302
American Association of Cancer Research, 369
American Joint Committee on Cancer (AJCC) staging system
    about, 302
    for posterior uveal melanomas, 231, 323–325, 324–325*t*, 330–331
    for retinoblastoma, 358, 359*t*, 360
Amiodarone, 104
Amyloidosis and amyloid deposits
    about, 158, 243, 244*t*
    in conjunctiva, 67–68, 68*f*
    in cornea, 109, 110*f*
    in eyelid, 243–245, 244*f*
    in orbit, 269
    of vitreous, 158–159, 159*f*
Anastomosis, 340–341, 341*f*
Androgen receptors, 236
Angiofibroma, 276
Angiomatosis retinae, 170, 170*f*, 341–344, 342*f*
Angiomatous tumors. *See* Vascular tumors
Angle-closure glaucoma, 121, 122*f*, 222
Angle recession (traumatic), 50*f*, 126
Aniridia, 216–217, 217*f*
Anterior border layer, of iris, 214, 214*f*
Anterior chamber, 117–128
    degenerations, 120–128
        iridocorneal endothelial (ICE) syndrome, 120–121, 123*f*, 308*t*
        primary congenital glaucoma, 91, 119, 119*f*
        secondary glaucoma, 122–128. *See also under* Glaucoma
    developmental anomalies, 118–120, 119–121*f*
    inflammation, 120, 122*f*, 143
    neoplasia, 128, 128*f*
    retinoblastoma and, 206
    topography, 117–118, 118*f*, 213
    trauma, 49, 50, 50*f*, 123–126, 125–126*f*
Anterior chamber angle
    deposits, 122, 126, 126*f*
    developmental anomalies, 91, 92*f*, 119–120, 119*f*
    glaucoma and, 121, 122, 122*f*, 125–127, 127*f*, 222, 309
    inflammation, 120–121, 122*f*, 143
    iris melanoma invasion into, 225, 305, 307*f*
    topography, 117, 118*f*
    trauma, 49
Anterior lens capsule
    deposits, 122, 124*f*, 143
    developmental anomalies, 140
    topography, 137, 138*f*
    wound repair, 47–48
Anterior lenticonus, 140
Anterior lentiglobus, 140
Anterior proliferative vitreoretinopathy (PVR), 52, 53*f*

Anterior segment dysgenesis, 91, 92f, 119–120, 120–121f
Anterior subcapsular fibrous plaques, 143–144, 144f
Anti–vascular endothelial growth factor agents, 182, 183f, 194, 329, 339, 343–344
Antibodies
    for flow cytometry, 33, 34f
    for immunohistochemistry, 29–32, 31f
Antiviral drugs, 98
Antoni A and B patterns, 281, 281f
APC gene, 171
Aphakia, congenital, 140
Aphakic bullous keratopathy, 101–102, 102–103f, 112, 114–115f
Apocrine glands, 88, 238
Apocrine hidrocystoma, 245, 246f
Arachnoid sheath, 285–286, 287f, 296, 297f
Argyrosis, 143
ARM2 gene, 191
ARN (acute retinal necrosis), 171, 172f
Arterial occlusions, 178, 178f, 183–185, 184f. See also Ischemia, of retina
Artifactitious clefts, 147
Ascending optic atrophy, 291
Aspergillus spp, 95, 173, 268–269, 268f
Asteroid bodies, 158, 220–221
Asteroid hyalosis, 157–158, 158f
Astrocytes
    optic atrophy and, 291
    of optic nerve, 285, 286–287f, 286t
    of retinal ganglion cell layer, 167
    retinal repair, 48, 156, 157f
Astrocytic hamartoma, 356, 356f
Astrocytomas
    of optic nerve, 295–296, 296f
    of retina, 356, 356f
Atopy, 105
Atrophia bulbi, 14–15
Atypical lymphoid hyperplasia (ALH), 273
Autoimmune disorders
    keratitis and, 98
    mucous membrane pemphigoid (MMP), 60–61, 60f
    noninfectious uveitis and, 219–221
Avellino dystrophy, 110, 112f, 113t
Axenfeld nerve loop, 130f
Axenfeld-Rieger syndrome, 119–120, 121f

B-cell lymphomas, 86, 87f, 160, 235, 274, 275f
B cells, 8, 32t
B-scan ultrasonography. See Standardized ultrasonography
B&B (Brown and Brenn) stain, 27t
B&H (Brown and Hopps) stain, 27t
Bacterial infections. See also specific bacteria
    of conjunctiva, 59, 59f
    of cornea, 92–93, 93f, 96–98, 97–98f
    of eyelid, 240
    inflammatory process, 8
    of lacrimal drainage system, 269
    of lens, 141, 142f
    of optic nerve, 288
    of orbit, 266
    of retina, 171
    staining, 27t

of uveal tract, 218, 218f
of vitreous, 152
Bacteroides spp, 266
Balloon cells, 226–227, 227f
Band keratopathy, 27t, 99–100, 100f
BAP1 (BRCA1-associated protein-1) gene, 32, 232, 313, 330
Bartonella henselae, 62, 288
Basal cell carcinoma (BCC), 249, 249–250f, 254, 380
Basal laminar (cuticular) drusen, 192t
Basedow disease, 264–266, 264f
Basement membrane
    of anterior chamber. See Descemet membrane
    of conjunctiva, 55, 60, 60f, 70–71, 71–72f, 74, 83t, 84
    of cornea, 89, 90f, 99, 103f, 107, 108f, 188
    of lens, 48, 137
    of retinal pigment epithelium
        in age-related macular degeneration, 191
        diabetic intraocular changes, 187, 189f
        neoplasia, 209, 210
        retinal detachment sequelae, 176
        topography, 167
Basophils (mast cells), 8, 10f
BAX proteins, 271–272
BCC (basal cell carcinoma), 249, 249–250f, 254, 380
Bcl-2 proteins, 271–272
Bear tracks, 320, 321f
"Beaten metal" appearance, of Descemet membrane, 112, 114f
Behçet disease, 221, 221f
Benign epithelial (complexion-associated) melanosis, 76, 77f, 78, 80–81f, 82t
Benign lymphoid hyperplasia, 85–86, 86f
Berger space, 150f
Bergmeister papilla, 151, 152f
Berlin edema, 52
Best disease, 198
β-blockers, 252
β-pleated sheet, 158, 243
Bladder (Wedl) cells, 143, 143f, 239, 239f
Blepharitis, 240
Blepharoconjunctivitis, 254f
Blindness. See Vision loss and impairment
Blood staining, of cornea, 104, 104f
Blood–retina barrier, 179–180, 187
Blue cells, 256, 257f
Blue nevus, 76, 257
Boat-shaped hemorrhage, 180, 181f
Bony orbit. See Orbit
Bony tumors. See Osteomas
Borrelia burgdorferi, 98
Botryoid variant, of rhabdomyosarcoma, 279
Bowman layer
    degenerations, 99, 99f, 188
    dystrophies, 107–110, 108–112f
    inflammation, 93f, 94f
    topography, 89, 90f
    wound repair, 45
BPD. See Butterfly-shaped pattern dystrophy
Brachytherapy
    for choroidal hemangiomas, 339
    for iris melanoma, 305

for posterior uveal melanoma, 301, 318*f*, 327–329, 328*f*, 331–332
for retinal capillary hemangioblastoma, 343
for retinoblastoma, 363
BRAF gene, 85
Branch retinal artery occlusion (BRAO), 185
Branch retinal vein occlusion (BRVO), 186–187
BRAO. *See* Branch retinal artery occlusion
BRCA1-associated protein-1 *(BAP1)* gene, 32, 232, 313, 330
Breast cancer, eye involvement and, 337, 372, 373*t*, 376–377*f*, 377
Breslow thickness, 260
Brown and Brenn (B&B) stain, 27*t*
Brown and Hopps (B&H) stain, 27*t*
Brown cells, 260*f*
Bruch membrane
    choroidal melanoma and, 228, 313
    choroidal neovascularization and, 196*f*
    degenerations, 191, 191*f*, 192*t*, 193, 193*f*
    glial scarring and, 48
    inflammation, 172*f*
    retinal degenerations and, 177, 177*f*, 187, 188*f*
    rupture of, 52–54
    staining, 27*t*
    topography, 162*f*, 163, 164*f*, 167
BRVO (branch retinal vein occlusion), 186–187
Bulbar conjunctiva, 55, 56*f*, 64*f*
Bullae, 60, 60*f*, 101
Bullous hemorrhage, 181*f*
Bullous keratopathy, 101–102, 102–103*f*, 112, 114–115*f*
Busacca nodules, 220
Butterfly-shaped pattern dystrophy (BPD), 197–198

C-MIN (conjunctival melanocytic intraepithelial neoplasia), 76–79, 77*f*, 83*t*
Calcific band keratopathy, 27*t*, 99–100, 100*f*
Calcific drusen, 192*t*
Calcific plaques, 134, 135*f*, 185
Calcium deposits
    lens and, 147, 147*f*
    optic nerve head drusen, 292–294, 294*f*
    in retinoblastoma, 349–350
Calcofluor white stain, 27*t*
Callender classification system (modified), 224, 230
CALT (conjunctiva-associated lymphoid tissue), 55
Canaliculitis, 269
Candida albicans, 173
Candida spp, 95, 173
Candlewax drippings, of sarcoidosis, 220
Capillary (infantile) hemangiomas, 57, 234, 252, 252*f*, 275, 341
Capsule, of lens. *See* Lens capsule
Carbohydrate sulfotransferase 6 *(CHST6)* gene, 110
Carboplatin, 361, 362
Carcinomas. *See also* Adenomas and adenocarcinomas; Metastatic carcinomas
    basal cell carcinoma, 249, 249–250*f*, 254, 380
    of conjunctiva, 74, 128
    Merkel cell carcinoma, 256
    sebaceous carcinoma, 27*t*, 116, 254–255*f*, 254–256
    sebaceous carcinoma in situ, 255*f*, 256
    spindle cell carcinoma, 74

squamous cell carcinoma, 70, 74, 84, 247–252, 254. *See also* Squamous cell carcinoma
    staining, 32*t*
Carotid occlusive disease, 178
Caruncle, 55, 56*f*, 254
Caseating granulomas, 11, 13*f*, 62
Cataracts, 143–147
    Alport syndrome and, 140
    aniridia and, 217, 217*f*
    of cortex, 145, 146*f*
    diabetes mellitus and, 188
    of epithelium, 143–145, 143–145*f*
    etiology, 51, 123, 143–144
    of nucleus, 145–147, 147*f*
    sectoral cataract, 304
    surgical complications, 101, 141
Cavernous hemangioma, 7, 275, 277*f*, 339–340, 340*f*
Cavernous optic atrophy, 27*t*, 292, 293*f*
CCM1/KRIT1 gene, 339
CCN1 gene, 280
CD (cluster of differentiation) antigens, 32, 32*t*
CD20 receptors, 264
CD25 receptors, 264
Cellulitis, 240, 241*f*, 266
Central nervous system (CNS)
    cells of, 48, 286*t*
    fungal infections spreading to, 268
    intraocular lymphoma extension to, 160
    metastasis mechanism, 372, 372*f*
    neurosensory retina and, 48, 163–164
    retinoblastoma extension to, 351–354, 368
    tumors of, 282, 339, 351–352, 380
Central retinal artery occlusion (CRAO), 183–185, 184*f*
Central retinal vein occlusion (CRVO), 185, 186*f*, 187
CFH gene, 191
CGH (comparative genomic hybridization), 35*t*
Chalazion, 63, 242*f*
Chalcosis, 143
Chamber angle. *See* Anterior chamber angle
Chandler syndrome, 120–121
Charged-particle radiation, 328–329
CHED (congenital hereditary endothelial dystrophy), 112, 114, 115*f*
Chemotherapy
    for posterior uveal melanoma, 330
    for retinoblastoma, 302, 361–362*f*, 361–363, 364
    types of, 361–362, 361–362*f*, 364
    for vitreous seeds, 361, 364
Children. *See also* Developmental anomalies
    axial myopia, 134
    combined hamartoma, 210–211
    conjunctivitis, 59
    juvenile xanthogranuloma, 221, 222*f*
    melanocytic nevus, 75, 75*f*, 76, 82*t*
    muscle differentiation tumors, 278–280, 279*f*
    orbital tumors, 269–270
    retinoblastoma, 347–348. *See also* Retinoblastoma
    scleral staphylomas, 134
    shaken baby syndrome, 189–191, 190*f*
    squamous papilloma, 69
    vascular tumors, 274–275, 276*f*
Children's Oncology Group (COG) clinical trials, 358, 360, 362, 368

Chlamydia spp, 27*t*, 59, 59*f*
Chloromas, 388
Cholesterol deposits, 52, 157, 169, 169*f*, 356
Cholesterol emboli, 185
Choriocapillaris, 167, 176–177, 216, 216*f*, 226
Chorioretinal nodules, 220
Chorioretinitis, 54, 173–174, 173*f*, 220–221
Chorioretinitis sclopetaria, 54
Chorioretinopathy, 321, 322*f*
Choristomas
  of conjunctiva, 57, 58*f*
  of cornea, 91
  defined, 7, 57
  of lens, 239, 239*f*
  lymphoid proliferation and, 234, 235, 235*f*
  types of, 57, 58*f*
Choroid. *See also* Choroidal neovascularization; Uveal
  tract
  amelanotic masses, 323, 323*t*, 337, 384*f*, 385
  blood supply, 167, 178*f*
  detachment, 320–321
  hemorrhage, 50, 52
  inflammation, 54, 54*f*, 173, 173*f*, 337
  metastases to, 373–377, 375–376*f*, 377*t*
  neoplasia
    fine-needle aspiration biopsy of, 40*f*
    hemangiomas, 233–234, 234*f*, 323, 335–339,
      336–337*f*
    leiomyoma, 236
    lymphoid proliferation, 235, 235*f*
    lymphomas, 161, 162*f*, 235, 235*f*
    melanocytomas, 309, 320
    melanomas, 226–232, 312–331. *See also* Posterior
      uveal melanoma
    metastasis to, 232–233, 233*f*
    neural sheath tumors, 236, 236*f*
    nevus, 225–226, 226*f*, 305, 308–309, 310*f*, 312*f*,
      313, 319–320
    osteomas, 234–235, 235*f*, 321–323, 322*f*, 337
    retinoblastoma invasion, 206–207, 208*f*, 354, 368
  topography, 164*f*, 213, 214*f*, 215–216*f*, 216*f*
  trauma, 52–54, 54*f*
  wound repair, 47
Choroidal neovascularization (CNV)
  choroidal neovascular membranes, 193, 196–197*f*
  choroidal nevus and, 226, 308
  diffuse drusen and, 191
  neoplasia and, 234
  polypoidal choroidal vasculopathy and, 195, 196*f*
  reticular pseudodrusen (RPD) and, 193
  trauma-related, 52, 54
  treatment, 182
Chromogens, 30–31, 31*f*
Chromogranin, 32, 32*t*
Chronic syphilis-related (luetic) interstitial keratitis, 97
CHRPE (congenital hypertrophy of the RPE), 170–171,
  171*f*, 320, 321*f*
CHST6 gene, 110
Cilia, 239
Ciliary arteries, 129*f*, 130
Ciliary body
  degenerations, 222, 223*f*
  deposits and, 158
  diabetic changes, 188, 189*f*
  metastases to, 373
  neoplasia
    adenoma, 210, 210*f*, 331
    leiomyoma, 236
    medulloepithelioma, 356–357, 357*f*
    melanoma, 226–232, 312–331. *See also* Posterior
      uveal melanoma
    neurofibromas, 236
    nevus, 305, 308–309
  topography, 118*f*, 138*f*, 213, 214*f*, 215, 215*f*
  trauma, 49, 50*f*, 53*f*
  wound repair, 47, 48
Ciliary epithelium
  acquired hyperplasia, 332
  diabetic changes, 188, 189*f*
  neoplasia, 209–211, 210*f*, 331
  topography, 153*f*, 163, 215*f*
Ciliary muscle, 49, 50–51*f*
Ciliochoroidal melanoma, 228
CIN (conjunctival intraepithelial neoplasia), 70, 71,
  71–73*f*, 74
Circumscribed choroidal hemangioma, 233–234,
  335–338, 336*f*
Circumscribed iris nevus, 304
Climatic droplet keratopathy, 100–101, 101*f*
Cloquet canal, 149, 150*f*
Clostridium spp, 266
Clump cells, 214
Cluster of differentiation (CD) antigens, 32, 32*t*
CME (cystoid macular edema), 156, 166–167, 180, 180*f*,
  183*f*, 338
CMV (cytomegalovirus), 32*t*, 171, 172*f*
CNS. *See* Central nervous system
CNV. *See* Choroidal neovascularization
Coats disease, 169, 169*f*, 350*f*, 355–356, 355*f*
Cobblestone degeneration, 176–177, 177*f*
Coccidioidomycosis, 288–289
COG (Children's Oncology Group) clinical trials, 358,
  360, 362, 368
Cogan-Reese iris nevus type, 120, 308*t*
Collaborative Ocular Melanoma Study (COMS), 301,
  323, 324, 327, 331–332
Collagen crosslinking, 106
Colloidal iron stain, 27*t*
Colobomas, 57, 131, 140, 217, 217*f*, 287, 288*f*
Colon polyps, 170–171
Combined hamartoma, 210–211, 211*f*, 333–334, 333*f*
Combined nevus, 257
Commotio retinae, 52
Communication, with pathologist, 19, 20, 30*t*, 161, 273
Comparative genomic hybridization (CGH), 35*t*
Complex choristomas, 57, 58*f*
Complexion-associated melanosis, 76, 77*f*, 78, 80–81*f*,
  82*t*
Compound nevus, 75*f*, 76, 258, 258*f*
Computed tomography (CT), 318, 321, 325, 325*t*, 352
COMS (Collaborative Ocular Melanoma Study), 301,
  323, 324, 327, 331–332
Cones, 164*f*, 165, 165*f*
Congenital (infantile) glaucoma, 91, 119, 119*f*
Congenital anomalies. *See* Developmental anomalies
Congenital aphakia, 140

Congenital hereditary endothelial dystrophy (CHED), 112, 114, 115*f*
Congenital hypertrophy of the RPE (CHRPE), 170–171, 171*f*, 320, 321*f*
Congenital melanocytic nevus, 257
Congenital ocular melanocytosis, 308*f*, 308*t*, 309, 310*f*, 313, 337
Congenital retinal arteriovenous malformations, 340–341, 341*f*
Congenital retinal macrovessel, 340, 341*f*
Congenital split nevus, 257, 257*f*
Congenital syphilis, 97–98, 98*f*
Congo red stain, 27*t*
Conjunctiva, 55–88
    degenerations, 64–69, 65–69*f*
    developmental anomalies, 57, 58*f*, 82*t*
    inflammation, 57–63, 59–65*f*, 78. *See also* Conjunctivitis
    neoplasia, 69–88. *See also specific neoplasias*
        carcinomas, 74, 128
        glandular, 88, 88*f*
        intraepithelial melanosis, 76–79, 77–78*f*
        lymphoid, 85–88, 86–87*f*
        melanocytic nevus, 75–76, 75–76*f*
        melanoma, 79, 84–85, 84–85*f*
        metastases to, 88
        other neoplasms, 88
        scleral involvement, 135
        squamous epithelial lesions, 69–74, 70–73*f*
    specimen handling and processing, 22–23, 23*f*, 69, 71
    topography, 55–56, 56*f*
    wound repair, 44*f*, 45–47
Conjunctiva-associated lymphoid tissue (CALT), 55
Conjunctival intraepithelial neoplasia (CIN), 70, 71, 71–73*f*, 74
Conjunctival melanocytic intraepithelial neoplasia (C MIN), 76–79, 77*f*, 83*t*
Conjunctival melanoma, 79, 82*t*, 84–85, 84–85*f*
Conjunctival melanosis, 76
Conjunctivitis, 57–63
    about, 57–59
    acute *vs* chronic, 59
    follicular, 61, 61–62*f*, 240, 242*f*
    granulomatous, 61–63, 63–64*f*
    infectious, 59, 59*f*, 62
    noninfectious, 60–61, 60*f*
    papillary, 61, 61–62*f*
    secondary acquired melanosis and, 78
Conjunctivochalasis, 68–69
Contact inhibition, 45
Contact lens use, 92, 95, 99
Contraction, of wounds, 43–44, 46*f*, 47
Copper deposits, 143
Cornea
    abrasions, 45, 188
    degenerations, 98–99, 99*f*, 101, 127
    deposits, 99–101, 100–101*f*, 104, 104*f*, 109–110, 110–112*f*. *See also* Cataracts
    developmental anomalies, 91, 92*f*
    dystrophies of, 106–115
        classification system, 106–107
        Descemet membrane, 114–115, 115*f*
        endothelial, 111–114, 114–115*f*

        epithelial and subepithelial, 107–110, 108–112*f*
        epithelial–stromal *TGFB1*, 106–107, 109*f*
        stromal, 110–111, 113*f*
    ectasias, 104–106, 105*f*
    embryonic development, 90
    graft failure, 102, 103*f*
    inflammation, 91–98. *See also* Keratitis
    neoplasia, 70, 71, 116
    topography, 89–91, 90*f*
    ulcers, 8, 45, 91, 92–93*f*, 93–95, 98
    wound repair, 45, 46*f*
Cornea plana, 91, 92*f*
Cornea verticillate, 104
Corneal deturgescence, 90
Corneal dystrophy of Bowman layer type I, 107, 108, 109*f*, 113*t*
Corneal dystrophy of Bowman layer type II, 108–110, 109–112*f*, 113*t*
Corneal intraepithelial neoplasia, 70, 71
Corneal melting, 98
Corneal pannus, 15, 99, 101, 102–103*f*, 107–108, 109*f*, 217
Cortex, of lens, 138*f*, 139, 145, 146*f*
Corticosteroid therapy, 95, 96–97, 97*f*, 290
Cotton-wool spots, 179, 185, 187, 376–377, 386
CRAO (central retinal artery occlusion), 183–185, 184*f*
CRVO (central retinal vein occlusion), 185, 186*f*, 187
Cryotherapy
    for retinal capillary hemangioblastoma, 343
    for retinal vasoproliferative tumors, 344
    for retinoblastoma, 302, 348, 363
Cryptococcosis, 288–289, 289*f*
Cryptococcus neoformans, 173
Crystalline lens. *See* Lens
CT (computed tomography), 318, 321, 325, 325*t*, 352
Cutaneous melanomas, 368
Cuticular (basal laminar) drusen, 192*t*
Cyclodialysis, 49–50, 51*f*, 126
Cysticercosis, 269
Cystoid macular edema (CME), 156, 166–167, 180, 180*f*, 183*f*, 338
Cystoid spaces
    corneal dystrophies, 108*f*
    optic atrophy, 292, 293*f*
    retinal degenerations, 174–175, 175*f*, 179–180*f*, 180
    retinal ischemia, 186*f*
Cysts
    of eyelid, 240, 245, 245–246*f*
    of iris, 308*f*, 308*t*
    of orbit, 262, 262*f*, 269
    with retinal protozoal infection, 174, 174*f*
    of vitreous, 151
Cytoid bodies, 179, 179*f*
Cytokeratins, 31, 32*t*, 115
Cytomegalovirus (CMV), 32*t*, 171, 172*f*
Cytospin preparation, 39

Dacryoadenitis, 263
Dacryocystitis, 269, 283
Dacryops, 245
Dalen-Fuchs nodules, 219
DALK. *See* Deep anterior lamellar keratoplasty
Decapitation secretion, 238

Deep anterior lamellar keratoplasty (DALK), 106
Degenerations
    about, 12, 14–15, 15*t*
    of anterior chamber, 120–128. *See also under* Anterior
        chamber
    of ciliary body, 222, 223*f*
    of conjunctiva, 64–69, 65–69*f*
    of cornea, 98–99, 99*f*, 101, 127
    defined, 12
    of iris, 120–121, 123*f*, 127, 222, 223*f*
    of lens, 91, 92*f*, 140, 141*f*
    of optic nerve, 291–294, 292–294*f*
    overview, 14–15, 15*t*
    of retina, 174–202. *See also* Retinal degenerations
    of sclera, 15, 15*f*, 134–135, 134–135*f*, 287, 288*f*
    stages of, 14–15, 15*t*
    of trabecular meshwork, 49, 122–123, 125–128,
        126–127*f*
    of uveal tract, 222, 223*f*
Degenerative retinoschisis, 175
DEM (diagnostic electron microscopy), 30*t*, 39
Demodex folliculorum, 240, 241
Demyelinating diseases, 289, 290*f*, 291
Dendritic nevus cells (branching), 224
Dendritic ulcer, 93–95, 94*f*
Deposits. *See also* Amyloidosis and amyloid deposits;
        Calcium deposits
    in anterior chamber angle, 122, 126, 126*f*
    in ciliary body, 158
    in cornea, 99–101, 100–101*f*, 104, 104–105*f*, 106,
        109–110, 110–112*f. See also* Cataracts
    defined, 12
    in eyelid skin, 243–245, 244*f*
    in muscles, 269
    at optic nerve head, 292–294, 294*f*
    in orbit, 269
    in retina, 158
    in vitreous, 157, 158–159, 159*f*
Dermal nevus, 258, 259*f*
Dermis, 237–238, 237*f*
Dermoids (dermoid cysts)
    conjunctival, 57, 58*f*
    corneal, 91
    defined, 7
    of eyelid, 240
    of orbit, 262, 262*f*
Dermolipomas, 57, 58*f*
Descemet membrane
    degenerations, 101, 102*f*
    developmental anomalies, 91, 92*f*, 119
    dystrophies, 111–115, 114–115*f*
    endotheliitis of, 94*f*, 95
    guttae and, 97, 111, 112, 113–114*f*
    inflammation, 97, 98*f*
    rupture of, 49, 49–50*f*, 105*f*, 106
    staining, 27*t*
    topography, 89–90, 90*f*, 117
    wound repair, 45, 46*f*
Desmin, 32, 32*t*
Developmental anomalies
    about, 6*t*, 7, 8*t*
    anterior chamber, 118–120, 120–121*f*
    conjunctiva, 57, 58*f*, 82*t*

cornea, 91, 92*f*
optic nerve, 150–151, 151–152*f*, 287, 287*f*
retina, 167–171, 168–171*f*
sclera, 130–131
trabecular meshwork, 118–120, 119–120*f*
Diabetes mellitus
    choroidopathy and, 187
    fungal infections and, 268
    macular edema and, 182
    other intraocular changes, 188, 189*f*
    retinal ischemia and, 178, 182, 185
    retinopathy and, 181*f*, 182*f*, 187
Diagnostic electron microscopy (DEM), 30*t*, 39
Dichroism, 67, 68*f*
Diffuse choroidal hemangioma, 234, 337–338, 337*f*
Diffuse choroidal melanoma, 232
Diffuse ciliary body melanomas, 228, 228*f*, 232, 313,
        314*f*
Diffuse drusen, 191, 193
Diffuse infiltrating retinoblastoma, 350
Diffuse iris nevus, 304, 308*f*, 308*t*
Diffuse photoreceptor dystrophies, 198, 202, 202*f*
Diffuse scleritis, 132, 133*f*
Dilator muscle, 214, 214*f*
Diode laser, 328, 338
Disciform (stromal) keratitis, 94*f*, 95
Distichiasis, 239
DLBCL. *See* Non-Hodgkin diffuse large B-cell
        lymphoma
DNA sequencing, 33–39, 35–36*t*, 37–38*f*
Dot-and-blot intraretinal hemorrhage, 180, 181*f*
Drusen
    choroidal nevus and, 226, 305, 308–309, 310*f*, 319
    clinical types of, 192–194*f*, 192*t*
    defined, 191
    of optic nerve head, 292–294, 294*f*, 356
Dry age-related macular degeneration, 193, 195*f*
Dry eye, 99
Ductal cysts, 245, 246*f*
Duplication cataract, 144, 144*f*
Dura, of optic nerve, 285–286, 286*f*
Dutcher bodies, 275*f*
Dyskeratosis, 238, 248
Dysplastic nevus, 257, 313
Dystopia, of globe, 261
Dystrophies
    about, 14
    of cornea, 106–115, 108–115*f*, 113*t*
    of macula, 196–198, 200–201*f*
    macular corneal dystrophy, 27*t*, 110–111, 113*f*, 113*t*
    retina, 198, 202, 202*f*

EBM (epithelial basement membrane), 89, 90*f*, 99, 103*f*,
        107, 108*f*, 188
EBMD (epithelial basement membrane dystrophy), 107,
        108*f*
EBRT. *See* External beam radiotherapy
Eccrine hidrocystoma, 245
Eccrine sweat glands, 238, 253, 253*f*
Echinococcus spp, 269
Echography. *See* Ultrasonography
Ectasias, 104–106, 105*f*, 132, 134
Ectropion uveae, 222, 223*f*, 304–305, 306*f*

Edema
    of cornea, 90*f*
    of macula. *See* Macular edema
    of optic nerve head, 291, 292*f*
    retinal ischemia and, 179–180
    trauma and, 52
EK (endothelial keratoplasty) graft, 102, 103*f*
Elastotic degeneration (solar elastosis), 65–66, 67*f*, 71,
        72*f*, 248, 248*f*
Electron microscopy, 30*t*
Ellipsoid zone (EZ), 164, 166*f*
ELM (external limiting membrane), 164*f*, 166*f*
Elschnig pearls, 144, 144*f*
Embolus, 185
Embryonal rhabdomyosarcoma, 278–279, 279*f*
Embryonic lens nucleus, 139
Emissary canals, 130, 130*f*, 228–229, 229*f*, 314*f*
Encephalofacial angiomatosis (Sturge-Weber
        syndrome), 234, 337
Endophthalmitis, 141, 142*f*, 152, 153*f*, 171, 364
Endophytic retinoblastoma, 350, 350*f*
Endothelial keratoplasty (EK) graft, 102, 103*f*
Endothelium, of cornea
    developmental anomalies, 91
    dystrophies, 97, 101, 102*f*, 111–115, 113–115*f*, 113*t*
    graft failures and, 102, 103*f*
    topography, 90, 90*f*
    wound repair, 45, 46*f*
Enhanced depth imaging (EDI) optical coherence
        tomography (EDI-OCT), 376, 385
Enhanced depth imaging (swept-source) OCT, 315, 316*f*
Enterobacteriaceae, 92
Enucleation
    for choroidal melanoma, 301, 331–332
    for posterior uveal melanoma, 231–232, 301, 327
    for retinoblastoma, 360–361
    trauma and, 54*f*
Eosinophils, 8, 10*f*
Ephelis (freckle), 258
Epibulbar dermoids, 7, 57, 58*f*
Epidermal neoplasms
    epidermal malignancies, 249–252
        basal cell carcinoma, 249, 249–250*f*, 254, 380
        squamous cell carcinoma (SCC), 249–252,
            250–251*f*. *See also* Squamous cell carcinoma
    keratoses
        actinic keratosis, 99, 247–249, 248*f*
        seborrheic keratosis, 245–246, 246–247*f*
Epidermis, 237–238, 237*f*
Epidermoid cysts, 245, 245*f*
Epiretinal membrane, 156
Episclera, 47, 129–130, 129*f*
Episcleral (sentinel) vessels, 84, 85*f*, 313, 314*f*
Episcleral space, 56
Episcleritis, 131
Epithelial basement membrane dystrophy (EBMD),
        107, 108*f*
Epithelial basement membrane (EBM), 89, 90*f*, 99, 103*f*,
        107, 108*f*, 188
Epithelial inclusion cysts, 68, 69*f*, 75, 75*f*
Epithelial ingrowth and downgrowth, 102, 103*f*
Epithelioid histiocytes, 11, 218, 219, 219–220*f*, 242*f*
Epithelioid melanoma cells, 224, 225*f*, 226, 227*f*, 230

Epithelioid nevus cells, 224
Epithelium
    of ciliary body, 53*f*, 215, 215*f*
    of conjunctiva, 45–47, 55, 56*f*
    of cornea, 45, 46*f*, 89, 90*f*, 91, 93*f*
    of eyelid, 238
    immunohistochemical testing for, 31
    of iris. *See* Iris pigment epithelium
    of lens, 47–48, 51, 137, 138*f*, 139, 239, 239*f*
    of retina, 48, 52, 53*f*. *See also* Retinal pigment
        epithelium
    of uveal tract, 47
Epstein-Barr virus, 98
Equatorial (bow) region, of lens, 138*f*, 139
Essential progressive iris atrophy, 120–121, 123*f*
Etoposide, 361
Exenteration, 330
Exfoliation syndrome (pseudoexfoliation syndrome),
        122–123, 124*f*, 147
Exophthalmos. *See* Proptosis
Exophytic retinoblastoma, 349, 350*f*
Exposure keratopathy, 99
External limiting membrane (ELM), 164, 164*f*, 166*f*,
        352*f*
External beam radiotherapy (EBRT)
    for choroidal hemangiomas, 339
    for choroidal melanoma, 301, 332
    for metastases, 387–388
    for posterior uveal melanoma, 301, 329
    for retinoblastoma, 302, 364, 368
Extranodal marginal zone B-cell lymphoma (MALT
        type), 86, 87*f*, 274, 275*f*, 383
Extraocular muscles
    degenerations, 269
    inflammation, 266
    thyroid eye disease and, 264, 265*f*
    wound repair, 48–49
Extravascular matrix patterns, 231, 231*f*
Exudative AMD. *See* Choroidal neovascularization
Eyelashes (cilia), 238
Eyelids, 237–260
    cysts, 245, 245–246*f*
    degenerations, 243, 243*f*
    deposits, 243–245, 244*f*
    developmental anomalies, 239–240, 239*f*
    inflammation
        infectious, 240–241, 241–242*f*
        noninfectious, 241, 242*f*, 266
    neoplasia, 245–260
        epidermal, 245–253
        melanocytic nevus, 257–259, 257–259*f*
        melanoma, 259–260
        Merkel cell carcinoma, 256, 257*f*
        of sebaceous glands. *See under* Sebaceous
            glands
        of skin, 256, 257*f*
        vascular tumors, 340
    special testing and procedures, 41, 41*f*
    specimen handling and processing, 22–23
    systemic associations, 244*t*, 247*t*
    topography, 237–238, 237*f*, 252
    wound repair, 48
EZ (ellipsoid zone), 164, 166*f*

FA. *See* Fluorescein angiography
FAF (fundus autofluorescence) imaging, 315, 316–317*f*
Familial adenomatous polyposis, 170–171, 320, 321*f*
Familial amyloid polyneuropathy (FAP), 158, 243
Familial amyloidosis, Finnish type, 243
Fetal lens nucleus, 139
Fibrillin, 139
Fibro-osseous dysplasia, 282, 283*f*
Fibroblasts, 43–44, 44*f*, 47–48, 156
Fibrocytes, 46*f*, 264–265
Fibrosing orbititis, 263–264, 264*f*
Fibrous (fibrovascular) proliferation, 52
Fibrous dysplasia, 282, 283*f*
Fibrous histiocytomas, 276, 278*f*
Fibrous ingrowth and downgrowth, 45, 67*f*, 102, 103*f*
Fibrovascular degenerative pannus, 102*f*
Fibrovascular plaques, 150, 151*f*
Fibrovascular proliferation, 52
Filariasis, 269
Fine-needle aspiration biopsy (FNAB)
    contradictions, 348
    for gene expression profile testing, 301
    indications, 320, 327, 334
    of metastases, 378–379
    procedure, 30*t*, 39–40, 40*f*, 334
FISH (fluorescence in situ hybridization), 35*t*
Fite-Faraco stain, 27*t*
5-fluorouracil, 47
Flame-shaped intraretinal hemorrhage, 180, 181*f*
Fleischer ring, 27*t*, 105*f*, 106
Fleurettes, 205, 206*f*, 207
Flexner-Wintersteiner rosettes, 204, 205, 206*f*, 209, 367
Flow cytometry, 30*t*, 33, 34*f*
Fluorescein angiography (FA)
    of cavernous hemangiomas, 340
    of choroid nevus, 309
    of choroidal hemangioma, 336*f*, 337
    of cystoid macular edema, 166–167
    of iris melanoma, 305
    of metastatic tumors, 375, 375–376, 381, 385
    of posterior uveal melanoma, 315, 319, 320, 322*f*
    of postnatal retinal vascular tumors, 342*f*, 343, 344, 345*f*
    of prenatal retinal vascular tumors, 340, 341*f*
    of retinoblastoma, 350, 355*f*
Fluorescence in situ hybridization (FISH), 35*t*
5-fluorouracil, 47
FNAB. *See* Fine-needle aspiration biopsy
"Foamy" histiocytes, 169, 169–170*f*, 170, 222*f*, 243*f*
Focal choroidal invasion, 207
Focal cortical opacifications, 145, 146*f*
Focal posttraumatic choroidal granulomatous
    inflammation, 54, 54*f*
Follicular conjunctivitis, 61, 61–62*f*, 240, 242*f*
Follicular lymphoma, 274
Foreign bodies
    choroid and, 54, 54*f*
    conjunctiva and, 63, 64*f*
    iris and, 308*t*
    lacrimal drainage system and, 269
    lens and, 145
    sclera and, 47
Foreign body giant cells, 11, 14*f*
Forkhead box C1 (*FOXC1*) gene, 91

Formalin, 21, 21*t*
Forniceal conjunctiva, 55, 56*f*
Fovea, 150*f*, 165–167, 165*f*
Foveal pseudocyst, 156
Foveola, 165, 165*f*
FOXC1 gene, 91
FOXE3 gene, 140
Freckle (ephelis), 258
Freckles (iris), 304, 306*f*, 308*t*
Frozen sections, 19, 27, 30*t*, 40–42, 41*f*
Fuchs adenoma, 210, 210*f*, 331
Fuchs endothelial corneal dystrophy, 97, 111–112, 114*f*
Fundus autofluorescence (FAF) imaging, 315, 316–317*f*
Fundus flavimaculatus, 196–197
Fundus photography, 315, 316–317*f*, 336*f*, 349, 350–351
Fundus pulverulentus, 197
Fungal infections
    of choroid, 173, 173*f*
    of cornea, 95, 96*f*
    of lacrimal drainage system, 269
    of lens, 141
    of optic nerve, 288–289, 289*f*
    of orbit, 266–269, 268*f*
    of retina, 173, 173*f*
    staining, 27*t*
    of uveal tract, 218, 218*f*
    of vitreous, 152, 153*f*
Fungemia, 173
Fusarium keratitis, 95, 96*f*
Fusarium staining, 27*t*

Ganglion cell layer (GCL), 164–165*f*, 165, 167, 183, 184*f*
Ganglion cells
    atrophy of, 291–292
    retinal ischemia and, 179
    topography, 285, 286*f*
Gardner syndrome, 170, 320, 321*f*
Gastrointestinal adenocarcinoma, 170, 246
Gastrointestinal tract, 372, 373*t*
GCA (giant cell arteritis), 289–290, 290*f*
GCL (ganglion cell layer), 164–165*f*, 165, 167, 183, 184*f*
Gelsolin amyloidosis, 243
Gene expression profile (GEP) testing, 36, 301–302
Genetic counseling, 365–367
Geographic atrophy, 177, 183*f*, 192–193, 195*f*, 200*f*
Geographic ulcer, 93–95
Ghost cell glaucoma, 125–126, 125*f*, 156
Ghost vessels, 97, 98*f*
Giant cell angiofibromas, 276
Giant cell arteritis (GCA), 289–290, 290*f*
Giant cells, 54*f*, 64*f*, 222*f*
Giant congenital melanocytic nevus, 257
Giant drusen, 356
Giemsa stain, 27*t*
Glands. *See also* Lacrimal gland
    accessory lacrimal glands, 88, 238
    eccrine sweat glands, 238, 253, 253*f*
    of Krause, 238
    meibomian, 62*f*, 99, 237*f*, 238–241, 252, 254
    of Moll, 238–239
    sweat glands, 55, 238–239, 252, 253, 253*f*
    of Wolfring, 238
    of Zeis. *See* Sebaceous glands

Glaucoma
 anterior chamber angle and, 121, 122, 122*f*, 125–127, 127*f*, 222, 309
 chronic, 294
 developmental anomalies and, 120
 optic atrophy and, 291–292, 293*f*
 primary congenital glaucoma (PCG), 91, 119, 119*f*
 secondary, 122–128
  angle-closure glaucoma, 121, 122*f*, 222
  with ciliary body melanoma, 313
  ghost cell glaucoma, 125–126, 156
  hemolytic glaucoma, 126, 126*f*
  iris melanocytomas and, 309
  iris melanoma and, 305
  melanomalytic glaucoma, 126, 127*f*, 128, 229, 230*f*
  neovascular glaucoma, 222, 329, 355, 357, 358, 361
  open-angle glaucoma, 125–127, 126*f*
  phacolytic glaucoma, 123, 124*f*, 143
  pigment dispersion associations, 126–128, 127*f*
  pseudoexfoliation syndrome, 122–123, 124*f*
  with retinoblastoma, 350
  Sturge-Weber syndrome and, 337
  trauma and, 49, 123–126, 125–126*f*
Glaukomflecken, 144–145
Glial cells
 hemangioblastomas and, 170
 for macula repair, 156, 157*f*
 of optic nerve, 285, 286–287*f*, 286*t*, 291–292, 293*f*
 of retina, 48, 156, 179, 185, 203
Glial scarring
 gliosis, defined, 179
 of macula, 156
 of optic nerve, 288, 291, 293*f*
 of retina, 48, 171, 173, 179, 187
Glioblastoma multiforme, 296
Gliomas
 of optic nerve, 295–296, 296*f*
 of retina, 356, 356*f*
Globe
 gross examination and dissection, 24, 25–26*f*
 proptosis of, 261
 specimen handling and orientation, 21–22, 22*f*
 trauma, 52–54, 54*f*
Glycosaminoglycans, 45, 46*f*
GMS (Grocott methenamine silver) stain, 27*t*
GNA11 gene, 232
GNAQ gene, 232
Goblet cells, 27*t*, 55, 56*f*
Goldenhar syndrome, 57
Golgi apparatus, 8, 12*f*
Gomori stain, 27*t*
Gonioscopy, 307*f*, 314*f*, 315
Graft failure (corneal), 97, 102, 103*f*
Gram stain, 27*t*
Granular corneal dystrophies, 27*t*, 107, 110, 111–112*f*, 113*t*
Granulocytic sarcoma, 388
Granulomas
 about, 11
 caseating, 11, 13*f*, 62
 of choroid, 337
 foreign bodies and, 63, 64*f*
 noncaseating, 11, 13*f*, 62–63, 63*f*, 220, 221*f*, 291, 291*f*

 of optic nerve, 289, 291*f*
 parasitic infections and, 356
 pyogenic, 63, 65*f*
 sarcoidosis and, 62–63, 63*f*, 220, 221*f*, 291, 291*f*
Granulomatous inflammation
 about, 11
 of choroid, 54, 54*f*, 337
 of conjunctiva, 61–63, 63–64*f*
 of eyelid, 242*f*
 of optic nerve, 289
 of orbit, 266, 268
 of retina, 172*f*, 173, 174*f*
 of sclera, 132, 133*f*
 of uveal tract, 218–221, 219–221*f*
 of vitreous, 152
Granulomatous panuveitis, 219
Graves disease, 264–266, 264*f*
Grocott methenamine silver (GMS) stain, 27*t*
Grouped pigmentation of the retina (bear tracks), 320, 321*f*
Guttae, 97, 111, 112, 113–114*f*

H&E (hematoxylin and eosin) stain, 26–27, 27*t*
Haemophilus influenzae, 266
Hamartomas
 about, 7, 57, 171
 congenital, 75
 conjunctival, 57
 of retina, 210–211, 211*f*, 333–334, 333*f*, 356, 356*f*
 of retinal pigment epithelium, 171, 210–211, 211*f*, 321*f*, 333–334, 333*f*
Hard drusen, 192*f*, 192*t*
Healing wounds. *See* Wound repair
Heinz bodies, 125*f*
Hemangiomas
 choroid, 233–234, 234*f*, 323, 335–339, 336–337*f*
 of eyelid, 252, 252*f*
 hemangioblastomas, 170, 170*f*, 340, 341–344, 342*f*
 of orbit, 275, 277*f*
 postnatal vascular tumors, 341–344, 342*f*, 345*f*
 prenatal vascular tumors, 339–340, 340–341*f*
Hemangiopericytomas, 276
Hematopoietic tissue, 33
Hematoxylin and eosin (H&E) stain, 26–27, 27*t*
Hemoglobin, 104, 104*f*
Hemolytic glaucoma, 126, 126*f*
Hemorrhage
 choroidal, 50, 52
 retinal, 172*f*, 180–181, 185, 186*f*, 190, 190*f*
 subdural, of optic nerve, 190, 190*f*
 subretinal, 52, 311*f*, 313, 318, 322*f*
 vitreous, 52, 154, 156–157, 186*f*
Hemosiderin, 104, 104*f*, 125–126, 126*f*
Hemosiderosis, 52, 126, 145, 185
Henle fiber layer, 165–166*f*, 166–167, 180, 194*f*
Herpes simplex virus (HSV)
 corneal epithelial keratitis and, 93–95, 94*f*
 immunohistochemical stains for, 32*t*
 interstitial keratitis and, 97
 optic nerve neuritis and, 288
 retinal infections caused by, 171
Herpes zoster virus, 32*t*
Heterochromia, of iris, 348

Hidrocystomas, 245, 246f
Histiocytes, 11, 13f, 47, 169, 169f
Histiocytomas, 276, 278f
Histochemical stains, 26–27, 27t
Histoplasmosis, 193
HIV infection/AIDS, 70, 171
HMB-45, 32, 32t
Hodgkin lymphoma, 85
Hollenhorst plaques, 185
Homer Wright rosettes, 204, 206f, 209
Hordeolum, 240
HSV. See Herpes simplex virus
Human papillomavirus (HPV), 69–70, 241, 241f
Hyaline deposits, 110, 111–112f
Hyalinization, of ciliary body, 222, 223f
Hyalocytes, 150
Hyaloid artery, 150, 151f
Hyaloid canal, 149, 150f
Hyaloideocapsular ligament, 149, 150f
Hyaluronic acid (hyaluronan), 264
Hydatid cyst, 269
Hydrops, in keratoconus, 105f, 106
Hypercalcemia, 100
Hyperglycemia, 188
Hyperkeratosis, 238, 240, 246, 248
Hyperlipoproteinemia, 243
Hypermelanosis, 78
Hyperplasia
  of ciliary body, 210, 331, 332
  of conjunctiva, 85–86, 86f
  of eyelid, 253, 253f
  lymphoid, 85–86, 86f, 272–274, 274f, 383–386
  of retinal pigment epithelium, 48, 170–171, 310f, 332, 333f
  of uveal tract, 235
Hyphema, 104, 125, 125f, 221, 348
Hypoplasia, of fovea, 217
Hypopyon, 95, 122f
Hypotony, 49, 52

ICE (iridocorneal endothelial) syndrome, 120–121, 123f, 308t
ICK (infectious crystalline keratopathy), 96–97, 97f
Idiopathic orbital inflammatory syndrome, 263–264, 263–264f
IgG4-RD. See Immunoglobulin G4–related disease
IHC. See Immunohistochemistry
IIRC (International Intraocular Retinoblastoma Classification), 357–358, 359t
IK. See Interstitial keratitis
ILM. See Internal limiting membrane
Immunocompromised patients
  bacterial infections and, 288, 289f
  fungal infections and, 173, 268–269
  infectious crystalline keratopathy and, 97
  keratoacanthoma and, 251
  ocular surface squamous neoplasia in, 70
  protozoal infection and, 173–174
  retinal viral infections, 171–173
Immunofluorescence assay, 60–61, 60f
Immunoglobulin G4–related disease (IgG4-RD), 264, 266, 267f
Immunohistochemistry (IHC), 29–32, 31f, 32t

Immunophenotyping, 33
Immunotherapy, 330
Index features, for differential diagnosis, 16–17
Indirect ophthalmoscopic examination, 315
Indocyanine green angiography, 315, 336f, 337–338
Infantile hemangiomas, 57, 234, 252, 252f, 275, 341
Infants, shaken baby syndrome and, 189–191, 190f
Infections. See also Bacterial infections; Fungal infections; Parasitic infections; Viral infections; specific infections
  of anterior chamber and angle, 120, 122f
  of Bowman layer, 93f, 94
  of choroid, 173, 173f
  of conjunctiva, 59, 59f, 62
  of cornea, 91–98
  exogenous vs endogenous, 218
  of lens, 141, 142f
  optic nerve neuritis, 288–289, 289f
  of orbit, 266–269, 268f
  of sclera, 131, 132f
  of uveal tract, 218–219, 218f
Infectious crystalline keratopathy (ICK), 96–97, 97f
Infectious endophthalmitis, 152
Inflamed juvenile conjunctival nevus, 76
Inflammation
  about, 6t, 8–12, 9–14f
  acute vs chronic, 8, 9f, 11–12
  of anterior chamber, 120, 122f, 143
  cell types associated with, 8, 9–14f, 11–12
  classification, 8
  of conjunctiva, 57–63. See also Conjunctivitis
  of cornea, 91–98. See also Keratitis
  of eyelids, 240–241, 241–242f, 266
  of lens, 141–143, 142f
  of optic nerve, 287–292. See also Optic neuritis
  overview, 6t, 8–12, 9–14f
  of retinoblastoma, 348
  of sclera, 131–134, 132–134f, 266
  of uveal tract, 218–221, 218–222f
Inner ischemic retinal atrophy, 178, 178f, 179, 185, 187
Inner nuclear layer (INL)
  blood supply, 167
  edema and, 180f
  retinal atrophy and, 178, 178f
  retinal hemorrhages and, 180, 181f
  retinal pigment epithelium atrophy and, 177
  topography of, 164f, 166f
  tumors of, 351
Inner plexiform layer (IPL), 164f, 166f, 167, 178f, 180
Intercellular bridges, 251
Interdigitation zone (IZ), 164, 166f
Internal limiting membrane (ILM)
  degenerations, 175, 176f
  glial scarring and, 48
  posterior vitreous detachment and, 154
  retinal hemorrhages and, 181f
  topography, 164f
Internal ulcer of von Hippel, 91, 92f
International Intraocular Retinoblastoma Classification (IIRC), 357–358, 359t
Interphotoreceptor retinoid-binding protein (IRBP), 203
Interstitial keratitis (IK), 94f, 95, 97–98, 98f, 99
Intradermal nevus, 258, 259f

Intraepithelial melanocytic proliferation, 76
Intraepithelial melanosis, 76–79, 77f
Intraepithelial nonproliferative melanocytic
    pigmentation, 76
Intraocular lymphoma, 39, 159–162, 160–162f, 235,
    380–383, 381–382f
Intraocular pressure, 48, 120
Intraocular silicone oil, 100
Intraretinal exudates, 180, 180f
Intraretinal microvascular abnormalities (IRMAs), 180f,
    182, 182f, 187
Intravitreal chemotherapy, 364
Invasive squamous cell carcinoma, 71–73f, 74
Iodine 125, 331–332, 363
IPL (inner plexiform layer), 164f, 166f, 167, 178f, 180
IRBP (interphotoreceptor retinoid-binding protein), 203
Iridocorneal endothelial (ICE) syndrome, 120–121,
    123f, 308t
Iridodialysis, 49, 50f, 126
Iridotomies, 47
Iris
    color, 214–215
    cysts, 308f, 308t
    degenerations, 120–121, 123f, 127, 222, 223f
    developmental anomalies, 91, 92f, 119, 121f, 168f,
        216–217, 217f
    hyphema and, 221
    metastases to, 373, 374f
    neoplasia
        fine-needle aspiration biopsy of, 39
        melanoma, 224–225, 225f, 304–305, 307–308f, 308t
        neurofibroma, 236
        nevus, 223–224, 224f, 304, 306f, 308f, 308t, 309
        vascular tumor, 341f
    neovascularization, 189f, 204, 205f, 222, 223f, 313
    topography, 118f, 138f, 213–215, 214f. See also Iris
        pigment epithelium
    trauma, 49, 50f, 51
Iris freckles, 304, 306f, 308t
Iris nevus syndrome, 120–121
Iris pigment epithelium
    degenerations, 222, 223f
    differential diagnosis, 308t
    lacy vacuolation, 188, 189f
    ocular trauma and, 51
    secondary glaucoma and, 122, 124f, 127f, 128
    topography, 213, 214f
Iris root, 118f, 119, 119f, 230f
Iris sphincter, 49
Iris strands, 91, 92f, 119, 121f
IRMAs (intraretinal microvascular abnormalities), 180f,
    182, 182f, 187
Iron deposits, 104, 104–105f, 106, 157
Iron foreign bodies, 145
Irritated seborrheic keratosis (inverted follicular
    keratosis), 246, 247f
Ischemia, of lens, 143–144
Ischemia, of retina, 177–188
    about, 177–178, 178f
    branch retinal artery occlusion, 185
    branch retinal vein occlusion, 186–187
    cellular responses to, 179, 179f
    central retinal artery occlusion, 183–185, 184f

central retinal vein occlusion, 185, 186f, 187
chronic, 181–182
diabetic choroidopathy, 187
diabetic intraocular changes, other, 188, 189f
diabetic retinopathy, 181f, 182f, 187
inner ischemic retinal atrophy, 178, 178f, 179, 185, 187
outer ischemic retinal atrophy, 178, 178f
vascular responses to, 179–182, 180–182f
IZ (interdigitation zone), 164, 166f

Junctional nevus, 76, 258, 258f
Juvenile ossifying fibroma, 282, 283f
Juvenile xanthogranuloma, 221, 222f, 308t

Keratin whorls (squamous eddies), 72f, 74, 246, 247f,
    251
Keratitis
    infectious
        bacterial, 92–93, 93f, 96–98, 97–98f
        corticosteroid use and, 95, 96–97, 97f
        fungal, 95, 96f, 97
        infectious crystalline keratopathy, 96–97, 97f
        interstitial keratitis (IK), 94f, 95, 97–98, 98f
        overview, 91
        protozoan, 95, 96f
        sequelae, 91
        viral, 93–95, 94f, 97–98
    noninfectious, 98, 101, 122f
Keratoacanthoma, 251–252, 251f
Keratoconjunctivitis sicca, 99
Keratoconus, 47, 49, 49f, 105–106, 105f
Keratocytes, 45, 46f
Keratoectasias, 104–106, 105f
Keratoepithelin, 107
Keratopathy, 27t, 94f, 95–97, 97f, 99–102, 100–103f, 112,
    114–115f
Ki-67 (proliferation marker), 66
Kissing nevus, 257, 257f
Klebsiella spp, 266
Koeppe nodules, 220
Krukenberg spindle, 127

Labrador keratopathy, 100–101, 101f
Lacrimal fossa, 270
Lacrimal gland
    cysts of, 245
    infections of, 269
    inflammation, 263, 266, 267f
    neoplasia, 17f, 270–272, 271–272f
    topography, 238, 261
Lacrimal sac, 269, 283
Lacy vacuolation, 188, 189f
Lamina cribrosa
    degenerations, 287, 288f
    optic atrophy and, 292
    topography, 129, 285, 286f
    vein occlusions and, 185
Lamina fusca, 129, 129f, 130, 130f, 215, 215f
Langerhans cells, 238
Langhans cells, 11, 14f
Large B-cell lymphoma, 17f, 274
Large cell (primary intraocular) lymphoma, 39,
    159–162, 160–162f, 235, 380–383, 381–382f

Laser photoablation, 362
Laser photocoagulation, 187, 363
Laser therapy, for retinoblastoma, 302
Lattice corneal dystrophy (LCD type 1), 27*t*, 109, 110*f*, 113*t*
Lattice degeneration, 110*f*, 112*f*, 155, 175, 176*f*
LCD type 1. *See* Lattice corneal dystrophy
Leaking vascular tumors, 341–344, 342*f*, 345*f*
Leiomyoma, 236, 280
Leiomyosarcoma, 280
Lens, 137–147
    degenerations, 14, 15*f*, 51, 127, 143–147, 143–147*f*.
        See also Cataracts
    developmental anomalies, 91, 92*f*, 140, 141*f*
    embryonic development, 137
    inflammation, 141–144, 142*f*
    ischemia and, 143–144
    neoplasia, 147
    shape abnormalities, 140, 150, 151*f*
    staining, 27*t*
    topography, 137–139, 138–139*f*
    trauma, 51, 141, 142*f*, 143–144
    wound repair, 47–48
Lens capsule
    degenerations, 143, 144–145, 144*f*
    developmental anomalies, 239
    staining, 27*t*
    topography, 137, 138–139*f*
    trauma, 51
Lens-induced granulomatous endophthalmitis, 141, 142*f*
Lenticonus, 140, 141*f*
Lentiglobus, 140
Lentigo maligna melanoma, 259–260, 260*f*
Leopard spots, 373
Leser-Trélat sign, 246
Leukemia, 386–388, 387*f*
Leukemic infiltration, 387–388, 387*f*
Leukocoria, 169*f*, 348, 348*f*, 354, 355*t*
Leukocyte common antigen, 32
Leukocytes, 33
Levator palpebrae superioris muscle, 238
Ligament of Weiger, 149, 150*f*
Lightbulb aneurysms, 355*f*
Limbal dermoid, 58*f*
Linear nevus sebaceous syndrome, 57
Lipid dropout spaces, 242*f*
Lipofuscin
    choroidal melanoma and, 313, 315, 317*f*
    choroidal nevus and, 308, 310*f*, 312*f*, 319
    macular dystrophies and, 198, 200–201*f*
    in retinal pigment epithelium, 167
Lipomas, 57, 58*f*, 282
Liposarcoma, 282
Lisch nodules, 308*f*, 308*t*
Liver metastases, 324
Loiasis, 269
Low-dose radiation. *See* Brachytherapy; External beam radiotherapy
Low-grade B-cell marginal zone mucosa-associated lymphoid tissue (MALT) lymphomas, 383
Lowe syndrome, 140
Lung cancer, 378, 378*f*
Lymphadenopathy, 62

Lymphangiomas, 274–275, 276*f*
Lymphocytes, 8, 9*f*, 11*f*, 32*t*
Lymphoid hyperplasia, 85–87, 86–87*f*, 273, 274*f*, 383–386
Lymphoid proliferation, 234, 235, 235*f*, 272–274, 274–275*f*
Lymphomas
    about, 380
    B-cell lymphomas, 86, 87*f*, 160, 235, 274, 275*f*
    classification, 85, 272–273
    of conjunctiva, 85–88, 86–87*f*
    defined, 85
    MALT lymphoma, 86, 87*f*, 274, 275*f*, 383
    non-Hodgkin lymphomas, 85, 273–274
    primary intraocular lymphoma, 39, 159–162, 160–162*f*, 235, 380–383, 381–382*f*
    primary uveal lymphoma, 383–386, 384*f*
    staining, 32*t*
Lynch syndrome, 254

Macrovessels, 340, 341*f*
Macula
    degenerations. *See* Age-related macular degeneration; Macular holes
    detachments, 287, 288*f*
    dystrophies, 196–198, 200–201*f*
    edema. *See* Macular edema
    topography, 164–166*f*, 165–167. *See also* Cystoid spaces
Macular corneal dystrophy (MCD), 27*t*, 110–111, 113*f*, 113*t*
Macular edema
    with central retinal vein occlusion, 185
    cystoid macular edema, 156, 166–167, 180, 180*f*, 183*f*, 338
    treatment, 182
Macular holes, 154, 156, 157*f*
Magnetic resonance imaging (MRI), 318, 351, 369, 376
Magnocellular nevus. *See* Melanocytomas
MALT. *See* Mucosa-associated lymphoid tissue
Mandible, 340
Mantle cell lymphoma, 274
Map-dot-fingerprint dystrophy, 107, 108*f*
Massive choroidal invasion, 206–207, 208*f*
Massively parallel sequencing, 36*t*
Masson trichrome stain, 27*t*
Mast cells (basophils), 8, 10*f*
MCC (Merkel cell carcinoma), 256, 257*f*
MCD. *See* Macular corneal dystrophy
Mean diameter (prognostic factor), 231–232
Measles virus, 171
Medulloepithelioma, 209–210, 209*f*, 356–357, 356*f*
Meibomian gland dysfunction (MGD), 99
Meibomian glands, 62*f*, 237*f*, 238–241, 252, 254
Melan A, 32, 32*t*
Melanin, 104, 127*f*, 214–215, 227
Melanocytes, 47, 238
Melanocytic tumors, 303–304. *See also* Melanocytomas; Melanomas; Nevus
Melanocytomas
    of choroid, 226, 309, 320
    of ciliary body, 309
    differential diagnosis, 320

of iris, 308*t*, 309
of optic nerve head, 294–295, 295*f*, 320
of uveal tract, 226
Melanoma-associated spongiform scleropathy, 134–135
Melanoma cell nucleoli, 231–232
Melanomalytic glaucoma, 126, 127*f*, 128, 229
Melanomas. *See also specific melanomas*
    about, 303–304
    of choroid and ciliary body, 226–232, 312–331. *See also* Posterior uveal melanoma
    congenital nevus and, 257
    of conjunctiva, 79, 82*t*, 84–85, 84–85*f*
    cutaneous, 304
    differential diagnosis, 323
    of eyelids, 257, 259–260, 260*f*
    of iris, 224–225, 225*f*, 304–305, 307–308*f*, 308*t*
    melanocytomas and, 226, 308*t*
    subtypes, 259–260, 260*f*
    of uveal tract, 226–229, 301
Melanosis, 76
Melanosomes, 167
Melphalan, 362, 364
Meningiomas, 32*t*, 282, 296–297, 297*f*
Meretoja syndrome, 243
Merkel cell carcinoma (MCC), 256, 257*f*
Merkel cell polyomavirus, 256
Mesectodermal leiomyoma, 236
Metaherpetic (trophic) ulcer, 93–95
Metastatic carcinomas
    about, 232–233, 233*f*, 371
    to choroid, 337, 373–377, 375–377*f*
    to ciliary body, 373
    clinical characteristics, 372–377
    diagnostic factors, 377–379
    differential diagnosis, 308*f*, 308*t*
    direct intraocular extension and, 380
    immunohistochemistry stains for, 32*t*
    to iris, 373, 374*f*
    mechanism of, 372, 372*f*
    to optic nerve, 373–377
    to orbit, 283
    primary tumor sites, 372, 373*t*
    prognosis and prognostic factors, 379
    to retina, 373–377, 378*f*
    sebaceous carcinoma, 256
    treatment, 379–380
Methotrexate, 383
MGD (meibomian gland dysfunction), 99
Microaneurysms, 182, 182*f*, 185
Microarrays
    clinical use of, 38–39
    overview, 36–38, 38*f*
    types of, 36*t*
Microcornea, 140
Microcysts, 101
Microglial cells, 179, 285, 286–287*f*, 286*t*
Microphthalmia, 131, 140, 150, 355
Middle limiting membrane (MLM), 164
Mitomycin C, 47
Mittendorf dot, 151
Mixed-cell type melanoma, 230
MLM. *See* Middle limiting membrane

MLPA (multiplex ligation-dependent probe amplification), 35*t*
MMP. *See* Mucous membrane pemphigoid
Modified Callender classification system, 224, 230
Mohs micrographic surgery, 41, 41*f*
Molecular pathology, 30*t*, 33–39, 35–36*t*
Molluscum contagiosum, 240, 242*f*
Monoclonal immunoglobulin, 67
Monocytes, 8, 11, 13*f*
Monosomy 3, 232, 330
Morgagnian cataract, 145, 146*f*
Morpheaform basal cell carcinoma, 249, 250*f*
MRI (magnetic resonance imaging), 318, 351, 369, 376
Mucoepidermoid carcinoma, 74
Mucor orbititis, 268, 268*f*
Mucormycosis, 266–268, 288–289
Mucosa-associated lymphoid tissue (MALT), 55, 85, 86, 87*f*, 274, 275*f*, 383
Mucous membrane pemphigoid (MMP) (ocular cicatricial pemphigoid), 60–61, 60*f*
Muir-Torre syndrome, 253–254, 253*f*
"Mulberry" lesion, 356, 356*f*
Müller cells, 48, 156, 157*f*, 165, 176
Müller muscle, 238
Multimodal imaging, 315, 316–317*f*, 318
Multinucleated giant cells, 11, 14*f*, 220, 221*f*, 259
Multiple myeloma, 244*f*
Multiple sclerosis, 289
Multiplex ligation-dependent probe amplification (MLPA), 35*t*
Muscle differentiation tumors, 278–280, 279*f*
Mutton-fat keratic precipitates, 219
MYCN oncogene, 203, 205, 207*f*, 366
Mycobacteria, 27*t*
Mycobacterium leprae, 27*t*, 98
Mycobacterium tuberculosis, 27*t*, 98, 288
Mycosis. *See* Fungal infections
Myelinated nerve fibers, 168
Myoglobin, 32, 32*t*
Myoid zone (MZ), 164, 166*f*
Myopia, 168
Myositis, 263, 263*f*
MZ. *See* Myoid zone

Nanophthalmos, 130–131
National Comprehensive Cancer Network (NCCN) clinical practice guidelines, 326
Necrobiosis, 131
Necrotizing granulomas, 289
Necrotizing orbitis, 266
Necrotizing retinitis, 171, 172–173*f*, 173, 174
Necrotizing scleritis, 132, 132–133*f*
Necrotizing ulcerative keratitis, 93*f*
Neoplasia, 6*t*, 16, 16*t*, 17*f*. *See also specific tumors and structures affected*
Neovascular glaucoma, 222, 329, 355, 357, 358, 361
Neovascularization
    age-related macular degeneration (AMD) and, 193–194, 196*f*, 320
    choroidal neovascularization (CNV). *See* Choroidal neovascularization
    of iris, 189*f*, 204, 205*f*, 222, 223*f*, 313
    of retina, 182, 183*f*, 185, 187

Nerve fiber layer (NFL)
  central retinal artery occlusion (CRAO) and, 184*f*
  degenerations, 175, 175*f*, 179, 179*f*
  developmental anomalies, 168
  retinal hemorrhages and, 180, 181*f*
  topography, 164–165, 164*f*, 166*f*, 167
Neurilemoma (schwannoma), 32*t*, 236, 236*f*, 281, 281*f*
Neuroendocrine carcinoma, 256, 257*f*
Neuroepithelial tumor, 209–210, 209*f*
Neurofibromas
  of iris, 236
  of orbit, 280–281, 280*f*
  of uveal tract, 236, 236*f*
Neurosensory retina, 48, 163–167, 164–166*f*
Neutrophils, 8, 9*f*, 44*f*, 45, 46*f*
Nevus (nevi)
  about, 227, 303
  cell types associated with, 258–259
  of choroid, 225–226, 226*f*, 305, 308–309, 310*f*, 312*f*, 313, 319–320
  of ciliary body, 305, 308–309
  congenital, 257, 257*f*
  of conjunctiva, 57, 74–76, 75–76*f*, 82*t*
  defined, 227
  differential diagnosis, 71
  of eyelids, 257–259, 257–259*f*
  of iris, 223–224, 224*f*, 304, 306*f*, 308*f*, 308*t*, 309
  iris nevus syndrome, 120–121, 123*f*
  magnocellular nevus. *See* Melanocytomas
  melanoma risk factor and, 313
  melanomas and, 257, 259
  of optic nerve head, 295, 295*f*
Next-generation sequencing, 36*t*
NFL. *See* Nerve fiber layer
NHLs. *See* Non-Hodgkin lymphomas
Nodular basal cell carcinoma, 249, 249*f*
Nodular drusen, 192*f*, 192*t*
Nodular episcleritis, 131
Nodular melanoma, 260, 260*f*
Nodular scleritis, 132, 132–133*f*
Non-Hodgkin diffuse large B-cell lymphoma (DLBCL), 380–382, 382*f*
Non-Hodgkin lymphomas (NHLs), 85, 273–274
Non-leaking vascular tumors, 339–340, 340–341*f*
Non-nevoid intraepithelial melanocytic proliferations, 78
Non-nevoid pigmented lesions of the conjunctiva, 80–81*f*, 82–83*t*
Noncaseating granulomas, 11, 13*f*, 62–63, 63*f*, 220, 221*f*, 291, 291*f*
Noninfectious inflammation
  chalazion, 241, 242*f*
  of conjunctiva, 60–61, 60*f*
  of cornea, 98, 101, 122*f*
  of eyelid, 241, 242*f*, 266
  lacrimal gland, 263, 266, 267*f*
  of lens, 141–143, 142*f*
  of optic nerve, 289–291, 290–291*f*
  of orbit, 263–265*f*, 263–266, 267*f*
  of orbital nerve, 266
  of retina, 174
  of sclera, 132–134, 132–134*f*
  of uveal tract, 152, 153*f*, 219–221, 219–222*f*

Nonmalignant melanocytic lesions, 82*t*
Nonnecrotizing granulomas, 220–221, 221*f*
Nonnecrotizing scleritis, 132–134
Nonneovascular (dry) age-related macular degeneration, 193, 195*f*
Nonspecific orbital inflammation (NSOI), 263–264, 263–264*f*
NSAIDs (nonsteroidal anti-inflammatory drugs), 98
NSOI. *See* Nonspecific orbital inflammation
Nuclear cataracts, 145–147, 147*f*
Nucleus, of lens, 138*f*, 139
Nystagmus, 168

OAL. *See* Ocular adnexal lymphoma
OCRL gene, 140
OCT. *See* Optical coherence tomography
OCTA (optical coherence tomography angiography), 178
Ocular adnexa, 48–49
Ocular adnexal lymphoma (OAL), 273
Ocular albinism, 167–168
Ocular cicatricial pemphigoid, 60–61, 60*f*
Ocular melanocytosis, 76, 76*f*, 82*t*
Ocular surface squamous neoplasia (OSSN), 66, 70–74, 71–73*f*, 116
Ocular toxocariasis, 356
Ocular toxoplasmosis, 173–174, 174*f*
Ocular trauma. *See* Degenerations; Foreign bodies; Trauma
Oculocerebrorenal syndrome, 140
Oculocutaneous albinism, 167–168
Oculodermal melanocytosis, 76, 82*t*
"Oil droplet," 140
Oil red O stain, 27, 27*t*
Oligodendrocytes, 285, 286*f*, 286*t*, 287*f*
Onchocerca volvulus, 98
Oncocytoma, 88, 88*f*
ONE Network online resource, 302
ONH. *See* Optic nerve head
ONL. *See* Outer nuclear layer
Open-angle glaucoma, 125–126, 126*f*, 127
Ophthalmic pathology
  about, 5
  organizational paradigm for, 6–7, 6*t*. *See also specific disease processes*
  specimen handling and processing, 5–6. *See also* Specimen handling and processing
  testing modalities, 6. *See also* Special testing and procedures
  wound repair, 6. *See also* Wound repair
Ophthalmoplegia, 269
OPL. *See* Outer plexiform layer
Optic atrophy, 291–292, 292–293*f*, 294
Optic disc, 285, 286*f*. *See also* Optic nerve head
Optic nerve, 285–297
  blood supply, 286
  degenerations, 291–294, 292–294*f*
  developmental anomalies, 150–151, 151–152*f*, 287, 287*f*
  hemorrhage, 190
  inflammation, 287–291. *See also* Optic neuritis
  leukemic infiltration, 387–388, 387*f*
  metastases to, 373–377

neoplasia
glioma, 295–296, 296f
hemangioblastomas, 170
immunohistochemistry stains for, 32t
intraocular lymphoma and, 161
medulloepithelioma, 357
melanocytoma, 294–295, 295f, 320
meningioma, 296–297, 297f
retinoblastoma invasion, 206, 208f
thyroid eye disease and, 265
topography, 285–286, 286f, 286t
wound repair, 49
Optic nerve head (ONH)
blood supply, 286
degenerations, 292–294, 294f
deposits, 292–294, 294f
edema, 291, 292f
neoplasia
glioma, 295–296, 296f
hamartomas, 356, 356f
melanocytoma, 294–295, 295f
retinoblastoma invasion of, 351–352, 354
vascular tumors, 342f, 343, 344
topography, 285–286
Optic neuritis
infectious, 288–289, 289f
noninfectious, 289–291, 290–291f
radiation neuropathy, 363, 364
Optic pits, 287, 288f
Optical coherence tomography angiography (OCTA), 178
Optical coherence tomography (OCT)
of astrocytomas, 356
of choroidal hemangioma, 336f, 337
of iris melanoma, 305
of macular holes, 156, 157f
of neurosensory retina, 164, 166f
for retinoblastoma, 350–351
types of, 178, 315, 316f
Ora serrata, 52, 52f, 167
Orbicularis oculi muscle, 48, 237–238, 237f
Orbit, 261–283
deposits, 269
developmental anomalies, 7, 8t, 262, 262f
drainage system. See Lacrimal gland
inflammation
infectious, 266–269, 268f
noninfectious, 263–265f, 263–266, 267f
neoplasia, 269–270, 272–283, 340. See also specific
neoplasm
topography, 261
wound repair, 48–49
Orbital lymphatic malformations, 274–275, 276f
Orbital nerve, 266
Orbital pseudotumor, 263–264, 263–264f
OSSN. See Ocular surface squamous neoplasia
Osteomas
of choroid, 234–235, 235f, 321–323, 322f, 337
of orbit, 282, 283f
Osteosarcoma (osteogenic sarcoma), 368
Outer ischemic retinal atrophy, 178, 178f
Outer nuclear layer (ONL), 164f, 167, 178f, 351
Outer plexiform layer (OPL), 164–165f, 167, 174, 175f,
178, 180, 180–181f, 351

"Owl's eye" inclusions, 172f
Oxyphilic adenoma, 88, 88f

p53 gene, 66, 70, 272–273
p63 gene, 66
Pagetoid spread, 256, 260
Paired box protein 6, 91
Palpebral conjunctiva, 55, 56f, 237, 237f, 238
PAM (primary acquired melanosis), 77–79, 77f, 80–81f,
82–83t, 84, 84f
Pannus
of conjunctiva, 65
of cornea, 15, 99, 101, 102–103f, 107–108, 109f, 217
differential diagnosis, 71
Panuveitis, 174, 219
Papillary conjunctivitis, 61, 61–62f
Papilledema, 292
Papillitis, 294
Papillomas, 240
Papillomatosis, 246
Paraffin tissue sections, 19, 24, 27
Parakeratosis, 238, 240, 248, 248f
Paranasal sinus, 240
Parasitic infections, 240, 241, 269, 356
Parinaud oculoglandular syndrome, 62
Pars plana, 52, 52f, 215, 215f
Pars plicata, 215, 215f
PAS (peripheral anterior synechiae), 121, 122–123f,
189f, 216–217, 222
PAS stain, 26, 27t
Pattern dystrophies, 197–198, 201f
Paving-stone degeneration, 176–177, 177f
PAX3-FOXO1 protein, 279
PAX6 gene, 91
PCG. See Primary congenital glaucoma
PCR. See Polymerase chain reaction techniques
PDT (photodynamic therapy), 329, 338–339, 343
Pediatric patients. See Children
Pedunculated papillomas, 69, 70f
PEHCR (peripheral exudative hemorrhagic
chorioretinopathy), 321, 322f
Pellucid marginal corneal degeneration (PMCD), 106
Penetrating keratoplasty (PK) graft, 96, 102, 103f, 106
Perifoveal vitreous detachment, 156
Periodic acid–Schiff (PAS) stain, 26, 27t
Peripapillary choroidal nevus, 312f
Peripapillary retina, 150, 157
Peripheral anterior synechiae (PAS), 121, 122–123f,
189f, 216–217, 222
Peripheral corneal vascularization, 99
Peripheral cystoid degeneration, 174–175
Peripheral exudative hemorrhagic chorioretinopathy
(PEHCR), 321, 322f
Peripheral nerve sheath tumors, 280–281, 280f
Periphlebitis, 220
Perls Prussian blue stain, 27t
Permanent sections, 19, 27, 40
Persistent fetal vasculature (PFV), 131, 140, 150, 152f,
354–355
Peters anomaly, 91, 92f
PFV. See Persistent fetal vasculature
Phacoantigenic uveitis, 141, 142f
Phacolytic glaucoma, 123, 124f, 143

Phacolytic uveitis, 143
Phakomatous choristoma, 239, 239f
Phlyctenular keratitis, 99
Photocoagulation, 343
Photodynamic therapy (PDT), 329, 338–339, 343
Photoreceptors
  atrophy of, 193
  dystrophies, 198, 202, 202f
Phthisis bulbi, 14, 15, 15f, 52
Pial sheath, 286, 287f
Pial vessels, 286
Pigment dispersion associations, 126–128, 127f
Pigment epithelial cyst, 308f, 308t
Pigmentary glaucoma, 305
Pilosebaceous units, 238, 239
Pinealoblastoma, 351–352, 353f, 367–368
Pinealoblastoma (primitive neuroectodermal tumor),
  351–352, 353f
Pinguecula, 64–66, 66f, 71, 72f
PIOL. See Primary intraocular lymphoma
PITX2 gene, 91
PK (penetrating keratoplasty) graft, 96, 102, 103f, 106
Planar xanthoma, 243, 243f
Plaque radiotherapy. See Brachytherapy
Plaques. See also Glial scarring
  anterior subcapsular fibrous plaques, 143–144, 144f
  calcific plaques, 134, 135f, 185
  fibrovascular plaques, 150, 151f
  Hollenhorst plaques, 185
  in vitreous, 150, 151f
Plasma cell myeloma, 67
Plasma cells, 8, 9f, 11, 12f
Plasmacytoma, 67
Platelet-fibrin emboli, 185
Pleomorphic adenoma (benign mixed tumor), 270, 271f
Pleomorphic rhabdomyosarcoma, 278
Plexiform neurofibromas, 280, 280f
Plica semilunaris, 55
Plump fusiform dendritic nevus cells, 226
Plump polyhedral nevus cells, 225
PMCD (pellucid marginal corneal degeneration), 106
PMNs (polymorphonuclear leukocytes), 8, 9f
PNET. See Primitive neuroectodermal tumor
Polymerase chain reaction (PCR) techniques
  clinical use of, 38–39
  overview, 34–36, 37f
  types of, 35t, 38
Polymorphonuclear leukocytes (PMNs), 8, 9f
Polypoidal choroidal vasculopathy, 195, 198–199f
PO section. See Pupil–optic nerve (PO) section
Posterior ciliary arteries, 167, 286, 290
Posterior embryotoxon, 119–120, 120f
Posterior lenticonus, 140, 141f
Posterior lentiglobus, 140
Posterior polymorphous corneal dystrophy (PPCD),
  114–115, 115f
Posterior subcapsular cataract, 143, 143–144f
Posterior synechiae, 47–48
Posterior uveal melanoma, 312–331
  about, 226, 312–313
  choroid melanoma
    about, 226
    classification, 324, 325t

    clinical characteristics, 226–229, 228f, 311f, 313
    diagnostic evaluation, 315, 317–318f
    differential diagnosis, 309, 332, 337
    prognosis and prognostic factors, 232
    risk factors, 309
    treatment, 301, 328–330, 328f
  ciliary body melanoma
    classification, 324, 325t
    clinical characteristics, 228, 313, 314f
    diagnostic evaluation, 230f, 309, 318
    differential diagnosis, 304, 332
    risk factors, 309
    treatment, 328
  classification, 323–324, 324–325t
  clinical characteristics, 226–229, 227–229f, 311–312f,
    313, 314f
  Collaborative Ocular Melanoma Study (COMS) on,
    301, 323, 324, 327, 331–332
  diagnostic evaluation, 312f, 314–315, 314f, 316–318f,
    318
  differential diagnosis, 224–225, 304, 309, 318–323,
    321–322f, 323t, 332, 337
  diffuse ciliary body melanomas, 228, 228f, 232, 313,
    314f
  metastatic evaluation, 231–232, 231f, 324–326, 325t
  prognosis and prognostic factors, 230–232, 325t,
    330–331
  risk factors, 309, 312–313, 319
  treatment, 327–330
    alternative treatments, 328f, 329–330
    brachytherapy with radioactive plaque, 301, 318f,
      327–328, 328f, 329
    charged-particle radiation, 328–329
    chemotherapy, 330
    enucleation, 301, 327
    exenteration, 330
    external beam radiotherapy, 301, 329
    immunotherapy, 330
    observation in management of, 327
    photodynamic therapy, 329
    radiation-associated complications, 329
    surgical excision, 328f, 329–330
    transpupillary thermotherapy (TTT), 329
Posterior vitreous detachment (PVD), 153–156,
  154–155f, 157
Postherpetic neurotrophic keratopathy, 94f, 95
Postnatal vascular (leaking) tumors, 341–344, 342f, 345f
Poxvirus, 240
PPCD. See Posterior polymorphous corneal dystrophy
PRAME gene, 232
PRB (protein), 365
Pre-Descemet stroma (Dua layer), 89, 90f
Prenatal vascular (non-leaking) tumors, 339–340,
  340–341f
Prepapillary vascular loops, 151
Preretinal hemorrhage, 181f
Preretinal membrane, 150, 155–156, 155f, 181f, 210–211
Presbyopia, 222
Preseptal cellulitis, 240, 241f
Presumed acquired retinal hemangiomas, 344, 345f
Primary acquired melanosis (PAM), 77–79, 77f, 80–81f,
  82–83t, 84, 84f
Primary aphakia, 140

Primary choroidal lymphomas, 235
Primary congenital glaucoma (PCG), 91, 119, 119*f*
Primary conjunctival lymphoma, 67
Primary intraocular lymphoma (PIOL), 39, 159–162, 160–162*f*, 235, 380–383, 381–382*f*
Primary uveal lymphoma, 383–386, 384*f*
Primary vitreoretinal lymphoma (PVRL), 39, 159–162, 160–162*f*, 235, 380–383, 381–382*f*
Primary vitreous, 149, 150
Primitive neuroectodermal tumor (PNET), 351–352, 353*f*, 367–368
Progesterone receptors, 236
Proliferative vitreoretinopathy (PVR), 52, 53*f*, 155–156, 155*f*
Propionibacterium acnes, 141, 142*f*
Proptosis (exophthalmos)
    fluctuating, 274–275
    of globe, 261
    leukemia and, 388
    metastases causing, 379
    thyroid disease and, 264, 265*f*
    tumors causing, 271*f*, 273, 274–275, 278, 279*f*, 280, 354, 354*f*
Proteus spp, 266
Proton beam therapy, 305
Protozoal infections, 173–174, 218, 218*f*
PRPH2 (peripherin 2) gene, 197
Psammoma bodies, 297, 297*f*
Pseudo–Roth spots, 386, 387*f*
Pseudoadenomatous hyperplasia, 210, 210*f*, 331
Pseudoelastosis (elastotic degeneration), 65–66, 67*f*, 71, 72*f*, 248, 248*f*
Pseudoexfoliation syndrome (exfoliation syndrome), 122–123, 124*f*, 147
Pseudoglands of Henle, 56*f*
Pseudohorn cysts, 246, 246*f*
Pseudohypopyon, 350, 351*f*
Pseudomonas aeruginosa, 92
Pseudopapilledema, 292
Pseudophakic bullous keratopathy, 101–102, 102–103*f*, 112, 114–115*f*
Pseudopolycoria, 119, 121*f*
Pseudorosettes, 204, 204*f*
Pterygium, 65–66, 67*f*, 71, 99
Ptosis, 269
Pulmonary carcinoma, 308*f*
Pulmonary infections, 289
Pulmonary metastases, 233*f*, 372, 373*t*
Punctum, 63
Pupil, 24, 25*f*, 213–214, 308*f*
Pupil–optic nerve (PO) section, 24, 25*f*
PVD (posterior vitreous detachment), 153–156, 154–155*f*, 157
PVR (proliferative vitreoretinopathy), 52, 53*f*, 155–156, 155*f*
PVRL. *See* Primary vitreoretinal lymphoma
Pyogenic granuloma, 63, 65*f*

Racemose hemangioma, 340–341, 341*f*
Racial primary (complexion-associated) melanosis, 76, 77*f*, 78, 80–81*f*, 82*t*
Radial keratoneuritis, 95
Radial perivascular lattice degeneration, 175, 176*f*

Radiation retinopathy, 178, 363, 364
Radiation therapy, 301
Radiotherapy. *See* External beam radiotherapy
"Railroad track"–like lesions, of Descemet membrane, 114, 115*f*
RB1 gene, 203, 301, 349*f*, 364, 365–367, 369
RBCD. *See* Reis-Bücklers corneal dystrophy
RCH. *See* Retinal capillary hemangioblastoma
Reactive lymphoid hyperplasia (RLH), 32*t*, 273, 274*f*
Real-time (quantitative) polymerase chain reaction (RT-PCR), 35*t*, 38
Recurrent corneal dystrophy, 109*f*
Recurrent pterygium, 65
Red reflex, 140
Reese-Ellsworth classification system, 357
Reis-Bücklers corneal dystrophy (RBCD), 107, 108, 109*f*, 113*t*
Remodeling phase, of wound repair, 43–44
Repair, defined, 43–44. *See also* Wound repair
Reticular degenerative retinoschisis, 175
Reticular dystrophy, 197–198
Reticular peripheral cystoid degeneration (RPCD), 175, 175*f*
Reticular pseudodrusen (RPD), 192–193, 192*t*, 194*f*
Retina
    blood supply, 167, 181–183. *See also* Ischemia, of retina
    degenerations, 174–202. *See also* Retinal degenerations
    deposits, 158
    detachment
        choroidal melanoma and, 228–229, 228*f*, 310*f*, 313, 329
        choroidal nevus and, 308
        Coats disease and, 355
        retinal degenerations and, 175
        retinal developmental anomalies and, 169, 169*f*
        retinoblastoma and, 350, 351*f*
        sequelae, 176, 177*f*
        Sturge-Weber syndrome and, 337
        vitreous detachments and, 154
    developmental anomalies, 167–171, 168–171*f*
    dystrophies, 198, 202, 202*f*
    hemorrhage
        abusive head trauma and, 190, 190*f*
        ischemia and, 180–181, 185, 186*f*
        subretinal, 52, 311*f*, 313, 318, 322*f*
        viral infections and, 172*f*
    inflammation
        infectious etiologies, 171–174, 172–174*f*
        noninfectious etiologies, 174
    metastases to, 373–377
    neoplasia. *See also specific neoplasms*
        hamartomas, 210–211, 211*f*, 333–334, 333*f*, 356, 356*f*
        invasion of, 211
        lymphomas, 161, 162*f*
        medulloepitheliomas, 209–210, 209*f*, 356–357
        retinoblastomas, 202–207, 347–370. *See also* Retinoblastoma
        vascular tumors, 170, 170*f*, 339–344, 340–342*f*, 345*f*
    neovascularization, 182, 183*f*, 185, 187
    ocular degeneration and, 14
    posterior uveal melanoma association with, 313

topography
  neurosensory retina, 163–167, 164–166f
  retinal pigment epithelium (RPE), 164, 167
trauma, 52, 52–53f, 54
vitreous detachment and, 154, 154f
wound repair, 48
Retinal angiomatous proliferation, 193
Retinal arteriovenous malformation, 340–341, 341f
Retinal artery and vein occlusions, 178, 178f, 181–182, 184f, 185–187, 186f
Retinal astrocytoma, 356, 356f
Retinal capillary hemangioblastoma (RCH), 170, 170f, 341–344, 342f
Retinal cavernous hemangioma, 339–340, 340f
Retinal degenerations, 174–202
  abusive head trauma, 189–191, 190f
  age-related macular degeneration (AMD), 191–195, 191–197f, 192t. See also Age-related macular degeneration
  detachment sequelae, 176, 177f
  ischemia, 177–188. See also Ischemia, of retina
  lattice degeneration, 175, 176f
  paving-stone degeneration, 176–177, 177f
  peripheral cystoid degeneration, 174–175
  polypoidal choroidal vasculopathy, 195, 201f
  retinoschisis, 175
  typical peripheral cystoid degeneration (TPCD), 175f
Retinal dialysis, 52, 52f
Retinal flecks, 140, 200f
Retinal pigment epithelium (RPE)
  amyloid deposits and, 158
  blood supply, 167, 216, 216f
  choroidal nevus and changes to, 226, 305, 308–309, 310f
  degenerations, 191–193, 191t, 192–194f
  developmental anomalies, 168f, 170–171, 171f
  inflammation, 172f
  intraocular lymphoma and, 160–161, 160f, 162f
  leopard spots and, 373
  macular dystrophies, 196–197, 200–201f
  neoplasia, 170, 171, 210–211, 211f, 331–334, 333f
  ocular degeneration and, 14, 15
  retinal degenerations and, 176–177
  retinal detachment sequelae and, 176
  retinal ischemia and, 178f
  topography, 164, 164–166f, 167, 216f
  trauma, 52, 53f
  wound repair, 48
Retinal vasoproliferative tumor (VPT), 344, 345f
Retinitis pigmentosa (RP), 151, 202, 202f
Retinoblastoma, 347–370
  about, 347–348
  associated conditions, 367–368
  chorioretinopathy, 321, 322f
  classification, 350, 357–358, 359t
  diagnostic evaluation, 348–357
    ancillary imaging, 350–354, 352–354f
    clinical examination, 348–350, 348–351f, 349t
    differential diagnosis, 354–357, 355t
    examination under anesthesia (EUA), 349, 350–351
  differential diagnosis, 16
  extraocular extension of, 352–354, 354f, 368
  genetic counseling and, 365–367
  histological features, 203–205, 204–207f

metastases of, 354, 368–369, 369t
neoplasia, 207, 209f
overview, 202–203, 301–302
pathogenesis, 203
presenting signs and symptoms, 349–350, 349–350f
prognosis and prognostic factors, 368–369, 369t
progression, 206–207, 208f
retinocytoma, 207, 209f
spontaneous regression of, 365
treatment, 358–364
  about, 358–360
  chemotherapy, 302, 361–362f, 361–363, 364
  enucleation, 360–361
  local consolidation therapy, 363–364
Retinoblastoma (RB1) gene, 203, 301, 349f, 364, 365–367, 369
Retinocytoma, 207, 209f, 367
Retinopathy
  chorioretinopathy, 321, 322f
  diabetes mellitus and, 181f, 182f, 187
  peripheral exudative hemorrhagic chorioretinopathy, 321, 322f
  of prematurity, 178
  proliferative vitreoretinopathy, 52, 53f, 155–156, 155f
  radiation-induced, 178, 363, 364
Retinoschisis, 175, 175f
Retrobulbar optic nerve, 129, 354
Retrocorneal membrane, 103f
Retrolaminar nerve, 286f
Reverse transcriptase-polymerase chain reaction (RT-PCR), 35t
Rhabdomyosarcoma, 17f, 32t, 183, 278–280, 279f
Rhegmatogenous retinal detachment (RRD), 155–156, 155f, 175
Rheumatoid arthritis, 98, 131, 133f
Rhinocerebral mucormycosis, 266–268
Rhizopus spp, 268
Rhodopsin (RHO) gene, 202
Ring infiltrate, 95, 96f
Ring melanoma (diffuse ciliary body melanomas), 228, 228f, 232, 313, 314f
Riolan muscle, 237–238
Rods, 164f, 202
Rosenthal fibers, 296, 296f
Roth spots, 386
RP. See Retinitis pigmentosa
RPCD (reticular peripheral cystoid degeneration), 175, 175f
RPD (reticular pseudodrusen), 192–193, 192t, 194f
RPE. See Retinal pigment epithelium
RRD (rhegmatogenous retinal detachment), 155–156, 155f, 175
Rubella, 140, 171
Rubeosis iridis, 222, 223f, 350
Russell bodies, 11, 12f
Ruthenium 106, 328, 363

S-100 protein, 32, 281
Salzmann nodular degeneration, 98–99, 99f
Sarcoidosis
  conjunctivitis and, 62–63, 63f
  optic nerve and, 289
  optic nerve neuritis and, 291, 291f
  of uveal tract, 220–221, 221f

Scarring
    of choroid, 174, 174*f*
    of conjunctiva, 47
    of cornea, 45, 46*f*, 90*f*, 94*f*
    of globe, 54
    laser photocoagulation and, 187, 188*f*
    of macula, 156
    of ocular adnexa, 48
    of optic nerve, 288
    of orbit, 48
    of retina, 48, 171, 173, 174, 174*f*, 179, 187
    of sclera, 47
    of uveal tract, 47
SCC. *See* Squamous cell carcinoma
Schaumann bodies, 220–221
Schlemm canal, 117
Schnabel cavernous optic atrophy, 292, 293*f*
Schwalbe line, 117, 118*f*, 119–120, 121*f*
Schwann cells, 280–281
Schwannoma (neurilemoma), 32*t*, 236, 236*f*, 281, 281*f*
Sclera, 129–135
    degenerations, 15, 15*f*, 134–135, 134–135*f*, 287, 288*f*
    developmental anomalies, 130–131
    embryonic development, 129
    inflammation, 131–134, 132–134*f*, 266
    neoplasia, 135, 228–229, 229*f*
    topography, 129–130*f*, 129–135, 216*f*, 285, 286*f*
    wound repair, 47
Scleral spur, 49–50, 50–51*f*, 117, 118*f*, 119, 119*f*, 130
Scleral staphyloma, 132, 134, 134–135*f*
Scleritis, 131–134, 132–134*f*, 266
Sclerocornea, 91, 92*f*
Scleromalacia perforans, 132
Sclerosing basal cell carcinoma, 249, 250*f*
Sclerosing orbititis, 264
Scotoma, 168
Sebaceous glands (of Zeis)
    inflammation, 240, 241, 242*f*
    neoplasia
        adenoma, 253–254, 253*f*
        carcinoma, 27*t*, 116, 254–255*f*, 254–256
        carcinoma in situ, 255*f*, 256
        hyperplasia, 253, 253*f*
    specialization of, 237, 238, 239
    topography of, 238
Seborrheic keratosis, 245–246, 246–247*f*
Sebum, 262, 262*f*
Secondary acquired melanosis, 78, 82*t*
Secondary aphakia, 140
Secondary glaucoma. *See under* Glaucoma
Secondary localized amyloidosis, 67
Secondary melanosis, 76
Secondary orbital meningiomas, 296
Secondary tumors
    leukemia, 386–388, 387*f*
    lymphoid tumors, 380–386. *See also* Lymphomas
    metastatic carcinoma, 371–380. *See also* Metastatic
        carcinomas
    overview, 301–302
    staging of, 302
Secondary vitreous, 149–150
Sectoral cataract, 304
Senile calcific plaque, 134, 135*f*

Sentinel (episcleral) vessels, 84, 85*f*, 313, 314*f*
Sessile papillomas, 69–70
Severe cytologic atypia, 79
Shaken baby syndrome, 189–191, 190*f*
Sickle cell retinopathy, 178
Siderosis, 145
Siderosis bulbi, 126
Silver deposits, 143
Simple episcleritis, 131
Simple epithelial (epidermoid) cyst, 262
Sinus infections (sinusitis), 269, 289
SLC4A11 gene, 112
Slender spindle nevus cells, 226, 226*f*
Slides. *See* Special testing and procedures; Specimen
        handling and processing
Slit-lamp biomicroscopy, 307*f*, 315
Small blue cell tumor, 203. *See also* Retinoblastoma
SNP oligonucleotide microarray analysis (SOMA), 36*t*
Soemmering ring secondary cataract, 144, 145*f*
Soft drusen, 192*t*, 193*f*
Soft-tissue sarcomas, 368
Solar elastosis (elastotic degeneration), 65–66, 67*f*, 71,
        72*f*, 248, 248*f*
Solitary fibrous tumor, 275–278, 277–278*f*
SOMA, 36*t*
Special testing and procedures, 29–42
    clinical use of, 38–39
    communication, with pathologist, 19, 20, 30*t*, 161,
        273
    diagnostic electron microscopy (DEM), 30*t*, 39
    for differential diagnosis, 17
    flow cytometry, 30*t*, 33, 34*f*
    FNAB, 30*t*, 39–40, 40*f*. *See also* Fine-needle aspiration
        biopsy
    frozen sections, 19, 27, 30*t*, 40–42, 41*f*
    immunohistochemistry (IHC), 29–32, 31*f*, 32*t*
    microarrays, 36–39, 36*t*, 38*f*
    molecular pathology, 30*t*, 33–39, 35–36*t*
    overview, 6, 29
    polymerase chain reaction (PCR) techniques, 34–36,
        35*t*, 37*f*, 38–39
Specimen handling and processing, 19–27
    communication, with pathologist, 19, 20, 30*t*, 161, 273
    for conjunctival neoplasia specimens, 69, 71
    for FNAB, 39. *See also* Fine-needle aspiration biopsy
    gross examination and dissection, 24
    orientation of specimen, 21–23, 22–23*f*
    overview, 5–6, 19
    slide preparation, 24, 26
    tissue preservation fixatives, 21, 21*t*
    tissue processing, 19, 24–25
    tissue staining, 26–27, 27*t*, 31–32, 32*t*
Spheroidal degeneration (actinic keratopathy), 100–101,
        101*f*
Sphincter muscle, 214, 214*f*
Spindle cell carcinoma, 74
Spindle cell melanoma, 227, 227*f*, 230
Spindle cells, 224, 236, 257, 281, 281*f*
Spindle-A and -B melanoma cells, 224, 226, 227*f*
Spitz nevus, 257
Squamous cell carcinoma (SCC)
    actinic keratosis and, 247–248, 249
    of conjunctiva, 70, 84

of eyelid, 249–252, 250–251f, 254
  invasive, 71–73f, 74
  in situ, 70, 71–72f, 74
Squamous eddies (keratin whorls), 72f, 74, 246, 247f, 251
Squamous epithelium, 103f, 238
Squamous papilloma, 69–70, 70f
Staghorn sinusoidal blood vessels, 276, 277f
Stains and staining techniques
  for histochemistry preparations, 26–27, 27t
  for immunohistochemistry testing, 31–32, 32t
Standardized ultrasonography
  about, 315
  of choroidal hemangioma, 336f, 337
  for posterior uveal melanomas, 315, 316–318f, 318, 328
  for retinoblastoma, 350–351
Staphylococcus aureus, 92, 240
Staphylococcus epidermidis, 141
Staphylococcus spp, 266
Staphyloma, 132, 134, 134–135f
Stargardt disease, 196–197, 200f
Sterile corneal ulceration, 98
Strabismus, 48–49, 168, 348, 348f
Streptococcus pneumoniae, 92
Streptococcus spp, 266
Streptococcus viridans, 96
Striate melanokeratosis, 78
Stroma
  of choroid, 216
  of ciliary body, 47
  of conjunctiva, 47
  of cornea
    dystrophies, 110–111, 113f
    ectatic disorders and stromal thinning, 104–106, 105f
    infections, 93f, 94f, 95
    topography, 89, 90f
    wound repair, 45
  of iris, 214, 214f, 224–225, 225f
  of sclera, 129–130, 129f
  of uveal tract, 47
Stromal (disciform) keratitis, 94f, 95
Stromal (subepithelial) nevus, 76
Stromal cyst, 308t
Sturge-Weber syndrome (encephalofacial angiomatosis), 234, 337
Stye (hordeolum), 240
Subepithelial (stromal) nevus, 76
Subhyaloid hemorrhages, 180
Subretinal drusenoid deposits, 192–193, 192t, 194f
Subretinal hemorrhage, 52, 311f, 313, 318, 322f
Substantia propria, 45–46
Superficial spreading melanoma, 260, 260f
Superficial temporal artery biopsy, 289, 290f
Suprachoroidal hemorrhage, 50, 51f
Surgery and surgical sites
  bullous keratopathy following, 101
  cataract surgery complications, 101, 141
  corneal graft failure, 97, 102, 103f
  epithelial inclusion cysts at, 68
  pyogenic granulomas at, 63, 65f
  sympathetic ophthalmia and, 219, 219–220f
Sweat glands, 55, 238–239, 252, 253, 253f
Swept-source (enhanced depth imaging) OCT, 315, 316f
Sympathetic ophthalmia, 219, 219–220f

Synaptophysin, 32, 32t
Syncytial growth pattern, 297, 297f
Syneresis, 153, 154f, 157
Syphilis, 97–98, 98f
Syringoma, 253, 253f
Systemic intravenous chemotherapy, 361, 361f
Systemic lymphoma, 67
Systemic neoplastic syndromes, 246, 247t

T-cell lymphomas, 160
T cells, 8, 32t
Taenia solium, 269
TAP trial, 338
Tarsal plate, 238
Tarsus, 237, 237f, 238, 239
TBCD. *See* Thiel-Behnke corneal dystrophy
Tears (of lacrimal gland), 238
TED. *See* Thyroid eye disease
Telangiectasias
  Coats disease and, 169, 169f, 355–356, 355f
  combined hamartoma and, 333, 333f
  IRMAs and, 180f, 182f, 187
  Merkel cell carcinoma and, 256
  retinoblastoma and, 351
Temporal artery, 27t, 290–291
Tenon capsule, 56
Tenon space, 56
10% neutral-buffered formalin, 21, 21t
Teratoid medulloepithelioma, 209
Teratomas, 7, 8t
Tertiary vitreous, 150
TGFB1 gene, 107, 109f
Thiel-Behnke corneal dystrophy (TBCD), 108–110, 109–112f, 113t
Thioflavin T (ThT) stain, 27t
Thyroid eye disease (TED), 264–266, 264f
Tingible body macrophages, 273
Tissue microarrays, 37, 38f
Tissue specimens. *See* Special testing and procedures; Specimen handling and processing
"Tomato ketchup" fundus, 337, 337f
Topical antimetabolites, 47
Topical medication toxicities, 98
Topography, 6–7, 6t, 17. *See also under specific structures*
Topotecan, 362, 364
Touton giant cells, 11, 14f, 222f
Toxocariasis, 356
Toxoplasmic retinochoroiditis, 173–174, 174f
TPCD. *See* Typical peripheral cystoid degeneration
Trabecular meshwork
  degenerations, 49, 122–123, 125–128, 126–127f
  developmental anomalies, 118–120, 119–120f
  glaucoma and, 143, 156
  neoplasia, 128, 128f, 229, 230f
  topography, 117–118, 118f
Trachoma, 67
Tractional retinal detachment, 52
Transillumination, 24, 25f, 318, 318f
Transpupillary thermotherapy (TTT), 329
Transthyretin, 158–159, 243
Trauma. *See also* Degenerations; Foreign bodies
  abusive head trauma, 189–191, 190f
  to anterior chamber, 49, 50f, 123–126, 125–126f

to ciliary muscle, 49
to cornea, 95, 100
Descemet membrane rupture, 49, 49–50f
to eyelid, 240
glaucoma and, 49, 123–126, 125–126f
infections resulting from, 95
to iris, 49, 50f
to lens, 51, 141, 142f, 143–144
to retina, 155–156
Treatment of Age-Related Macular Degeneration With
Photodynamic Therapy (TAP) trial (1999), 338
Treponema pallidum, 97–98, 98f, 288
Triamcinolone acetonide, 182
Trilateral retinoblastoma, 351–352, 353f, 367
TTT (transpupillary thermotherapy), 329
Tubercles, 11, 13f, 62–63, 63f, 220, 221f, 291, 291f
Tuberculosis, 266
Tuberous sclerosis, 356
Tumor necrosis, 204, 205f
Tumor suppressor genes, 66
Tunica vasculosa lentis, 151
Typical degenerative retinoschisis, 175
Typical peripheral cystoid degeneration (TPCD),
174–175, 175f

UBM. *See* Ultrasound biomicroscopy
Ulcers (corneal), 8, 45, 91, 92–93f, 93–95, 98
Ultrasonography (echography)
of choroidal hemangioma, 336f, 337
of iris melanoma, 305
of metastatic tumors, 375–376, 376f
of posterior uveal melanoma, 315, 316–318f, 318, 328
for retinoblastoma, 349, 350–351, 353f
Ultrasound biomicroscopy (UBM), 307f, 315
Ultraviolet (UV) radiation
actinic keratopathy, 100
actinic keratosis, 248f
posterior uveal melanomas, 313
Utcrine fibroid, 236
Uveal lymphoid infiltration (hyperplasia), 235
Uveal lymphoma, 383–386, 384f
Uveal melanoma, 16, 82t, 84, 126
Uveal tract neoplasia, 134–135, 301
Uveal tract (uvea). *See also* Choroid; Ciliary body; Iris
degenerations, 134–135, 222, 223f
developmental anomalies, 216–217, 216–217f
inflammation, 218–221, 218–222f. *See also* Uveitis
neoplasia. *See* Posterior uveal melanoma
topography, 130, 213–216, 214–216f
trauma, 50
wound repair, 47
Uveitis, 218–221
infectious, 218–219, 218f
noninfectious, 152, 153f, 219–221, 219–222f
phacoantigenic uveitis, 141–143, 142f
vitreous and, 151, 152, 153f
UV radiation. *See* Ultraviolet (UV) radiation

Varicella-zoster virus (VZV), 171, 288
Varix, of the vortex vein, 322f, 323
Vascular developmental anomalies, 169–170
Vascular endothelial growth factor (VEGF), 182, 185,
194, 343

Vascular endothelial growth factor (VEGF) inhibitors,
182, 183f, 194, 329, 339, 343–344
Vascular tumors, 335–346
about, 335, 339
choroidal hemangiomas, 335–339, 336–337f
of eyelid, 340
of iris, 340–341, 341f
of optic nerve head, 342f, 343, 344
of orbit, 274–275, 276–277f, 340
retinal
about, 339
postnatal (leaking), 339, 341–344, 342f, 345f
prenatal (non-leaking), 339–340, 340–341f
Vasculitis, 8, 178
Vasculopathies. *See* Degenerations
Vasoproliferative tumors (VPTs), 344, 345f
VEGF. *See* Vascular endothelial growth factor
Vellus hairs, 238, 239
Venous occlusion, 178, 178f, 185–187, 186f. *See also*
Ischemia, of retina
Verhoeff–van Gieson (elastin) stain, 27t
Vernal keratoconjunctivitis, 99
Verruca vulgaris (wart), 240, 241f
Verteporfin, 338
Verteporfin in Photodynamic Therapy (VIP) trial
(2001), 338
VHL gene, 170, 170f
VHL syndrome. *See* Von Hippel–Lindau (VHL)
syndrome
Vimentin, 281
Vincristine, 361
VIP trial. *See* Verteporfin in Photodynamic Therapy
(VIP) trial
Viral infections. *See also specific viruses*
conjunctival neoplasia and, 69, 70
conjunctivitis and, 59
of cornea, 93–95, 94f, 97–98
of eyelid, 240
of lacrimal drainage system, 269
optic nerve neuritis, 288
of retina, 171–173, 172f
of uveal tract, 218, 218f
Vision loss and impairment
age-related macular degeneration, 191–195. *See also*
Age-related macular degeneration
with diabetes mellitus, 187
management resources, 302
optic nerve trauma, 49
stages of, 14–15
Vitamin A deficiency, 71
Vitrectomy, 344
Vitreoretinal (primary intraocular) lymphoma, 39,
159–162, 160–162f, 235, 380–383, 381–382f
Vitreous, 149–162
degenerations, 153–155f, 153–158, 157–158f
deposits, 157, 158–159, 159f
detachment of, 153–156, 154f
developmental anomalies, 150–151, 151–152f
embryonic development, 149–150
hemorrhages of, 52, 154, 156–157, 313
inflammation, 152, 153f, 160, 160f
neoplasia, 159–162, 160–162f
posterior uveal melanoma association with, 313

retinal lattice degeneration and, 175, 176f
topography, 149–150, 150f, 164f
wound repair, 48
Vitreous amyloidosis, 158–159, 159f
Vitreous base, 52, 52–53f, 150f, 153f, 155, 155f
Vitreous hemorrhage, 52, 154, 156–157
Vitreous seeds
chemotherapy for, 361, 364
in choroidal melanoma, 311f, 313
metastases and, 377
in retinoblastoma, 204, 350, 351, 351f, 353f
retinoblastoma classification and, 357
Vitritis, 152
Vogt-Koyanagi-Harada (VKH) syndrome, 219,
220
Von Hippel lesions, 341–343
Von Hippel–Lindau (VHL) syndrome, 170, 170f,
341–343
Von Kossa stain, 27t
Vortex veins, 50, 130, 167
Vossius ring, 51
VPTs (vasoproliferative tumors), 344, 345f
VZV. See Varicella-zoster virus

Wallerian degeneration, 291
Wedl (bladder) cells, 143, 143f, 144, 239, 239f
Well-differentiated squamous cell carcinoma with
keratoacanthoma-like differentiation, 251–252,
251f
Wet AMD. See Choroidal neovascularization
White-centered hemorrhages (Roth spots), 180–181
World Health Organization (WHO), 78, 270, 273

Wound repair, 43–54
of conjunctiva, 44f, 45–47
of cornea, 45, 46f
of extraocular muscles, 48–49
of lens, 47–48
of ocular adnexa, 48–49
of optic nerve, 49
of orbit, 48–49
overview, 6, 43–44, 44f
pathologically apparent sequelae of ocular trauma,
49–54, 49–54f
phases of, 43–44, 44f
of retina, 48
of sclera, 47
of uveal tract, 47
of vitreous, 48
Wright-Giemsa stain, 27t
Wyburn-Mason syndrome (Bonnet-Dechaume-Blanc
syndrome), 340

Xanthelasma, 243, 243f
Xanthomas, 243
Xanthophyll pigment, 167
Xeroderma pigmentosum, 70

Yeasts. See Fungal infections

Ziehl-Neelsen stain, 27t
Zimmerman tumor, 239, 239f
Zonal granuloma, 141, 142f
Zonular fibers (zonule of Zinn), 51, 138f, 139, 150
Zygomycosis, 266–268, 288–289